Auditory Brainstem Evoked Potentials

Clinical and Research Applications

Editor-in-Chief for Audiology
Brad A. Stach, PhD

Auditory Brainstem Evoked Potentials

Clinical and Research Applications

Ananthanarayan Krishnan, PhD, CCC-A

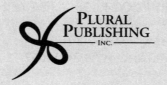

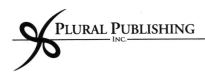

5521 Ruffin Road
San Diego, CA 92123

e-mail: information@pluralpublishing.com
Website: https://www.pluralpublishing.com

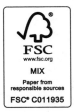

Copyright © 2023 by Plural Publishing, Inc.

Typeset in 10.5/13 Palatino by Flanagan's Publishing Services, Inc.
Printed in the United States of America by McNaughton & Gunn

All rights, including that of translation, reserved. No part of this publication may be reproduced, stored in a retrieval system, or transmitted in any form or by any means, electronic, mechanical, recording, or otherwise, including photocopying, recording, taping, Web distribution, or information storage and retrieval systems without the prior written consent of the publisher.

For permission to use material from this text, contact us by
Telephone: (866) 758-7251
Fax: (888) 758-7255
e-mail: permissions@pluralpublishing.com

Every attempt has been made to contact the copyright holders for material originally printed in another source. If any have been inadvertently overlooked, the publisher will gladly make the necessary arrangements at the first opportunity.

Library of Congress Cataloging-in-Publication Data

Names: Krishnan, Ananthanarayan, author.
Title: Auditory brainstem evoked responses : clinical and research
  applications / Ananthanarayan Krishnan.
Description: San Diego, CA : Plural Publishing, Inc., [2023] | Includes
  bibliographical references and index.
Identifiers: LCCN 2021017661 (print) | LCCN 2021017662 (ebook) | ISBN
  9781635502398 (paperback) | ISBN 9781635502527 (ebook)
Subjects: MESH: Evoked Potentials, Auditory, Brain Stem—physiology |
  Audiometry, Evoked Response | Auditory Diseases, Central—diagnosis
Classification: LCC RC386.6.E86 (print) | LCC RC386.6.E86 (ebook) | NLM
  WV 270 | DDC 616.8/047547—dc23
LC record available at https://lccn.loc.gov/2021017661
LC ebook record available at https://lccn.loc.gov/2021017662

CONTENTS

Preface	*xi*
Reviewers	*xiii*

1 Overview of the Neuroanatomy of Auditory Periphery and Brainstem — 1
    Scope — 1
  I. Auditory Periphery: Cochlear and Auditory Nerve Neuroanatomy — 1
      Cochlea: Structure and Functional Implications — 1
      Afferent Innervation of the Cochlea — 4
      Formation of the Auditory Nerve — 5
  II. Neuroanatomy of the Auditory Brainstem — 5
      Salient Features of Organization of Brainstem Structures and Pathways — 5
      Cochlear Nucleus (CN) — 7
      Superior Olivary Complex (SOC) — 9
      Nuclei of Lateral Lemniscus (NLL) — 11
      Inferior Colliculus (IC) — 12
  III. Efferent Pathways — 14
      Efferent Innervation of the Cochlea — 14
      Efferent Innervation of the IC — 14
  IV. Summary — 16
  V. Recommended Readings — 17
      Excellent Reviews With Sufficient Detail — 17
    References — 17

2 Neural Activity Underlying Scalp-Recorded Evoked Potentials — 19
    Scope — 19
  I. Neuronal Physiology — 19
      Structure of a Neuron — 19
      Requirements for Neural Signaling — 19
      Generation and Maintenance of the Resting Membrane Potential (RMP)-Polarized Cell — 20
      Action Potential: Generation, Propagation, and Synaptic Transmission — 21
  II. Neural Bases of Evoked Potentials — 24
  III. Auditory Evoked Potentials (AEP): Classification and Types — 27
  IV. Summary — 30
  V. Recommended Readings — 30
      Excellent Review of Dipoles and Overview of Neuronal Physiology — 30
    References — 30

vi   *Auditory Brainstem Evoked Potentials: Clinical and Research Applications*

3 Stimuli and Data Acquisition Principles — 31

- Scope — 31
- I. Stimulus Section — 31
  - Stimulus Type — 31
  - Transducer Type — 34
  - Calibration of Stimulus Intensity — 35
  - How Do These SPL Measures Translate to the dB nHL Scale? — 36
- II. Analog Signal Conditioning and Preprocessing Section — 38
- III. Digital Signal Processing Section — 41
- IV. Summary — 45
- V. Recommended Readings — 46
  - Excellent Chapters With More Details — 46
- References — 46

4 Normative Aspects of the Auditory Evoked Responses From the Brainstem — 47

- Scope — 47
- I. Auditory Brainstem Responses (ABRs) — 47
  - ABR Components and Response Morphology — 47
  - Neural Generators of the ABR Components — 48
  - Latency Correspondence Between Intracranial and Scalp-Recorded ABR Components — 50
  - Identification of ABR Generators in Individuals With Confirmed Focal Brainstem Lesions — 51
  - ABR Indices — 52
  - What Are the Physiological Determinants of ABR Latency and Amplitude? — 53
  - Response Amplitude — 53
  - Effects of Stimulus Factors — 54
  - Effects of Recording Factors — 64
  - Effects of Subject Factors — 70
- II. Summary — 74
- References — 75

5 Clinical Applications of the Auditory Brainstem Responses: Audiologic Applications for Hearing Screening and Threshold Estimation — 83

- Scope — 83
- I. Hearing Screening — 83
  - Hearing Screening: Factors Determining Optimal Implementation — 83
  - Hearing Screening Protocols — 86
- II. Frequency-Specific Threshold Estimation Using Auditory Brainstem Responses — 95
  - Frequency and Place Specificity — 96
  - Derived Narrowband Responses Using High-Pass Masking Noise on Click-Evoked ABRs — 96
  - Notched Noise Masking to Ensure Place Specificity of the ABR — 98
  - Estimation of the Air-Conduction Threshold Using ABRs Elicited by Frequency-Specific Tone Bursts — 100
  - Estimation of the Bone-Conduction Threshold Using ABRs Elicited by Frequency-Specific Tone Bursts — 103

		Page
	AC-ABR and BC-ABR Protocols for Threshold Estimation	106
	Preliminary Considerations	106
	ABR-AC and ABR-BC Threshold Estimation Procedure	108
	Click ABR Protocol to Identify Auditory Neuropathy	110
	Emergence of Narrowband Chirp Stimuli to Estimate AC-ABR and BC-ABR Thresholds	111
III.	Frequency-Specific Threshold Estimation Using the Brainstem Auditory Steady-State Response (ASSR)	112
IV.	Summary	116
	References	117

6 Clinical Applications of the Auditory Brainstem Response: Differential Diagnosis   125

		Page
	Scope	125
I.	ABR in Conductive Hearing Loss (CHL)	125
	Effects on ABR Characteristics	125
	Effects of Chronic Middle Ear Infection on the Brainstem Response	129
	CHL Causes Structural and Functional Changes in the Auditory Brainstem	130
II.	ABR in Cochlear Hearing Loss	133
	Effects on ABR Characteristics	133
	Relationship Between Magnitude of Latency Shift and Degree and Configuration of Cochlear Hearing Loss	133
	Relationship Between Slope of Wave V Latency-Intensity Function and Degree and Configuration of Cochlear Hearing Loss	135
	Effects of Cochlear Hearing Loss on ABR Interpeak Latencies	138
III.	ABR in Auditory Nerve and Brainstem Lesions	139
	Effects on ABR Characteristics	139
	Effects of Auditory Nerve and Lower (Caudal) Brainstem Lesions on the ABR	139
	Abnormal Interpeak Latencies (IPL: I–III, I–V, and III–V)	141
	Abnormal Interaural Latency Difference in Wave V (ILDv)	142
	ABR Sensitivity Is Reduced in the Detection of Small Auditory Nerve Tumors	143
	Stacked ABR as a Method to Improve Detection of Small Acoustic Tumors	145
	Relationship Between ABR and Auditory Nerve Tumor Size	151
	Bilateral Effects of Auditory Nerve and Lower Brainstem Lesions	151
	Use of V/I Amplitude Ratio in the Detection of Auditory Nerve and Lower Brainstem Lesions	152
IV.	ABR in Auditory Neuropathy (AN) and Cochlear Synaptopathy	153
	Introduction	153
	ABRs in Auditory Neuropathy	153
	ABRs in Cochlear Synaptopathy	155
V.	ABR in Upper (Rostral) Brainstem Lesions	161
	ABR Characteristics	161
VI.	ABR Test Strategy for Neurodiagnostic Evaluation of Site(s) of Lesion	162
	Choice of Stimulus Parameters	162
	Choice of Recording Parameters	163
VII.	Summary	164
	References	165

7 Neurotologic Applications: Electrocochleography (ECochG) and Intraoperative Monitoring (IOM) — 175

- Scope — 175
- I. Electrocochleography (ECochG) — 175
  - Cochlear Microphonic (CM) — 176
  - Clinical Applications of the CM — 178
  - Summating Potential (SP) — 180
  - Clinical Applications of SP — 182
  - Whole-Nerve Compound Action Potential (CAP) — 184
- II. ABR Diagnostic Measure for Cochlear Hydrops: Cochlear Hydrops Analysis Masking Procedure (CHAMP) — 190
- III. The Electrical Compound Action Potential (eCAP) and Its Application in Cochlear Implants: Intracochlear ECochG — 191
  - Response Characteristics — 191
  - Clinical Applications — 193
- IV. Electrical ABR (eABR) and Its Application in Cochlear Implant Evaluation — 194
  - Response Characteristics of the Normal eABR — 195
  - Methods to Record and Analyze the eABR — 197
- V. Application of Auditory Nerve and Brainstem Responses in Intraoperative Monitoring — 198
  - Introduction and Rationale — 198
  - Surgical Approaches — 199
  - Commonly Used Measures for IOM — 200
  - IOM Procedures and Interpretation of Changes in Response During Surgery — 204
  - Stimulus — 204
  - Response Recording — 205
  - Response Interpretation and Reporting — 206
  - Hearing Preservation (HP) in IOM — 206
- VI. Summary — 207
- References — 210

8 Brainstem Evoked Responses to Complex Sounds: Characteristics and Clinical Applications — 219

- Scope — 219
- I. Envelope Following Response (EFR) — 220
- II. Response Characteristics of EFRs Elicited by SAM Tones — 222
  - Effects of Intensity — 223
  - Effects of Carrier Frequency — 224
  - Effects of Modulation Rate — 225
  - Effects of Age — 226
- III. Use of EFR in Auditory Threshold Estimation — 227
  - Air-Conduction Threshold Estimation in Adults and Infants With Normal Hearing (AC-EFR) — 227
  - Threshold Estimation in Adults and Infants With Sensorineural Hearing Loss — 229
  - Bone-Conduction Threshold Estimation in Normal and Hearing-Impaired Individuals (BC-EFR) — 231
- IV. EFRs Elicited by Speech Sounds — 232
  - Characteristics of Speech Stimuli — 232
  - Response Characteristics of the EFR to the CV Syllable /da/ — 234

	Effects of Stimulus Polarity on Speech-Evoked EFR	235
	Test-Retest Reliability of the EFRs	235
	Stimulus Specificity of the EFR	235
	Potential Clinical Applications of EFRs	237
	Effects of Cochlear Impairment on Envelope Encoding	237
	Utility of EFR in Hearing Aid Outcome Measure	238
V.	Frequency Following Response (FFR)	240
	General Description	240
	Response Characteristics	241
	Effects of Stimulus Level	241
	Effects of Stimulus Frequency	243
VI.	Frequency Following Responses to Complex Sounds	244
	Frequency Following Responses Representing Cochlear Nonlinearity	244
	FFRs Elicited by Time-Variant Speech-Like and Speech Sounds	249
VII.	Cochlear Regions Contributing to the FFR	250
VIII.	How Is the Population Response Reflected in the FFR Related to Single-Neuron Activity?	253
IX.	Neural Generators of the EFR/FFR	254
	Early Research Supporting Brainstem Origin of the FFR	254
	Current Views on the Neural Generators of the FFR	255
X.	Clinical Applications of the FFR	257
XI.	Recording and Analysis of EFR and FFR	261
	Electrode Montage	261
	Time-Domain Measures	264
	Response Latency	264
	Autocorrelation	266
	Autocorrelogram (ACG)	266
	Pitch Tracking Accuracy Using Autocorrelation	266
	Phase Coherence	266
	Frequency-Domain Measures	267
XII.	Summary	268
	References	269

9 Research Applications of the Frequency Following Response — 281

	Scope	281
I.	Pitch: an Important Perceptual Attribute	281
	Hierarchical Nature of Pitch Processing	283
II.	Neural Representation of Pitch-Relevant Information of Complex Sounds	283
	Neural Correlates of Pitch of Harmonic, Inharmonic, and Frequency-Shifted Sounds	283
	Neural Correlates of Resolved Versus Unresolved Complex Sounds	287
	Relative Roles of Envelope and Temporal Fine Structure in Pitch	291
	Neural Correlates of Pitch Salience	294
	Neural Representation of Speech in Adverse Listening Conditions	296
	Effects of Reverberation	296
	Effects of Background Noise	298
III.	Neural Representation of Linguistic Pitch-Relevant Information in the Brainstem	300
	Perceptual Attributes of Pitch in Tonal Languages	300
	Language Experience–Dependent Plasticity in Pitch Processing in the Brainstem	301
	Language Experience–Dependent Effects in the Brainstem Are Feature Specific	303

Domain Specificity of the Experience-Dependent Effects in the Brainstem		304
Experience-Dependent Effects Are More Resilient to Signal Degradation		306
Structural Versus Functional Asymmetries in Neural Representation		309
Hierarchical Processing as a Basis of Experience-Dependent Pitch Processing		311
IV. FFR Correlates of Binaural Processing		314
FFR Correlates of Binaural Interaction		314
FFR Correlates of Binaural Masking Level Difference (BMLD)		314
FFR Correlates of Spatial Release From Masking		317
Neural Representation of Vocoded Speech Sounds		318
EFR/FFR Applications in Different Populations—Potential for Development of Clinical Measures		324
V. Summary		324
References		325

10 Auditory Brainstem Responses Laboratory Exercises — 337

Scope	337
Preliminary Considerations for Recording Auditory Brainstem Responses	337
I. Effects of Stimulus Factors on the ABR Components	338
Lab 1. Effects of Stimulus Intensity of Click-Evoked ABR	338
Lab 2. Effects of Stimulus Intensity on the Broadband Chirp-Evoked ABR	340
Lab 3. Effects of Stimulus Frequency on Tone Burst-Evoked ABR	340
Lab 4. Effects of Stimulus Repetition Rate on the ABR	341
Lab 5. Effects of Stimulus Rise-Fall Time	342
Lab 6. Effects of Stimulus Onset Polarity on the ABR	343
II. Effects of Recording Parameters on the ABR	344
Lab 7. Effects of Number of Sweeps on Averaging the ABR	344
Lab 8. Effects of Recording Electrode Montage	345
Lab 9. Effects of High-Pass and Low-Pass Analog Filter Settings on the ABR	345
III. Threshold Estimation Using the ABR	346
Lab 10. Estimation of Air-Conduction Threshold Using Simulated Conductive Hearing Loss	346
IV. Threshold Assessment in Babies (Birth to Six Months)	347
Example of an ABR Protocol for Threshold Estimation in Babies	347
Lab 11. Identification and AC-ABR Threshold Estimation From ABR Waveforms Recorded From Infants	349
V. Interpretation of ABRs to Determine the Site of Lesion	356
Lab 12. Unmarked ABR Waveform Data (audiograms in some cases)	356
VI. Recording of Auditory Steady-State Response, Envelope Following Response, and Frequency Following Response	359
Lab 13. Recording and Analysis of ASSR	359
Lab 14. Recording and Analysis of EFRs and FFRs	359
VII. Protocol Consideration for Electrocochleography (ECochG)	360
VIII. Summary	360
IX. Recommended Reading	363

Index — 365

PREFACE

I have been teaching auditory electrophysiology to graduate students and conducting research using electrophysiologic measures for over 30 years now. My complaining about the appropriateness of the available textbooks for my classes (in terms of the organization of the content, the appropriate level, the appropriate depth, and the right balance between theory and clinical applications most relevant to the students) has steadily increased over the years. Finally, I thought it was time to stop complaining and do something about it. Thus, this undertaking is an *attempt* to address my objectives and to stop my decades-long complaining. However, this attempt should not be construed as a negative reflection on several excellent resources already provided by my colleagues in the field.

This book is primarily intended to serve as a prescribed textbook for graduate-level electrophysiology course(s) for AuD and PhD students. However, its contents should also be of interest to researchers using auditory evoked potentials to complex sounds (envelope following response [EFR] and frequency following response [FFR]) to address questions relevant to the neural representation of complex sounds and how they may be altered by experience, training, and hearing impairment. The main aim is to provide an organized, coherent, sufficient, and reasonably up-to-date (but not exhaustive) account of relevant literature about the principles related to the neural bases, response characteristics, and specific clinical and research applications of the auditory evoked brainstem potentials. The goal is twofold: (a) to foster an understanding of how these measures reflect the neuroanatomical and functional organization of the auditory system from the periphery through the brainstem, and (b) to develop an appreciation for the structure-function relationship and the consequences of an impairment on this relationship that may be reflected in these measures. It is my firm belief that such knowledge integrated into the clinical practice is essential to be able to "practice at the top of your license," rather than merely be a technician. Finally, the level of technical detail presented was deliberately reduced (without filtering out important information) to encourage the reader to remain focused on learning the essentials of the relevant information. However, inquiring minds can always pursue the listed references to quench their thirst.

The contents are organized in a coherent manner by first providing a sufficient overview of the nature of the neuroanatomical organization of the structures and pathways in the auditory periphery and the brainstem (Chapter 1) followed by a review of neuronal physiology and the neural bases of auditory evoked potentials (Chapter 2). Since structure and function are closely related, knowledge of the structural organization and the neural bases of these responses will help the clinician to understand the functional consequences of a structural abnormality, enabling the development of better clinical management strategies. Chapter 3 provides a complete description of stimulus characteristics and principles of evoked potential data acquisition. This is followed by a description of the normative aspects of the auditory brainstem response (ABR) as it relates to stimulus, recording, and subject factors (Chapter 4). This knowledge is a prerequisite to set up the normative database required to interpret these responses as normal or abnormal in clinical diagnosis. A complete description of audiologic applications of the ABR for hearing screening for early identification of hearing loss and frequency-specific estimation of hearing thresholds or minimum hearing levels is provided in Chapter 5. While there is no single standard protocol for each application across clinics to date, the latest developments relevant to hearing screening and frequency-specific threshold estimation move toward the development of effective and efficient protocols that employ next-generation technology to both increase accuracy and reduce test time.

Chapter 6 examines the clinical utility of the ABR to differentiate hearing losses resulting from structural abnormalities in the conductive mechanism, sensory-to-neural transduction in the cochlea, and synaptic processing and neural transmission in the auditory nerve and brainstem. In terms of neuro-otologic applications, the use of cochlear receptor potentials (cochlear microphonic [CM] and summating potential [SP]) and the auditory nerve compound action potential (AN-CAP) to evaluate the functional integrity of the inner ear outer hair cell subsystem and the auditory nerve for differential diagnosis, and for neural function monitoring during surgeries that involve the auditory nerve and the brainstem, is examined in Chapter 7. This includes a description of the use of AN-CAP recorded directly from the auditory nerve and/or the cochlear nucleus, and the scalp-recorded ABR in intraoperative monitoring to minimize surgically induced permanent injuries, and to attempt preservation of hearing. In the next two chapters (Chapters 8 and 9), the clinical utility and research utility of the emerging brainstem evoked potentials generated by complex sounds (EFR and FFR) including speech are described. Since both these responses provide information about the nature of the temporal neural encoding of certain acoustic features important for the perception of complex sounds, they can potentially serve as effective electrophysiologic measures to evaluate the nature of degradation of these features in individuals with hearing impairment consequent to cochlear and/or retrocochlear pathologies; monitor treatment outcomes with amplification; evaluate effects of auditory retraining; and test and evaluate optimal signal processing strategies for hearing prosthetic devices. There is no substitute for sufficient hands-on experience to develop sound skills to record, analyze, and interpret the auditory brainstem responses from real people. This essential requirement not only reinforces the understanding of concepts relevant to the effects of various stimulus and recording factors on the ABR response components presented in the classroom but also facilitates learning and reinforcing practical skills necessary to accurately record and interpret the responses for optimal clinical application (Chapter 10). Finally, the accompanying online PowerPoint lectures on the PluralPlus companion website should be useful for both students and instructors in preparation of the course.

Although my initial intent was to gear the content of this book to a single course limited to the clinical and research applications of the transient auditory brainstem response (ABR), the more expanded content presented is unlikely to be covered in a single-semester course. Thus, this book can be used in a two-course sequence, wherein the first course covers the basic clinical applications (hearing screening, threshold estimation, and the use of ABR in differential diagnosis) and the second course covers the use of ABR in intraoperative monitoring, sustained brainstem responses to complex sounds and their clinical applications, and the use of sustained brainstem responses to complex sounds in research to understand the neural representation of complex sounds in normal and impaired ears.

I would like to thank the multiple reviewers (who provided helpful feedback that has made the final product better), colleagues in the profession, and graduate students who have helped shape this book. I am deeply indebted to my wife Lata Krishnan (sadly, I was not able to convince her to be a co-author) for painstakingly editing the manuscript. It was a pleasure working with the editorial staff at Plural Publishing (Christina Gunning, in particular, who was patient and helpful), and I appreciate their cooperation during times when my progress was hampered. While I have received quite a bit of help from my colleagues, all omissions and errors that persist are my own.

This book is a product developed during the isolation forced by the COVID-19 pandemic. While the isolation (which trapped me in India) forced me to work on it, encouraged on by my undergraduate classmates (AIISH batch of 1970), I do feel sad about the terrible devastation visited upon (unfortunately continuing to date and postponing a planned trip to India next week) humankind by this pandemic. I fervently hope that we come out of this soon and revert to some semblance of a normal life. Godspeed everyone.

Ravi Krishnan
West Lafayette
April, 2021

REVIEWERS

Plural Publishing and the author thank the following reviewers for taking the time to provide their valuable feedback during the manuscript development process. Additional anonymous feedback was provided by other expert reviewers.

Samira Anderson, AuD, PhD
Associate Professor
Department of Hearing and Speech Sciences
University of Maryland
College Park, Maryland

Gavin Bidelman, PhD
Associate Professor
School of Communication Sciences and Disorders
University of Memphis
Memphis, Tennessee

Brenda Fields Cross, AuD
Assistant Clinical Professor
Department Chair, Communication Disorders
West Texas A&M University
Canyon, Texas

Hannah Ditmars, AuD, CCC-A
Assistant Professor
Department of Special Education and Communication Disorders
College of Education and Human Sciences
University of Nebraska–Lincoln
Lincoln, Nebraska

Kate Dunckley, PhD, CCC-A
Assistant Professor
Rush University Medical Center
Chicago, Illinois

Jason Tait Sanchez, PhD, CCC-A, FAAA
Associate Professor and Director of Graduate Studies
Department of Communication Sciences and Disorders
Department of Neurobiology
Northwestern University
Evanston, Illinois

Lauren A. Shaffer, PhD, CCC-A
Associate Professor
Ball State University
Muncie, Indiana

Thomas R. Zalewski, PhD
Professor of Audiology
Bloomsburg University
Bloomsburg, Pennsylvania

This book is dedicated to my parents, family, mentors, colleagues, friends, and students who have all contributed to my knowledge and hopefully have instilled some wisdom in me.

*"The way of devotion is not different from the way of **knowledge or gnyaana**. When intelligence matures and lodges securely in the mind, it becomes **wisdom**. When wisdom is integrated with life and shoots out in action, it becomes **bhakti**. Knowledge, when it becomes fully mature, is bhakti. If it does not get transformed into bhakti, **such knowledge is useless tinsel**. To believe that gnyaana and bhakti, **knowledge and devotion, are different from each other, is ignorance**."*

—Bharath Rathna Sri Chakravarti Rajagopalachari

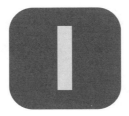

Overview of the Neuroanatomy of Auditory Periphery and Brainstem

SCOPE

The overview in this chapter is primarily intended to provide a sufficient, if not exhaustive, foundation of the nature of the neuroanatomic organization of the structures and pathways in the auditory periphery and the brainstem. This knowledge is important because neural elements and tracts in these structures contribute to the generation of the cochlear, auditory nerve, and brainstem evoked responses we use clinically to determine the functional integrity of the peripheral and brainstem auditory system. Without this knowledge, our ability to record and interpret these responses will be less than optimal. Since structure and function are closely related, knowledge of the structural organization will help the clinician to understand the functional consequences of a structural abnormality, enabling the development of better clinical management strategies—essentially becoming a better clinician. Consistent with convention, the cochlear and auditory nerve neuroanatomy is treated as peripheral, and the brainstem includes a description starting with cochlear nucleus and including superior olivary complex, nuclei of lateral lemniscus, and inferior colliculus.

I. AUDITORY PERIPHERY: COCHLEAR AND AUDITORY NERVE NEUROANATOMY

Cochlea: Structure and Functional Implications

The mammalian cochlea in the inner can be characterized as a spiral duct with an inner membranous part (membranous labyrinth) and an outer bony part (osseous labyrinth) that is partitioned into three fluid-filled spaces, namely, the perilymph (high sodium ion [Na^+] concentration and low potassium ion [K^+] concentration) filled scala vestibuli and scala tympani, and the endolymph (high K^+ and low Na^+) filled scala media (Figure 1–1). Epithelial cells with tight junctions surrounding the membranous portion help maintain this ionic difference (Smith, 1978). The self-contained membranous scala media houses the organ of Corti that in turn sits on the basilar membrane. The basilar membrane partitions the cochlear duct into scala vestibuli and scala tympani and also forms the floor of the organ of Corti. The Reissner's membrane separates the scala media from the scala vestibuli. The hair cells and their supporting cells rest on the

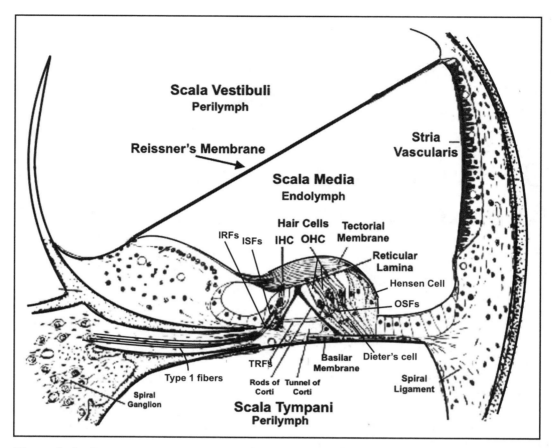

Figure 1–1. Cross-section of cochlea showing the three fluid-filled partitions (scala vestibuli, scala tympani (perilymph), and scala media (endolymph)) and the organ of Corti with outer hair cells (OHCs) and inner hair cells (IHCs), stereocilia, basilar membrane, tectorial membrane, and stria vascularis (the cochlear battery). Also shown are both the afferent fibers of the OHCs (outer spiral fibers [OSFs]) and IHCs (inner radial fibers [IRFs]) and the efferent fibers of the IHCs (inner spiral fibers [ISFs] and the OHCs (tunnel radial fibers [TRFs]). Type 1 myelinated fibers from the IHCs are shown coursing toward the cells in the spiral ganglion.

basilar membrane, and have an overhanging gelatinous suprastructure called the tectorial membrane (see Figure 1–1). It can be seen in Figure 1–1 that only the stereocilia of the outer hair cells (OHCs) contact the undersurface of the tectorial membrane.

The *basilar membrane*, attached medially to the osseous spiral lamina and laterally to the spiral ligament, extends from the base to the apex of the cochlea (about 35 mm) where the perilymphatic spaces communicate via the helicotrema. The change in the *stiffness gradient* (resulting from the relatively denser network of radial and longitudinal fibers underneath the basilar membrane in the base, and relatively sparse network of these fibers in the apex [Figure 1–2, bottom right]) and the membrane width, going from narrow at the base (100 μM) to wide (500 μM) at the apex (see Figure 1–2), contribute significantly to the frequency for place transformation. That is, the traveling wave generated by the back-and-forth motion of the stapes in the oval window upon sound stimulation progresses in an apical direction, with its envelope gradually reaching a maximum at a place determined by the frequency of the stimulus and quickly decreasing in amplitude thereafter (Figure 1–3). The location of the peak of the displacement shifts to the left (toward the base of the cochlea) with increasing frequency. It should be noted here that von Bekesy's (1960) experiments were on cadavers using high stimulus levels; therefore, the displace-

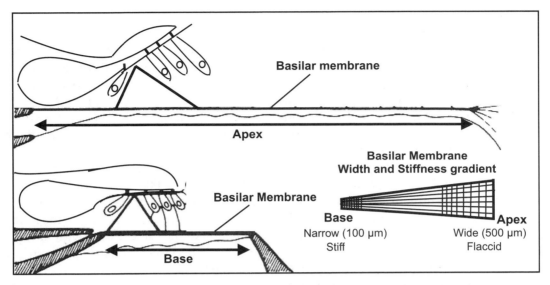

Figure 1–2. The changes in the width and stiffness of the basilar membrane from base to apex. The basilar membrane is wider at the apex and more flaccid, whereas it is narrower at the base and exhibits greater stiffness (see lower right).

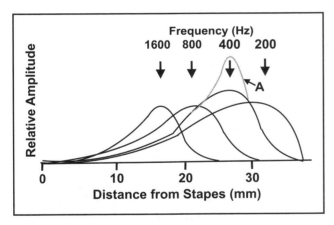

Figure 1–3. A family of Bekesy traveling wave envelopes showing frequency for place transformation. Traveling wave maxima progressively shift from apex to base (that is, to the left) as frequency is increased. Note the amplification in the maximum amplitude for 400 Hz (*arrow pointed by A*) reflecting cochlear amplification using the active process. The frequency corresponding to each traveling wave is identified at the top. Traveling waves approximately reflect data from G. von Bekesy, 1960, *Experiments in Hearing*. New York, NY: McGraw-Hill, Figure 11.49.

ment patterns shown here reflect only the passive physical response minus the cochlear active processes (also referred to as the cochlear amplifier associated with the outer hair cell subsystem) that further improve sensitivity and frequency selectivity substantially. The effects of the active process are illustrated by the larger and sharper peak of the basilar membrane displacement for the 400-Hz traveling wave (arrow A in Figure 1–3). The electromotility (length changes in the OHCs with stimulation) is thought to supply the mechanical feedback process that amplifies low-level sound (Brownell, Bader, Bertrand, & de Ribaupierre, 1985; Dallos, 1992). The cochlear amplification derived from the electromotility of OHCs increases the sensitivity to soft sounds by 40 to 60 dB (Dallos, 1992, 2008). The electromotility, thought to produce the cochlear amplification of OHCs, is presumably driven by prestin, a motor protein expressed in the mammalian OHCs. Cochlear amplification is essential for normal hearing in adult animals. The property of frequency for place transformation becomes particularly relevant when we later discuss considerations of specific stimulus properties to obtain cochlear place-specific responses to estimate audiogram-like hearing thresholds using the auditory brainstem response (ABR).

The *organ of Corti* sits on the basilar membrane and consists of two structurally and functionally distinct receptor cells (OHCs and inner hair cells [IHCs]), lateral support cells (Hensen's cells), and vertical alignment cells (Deiters' cells, phalangeal processes of the Dieters' cells and the reticular lamina) (see Figure 1–1), and the afferent and efferent fibers with distinct innervation patterns for each receptor type. The highly vascular stria vascularis on the outer wall of the scala media serves to power the metabolic processes involved in the +80-mV endolymphatic potential needed to mediate the transduction mechanisms of the hair cell and is also involved in recovering the K+ expelled during transduction (Wangemann, 2002).

The test tube–shaped **OHCs** (9,000–12,000 in number and arranged in three to five rows along the length of the cochlea) are located on the lateral portion of the outer pillar of Corti, slanted toward the outer pillar (see Figure 1–2). The six to seven rows of stereocilia on the apex of each OHC are arranged in a V or W pattern (Figure 1–4, bottom), with the tallest ones on the most lateral row (toward the outer wall). The length of the OHC stereocilia also increases along the longitudinal axis of the cochlear partition (from about 2 μm in the base to about 8 μm in the apex). In addition, the height of the OHC increases from about 10 μm in the base to about 80 μm in the apex. Both physical changes in the OHCs are thought to contribute to the cochlear frequency for place transformation —the taller hair cells with their longer stereocilia in the apical regions are more selective to low frequencies. The stereocilia are cross-linked, both within each row and between rows (Pickles, Comis, & Osborne, 1984), which aids in the opening and closing of potassium channels at the tip of the stereocilia to facilitate excitation and inhibition of the hair cells, respectively.

The flask-shaped, relatively bigger single row of **IHCs** (about 3,000–4,000 in number) are located on the medial side of the inner pillar of Corti (see Figure 1–2), again slanted toward the inner pillar of Corti. Unlike the OHCs, the height and the length of the IHCs and their stereocilia remain unchanged along the longitudinal axis of the cochlear partition. The two to four rows of stereocilia on the top of each IHC form a crescent shape (Figure 1–4, top). Like the OHCs, the stereocilia of the IHCs have similar cross-links.

Afferent Innervation of the Cochlea

The cell bodies of the afferent neurons form the spiral ganglion located in the central core of the cochlear spiral called the modiolus. The peripheral portion of the afferent bipolar neurons enters the cochlea through the habenula perforata and synapses at the base of each hair cell. The peripheral portions innervating the OHCs, called the outer spiral fibers (OSFs), enter the cochlea through the habenula perforata in the osseous spiral lamina and cross along the floor of the tunnel of Corti toward the OHCs. As they spiral around the cochlea in an apical-to-basal direction, each OSF synapses with 10 to 15 OHCs (starting with the OHCs in the inner row, then the middle row, and finally the outermost row—see Figure 1–5). Thus, the output of many OHCs converges on one OSF, suggesting integration of information from many OHCs spread across the cochlear partition. These unmyelinated OSFs are also referred to as Type II fibers (smaller diameter and slower conducting) and form only about 5% to 10% (Spoendlin, 1978) of the 30,000 auditory nerve fibers in humans. While the peripheral fibers innervating the IHCs follow a similar path from the spiral ganglion, the innervation pattern is very different (see Figure 1–5). The peripheral portion of

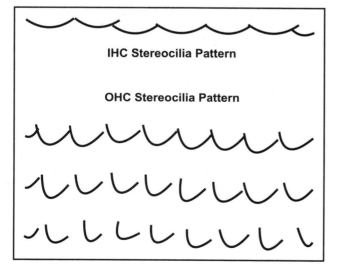

Figure 1–4. Stereocilia pattern for the inner hair cells (IHCs) and outer hair cells (OHCs) in a surface view of the normal organ of Corti. The crescent pattern for the single row of IHC stereocilia (*top*) and the V or W pattern for the three rows of OHC stereocilia (*bottom*) are clearly evident. Top in each is the modiolar side, and the bottom is the outer wall side.

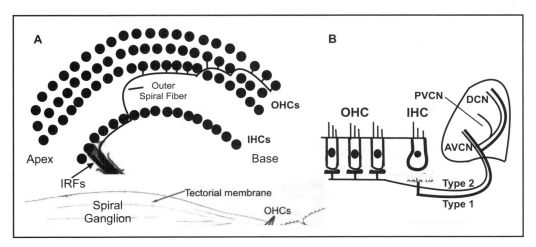

Figure 1–5. Afferent innervation pattern of the outer hair cells (OHCs) and inner hair cells (IHCs). Panel A illustrates the afferent innervation pattern of the cochlear OHCs and IHCs. Panel B shows the nature of the afferent synapses on the IHCs and OHCs.

the fibers innervating the IHCs is called the inner radial fiber (IRF). Unlike the OSF, these myelinated fibers, called Type I fibers (larger diameter and faster conducting), enter the cochlea through the habenula perforata (as many as 20 fibers through each radial canal, travel radially and synapse the nearest IHC at its base). Unlike each OSF, each IRF innervates only one IHC. However, as many as 30 IRFs innervate one IHC, thus providing a diverging output from one IHC. These IRFs form 90% to 95% of the total number of afferents in the auditory nerve.

Formation of the Auditory Nerve

The central axons of the spiral ganglion cells twist to form the auditory nerve bundle, and along with the central axons of the vestibular branch form the VIII cranial nerve (Figure 1–6, left panel). The VIII cranial nerve exits the temporal bone via the internal auditory meatus and enters the brainstem at the lateral aspect of the pontomedullary junction and bifurcates into an anterior and a posterior branch. The anterior branch courses anteriorly and terminates in the neurons forming the anterior ventral cochlear nucleus (AVCN). The posterior branch sends off collaterals to innervate neurons in the posterior ventral cochlear nucleus (PVCN) as it proceeds posterodorsally to terminate in the neurons of the dorsal cochlear nucleus (DCN) (Figure 1–6, right panel). The individual fibers forming the auditory nerve are organized systematically such that apical (low-frequency cochlear regions) fibers are toward the core, and basal (high-frequency cochlear regions) are increasingly on the surface of the auditory nerve bundle. This orderly arrangement representing cochlear place (and therefore frequency) provides the framework for the development of tonotopic organization at the terminal points of the auditory nerve in the cochlear nucleus (see Figure 1–6, right panel—see the frequency arrangement, **L** [low], **M** [mid], and **H** [high], in the AVCN).

II. NEUROANATOMY OF THE AUDITORY BRAINSTEM

Salient Features of Organization of Brainstem Structures and Pathways

For the purpose of discussion here, the auditory brainstem extends from the medullary-level cochlear nucleus to the midbrain-level inferior colliculus, including the caudal pontine–level superior olivary complex (SOC) and nuclei of the lateral lemniscus, and the midbrain inferior colliculus (Figure 1–7, left panel). The neuroanatomic organization of each nucleus along the auditory brainstem

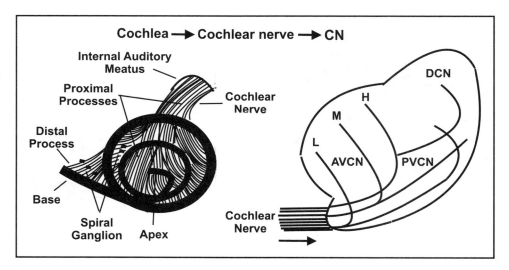

Figure 1–6. Origin and termination of the auditory nerve in the subdivisions of cochlear nucleus. Innervation and exit of the cochlear nerve from the cochlea are shown on the left. Course and termination points of the auditory nerve in the cochlear nucleus are shown on the right. Distal and proximal portions originating from the cochlear spiral (*left*) of the afferent fibers are identified. The bifurcation of the auditory nerve fibers into anterior and posterior branches is also illustrated.

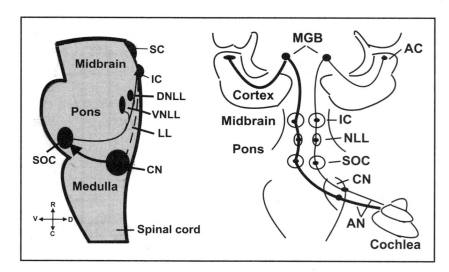

Figure 1–7. Schematic lateral view of the brainstem and midbrain showing auditory nuclei along the brainstem and their anatomic levels. Nuclei identified are cochlear nucleus (CN) and superior olivary complex (SOC) at the medullary and pontine levels; ventral nucleus of lateral lemniscus (VNLL) and dorsal nucleus of lateral lemniscus (DNLL) at the rostral pontine level; ascending lateral lemniscus (LL) fibers through the brainstem; and inferior colliculus (IC) at the midbrain level; the superior colliculus (SC), the visual midbrain nucleus, is also identified.

shares certain characteristics that include bilateral structures, contralateral dominant afferent pathways (Figure 1–7, right panel), core (with exquisite representation of the cochlear frequency map-tonotopic organization) and belt (nontonotopic, multisensory, efferent recipients) subdivisions, efferent pathways, and the presence of binaural neurons past the cochlear nucleus. The following description of the neuroanatomic organization of each brainstem structure includes information about location, subdivisions, cell types, inputs, outputs, and orientation of the tonotopic map. The intent here is to provide an introduction to the neuroanatomic organization of nuclei and tracts along the auditory pathway(s) in the brainstem.

Cochlear Nucleus (CN)

Location: The cochlear nucleus (CN) is located on the dorsolateral aspect of the pontomedullary junction proximal to the root entry zone of the auditory nerve (see Figure 1–7, left panel).

Subdivisions: It is a rather complex nucleus with a broad diversity in cell types that forces consideration of division into multiple subdivisions (Adams, 1986; Brawer, Morest, & Kane, 1974; Cant, 1992; Moore & Osen, 1979; Osen, 1969). However, the scope here is to consider just the two main subdivisions—ventral cochlear nucleus (VCN) and DCN. The VCN is further subdivided (see Figure 1–6, right panel) into an AVCN and a PVCN.

Cell types: The anterior portion of AVCN contains large spherical bushy cells (the principal cell type here with short bushy dendrites) and medium-sized stellate or multipolar cells. The posterior portion of the AVCN contains small spherical bushy cells, globular bushy cells, and large stellate cells. These large stellate cells are also found in the anterior PVCN. The posterior PVCN is characterized by the presence of octopus cells. The cell types in the laminar DCN include stellate, fusiform, granule, and giant cells. These morphologically distinct cell types (Figure 1–8) also show different response properties, suggesting differences in their functional roles (Young et al., 1988).

Inputs: All Type I and II fibers of the auditory nerve form the afferent inputs to the subdivisions of the CN (Raphael & Altschuler, 2003; Robertson, 1984; Ryugo, 1992). As described earlier, the AN bifurcates upon entering the CN into an anterior and a posterior branch. The anterior branch courses anteriorly and terminates in the AVCN. The posterior branch courses posteriorly and dorsally sending collateral terminals to the PVCN and continuing on to terminate in the DCN (see Figures 1–6, right panel, and Figure 1–8). While the trajectory of AN inputs to the CN from all portions of the cochlea are similar, the location of bifurcation in the CN systematically moves from ventral for fibers innervating the apical cochlear regions to dorsal for fibers innervating the basal cochlear regions

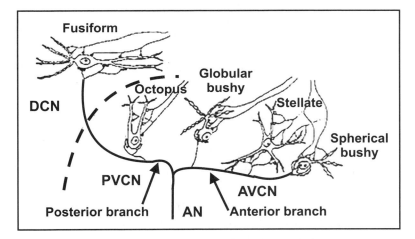

Figure 1–8. Auditory nerve bifurcation into an anterior and posterior branch in the cochlear nucleus (CN) and prominent cell types in anterior ventral cochlear nucleus (AVCN), posterior ventral cochlear nucleus (PVCN), and dorsal cochlear nucleus (DCN). Note the large calyx of Held–type synapses engulfing the soma of the spherical and globular bushy cells.

(Lorente de No, 1933). This pattern sets up the dorsal, high-frequency and ventral, low-frequency tonotopic map in each of the three subdivisions of the CN. While the AVCN receives several intrinsic and extrinsic inhibitory inputs, what is characteristic here are the large excitatory end bulb of Held synapses between the anterior branch of the auditory nerve and the spherical and globular bushy cells in AVCN. These complex synapses provide a coordinated release of neurotransmitter onto these CN cells. It should be noted here that the globular cells in comparison have relatively smaller synapses. The auditory nerve innervates the fusiform cells in the DCN on their basal dendrites and not the soma.

Outputs: The ipsilateral and the dominant contralateral outputs of the three subdivisions of the CN are carried by three major pathways, each primarily dedicated to one of the three subdivisions (Figure 1–9) The largest of the three, the ventral acoustic stria (VAS) or the trapezoid body (TB), carries excitatory outputs from the spherical bushy cells in the AVCN and runs along the ventral portion of the brainstem and projects to the ipsilateral medial superior olive (MSO) via the lateral dendrites, and the contralateral MSO via the medial dendrites (Cant, 1992). The contralateral input to the lateral superior olive (LSO) originates in the globular cell region of the AVCN, which projects excitatory outputs via the TB to the contralateral medial nucleus of the trapezoid body (MNTB) using the giant calyx of Held synapse that almost engulfs the MNTB. The calyx of Held allows the principal neurons in the MNTB to provide a well-timed and sustained inhibition to the LSO as well as to many other auditory nuclei (i.e., provides the contralateral inhibitory input to the binaural neurons in the LSO). The MNTB in turn projects an inhibitory input to the medial side of the ipsilateral LSO. The TB fibers from the multipolar cell regions (primarily PVCN) also ascend as the lateral lemniscus along the contralateral brainstem and send out collaterals to the ventral (VNLL) and dorsal nuclei of the lateral lemniscus (DNLL) before terminating in the central nucleus of the inferior colliculus (CNIC). The larger multipolar cells in the PVCN project only to the contralateral CN via the intermediate acoustic stria (IAS). Octopus cells in the PVCN project to the periolivary region in the SOC

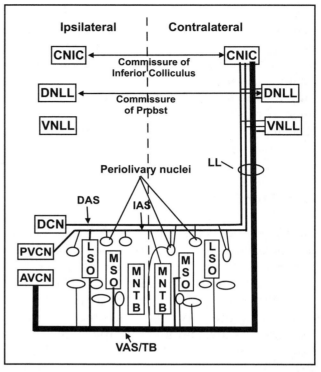

Figure 1–9. Outputs of the subdivisions (anterior ventral cochlear nucleus [AVCN], posterior ventral cochlear nucleus [PVCN], and dorsal cochlear nucleus [DCN]) of the cochlear nucleus. Three major output pathways are the dorsal acoustic stria (DAS) from the DCN; intermediate acoustic stria (IAS) from the PVCN; and the ventral acoustic stria (VAS) or trapezoid body (TB). Targets include lateral superior olive (LSO), medial superior olive (MSO), and medial nucleus of the trapezoid body (MNTB) in the superior olivary complex (SOC); ventral and dorsal nuclei of lateral lemniscus (VNLL and DNLL); and the central nucleus of inferior colliculus (CNIC). All of these fibers together form the lateral lemniscus as they ascend from the CN to the CNIC.

and to the contralateral VNLL (Warr, 1982). Finally, the dorsal acoustic stria (DAS) carries information from the DCN (fusiform and giant cells) to the contralateral CNIC bypassing the SOC (Warr, 1982).

Tonotopic Organization: Refers to the spatial representation of the cochlear frequency map in a given three-dimensional nucleus. In each of the three subdivisions of the cochlear nucleus, neurons tuned to low frequencies are in the ventral portion, and neurons tuned to progressively higher frequencies are located in progressively dorsal regions as you track along a ventral-to-dorsal direction (Figure 1–10).

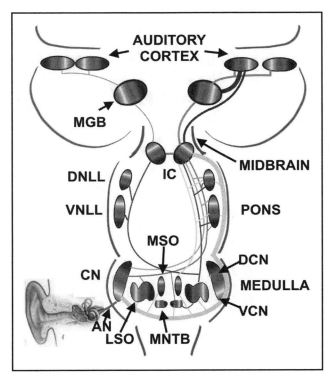

Figure 1–10. Nuclei along the ascending (*lighter lines*) and descending (*darker lines*) auditory pathways showing the orientation of the tonotopic maps in each nucleus (*low frequency: lighter color; high frequency: darker color*).

Superior Olivary Complex (SOC)

Location: The SOC is a nuclear mass located on the ventral portion of the caudal pons, medial and ventral to the CN, and represents the first point of information convergence from the two ears (see Figure 1–10). The human SOC has about 5,871 neurons (LSO: 1,980 neurons; MSO: 3,891 neurons with no well-defined MNTB) (Hilbig, Beil, Hilbig, Call, & Bidman, 2009).

Subdivisions: The SOC is divided into three subdivisions, the most lateral and S-shaped structure, the LSO; the banana-shaped structure, medial and slightly dorsal to the LSO, the MSO; and the most medial and ventral subdivision, the MNTB (see Figure 1–10). The MNTB neurons are embedded in the TB fibers. The LSO and the MSO are thought to be a single functional unit. However, given that the MNTB is almost nonexistent in humans (Masterton, Thompson, Bechtold, & RoBards, 1975), its role in the binaural processing of interaural intensity cues for localization is doubted—at least in humans. While the LSO/MNTB is specialized for processing interaural intensity differences, the MSO is specialized to process interaural time differences relevant for sound localization in the horizontal plane. The size of the MSO varies with head size (smaller heads, smaller MSO and more dominant LSO) and appears to indicate the relative usefulness of interaural cues for localization in each animal (Hilbig et al., 2009; Masterton et al., 1975). Except for humans, the LSO is the most prominent and well-differentiated nucleus in most other species. Like a belt around the three main subdivisions are neurons that are collectively called the periolivary nuclei that are thought to be part of the efferent system (Hilbig et al., 2009).

Cell types: In the MSO, there are essentially three types of principal cells: bipolar disc-shaped cells oriented in a rostrocaudal direction, multipolar cells with a distributed dendritic tree, and marginal cells along the medial and lateral surface with dendrites covering the MSO surface. The orientation of the principal disc-shaped cells allows for binaural inputs to project to the MSO laterally from the ipsilateral CN and medially from the contralateral CN. The prominent LSO cell types include disc-shaped principal cells (referred to as elongate fusiform cells) similar in orientation to the MSO principal cells, and multipolar cells that span the cell surface but with no clear orientation of the dendrites. The predominant cell type in the MNTB is the principal globular cell. In addition, multipolar cells and elongate fusiform cells are found in the MNTB.

Inputs: The afferent inputs to the MSO, LSO, and MNTB are primarily the outputs of the AVCN described in the CN output section (Figure 1–11, bottom portion). To refresh, the MSOs receive binaural excitatory inputs from the AVCN spherical cells with the lateral dendrites carrying the ipsilateral inputs and the medial dendrites carrying the contralateral inputs. The MSO marginal cells receive inhibitory inputs from the MNTB and excitatory inputs from the CN, similar to the MSO. In contrast, the LSO receives excitatory ipsilateral inputs laterally from the spherical bushy cells in AVCN and contralateral inhibitory inputs through the ipsilateral MNTB, which converts the excitatory inputs it receives from the globular bushy cells in

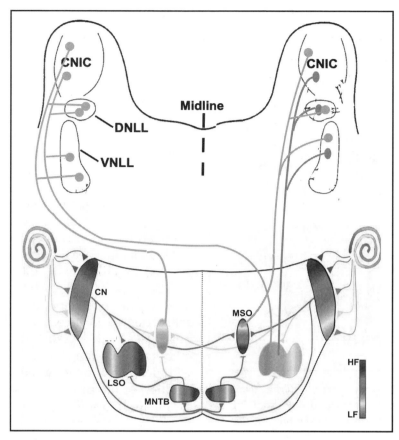

Figure 1–11. Binaural inputs from the cochlear nucleus to the lateral superior olive (LSO) and medial superior olive (MSO) (*bottom*), and outputs to higher brainstem nuclei from LSO and MSO.

the contralateral AVCN. The MNTB synapse is a very large secure calyx of Held synapse.

Outputs: The outputs of the MSO principal and marginal cells on each side ascend ipsilaterally via the lateral lemniscus (Figure 1–11, top portion) sending out collaterals to the DNLL before terminating in the CNIC. Unlike the MSO, the outputs from each LSO project bilaterally along the lateral lemniscus to the CNIC. The outputs to the ipsilateral CNIC are inhibitory (Saint Marie, Ostapoff, Morest, & Wenthold, 1989), and the outputs to the contralateral CNIC are excitatory. Collaterals along the way are also projected to both the DNLL and the VNLL. The MNTB primarily projects to the LSO on the same side; however, it is likely that collaterals send projections to VNLL and IC (Kuwabara, DiCaprio, & Zook, 1991). Although the organization of nuclei and tracts are similar across animal models, there are individual differences in the projection strengths and targets.

Tonotopic organization: While the MSO, LSO, and MNTB are tonotopically organized, it is likely that the MSO is low-frequency biased and the LSO is high-frequency biased to optimally process interaural time and intensity differences, respectively. In the MSO, low frequencies are represented in the dorsal part and high frequencies are represented in the ventral part. In both the LSO and the MNTB, low frequencies are represented in the lateral portion and high frequencies are represented in the medial portion (see Figures 1–10 and 1–11). In addition, for each frequency region, it is likely that an orthogonal spatial map exists in the SOC to represent interaural differences and therefore the location of the sound source in the horizontal plane.

Nuclei of Lateral Lemniscus (NLL)

Location: The lateral lemniscus is a large fiber bundle that ascends bilaterally on the lateral aspect through the medulla and pons and terminates in the inferior colliculus (IC) on each side at the midbrain level. At its terminal point, it carries outputs from all caudal auditory structures in the brainstem. Groups of cells scattered among the ventral and dorsal portions of the lateral lemniscal fibers, at the mid to rostral pontine level (and just caudal to the IC), form the nuclei of lateral lemniscus (Figures 1–10, 1–11, and 1–12).

Subdivisions: Three subdivisions are identified for the nuclei of lateral lemniscus (see Figure 1–12). The most ventral subdivision is the ventral nucleus of lateral lemniscus (VNLL). The VNLL is distinct in all nonprimates but is poorly defined in humans. The VNLL is thought to mediate the acoustic startle reflex via connections to the brainstem reticular formation (Berg & Davis, 1985; Lee, Lopez, Meloni, & Davis, 1996). The most dorsal subdivision is the dorsal nucleus of lateral lemniscus (DNLL). In some animals (not seen in humans), an intermediate group of cells form the intermediate nucleus of lateral lemniscus (INLL) (Glendenning, Brunso-Bechtold, & Thompsonn, 1981).

Cell types: In the VNLL, multipolar cells show a dense columnar organization in one region and a less dense dispersion in another region. The DNLL has a richer diversity of cell types (including elongate and multipolar cells) that form horizontal sheets, varying in size, shape, orientation, and dendritic patterns (Kane & Barone, 1980). Similar cell types as in the DNLL are present in the INLL.

Inputs: The primary inputs to the VNLL are from the contralateral PVCN (octopus cells and multipolar cells) via the IAS and lateral lemniscus. The cells in the contralateral AVCN and DCN also project to the VNLL via the DAS and TB, respectively (Hilbig et al., 2009). The VNLL also receives input from the ipsilateral SOC, primarily the LSO and MNTB (Glendenning, Hutson, Nudo, & Masterton, 1985). The DNLL receives excitatory inputs from the ipsilateral MSO and contralateral LSO, and inhibitory inputs from the ipsilateral LSO. Other inputs include the contralateral DNLL (via the commissure of Probst), ipsilateral VNLL, contralateral DCN, superior colliculus, and efferents from the IC (Adams, 1979; Brunso-Bechtold, Thompson, & Masterton 1981; Glendenning et al., 1985; Kudo, 1981). The main inputs to the INLL are from the contralateral VCN and the MNTB.

Outputs: The VNLL has a prominent projection to the ipsilateral CNIC. There are some minor projections to the DNLL on the same side and contralateral IC (Brunso-Bechtold, Thompson, & Masterton, 1981; Kudo, 1981). Like the VNLL, the DNLL also has a major projection to the IC—but unlike the VNLL, it projects to both the ipsilateral and contralateral IC. The DNLL also has a reciprocating output to the superior colliculus. Unlike the VNLL (which largely behaves like a monaural pathway), most DNLL neurons provide binaural inhibitory inputs. The outputs of the INLL are similar to the VNLL outputs.

Tonotopic organization: In all three subdivisions of the nuclei of lateral lemniscus, the low frequencies are represented in the dorsal portion and high frequencies in the ventral portion, similar to the tonotopic map in the MSO (see Figure 1–10).

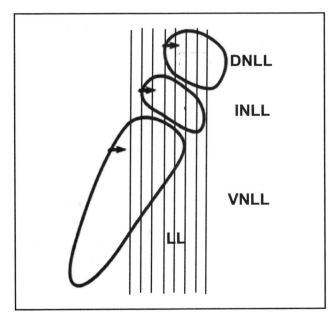

Figure 1–12. Nuclei of lateral lemniscus: dorsal nucleus of lateral lemniscus (DNLL), intermediate nucleus of lateral lemniscus (INLL), and ventral nucleus of lateral lemniscus (VNLL). The vertical lines through the nuclei represent the fibers of the lateral lemniscus.

Inferior Colliculus (IC)

Location: The IC appears as a pair of large spherical protrusions on the dorsal surface of the caudal midbrain, inferior to the midbrain visual nucleus—the superior colliculus (see Figures 1–7 and 1–10). In humans, the IC is about 3 to 3.5 cm rostral to the pontomedullary junction. This is the first point along the auditory pathway for the clear emergence of a tonotopic core and a surrounding nontonotopic belt organization that may be coordinating auditory with nonauditory motor and multisensory functions. The IC is the recipient of most of the ascending fibers from caudal structures and descending fibers from the auditory cortex, suggesting that it plays an important role in shaping signal representation via interplay of bottom-up and top-down influences.

Subdivisions: The IC is subdivided into a central core region called the central nucleus of inferior colliculus (CNIC) and several distinct subdivisions forming a belt around the CNIC (Figure 1–13). The belt subdivisions include the lateral nucleus (LN), dorsal cortex (DC), dorsomedial nucleus (DM), and ventral central gray (CG) region. The primary focus here is the description of the tonotopically organized core CNIC, since the specific roles of the belt regions are not well understood. However, it should be noted that the dorsal cortex is the major recipient of the corticocollicular pathways that play an important role in shaping the response properties of the CNIC neurons. The description of this efferent pathway is considered in the section on efferent innervation.

Cell types: Disc-shaped principal cells, representing 75% to 85% of the total number of cells in the CNIC, are arranged in distinct sheets (forming a laminar structure) oriented at a slight angle (Morest & Oliver, 1984), with each sheet extending from a dorsomedial to a ventrolateral direction (see Figure 1–13). Axons run parallel (see Figure 1–13a) to the cells within each lamina (banded axons). Simple and complex stellate cells make up the remaining 15% to 25% of the population. In contrast to the disc-shaped principal cells, the axons and dendrites run across the laminar structure (see Figure 1–13b, c, d). All four layers of the dorsal cortex are dominated by stellate-type cells with no laminar struc-

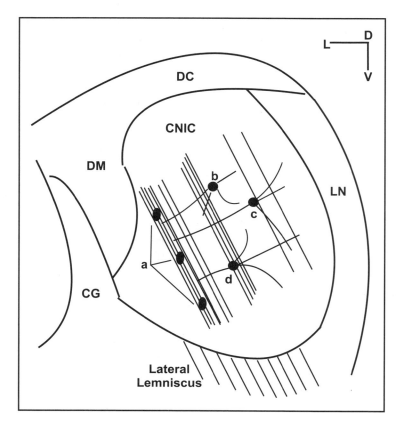

Figure 1–13. Subdivisions of the inferior colliculus (IC) including the core region, central nucleus of inferior colliculus (CNIC), and the surrounding belt regions including the multilayer dorsal cortex (DC), dorsomedial nucleus (DM), lateral nucleus (LN), and the central gray (CG). The isofrequency laminar organization (*parallel lines*) in the CNIC and the organization of the principal cells (a) and multipolar cells (b, c, d) are illustrated. While the axons of the principal cells run parallel to cells within each lamina, the multipolar cells send their dendrites across laminae..

ture. The dorsomedial nucleus is characterized by large multipolar cells. In humans, this belt region is regarded as a tegmental (motor) nucleus rather than a tectal (sensory) nucleus. The lateral nucleus contains both tectal and tegmental cells. Thus, the CNIC is optimally organized for processing auditory stimuli ascending from the lateral lemniscus, whereas most of the belt regions appear to be organized for coordination of auditory and nonauditory processes (Oliver & Huerta, 1992).

Inputs: As indicated earlier, the IC is the recipient of projections from almost all nuclei in the brainstem as well as the corticocollicular inputs from deep layers of the auditory cortex. The orderly overlapping and well-segregated projections (with tonotopic information preserved) from the brainstem structures target the appropriate frequency lamina in the CNIC (Oliver & Huerta, 1992). The CNIC also receives inputs from the contralateral CNIC via the commissure of the inferior colliculus. In addition, the CNIC receives direct and indirect efferent inputs from the corticocollicular pathways. The dorsal cortex of the IC receives inputs mainly from the auditory cortex (corticocollicular pathway) and sparse inputs from the brainstem excluding the SOC (Oliver & Huerta, 1992). The lateral nucleus receives significant inputs from the somatosensory system and the auditory cortex but little or no input via the lateral lemniscus. The dorsomedial nucleus receives some afferent inputs via the lateral lemniscus and some descending inputs from the auditory cortex.

Outputs: The primary output from the CNIC is to the tonotopically organized core of the medial geniculate body (MGB)—the ventral subdivision of the MGB (MGB$_V$) and a smaller projection to the medial subdivision of MGB (MGB$_M$) via the brachium of the IC (Figure 1–14). The CNIC also projects to the contralateral CNIC via the commissure of the IC. The dorsal cortex has a diffuse projection to the dorsal subdivision of the MGB (MGB$_D$). The lateral nucleus and the dorsomedial nucleus project polysensory information to the MGB$_M$. Thus, the core-to-core and the belt-to-belt projections reflect segregated parallel processing.

Tonotopic organization: The exquisite laminar organization in the CNIC provides a robust framework for its highly tonotopic organization. Isofrequency sheets, representing each lamina, consist of neurons responding to the same or a very

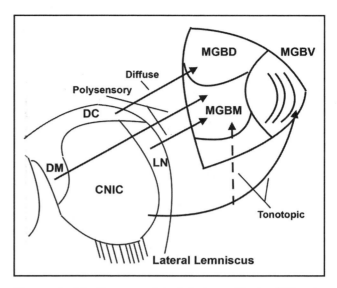

Figure 1–14. Outputs of the inferior colliculus (IC) core (central nucleus of inferior colliculus [CNIC]) and IC belt regions to the medial geniculate body core (MGB$_V$) and the belt areas MGB$_D$ and MGB$_M$, respectively. Note the tonotopic core-to-core projection and the nontonotopic polysensory projections.

narrow range of frequencies (Malmierca, Rees, Le Beau, & Bjaalie, 1995; Schreiner & Langner, 1997). Consistent with the angular orientation of the isofrequency sheets, low frequencies are represented in the dorsolateral sheets, and high frequencies are represented in the ventromedial sheets (Figures 1–10 and 1–15). Interestingly, CNIC neurons also exhibit a sound source location map. Neurons responding best to sound location toward the midline are located in the caudal regions, and rostrally located neurons respond best to sounds from the side.

It is relevant to point out that some of the cell types described here have been implicated in the generation of the ABR components from different structures along the auditory pathway in the cat brainstem. Melcher and Kiang (1996) examined the relationship between different brainstem cell types and generator sources for the scalp-recorded ABR by combining information from models (models relating the ABR to underlying neural activity) and experimental data from different levels in the brainstem. Based on this analysis, they proposed that P1 (wave 1) is generated by spiral ganglion cells of the AN; P2 (wave II) primarily by the globular bushy cells in the ipsilateral CN; P3 (wave III) partly from

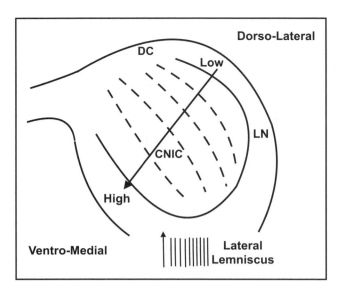

Figure 1–15. Tonotopic map using the laminar organization in the central nucleus of the inferior colliculus (CNIC). The isofrequency sheets progress from low frequencies in the dorsolateral portion and high frequencies in the ventromedial portions.

the spherical bushy cells in the CN and cells receiving inputs from the globular cells; P4 (wave IV or the IV–V complex) mostly by the principal cells in the MSO which in turn are driven by CN spherical cells; and P5 (wave V) driven by MSO principal cells. Based on these results, these authors infer that the ABR components in cats reflect neural activity driven by two distinct parallel pathways—one originating with globular cells and the other with spherical cells. They also suggest that the human ABR is largely generated by brainstem neurons along the spherical cell pathway given the poor representation of the globular cell pathway in humans.

III. EFFERENT PATHWAYS

Just like ascending pathways carry information from the auditory periphery to the cortex in a highly organized fashion, there are also descending pathways carrying information from the cortex to the cochlea. Given the focus of this book on the brainstem, the discussion here is limited to the efferent innervation of the cochlear OHCs and IHCs by the medial and lateral efferents arising in the SOC, and the corticocollicular projections arising in the deep layers of the auditory cortex and projecting to the subdivisions of the IC.

Efferent Innervation of the Cochlea

Similar to the afferent innervation of the cochlea, separate fibers and distinct innervation patterns are also observed for the efferents innervating the OHCs and IHCs (Figure 1–16). For each hair cell subsystem, there is an ipsilateral (uncrossed) and a contralateral (crossed) point of origin from the superior olivary complex in the caudal brainstem (Warr & Guinan, 1979). The fibers innervating the OHCs, called the medial efferents (medial olivocochlear bundle or Rasmussen's bundle), have an ipsilateral (10% of the total) and a dominant contralateral (30% of the total) component originating in the periolivary nuclei surrounding the MSO. The crossed component, called the medial efferents, joins the uncrossed component in the dorsal portion of the brainstem and descends through the cochlear nucleus and the vestibular portion of the VIII cranial nerve, enters the cochlea through the habenula perforata, crosses the cochlear tunnel diagonally as tunnel radial fibers, and innervates the OHCs at their base. The innervation density of the medial efferents is greater in the base compared to the apex. The lateral efferents, predominantly originating from the ipsilateral LSO, follow the same course to the cochlea as the uncrossed medial efferents (see Figure 1–16). Once in the cochlea, these fibers, called the inner spiral fibers, spiral around the cochlea before innervating the IHCs on their afferent synapse (see Figure 1–8). Innervation density is broader compared to the medial efferents. Since these efferents appear to modulate the gain of the cochlear amplifier associated with the OHC subsystem, there is considerable interest in their role in improving hearing in adverse listening conditions.

Efferent Innervation of the IC

The corticocollicular fibers originate from cells in Layer V of the auditory cortex, bypass the MGB in the thalamus, and project primarily to the ipsilateral dorsal cortex (Figure 1–17) of the IC with smaller projections to the CNIC and the belt regions

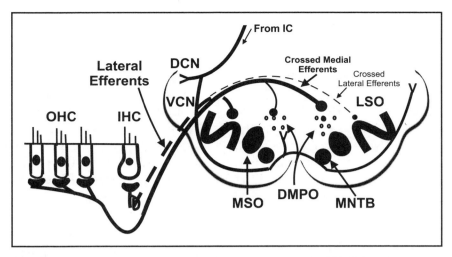

Figure 1-16. Efferent innervation of the outer hair cells (OHCs) and the inner hair cells (IHCs). The crossed and uncrossed components of lateral (*dashed line*) and medial efferents (*solid line*) are identified. Collectively, the olivocochlear bundle is illustrated as the thick black track. Note the difference in both the point of origin (lateral: lateral superior olive [LSO]; medial: periolivary region around medial superior olive [MSO]) and the location of the synapse for the medial efferents (on the OHC cell body) and the lateral efferents (on the afferents of the IHC).

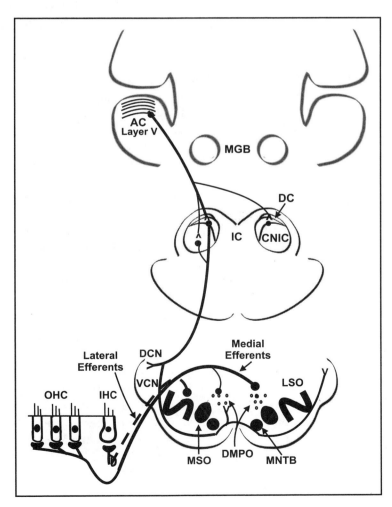

Figure 1-17. Corticocollicular pathway originating in Layer V of the auditory cortex and terminating in the dorsal cortex (DC), central nucleus of inferior colliculus (CNIC), and lateral nucleus (LN) of the inferior colliculus (IC), including segments extending to the periolivary region of the superior olivary complex (SOC)—the point of origin of the olivocochlear bundle. Medial and lateral efferents, part of the olivocochlear bundle, terminate in the outer hair cells (OHCs) and inner hair cells (IHCs), respectively. Dashed lines illustrate the afferent pathways.

of the IC. From the IC, there are also components of this corticofugal pathway that descend down the brainstem bilaterally and innervate the cells in the periolivary region on each side—the point of origin of the medial and lateral efferents to the OHCs and IHCs, respectively (see Figure 1–17). Both neuroanatomic (Lim & Anderson, 2007; Saldana, Feliciano, & Mugnaini, 1996) and compelling physiologic evidence show that descending cortical inputs to the IC influence shaping of the response properties (e.g., changes in frequency selectivity) in the CNIC (Bajo, Nodal, Moore, & King, 2010; Yan & Suga, 1998; Yan, Zhang, & Ehret, 2005).

IV. SUMMARY

- The structure, afferent and efferent innervation pattern, and functional roles of the OHCs and IHCs are very different. For example, the OHCs are both structurally and functionally more like muscle cells and exhibit motility, while the IHCs are more like sensory receptors; OHCs have a converging afferent innervation (output of many OHCs carried by a single OSF), while the IHCs have a divergent afferent innervation (one inner IRF to one IHC); medial efferents target the OHCs while the lateral efferents target the IHCs; and functionally, the IHCs provide the primary drive (sensory transduction) to the auditory nerve given that 95% of the AN fibers innervate the IHCs. On the other hand, the OHCs assume the role of a mechanoelectric amplifier by feeding back energy to selectively increase the amplitude of basilar membrane displacement in a frequency-specific manner. It is believed that this amplification is somehow detected by the IHCs and transmitted to the central auditory system. Clinical measures assessing the functional integrity of the OHCs include the cochlear microphonics (CM), summating potential (SP), and otoacoustic emissions (OAEs), and will be discussed later.

- The auditory nerve is systematically organized into a bundle that carries low-frequency fibers at its core and increasingly higher-frequency fibers toward the surface. The high-frequency and low-frequency fibers of the AN terminate in the dorsal portions and ventral portions of the CN subdivisions, respectively. Clinical measures assessing the functional integrity of the IHC transduction process and the function of the auditory nerve include electrocochleography and the evaluation of Wave I of the ABR and will be discussed later.

- The diversity of cell types in the CN across its subdivisions suggests a functional hierarchy moving from auditory nerve–like responses in the AVCN to more complex responses governed by inhibition in the DCN. The segregated outputs of the CN carried by three different pathways project to almost all brainstem structures before terminating in the IC. Each of the subdivisions of the CN is highly tonotopic with high frequencies represented in the dorsal portion and low frequency in the ventral portion. Components I, II, and III of the ABR may represent neural activity originating in the CN.

- The SOC is the first point along the auditory pathway where the outputs from both ears converge. The MSO is specialized for processing the interaural time difference, and the LSO/MNTB are specialized to process the interaural intensity differences used in representing the location of a sound source in the horizontal plane. The outputs of this initial binaural processing are passed on to the nuclei of LL and the CNIC. The MSO has a dorsal low-frequency and a ventral high-frequency tonotopic map. The LSO/MNTB have a lateral low-frequency and medial high-frequency tonotopic map. Wave III of the ABR is thought to reflect neural activity originating in the SOC, primarily on the contralateral side.

- The IC is a major midbrain auditory nucleus where almost all ascending and descending information converges. It is also the first level along the auditory pathway where the nucleus is organized into a core (CNIC) tonotopic, primarily auditory processor and a surrounding nontonotopic belt that appears to be more a coordinator of the auditory processing of the CNIC with visual, motor, and somatosensory systems. The laminar organization in the CNIC provides for a robust framework to achieve a highly tonotopic map with dorsolateral isofrequency sheets representing low frequencies and the medioventral isofrequency sheets representing high frequencies. In addition, the CNIC has a spatial map with caudal neurons responding best to sounds along the midline, while the rostral neurons respond best to sounds from the side. There is an orderly tonotopic core-to-core, and nontonotopic polysensory projections to the core and belt regions, respectively of the MGB. Waves IV and V of the ABR are thought to reflect neural activity in the lateral lemniscus and the IC. The sustained frequency following response with a latency of about 6 to 9 ms is also thought to be of IC origin.

V. RECOMMENDED READINGS

Excellent Reviews With Sufficient Detail

Harrison, A. V. (2007). Anatomy and physiology of the auditory periphery. In B. F. Burkard, M. Don, & J. J. Eggermont (Eds.), *Auditory evoked potentials: Basic principles and clinical application* (Chapter 7, pp. 140–158). Baltimore, MD: Lippincott Williams & Wilkins.

Palmer, A. R. (2007). Anatomy and physiology of the auditory brainstem. In B. F. Burkard, M. Don, & J. J. Eggermont (Eds.), *Auditory evoked potentials: Basic principles and clinical application* (Chapter 8, pp. 200–228). Baltimore, MD: Lippincott Williams & Wilkins.

REFERENCES

Adams, J. (1979). Ascending projections to the inferior colliculus. *Journal of Comparative Neurology, 183*, 519–538.

Adams, J. (1986). Neuronal morphology of the human cochlear nucleus. *Archives of Otolaryngology-Head and Neck Surgery, 112*, 1253–1261.

Bajo, V. M., Nodal, F. R., Moore, D. R., & King, A. J. (2010). The descending corticocollicular pathway mediates learning-induced auditory plasticity. *Nature Neuroscience, 13*(2), 253–260.

Berg, W. K., & Davis, M. (1985). Associative learning modifies startle reflexes at the lateral lemniscus. *Behavioral Neuroscience, 99*(2), 191–199.

Brawer, J. R., Morest, D. K., & Kane, E. C. (1974). The neuronal architecture of the cochlear nucleus of the cat. *Journal of Comparative Neurology, 155*, 251–300.

Brownell, W. E., Bader, C. R., Bertrand, D., & de Ribaupierre, Y. (1985). Evoked mechanical responses of isolated cochlear outer hair cells. *Science, 277*(4683), 194–196.

Brunso-Bechtold, J., Thompson, G., & Masterton, R. (1981). HRP study of the organization of auditory afferents ascending to the central nucleus of inferior colliculus. *Journal of Comparative Neurology, 197*, 705–722.

Cant, N. B. (1992). The cochlear nucleus: Neuronal types and their synaptic organization. In B. Webster, A. N. Popper, & R. R. Fay (Eds.), *The mammalian auditory pathway: Neuroanatomy* (pp. 63–117). New York, NY: Springer-Verlag.

Dallos, P. (1992). The active cochlea. *Journal of Neuroscience, 12*(12), 4575–4585.

Dallos, P. (2008). Cochlear amplification, outer hair cells and prestin. *Current Opinion in Neurobiology, 18*(4), 370–376.

Glendenning, K. K., Brunso-Bechtold, J. K., & Thompsonn, C. C. (1981). Ascending auditory afferents to the nuclei of lateral lemniscus. *Journal of Comparative Neurology, 197*, 673–703.

Glendenning, K. K., Hutson, K. A., Nudo, R. J., & Masterton, R. B. (1985). Acoustic chiasm: II. Anatomical basis of binaurality in lateral superior olive of cat. *Journal of Comparative Neurology, 232*, 261–285.

Hilbig, H., Beil, B., Hilbig, H., Call, J., & Bidman, H.-J. (2009). Superior olivary complex organization and cytoarchitecture may be correlated with function and catarrhine primate phylogeny. *Brain Structure and Function, 213*(4), 489–497.

Kane, E. S., & Barone, L. M. (1980). The dorsal nucleus of the lateral lemniscus in the cat: Neuronal types and their distributions. *Journal of Comparative Neurology, 192*, 797–826.

Kudo, M. (1981). Projections of the nuclei of lateral lemniscus in the cat: An autoradiographic study. *Brain Research, 221*, 57–69.

Kuwabara, N., DiCaprio, R. A., & Zook, J. M. (1991). Afferents to the medial nucleus of the trapezoid body and their collateral projections. *Journal of Comparative Neurology, 314*, 684–706.

Lee, Y., Lopez, D. E., Meloni, E. G., & Davis, M. (1996). A primary acoustic startle pathway: Obligatory role of cochlear root neurons and the nucleus reticularis pontis caudalis. *Journal of Neuroscience, 16*(11), 3775–3789.

Lim, H. H., & Anderson, D. J. (2007). Antidromic activation reveals tonotopically organized projections from primary auditory cortex to the central nucleus of the inferior colliculus in guinea pig. *Journal of Neurophysiology, 97*(2), 1413–1427.

Lorente de No, R. (1933). Anatomy of the eighth nerve: The central projections of the nerve endings of the internal ear. *Laryngoscope, 43,* 1–13.

Malmierca, M. S., Rees, A., Le Beau, F. E. N., & Bjaalie, J. G. (1995). Laminar organization of frequency-defined local axons within and between the inferior colliculi of the guinea pig. *Journal of Comparative Neurology, 357,* 124–144.

Masterton, B., Thompson, G. C., Bechtold, J. K., & RoBards, M. J. (1975). Neuroanatomical basis of interaural phase-difference analysis for sound localization: A comparative study. *Journal of Comparative Psychology, 89,* 379–386.

Melcher, J. R., & Kiang, N. Y. S. (1996). Generators of the brainstem auditory evoked potential in cat III: Identified cell populations. *Hearing Research, 93,* 52–71.

Moore, J. K., & Osen, K. K. (1979). The cochlear nuclei in man. *American Journal of Anatomy, 154,* 393–417.

Morest, D. K., & Oliver, D. L. (1984). The neuronal architecture of the inferior colliculus in the cat: Defining the functional anatomy of the auditory midbrain. *Journal of Comparative Neurology, 222,* 209–236.

Oliver, D. L., & Huerta, M. F. (1992). Inferior and superior colliculi. In D. B. Webster, A. N. Popper, &, R. R. Fay (Eds.), *The mammalian auditory pathway: Neuroanatomy* (pp. 168–221). New York, NY: Springer-Verlag.

Osen, K. K. (1969). Cytoarchitecture of the cochlear nuclei in cat. *Journal of Comparative Neurology, 136*(4), 453–483.

Pickles, J. O., Comis, S. D., & Osborne, M. P. (1984). Cross-links between stereocilia in the guinea pig organ of Corti and their possible relation to sensory transduction. *Hearing Research, 15*(2), 103–112.

Raphael, Y., & Altschuler, R. A. (2003). Structure and innervation of the cochlea. *Brain Research Bulletin, 60,* 397–422.

Robertson, D. (1984). Horseradish peroxidase injection of physiologically characterized afferent and efferent neurons in the guinea pig spiral ganglion. *Hearing Research, 15,* 113–121.

Ryugo, D. K. (1992). The auditory nerve: Peripheral innervation, cell body morphology and central projections. In D. B. Webster, A. N. Popper, & R. R Fay (Eds.), *The mammalian auditory pathway: Neuroanatomy* (pp. 22–64). New York, NY: Springer-Verlag.

Saint Marie, R. L., Ostapoff, E. M., Morest, D. K., & Wenthold, R. J. (1989). Glycine immunoreactive projection of the cat lateral superior olive: Possible role in the midbrain ear dominance. *Journal of Comparative Neurology, 279,* 382–396.

Saldana, E., Feliciano, M., & Mugnaini, E. (1996). Distribution of descending projections from primary auditory neocortex to inferior colliculus mimics the topography of intracollicular projections. *Journal of Comparative Neurology, 371*(1), 15–40.

Schreiner, C. E., & Langner, G. (1997). Laminar fine structure of frequency organization in auditory midbrain. *Nature, 388,* 383–386.

Smith, C. A. (1978). Structure of the cochlear duct. In R. F. Naunton & C. Fernandez (Eds.), *Evoked electrical activity in the auditory nervous system* (pp. 3–19). New York, NY: Academic Press.

Spoendlin, H. (1978). The afferent innervation of the cochlea. In R. F. Naunton & C. Fernandez (Eds.), *Evoked electrical activity in the auditory nervous system* (pp. 21–39). New York, NY: Academic Press.

von Bekesy, G. (1960). *Experiments in hearing.* New York, NY: McGraw-Hill.

Wangemann, P. K. (2002). K^+ cycling and the endocochlear potential. *Hearing Research, 165,* 1–9.

Warr, W. B. (1982). Parallel ascending pathways from the cochlear nucleus: Neuroanatomical evidence of functional specialization. In W. D. Neff (Ed.), *Contribution to sensory physiology* (Vol. 7, pp. 1–38). New York, NY: Academic.

Warr, W. B., & Guinan, J. J. (1979). Efferent innervation of the organ of Corti: Two separate systems. *Brain Research, 173,* 152–155.

Yan, J., Zhang, Y., & Ehret, G. (2005). Corticofugal shaping of frequency tuning curves in the central nucleus of the inferior colliculus of mice. *Journal of Neurophysiology, 93*(1), 71–83.

Yan, W., & Suga, N. (1998). Corticofugal modulation of the midbrain frequency map in the bat auditory system. *Nature Neuroscience, 1*(1), 54–58.

Young, E. D., Shofner, W. P., White, J. A., Robert, J.-M., & Voigt, H. F. (1988). Response properties of the cochlear nucleus neurons in relationship to physiological mechanisms. In G. M. Edelman, W. E. Gall, & W. M. Cowan (Eds), *Auditory function: Neurobiological basis of hearing* (pp. 277–312). New York, NY: Wiley.

2

Neural Activity Underlying Scalp-Recorded Evoked Potentials

SCOPE

A good understanding of the basic structure and function of sensory neurons in the central nervous system is an essential prerequisite to understand the neural basis of evoked potentials. With the knowledge of neuronal physiology, we can begin to understand how the tiny (nanovolt to microvolt) stimulus-elicited electrical voltages from a population of neurons (therefore the name *evoked potentials*) are transmitted from generator sources deep within the brainstem to electrodes at the surface of the head. Once the neural basis of evoked potentials is understood, we can begin to classify the evoked potentials based on how they are recorded, whether they reflect an onset or a sustained response, their latency/generator site(s), and whether they reflect activity from sensory neurons or from muscles. The aim here is to provide the clinician with a strong theoretical background to be able to optimally record and interpret these responses.

I. NEURONAL PHYSIOLOGY

Structure of a Neuron

The human brain consists of about 86 billion (Herculano-Houzel, 2017) neurons plus supporting neuroglial cells. Each sensory neuron consists of a cell body (*soma*) with a nucleus inside and several branched processes called *dendrites* and an unbranched long process called the *axon* that extend from the soma (Figure 2–1). While the dendrites transmit information toward the cell, the axons arising at the axonal hillock carry information away to other cells with the axonal terminals forming the presynaptic region. These axons can be either fast conducting myelinated (covered by a myelin sheath formed by layers of Schwann cells) or slow conducting unmyelinated.

Requirements for Neural Signaling

There are at least four essential requirements for a neuron to be able to generate and transmit information. First, the neuron has to be in a polarized state. That is, it should be able to generate and maintain a charge difference across the neuronal membrane, the *membrane potential*. Second, there should be a rapid depolarization followed by repolarization to generate the excitatory spike or *action potential* (AP). Third, the neuron should be able to propagate the APs from the cell body along the axons. Fourth, signals should be transmitted from one cell to another via *synapses* to produce either an *excitatory postsynaptic potential* (EPSP) or an *inhibitory postsynaptic potential* (IPSP).

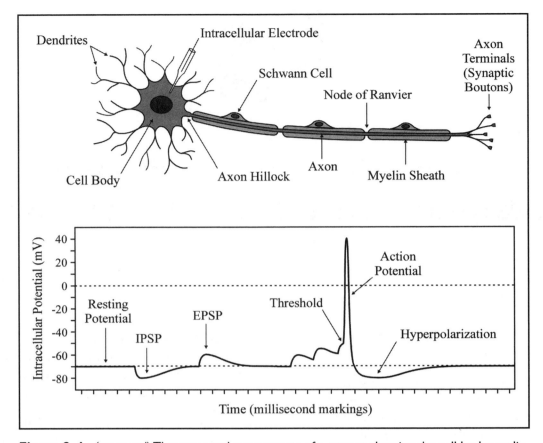

Figure 2–1. (*top panel*) The structural components of a neuron showing the cell body, myelinated axon, and axon terminals. (*bottom panel*) The temporal evolution of an action potential (AP) including the resting potential, inhibitory and excitatory postsynaptic potentials (IPSP and EPSP), depolarizations leading to AP, and the hyperpolarization phase of the AP before returning to resting state. Adapted from *Human Auditory Evoked Potentials* (p. 96) by Terence W. Picton. Copyright 2011 Plural Publishing, Inc. All rights reserved.

Generation and Maintenance of the Resting Membrane Potential (RMP)-Polarized Cell

In order to generate and maintain an RMP (be in a polarized state), a charge difference between the inside and the outside of the cell has to be created and maintained. This is accomplished by essentially two mechanisms: (1) a passive mechanism that combines the ionic concentration gradient across the cell and the selective permeability of the cell membrane to potassium ions; and (2), an active process that expends energy to move the ions against their concentration gradients. Specifically, the concentration of sodium (Na$^+$) ions is greater on the outside of the cell compared to the inside; the concentration of the potassium (K$^+$) ions is greater inside compared to the outside. Therefore, these ions will passively tend to diffuse along their concentration gradients through Na$^+$ and Ka$^+$ channels, respectively. However, at rest, the selective permeability of the cell membrane to K$^+$ ions and the relatively greater number of K$^+$ channels will expel more positively charged K$^+$ ions than the number of positively charged Na$^+$ coming in. The result is that the inside of the neuron has a negative charge relative to the outside. Additionally, in order to move out the Na$^+$ ions leaking in, and to maintain the RMP, the active Na$^+$/K$^+$ pump expels three Na$^+$ ions and reclaims two K$^+$ ions working against the concentration gradient and expending energy (Figure 2–2). Importantly, this difference

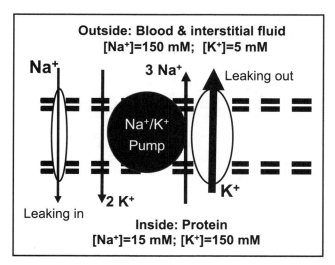

Figure 2–2. Sodium (Na⁺) and potassium (K⁺) ion concentrations within and outside a neuron. Note the greater concentration of the Na⁺ ions on the outside relative to the inside and the opposite gradient for the K⁺ ions. Also shown are the larger leak channels of the K⁺ ions to the outside compared to the smaller leak channels of the Na⁺ ions into the neuron reflecting the greater membrane permeability to K⁺ ions. The active Na⁺/K⁺ pump, working against the concentration gradient, brings in two K⁺ ions for every three Na⁺ ions that are expelled.

in charge is associated with an electrical gradient that is important for the generation of the RMP of −70 mV inside the neuron with respect to the outside. Now the membrane is said to be polarized and ready to elicit a stimulus-driven AP.

Action Potential: Generation, Propagation, and Synaptic Transmission

Generation: Rapid changes (in the 1–2 ms range) in the membrane potentials are essential for neural signaling using the AP. Application of an electrical or chemical stimulus that can open/close specific ion channels can begin to produce these changes that will eventually generate the AP. The preamble to the generation of the all-or-none AP includes the graded potentials (small depolarizations well below the threshold for AP generation) that steadily grow with increase in stimulus intensity nudging the RMP to lesser negative values (only some Na⁺ channels become active). When the stimulus has sufficient strength to move the graded potentials to about −55 mV, the threshold potential for AP generation is reached. Now, many voltage-gated Na⁺ channels open, resulting in a rapid influx of Na⁺ ions into the cells (*depolarizing phase* of the AP characterized by a potential change that momentarily reaches a maximum of **40 mV: overshoot**). During this overshoot, the voltage-dependent Na⁺ ion channels rapidly close, reversing the direction of the electrical potential change and limiting further Na⁺ influx. Almost at the same time, the voltage-gated K⁺ channel starts to open, leading to the *repolarization phase* (return of the voltage toward the RMP) characterized by an efflux of K⁺ ions resulting in a net decrease in positive charge within the cell. Since the potassium channels take a longer time to close, a *hyperpolarization (undershoot)* is observed before the RMP is reestablished. These rapid temporal changes in membrane potential characterized by depolarization (overshoot), repolarization, and hyperpolarization (undershoot) describe the all-or-none AP (Figure 2–3). The AP is not a graded response; it occurs only when threshold is reached, and it is independent of stimulus strength; therefore, it is referred to as an all-or-none response.

The ability to generate and propagate these rapid changes in membrane potential is limited by the *absolute* and *relative refractory period*. Absolute refractory period refers to the transient temporal period of depolarization during AP generation when voltage-gated Na⁺ channels are still open when another AP cannot be generated. That is, another stimulus occurring in this time window will not be able to produce a second AP (see Figure 2–3). The relative refractory period refers to a slightly longer time window during the repolarization phase of the AP when voltage-gated K⁺ channels are open (remember, the Na⁺ channels remain closed). During this phase, a second AP may be generated provided stimulus strength exceeds the threshold for AP generation. The later in time during this phase that another stimulus occurs, the greater will be the probability to generate a second AP.

Propagation: APs propagate along unmyelinated and myelinated axons through a process of spread of depolarization to adjacent segments that result in new APs along the length of the axon (Figure 2–4). However, the manner of propagation is different in unmyelinated and myelinated

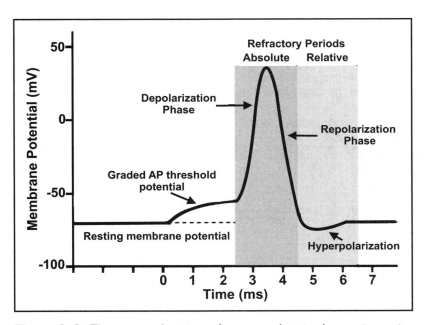

Figure 2–3. The temporal course of transmembranic changes in resting membrane potential (RMP) associated with the generation of the action potential (AP). The RMP is at −70 mV prior to stimulation. The phases of the membrane potential changes (AP) associated with depolarization (Na^+ influx following opening of voltage-gated NA^+ channels), repolarization (K^+ channels opening), and hyperpolarization (slow closing of K^+ channels) before returning to resting state.

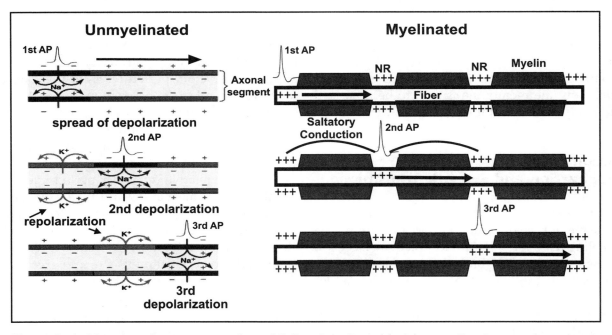

Figure 2–4. Neural conduction in unmyelinated (*left*) and myelinated (*right*) axons. For the unmyelinated axon, the AP is regenerated along the axon due to the spread of depolarization along adjacent segments of the axon which creates an impression of the AP moving along the axon from left to right. For the myelinated axon, APs are only regenerated at the nodes of Ranvier (NR), where Na^+ channels are available. The AP appears to jump from one node to the next, a process referred to as saltatory conduction. This results in a faster neural conduction along a myelinated axon compared to the unmyelinated axon.

fibers. For the unmyelinated fiber (Figure 2–4, left panel), initial depolarization producing the first AP spreads to adjacent membrane regions to the right causing voltage-gated Na⁺ channels to open to produce the second AP in that region. As this process repeats along the axon, new APs are generated that appear to move along the axon indicated by the long arrow (see second and third segments in Figure 2–4). While the depolarization spreads to the right, it leaves behind a region that is in refractory state (Na⁺ channels still closed), thus allowing the APs to propagate in only one direction. It should be noted here that there is indeed bidirectional spread at the active region, but impulse transmission is only toward the axonal terminals. Since APs are generated in adjacent sections in a continuous manner in unmyelinated fibers (like a centipede inching along), the conduction velocity is much slower than observed for the myelinated fibers, which take advantage of saltatory conduction (like a kangaroo in full stride). Myelinated axons have periodic gaps in the myelin sheath called nodes of Ranvier. In saltatory conduction, APs only arise in the axon membrane at the nodes of Ranvier because voltage-gated Na⁺ channels essential for AP generation are concentrated here. The high electrical resistance of the myelin sheath ensures that APs propagating with almost uniform velocity jump from node to node (Figure 2–4, right panel), thus increasing the conduction velocity. Also, this high resistance ensures that the depolarization current travels with enough strength to the next node of Ranvier. The diameter of the fiber and myelinization are the two determinants of conduction velocity. Axons with larger diameters retain more Na⁺ ions, have larger depolarizations, and therefore exhibit faster conduction velocity. Myelinization insulates and prevents dissipation of depolarizations in small axons, and with the mechanism of saltatory conduction greatly increases conduction velocity. In demyelinating disorders, the loss of myelin could block or slow down conduction, which in turn may disrupt neural synchrony in a population of neurons.

Synaptic transmission: A synapse is a functional coupling between neurons where electrical impulses at the axonal terminal (presynaptic region of presynaptic neuron) are transmitted chemically to the soma or dendrite of a postsynaptic neuron. The enlarged axonal presynaptic terminal contains numerous synaptic vesicles (which contain neurotransmitters—the effective chemical stimuli for postsynaptic events). The presynaptic terminal and the postsynaptic dendrite/soma are separated by a gap called the *synaptic cleft*. Depolarization of the presynaptic terminal by the AP along the axon engages voltage-gated calcium channels causing an influx of calcium ions, which in turn causes vesicles containing the neurotransmitter to fuse with the presynaptic membrane and then to release the neurotransmitter into the synaptic cleft. From the synaptic cleft, the neurotransmitter diffuses to the postsynaptic membrane where it binds to receptors specific to that neurotransmitter. Whether the postsynaptic response is excitatory or inhibitory is dependent on both the type of neurotransmitter and the receptor (Goodlett & Horn, 2001). For example, acetylcholine is excitatory when it binds with one type of receptor but inhibitory when it binds with another receptor type. Assuming an excitatory neural transmitter and receptor, and sufficient release of neurotransmitters to reach threshold, an AP will be generated and propagated in the postsynaptic neuron (Figure 2–5). Neurotransmitters that depolarize the postsynaptic membrane

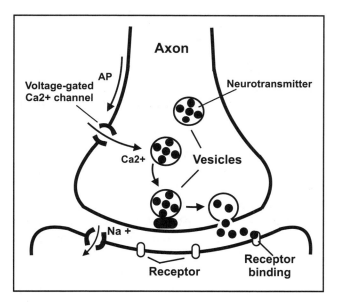

Figure 2–5. Axonal synaptic terminal showing the presynaptic membrane with voltage-gated Ca²⁺ channel, and neurotransmitter vesicles; synaptic cleft (the gap between the pre- and postsynaptic membrane); and the postsynaptic membrane with voltage-gated Na⁺ channels and receptors.

tend to produce EPSPs and therefore promote generation and transmission of APs postsynaptically. Acetylcholine and glutamate are examples of excitatory neurotransmitters in the auditory system. In contrast, neurotransmitters that hyperpolarize (increase negativity of the membrane potential by increasing permeability to K^+) are less likely to generate and propagate an AP postsynaptically. Gamma aminobutyric acid (GABA) and glycine are examples of inhibitory neurotransmitters in the auditory system. Traditionally, the axon hillock (a hill-like prominence on the cell body as it slopes into the axon) has been thought of as the trigger zone for initiation of APs. Specifically, propagated membrane potentials from synaptic inputs are summated to generate an AP in this region. However, increasingly it is believed that the earliest site of AP initiation is in the initial segment of the axon past the axon hillock. We have described the events leading to the generation and propagation of neural activity in a single neuron. Next, we consider properties of neural activity from a population of neurons that can be recorded with electrodes placed on the scalp, called evoked potentials.

II. NEURAL BASES OF EVOKED POTENTIALS

Definition of an evoked potential: Evoked potentials represent the sum of time-locked (precise latency implied) synchronous *neural activity (AP or postsynaptic potentials)* in a population of neural elements *evoked* by an external (exogenous, e.g., click) or an internal (endogenous, e.g., brain processes not solely dependent on the physical characteristics of the stimulus) stimulus that are *volume conducted* (passive conduction of the electrical field created by neural activity from the generator source to the scalp through a medium of brain tissue and cranial bones) and recordable at the scalp using electroencephalograph (EEG)-type disc electrodes. Stimuli evoking these responses could be of different modalities: auditory, visual, or somatosensory, for example.

Neural basis of evoked potentials: The transmembranic flow of ionic current in the cell is the genesis of voltage potentials that underly the generation of scalp-recorded evoked responses. When the cell is depolarized with an effective stimulus, positive ions enter the cell, and the net extracellular charge in the vicinity of the cell will be negative (referred to as a *sink*). In the next phase when the currents flow out to the extracellular space (during hyperpolarization of the cell), the net charge in this region will be positive (referred to as a *source*). This sequence of depolarization (sink) and hyperpolarization (source) associated with transmembranic ionic current flow in the cell produces a net negative and positive charge, respectively, in the extracellular space. Thus, a dipole source is set up with a positive and a negative electric field. The distribution of this current flow in the extracellular space creates a potential field. The passive transmission of the resulting electric field outward toward the scalp through brain tissue, extracellular space, skull, and scalp is called *volume conduction*.

Factors affecting volume conduction: The effectiveness of volume conduction is determined by several factors including distance of the recording electrode from the dipole source, geometric orientation of the dipoles, and temporal synchronization and spatial summation of the volume-conducted electrical field (Scherg, 1990).

Distance of recording electrode from the dipole source: Volume conduction in the EEG domain is thought to occur in a purely resistive medium; therefore, the amplitude of the electrical field decreases precipitously as the electrode distance from the source increases (Figure 2–6). It can be seen in Figure 2–6 that the magnitude of the surface-recorded somatosensory electrical potential is less than 5% of the total amplitude for recordings made near the dipole source. In fact, the higher resistance of the skull to current flow contributes largely to the small magnitude of the scalp-recorded potentials. Moving the electrode away from the source also decreases the spatial resolution of the recorded evoked potential (Figure 2–7). It can be seen in Figure 2–7 that for both a single dipole and two overlapping dipoles, recordings from the nearer electrode (a) show clear, sharply resolved peaks compared to the broad and smaller amplitude peaks for the distant electrode (b). Thus, increasing distance of the electrode from the dipole source decreases response amplitude and spatial resolution of the measured response.

Geometric orientation of the dipoles: Geometric orientation refers to the arrangement of the

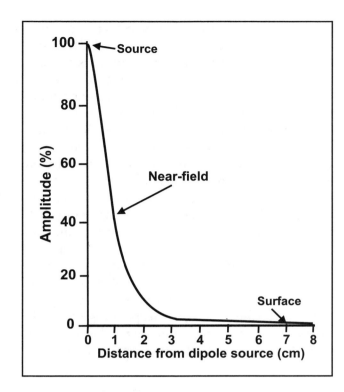

Figure 2–6. Effects of increasing the distance of the recording electrode from a dipole source on the amplitude of the volume-conducted potentials. The amplitude of the response decreases precipitously as the electrode is moved farther away from the source. Recordings made near the source (near field recordings) have significantly larger amplitude compared to surface recording (like recording from the scalp). Note that the amplitude of the surface recording is about 1% of the magnitude of response recorded at the source. Figure created using data from C. C. Wood & T. Allison. (1981). *Canadian Journal of Psychology, 35*(2), 113–115 (Figure 8).

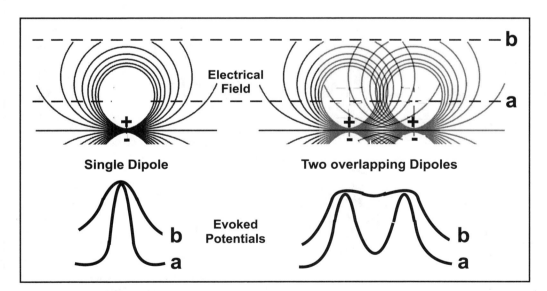

Figure 2–7. Effects of increasing the distance of the recording electrode from a dipole source on the amplitude and spatial resolution of the volume-conducted potentials. The electrical fields (*top row*) for a single dipole (*left*) and two dipoles (*right*) with overlapping electrical fields. Shown in the bottom row are the evoked potentials for electrode locations (a) and (b) for both dipoles. For the single dipole, both the amplitude and the spatial resolution decrease as the electrode is moved farther from the source (b). Similarly, for the overlapping dipoles, amplitude decreases, and more dramatically, spatial resolution showing distinct response peaks reflecting activity from the two sources (a) changes to a single broad peak as the electrode is moved farther from the source (b).

activated neurons and their dendritic field within a population of neurons. If the neurons are arranged in a parallel fashion with the same geometric orientation, it creates an open field (effectively behaving like one *equivalent dipole*), which allows the current from the neural elements to sum optimally, and the volume-conducted potential to be recorded at the scalp (top in Figure 2–8). In contrast, if the neurons are arranged with random orientations, it creates a closed field where the current from the neural elements will cancel out close to the generating site and cannot be detected at the scalp (bottom in Figure 2–8).

Temporal synchronization and spatial summation: Volume conduction is best when the neural activity across individual neurons in the population is well synchronized temporally. Temporal synchronization of extracellular field potentials requires sustained neural activity and is reduced for rapid transient transmembranic current flow. If transmembranic current flow is restricted to a small region of the active neurons, then the ability to spatially sum neural activity across neurons is reduced. The result is that the strength of the volume-conducted potential will be reduced. Thus, for optimal volume conduction, the changes in voltage have to be widespread and of longer duration. Relevant to note here is that the postsynaptic potentials (PSPs) last appreciably longer than the APs along an axon. Since neurons in the central nervous system receive many inputs, greater synchrony of these synaptic inputs will result in larger PSPs that are more likely to be detected at the scalp via volume conduction. Similarly, whole nerve APs (like the compound action potential [CAP] of the auditory nerve) represent the summed activity of a population of axons. Several factors determine synchrony, including temporal synchrony among the responding fibers (the greater the synchrony, the stronger the response), amount of temporal jitter (the small variability in

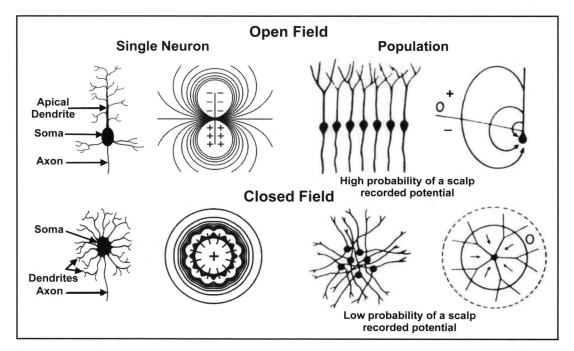

Figure 2–8. Effects of geometric orientation on the electrical field of a single neuron (*left*) and a population of neurons (*right*) and its potential to generate a volume-conducted evoked potential. In an open field (*top row*), since the single neuron and the population of neurons are oriented similarly (forming a single equivalent dipole), the generated electrical field in the extracellular space can be volume conducted to produce a recordable evoke potential at the scalp. In contrast, in the case of the closed field (*bottom row*), since the dendrites on the single neurons are oriented randomly, and the neurons in population are oriented randomly, the electrical fields are cancelled, thereby reducing the probability of a recordable volume-conducted evoked potential at the scalp. The left two columns of the figure were re-created using data from Picton (2011).

the timing of neural discharges) between discharges (the smaller the jitter, the greater the response coherence and magnitude), and conduction velocity differences among the contributing axons that could disrupt the timing and summation of the response. It is relevant to consider these determinants of volume conduction because the components of the auditory brainstem response (ABR) likely involve both axonal and PSP contributions and are therefore affected by these factors. Relating this to the neural bases of the ABRs the population neural activity from the auditory nerve and brainstem fiber tracts deep within the brainstem are volume conducted and picked up as small (nano- to submicrovolt range) evoked potentials via scalp electrodes. With this basic review of what evoked potentials are and the neural bases for their generation, we now begin to focus on types of evoked potentials elicited by auditory stimuli and their classification based on response latency and generator site(s) along the ascending auditory pathway.

III. AUDITORY EVOKED POTENTIALS (AEP): CLASSIFICATION AND TYPES

Temporal sequence of the AEPs: When a brief auditory stimulus like a click is presented to the ear, it excites hair cells over a broad extent of the cochlear spiral, which in turn triggers neural activity in the auditory nerve and "sequentially" along the nuclei and tracts in the brainstem, midbrain, and auditory cortex. The volume-conducted neural activity from these relay nuclei and tracts can be detected by scalp electrodes as a temporal unfolding of electrical events indexing certain aspects of the acoustic features of the click stimulus (Picton, Hillyard, Krausz, & Galambos, 1974). A visual representation of a series of biphasic electrical potentials and their time of occurrence poststimulus is presented in Figure 2–9. The peak or absolute latency in milliseconds is the measure of the temporal delay of the response from the stimulus onset. By convention,

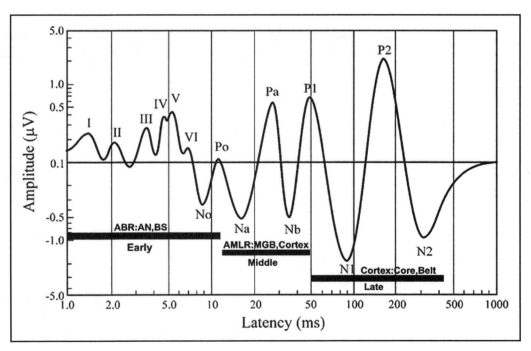

Figure 2–9. Auditory evoked potentials to click stimulus recorded over a 1000-ms analysis window showing early (auditory nerve and brainstem components: ABR) components in the first 10 ms poststimulus onset; middle latency components (thalamic and cortical components: AMLR) in the time window 10–60 ms; and the late auditory evoked potentials (core and belt cortical regions) in the 60–700 ms range. Figure adapted and modified from Picton (2011), Figure 1–2. Adapted from *Human Auditory Evoked Potentials* (p. 3) by Terence W. Picton. Copyright 2011 Plural Publishing, Inc. All rights reserved.

the early response components (from stimulus onset to about 15 ms) are identified by their positive peaks using roman numerals (I–VI), and the components that follow are identified by their positive and negative peaks. For each class of the later AEPs, a letter or number subscript is added to the nomenclature to further differentiate the components within the class (e.g., the first positive peak in the class of components occurring in the time window spanning from 10 to 50 ms would be Pa; the first negative peak would be Na). Also note that the amplitude of the response progressively increases from the early time window to the later time windows.

Classification of AEPs based on latency/generator site(s): The sequence of latencies from short to long is not sufficient to distinguish the response components of the AEP. The first attempt at classification into categories (based on response latency) was provided by Davis (1976) and included first, fast, middle, slow, and late responses (Table 2–1).

More recent latency-based categories include very early (response components occurring in the first 5 ms), early (10–15 ms), middle (10 and 50 ms), and late (50–1000 ms). In order to associate these temporal windows with the presumed anatomical generator(s) of these components, the nomenclature was further changed. The very early response is called the electrocochleogram (ECochG) and includes the cochlear receptor potentials (cochlear microphonic [CM], summating potential [SP]), and VIII nerve CAP. The early response is the ABR indexing neural activity from the auditory nerve and the brainstem structures including the midbrain level inferior colliculus; the auditory middle latency response (AMLR), presumably reflecting neural activity in the medial geniculate body, thalamocortical projections, and the auditory cortex; and the late auditory evoked potential (LAEP), presumably reflecting activity from the primary auditory cortex progressing to include endogenous components whose very long latencies may reflect

Table 2–1. Classification of Auditory Evoked Potentials Based on Latency/Generator(s)

Latency	Transient (Onset)	Steady-State	Sustained
First (0–5 ms) *Cochlea/auditory nerve*	Cochlear nerve Compound action potential (CAP: N1, N2)	Cochlear microphonic (CM) Phase locked	Summating potential (SP)
Fast (1–15 ms) *Auditory nerve/ brainstem*	Auditory brainstem response (ABR: I–VII)	Frequency following response (FFR); Envelope following response (EFR); Fast (>70 Hz) Auditory steady-state response (ASSR)	Pedestal of FFR
Middle (10–50 ms) *Thalamus/cortex*	Middle-latency response (AMLR: Na, Pa, Nb)	40-Hz potential	
Slow (30–500 ms) *Cortex*	Vertex potential (P1, N1, P2, N2)	Slow (<30 Hz) Auditory steady-state response (ASSR)	Cortical sustained potential (SP)
Late (200–1,000 ms) *Cortex*	Mismatch negativity (MMN); processing negativity; late positive waves (P3 or P300)		Contingent negative variation (CNV)

Source: Adapted from *Human Auditory Evoked Potentials* (p. 5) by Terence W. Picton, 2011. Copyright 2011 Plural Publishing, Inc. All rights reserved.

processing time rather than simply travel time to a given physical generator site. This latter classification is preferable since it provides information about both time window and site of generation.

Classification of AEPs based on type of neural activity: In addition to the above classification scheme, AEPs can also be described based on the temporal characteristics of the response, and the location of the recording electrode. AEPs that reflect neural activity that is synchronized only to the onset of the stimulus are referred to as transient onset responses. Almost all of the AEPs described in the preceding section would fall under this type. If the receptor or neural activity persists over the duration of the stimulus, then they are called sustained potentials. Examples of sustained AEPs include the receptor potentials, CM and SP; the brainstem and cortical components of the auditory steady-state response (ASSR); and the sustained phase-locked neural activity reflected in the brainstem envelope following response (EFR) and frequency following response (FFR). When responses are recorded with electrodes in close proximity to the generator, they are referred to as near-field responses, while the scalp-recorded responses are called far-field responses. Considering the volume conduction properties, near-field responses will be appreciably larger in magnitude with greater spatial resolution compared to the scalp-recorded far-field responses. Recording of the VIII nerve CAP using an electrode placed on the lateral wall of the cochlea (promontory) is an example of a relatively near-field recording. AEPs that primarily exhibit stimulus-dependent properties are referred to as exogenous potentials (examples include ABR and AMLR), and AEPs that reflect some aspect of brain processing and are not simply dependent on the physical attributes of the stimulus are endogenous evoked potentials (examples include the late potentials P300 and N400). Myogenic (muscle) evoked potentials, which are several orders of magnitude larger than the neurogenic (neural) evoked potentials, can overlap and contaminate the smaller neural potentials (see Table 2–2 on the latencies of different myogenic components). The usual culprit in the recording of the ABR is the postauricular muscle potential, particularly at high stimulus presentation levels.

Table 2–2. Types and Characteristics of Myogenic Evoked Potentials

Muscle	Response Characteristics
Postauricular (PAM)	Large, broad component with negative peak at about 11–12 ms followed by a positive peak at 14–16 ms. Can distort ABR wave V elicited by low-frequency stimulus and sustained EFR and FFR. In automated scale based on largest components can flatten and obscure the ABR components and affect its detectability. Variable presence. If persistent, having the individual relax or using an earlobe or C7 reference electrode might alleviate the problem.
Temporalis	Negative peak at 15–17 ms followed by a positive peak at 23 ms. Does not pose a problem for the ABR but distorts sustained responses like the EFR and FFR. Easily recorded when teeth are clenched. Instruct to relax.
Neck	Complex waveform with multiple peaks (negative peaks at 11 and 25 ms; positive peaks at 17 and 34 ms. Prominent at the inion electrode and does not pose a serious threat for ABR recording but might still distort the sustained EFR and FFR.
Frontalis	Positive peak at about 30 ms and highly variable. Does not pose a problem for ABR recording.

IV. SUMMARY

- Neural signaling requires the neuron to generate and maintain a polarized state with an RMP of –70 mV; change this potential rapidly via depolarization and repolarization to generate an AP; transmit this AP along the axon efficiently to other neurons through a functional chemical coupling—the synapse. A problem in any of these elements of neuronal physiology will compromise neural signaling and information transfer.

- Evoked potentials reflect stimulus-elicited synchronous neural activity (AP or PSPs) in a population of neural elements that is volume conducted away from the source and recordable using EEG-type scalp electrodes. The efficiency of volume conduction depends on the distance of the electrode from the source—the farther the electrode, the smaller is the response and the poorer is the spatial resolution; geometric orientation of the dipoles—open fields are more conducive to volume conduction, and cancellation of electrical fields in closed fields makes it unlikely to detect evoked potentials at the scalp; and neural synchrony—the greater the temporal synchrony of the neural activity, the stronger is the volume-conducted potential.

- Auditory evoked potentials may be classified based on latency and location of generator(s) into very early (0–5 ms) cochlear and auditory nerve responses; early (0–15 ms) auditory brainstem responses of the onset response type (ABR) or the sustained phase-locked activity to the stimulus envelope periodicity (ASSR and EFR) or its temporal fine structure (FFR); middle (10–50 ms) thalamic and cortical responses; and late (50 ms and later) cortical exogenous and endogenous evoked potentials.

- Several auditory stimulus-dependent, large myogenic evoked potentials arising from the postauricular muscle, temporal muscle, neck muscles, and frontalis muscles can potentially contaminate the auditory evoked responses. Therefore, care should be taken to eliminate or minimize the presence of these nonneural evoked potentials.

V. RECOMMENDED READINGS

Excellent Review of Dipoles and Overview of Neuronal Physiology

Picton, T. W. (2011). Finding sources: Forward and backward. In T. W. Picton (Ed.), *Human auditory evoked potential* (Chapter 4, pp. 94–104). San Diego, CA: Plural Publishing.

Eggermont, J. J. (2007). Electric and magnetic fields of synchronous neural activity: Peripheral and central origins of auditory evoked potentials. In R. E. Burkard, M. Don, & J. J. Eggermont (Eds.), *Auditory evoked potentials: Basic principles and clinical application* (Chapter 1, pp. 2–11). Baltimore, MD: Lippincott Williams & Wilkins.

REFERENCES

Davis, H. (1976). Principles of electric response audiometry. *Annals of Otology, Rhinology, and Laryngology, 85*(Suppl. 28), 1–96.

Goodlett, C. R., & Horn, K. H. (2001). Mechanisms of alcohol-induced damage to the developing nervous system. *Alcohol Research and Health, 25,* 175–184.

Herculano-Houzel, S. (2017). Number of neurons as biological correlates of cognitive ability. *Current Opinions in Behavioral Sciences, 16,* 1–7.

Picton, T. W., Hillyard, S. A., Krausz, H. L., & Galambos, R. (1974). Human auditory evoked potentials. I. Evaluation of components. *Electroencephalography and Clinical Neurophysiology, 36,* 179–190.

Scherg, M. (1990). Fundamentals of dipole source potential analysis. In F. Grandori, M. Hoke, & G. L. Romani (Eds.), *Advances in audiology, Vol. 6. Auditory evoked magnetic fields and electric potentials* (pp. 44–67). New York, NY: Karger.

Wood, C. C., & Allison, T. (1981). Interpretation of evoked potentials: A neurophysiological perspective. *Canadian Journal of Psychology, 35*(2), 113–135.

3

Stimuli and Data Acquisition Principles

SCOPE

In the previous chapter, we learned that the volume-conducted ensemble neural activity originating from nuclei and tracts deep within the brainstem in response to *auditory stimuli* can be detected and *measured* at the scalp using electroencephalograph (EEG)-type electrodes. Here we focus on two questions. First, what are the characteristics of stimuli and their parameters used to evoke these responses? Second, how is the evoked potential data acquired? To answer these questions, we first introduce the reader to the common types of stimuli and transducers used, their spectrotemporal characteristics, and the stimulus parameters that change the response indices (latency and amplitude). Next, we consider the analog and digital components of evoked potential *data acquisition* and their *principles of operation*. The goal is to help the reader understand the nature of the stimuli required, stimulus parameters to consider, and the principles of data acquisition operations involved in the recording of auditory evoked potentials in general, and the auditory brainstem response (ABR) in particular. A variety of auditory evoked potentials can be recorded using most commercially available evoked potential systems by using appropriate stimuli and recording parameters. However, the focus henceforth is on the ABR.

I. STIMULUS SECTION

Stimulus Type

A schematic representation of the organization of the stimulus, analog processing, and digital processing sections of an evoked potential system is shown in Figure 3–1. The *stimulus section* identifies the stimulus types, transducer types, stimulus parameters that can be manipulated, stimulus routing, and the output carrying stimulus trigger(s) to be synchronized with the onset of digitization (response averaging, see arrow from the stimulus section). Most systems can play a range of digitally stored calibrated stimulus files and afford the flexibility of importing custom-made stimuli for specific purposes (e.g., complex tones to evaluate pitch-relevant information contained in the brainstem response). Stimuli are most commonly routed to insert earphones (ER3A or ER2) or speaker(s). The selection of stimulus type; transducer type; control of stimulus parameters such as intensity, frequency, repetition rate, onset polarity, and the ear to be stimulated are software controlled and menu-driven on the acquisition window.

The choice of a specific stimulus type depends on the clinical application. For hearing screening (more details in Chapter 5) and a quick check of the functional integrity of the peripheral and

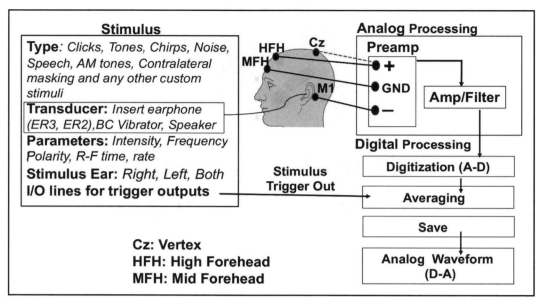

Figure 3–1. The components of the auditory evoked potential stimulus generation and data acquisition system. The stimulus section includes stimulus type, transducer type, stimulus parameters, and routing of signals. The initial low-level analog processing stage includes differential amplification and filtering. The digital processing stage includes digitization (A-D conversion) and response averaging over a chosen time epoch. The onset of response averaging is synchronized to the stimulus onset using trigger pulses from the stimulus section.

brainstem structures (more details in Chapter 6), clicks are routinely used. However, there is a slow movement toward replacing clicks with broadband chirps as they have been shown to elicit relatively more robust responses. For obtaining "audiogram-like" information, *frequency-specific* tone bursts or more recently narrowband chirps are considered. A description of the spectrotemporal characteristics of these stimuli is helpful here.

Clicks: Clicks are generated by driving a transducer (let us assume the ER3A insert earphone) with a very brief electrical pulse (100 μs in duration). They are most commonly used because their instantaneous rise time (ideal for robust onset synchronization of the neural activity generating the ABR components) and the resulting broad spectrum (recruits more neurons) combine to produce a very robust response. The waveforms and spectra of an electrical pulse (A) and the acoustic click through an ER3A insert earphone (B) are superimposed in Figure 3–2. Note that the spectrum of the electrical pulse (A) has a broader spectrum, out to the first null point at 10 kHz—the reciprocal of the 100-μs pulse width. In contrast, the spectrum of the acoustic click (B) is relatively flat (with a few resonance peaks, characteristic of the transfer function of this particular transducer and that of the 2 cc coupler) and extends to only about 3 to 4 kHz, and then the magnitude drops at a rate of 20 to 30 dB/octave. Note also that the acoustic click waveform (B) shows damped ringing and a delay corresponding to the travel time (approximately 1 ms) in the tubing from the transducer to the ear tip.

Broadband Chirps: Like the click, the chirp is also a brief stimulus with a spectrum ideal to evoke the ABR. Unlike the click, whose cochlear regional activation is latency bound (different cochlear regions respond at different times because of the traveling wave delay) and therefore could potentially smear the sum of regional contributions resulting in a less than optimal response, chirps were designed to overcome this problem by constructing a novel complex transient stimulus where individual frequencies occur at different times to reduce or eliminate the influence of the traveling wave delay. Specifically, the cochlear response time of each of the frequency components is adjusted (low frequencies with longer cochlear delays start earlier than the high frequencies) to compensate for the traveling wave delay so that cochlear regional contributions to the neural activity producing the ABR occur simultaneously (Dau, Wagner, Mellert, & Kollmeier, 2000; Elberling, Callo, & Don, 2010; Elberling & Don, 2008; Fobel & Dau, 2004). As expected, empirical evidence shows that the chirp-evoked ABRs are sharper and more robust than their click-evoked counterparts (Elberling, Callo, & Don, 2010). While the spectra of the click and the chirp are almost identical, the stimulus waveforms are longer for chirps and appear frequency modulated—changing from low to high frequency (Figure 3–3, right panel). Since chirps produce a larger

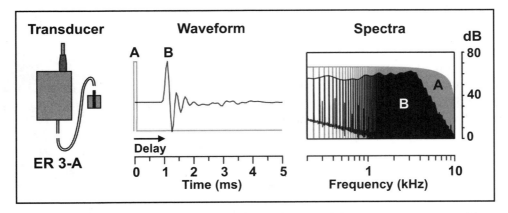

Figure 3–2. Electrical (A) and acoustic (B) waveforms and their respective spectra. Note that the acoustic spectrum of the click at the ER3A transducer output rolls-off around 4000 Hz, while the spectrum of the 100 μs electrical pulse extends past 10 kHz. Adapted from *Human Auditory Evoked Potentials* (p. 126) by Terence W. Picton. Copyright 2011 Plural Publishing, Inc. All rights reserved.

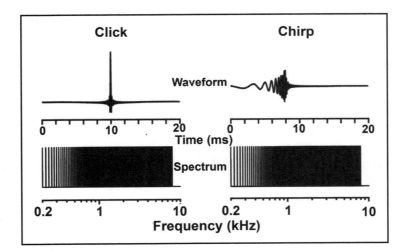

Figure 3–3. Comparison of acoustic waveforms and spectra of a click (*left*) and a broadband chirp (*right*). Both stimuli contain frequencies across the audible frequency range. For the chirp stimulus, the relative timing of the frequency components within the stimulus are adjusted to compensate for the normal cochlear delay to activate different cochlear regions simultaneously to enhance neural synchrony. Note that while the temporal course of these stimuli is different, their spectra are nearly identical. Adapted from *Human Auditory Evoked Potentials* (p. 141) by Terence W. Picton. Copyright 2011 Plural Publishing, Inc. All rights reserved.

ABR response even at lower intensities, there is considerable interest in adopting *narrowband chirp* stimuli to improve frequency-specific estimates of behavioral thresholds.

Tone Bursts: Since clicks and broadband chirp ABRs represent primary activity over a wide range of frequency regions on the cochlear partition, they are not ideal for recording frequency-specific (more accurately, place-specific) ABRs to obtain audiogram-like information for threshold estimation. Also, the ABR components reflect neural activity synchronized to the onset of a stimulus; therefore, longer tones used in behavioral audiometry are not ideal for recording the ABRs. Thus, we arrive at a compromise stimulus, the tone burst. The tone burst is essentially a brief (about 5-ms long) tone with relatively rapid rise-fall times (typically two cycles of rise, two cycles fall, and a plateau of one cycle—the 2-1-2 tone). Unlike pure tones, the spectra of these brief tone bursts show maximum energy at the nominal frequency of the tone (e.g., 1000 Hz in Figure 3–4) and appreciable energy in the sidebands above and below this frequency. This spectral splatter is due to the brief signal duration and its rapid rise time (see Figure 3–4). One way to reduce this spectral splatter is to turn these brief signals on and off more gradually (i.e., by using time windowing or gating functions that allow a more gradual growth of stimulus amplitude to its maximum). Two nonlinear gating functions (cosine-squared or Blackman windows) are commonly utilized to limit the spectral splatter in an attempt to make the stimulus more frequency specific. These functions are mathematical spectral limiting manipulations utilizing linear or nonlinear rise and fall times. It can be seen in Figure 3–4 that the energy in the sidebands decreases appreciably as the rise-fall time is increased. Tone bursts created with these specifications meet two important requirements: (a) the rise-fall time is gradual enough to produce a frequency-specific stimulus (which in turn will produce a place-specific response), and (b) the rise-fall time is fast enough to engage the brainstem neurons to produce a synchronized onset response. Frequency-specific stimuli, however, do not always guarantee place-specific ABR (i.e., primary activity generating the ABR localized to the cochlear place corresponding to the frequency of the tone burst). Independent of

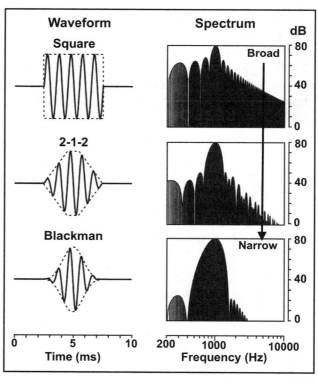

Figure 3–4. Waveform (*left*) and spectra of three brief (5 ms) 1000-Hz tone bursts with different envelopes: instantaneous rise and fall times (*top*), a 2-1-2 cosine squared gating window (*middle*); and a Blackman window. As expected, the tone burst with the rapid rise-fall time shows a large spread of energy beyond 1000 Hz. While spread is reduced for the 2-1-2 tone burst, the Blackman gated tone clearly shows that much of its energy is restricted to 1000 Hz with great attenuation of energy at other frequencies. Adapted from *Human Auditory Evoked Potentials* (p. 132) by Terence W. Picton. Copyright 2011 Plural Publishing, Inc. All rights reserved.

the frequency-specific acoustic spectrum presented to the ear, intensity-dependent changes in cochlear regions contributing to the response, as dictated by cochlear mechanics, will limit place specificity of the recorded ABRs. We return to a more detailed consideration of the concepts of frequency and place specificity and their utility in ABR recordings for clinical applications in Chapter 5.

Transducer Type

In clinical applications, stimuli are presented via tubal insert earphones to record air conduction

ABR (AC-ABR) and via a bone vibrator to record bone conduction ABR (BC-ABR). Just as in pure-tone audiometry, AC-ABR and BC-ABR are compared to evaluate the status of the middle ear (i.e., the presence/absence of an electrophysiologic estimate of an air-bone gap). Frequency and intensity are two major stimulus factors that alter the characteristics of the ABR predictably. Therefore, it is important to know if these physical attributes are optimally presented to the auditory system by examining the frequency response and output characteristics of the transducers used to record the ABR. The two commonly used insert phones for air conduction stimulation are the Etymōtic tubal insert phones ER3A (recently replaced by ER-3C, which has the same frequency response as ER-3A) and ER2. The frequency response and the output values are different for the two insert earphones. While the frequency response (as measured in the Zwislocki coupler) is essentially flat out to 10 kHz for the ER2, the output for ER3A rolls-off around 4 kHz and continues to decrease at the rate of about 30 dB/octave (Figure 3–5). However, it takes greater current to drive the ER2s, and their outputs are about 20 to 30 dB lower compared to the ER3As. To compensate for this and to ensure that the output is not distorted, some systems provide a 20 dB boost to drive the ER2s. The higher-frequency extension of the frequency response for the ER2 enables the recording of ABRs with contributions from the more synchronous, higher-frequency cochlear regions (Elberling, Kristensen, & Don, 2012). Two bone vibrators (the more commonly used RadioEar B71, and the relatively newer B81) are used for bone conduction stimulation. The frequency response of these two transducers is nearly identical (Figure 3–6), and they show damped resonance peaks between 375 and 450 Hz, 1300 to 1450 Hz, and 4000 to 4125 Hz with outputs continuing to decrease above about 1500 Hz at a rate of about 20 dB/octave (Jansson, Hakansson, Johannsen, & Tengstrand, 2015). These authors found that the maximum output levels for these two transducers were 85 to 90 dB HL between 1000 and 4000 Hz. Below 1500 Hz, the output of the B81 is about 11 to 22 dB higher than the output for the B71. They also reported significantly higher total harmonic distortion for the B71 at low frequencies, which limits the usable output range.

Calibration of Stimulus Intensity

As with any measurement, it is critical to accurately specify the stimulus output (level) to ensure test validity, interpretation, replicability, and transportability of results. The expression of stimulus level in decibels (dB) for the brief stimuli used to elicit auditory evoked potentials is a *variant* of the actual decibel sound pressure level (dB SPL), decibel

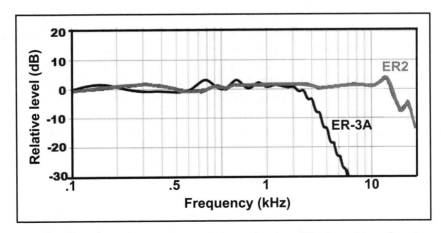

Figure 3–5. Amplitude response (relative level in dB) plotted as a function of frequency for ER2 (*gray line*) and ER3A (*black line*). Note the relatively flat and extended frequency response for the ER2 compared to the ER3A, which begins to roll-off around 4000 Hz.

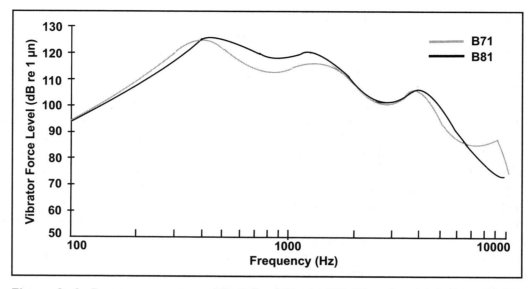

Figure 3–6. Frequency response of RadioEar B81 and B71. Note the slightly (about 5 dB) greater output in the 400 to 1500 Hz frequency for the B81 bone vibrator. Specification data from RadioEar.

normal hearing level (dB nHL), and decibel sensation level (dB SL) applied to output specification of longer signals used for pure-tone audiometry. All three measures are relative since they imply a reference to the behavioral threshold for the specific stimuli used to elicit the auditory evoked potential. Sound level in dB SPL may be defined as a logarithmic ratio of the measured absolute sound pressure (where Sound pressure = Force/Area) and a reference which by convention is 20 µPa (micropascals)—the smallest audible pressure that corresponds to thresholds in the range of 1000 to 4000 Hz. Reduced to an equation, dB SPL = *20 log P/P_o*, where *P* is the measured pressure, and P_o is the reference pressure. The decibel logarithmic scale is used to compress the rather unwieldy, broad range of sound pressure (10^{14}) spanning the dynamic range of hearing. For the longer duration stimuli used in pure-tone audiometry, the SPL developed in a 2-cc acoustic coupler can be easily measured by sound level meters (SLMs) in terms of its root-mean-square (RMS) value, which is an accurate representation of the effective level of the stimulus. However, calculations of RMS value using an SLM for the brief (1–4 ms long) stimuli used in auditory evoked potential measurements are not accurate, as most SLM responses are not fast enough and therefore may not provide the real equivalent power of these stimuli. Commonly used options include a measure of the peak SPL (pSPL) or a peak-to-peak equivalent SPL (peSPL). The pSPL measure, as the name implies, corresponds to the peak dB SPL registered on the SLM (Figure 3–7, arrow A). The peSPL, a more complicated measure, is essentially the RMS SPL of a continuous tone whose peak-to-peak amplitude is equal to that of the brief stimulus (Figure 3–7, arrow peSPL). It should be noted here that the pSPL measure may be more susceptible to level changes (as much as 3.5 dB [Burkard, 1984; Durrant & Boston, 2007; Picton, 2011]) if the stimulus waveform is not symmetric about its zero crossings, and when there are small adjustments in the coupling of the insert earphone to the ear. The use of just peak SPL measures (as opposed to peak-to-peak equivalent) is not recommended. The advantage to using the peSPL measure is that it is easily applicable and therefore replicable across labs and clinics, and it is similar to the pure-tone calibration method.

How Do These SPL Measures Translate to the dB nHL Scale?

The use of dB nHL to express the intensity of stimuli used to record auditory evoked potentials in

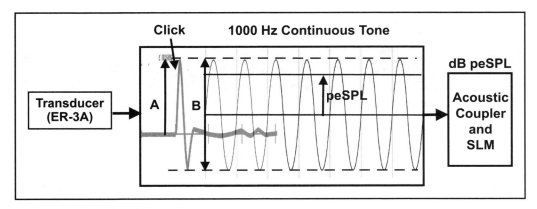

Figure 3–7. Peak amplitude of click (A) and peak-to-peak amplitude (B) of a 1000-Hz continuous tone equal in peak-to-peak amplitude to the click delivered by an Etymōtic Research ER3A insert earphone. The root-mean-square level of this tone is then measured in the acoustic coupler to yield the dB peSPL. Adapted from *Human Auditory Evoked Potentials* (p. 70) by Terence W. Picton. Copyright 2011 Plural Publishing, Inc. All rights reserved.

principle follows the rationale for the dB HL scale used in pure-tone audiometry. The expression *dB HL* can be defined as the level in decibels by way of the *audiometric zero*. Audiometric zero is, in turn, derived from the minimum audible pressure (MAP) curve. The MAP curve represents the average hearing threshold in dB SPL in a group of young, normal-hearing individuals. The arbitrarily picked pure-tone audiometric zero in the dB HL scale simply represents a flattening of the MAP curve by applying the different reference equivalent threshold SPL for each frequency. That is, 0 dB HL corresponds to a different reference equivalent threshold level in dB SPL for each frequency, since pure-tone thresholds change as a function of stimulus frequency. For example, 0 dB HL for a 1000 Hz pure tone using a Telephonics TDH49 earphone with MX41/AR cushion is about 7 dB SPL. Since the RMS SPL can be measured easily in an acoustic coupler, for the longer pure-tone stimuli used in audiometry, this is a fairly simple exercise to determine the reference equivalent SPL. So, *dB HL = Presentation level setting + Reference equivalent threshold SPL*. The dB nHL expression used for specifying the level of auditory stimuli used to record auditory evoked potentials essentially tries to mimic this approach. That is, measure the behavioral threshold for each stimulus type used in eliciting the evoked response in a group of normal-hearing individuals to develop what could be the *auditory evoked potential zero*. Then determine the peak-to-peak equivalent (peSPL) level that corresponds to the equivalent reference threshold SPL for each stimulus to establish the dB nHL scale. The International Organization for Standardization (ISO) standard 389-6 (Reference threshold of hearing for test signals of short duration), first approved in 2007 and then reapproved in 2015, recommends the use of the peak-to-peak equivalent method to calibrate and to determine the reference threshold for clicks and tone bursts. Further, it recommends specific reference equivalent threshold SPLs (peRETSPL) for specific transducers to promote the use of a uniform standard in estimates of hearing threshold using auditory evoked potentials (Table 3–1). Data for this standard are largely derived from the work of Richter and Fedtke (2005). For example, for clicks, 0 dB nHL = 35 dB peSPL. These peRETSPL are generally close to the values provided by manufacturers of several commonly used evoked potential systems.

We have seen that the establishment of reference levels for the development of the dB nHL scale is a rather complicated and confusing task. Durrant and Boston (2007) have rightly pointed out several factors in this endeavor that could potentially alter the measured value. These include the number of subjects needed, the appropriate environment, optimal stimulus parameters to consider for the measure, and the appropriate coupler to use. All of

Table 3–1. ISO 389-6 (2007) Recommended peRETSPLs for Clicks and Tone Bursts Presented at 20/Sec With Train Duration of 1 Sec Using a Peak-to-Peak Equivalent SPL Measure

Transducer Type	Ear Simulator	Stimulus	peRETSPL (re 20µPa)
Etymōtic Research ER-3A	IEC 60318-4	Click	35.5
Etymōtic Research ER-2	IEC 60318-4	Click	43.5
Etymōtic Research ER-3A	IEC 60318-4	Tone burst (250 Hz)	28.0
		(500 Hz)	23.5
		(1000 Hz)	21.5
		(2000 Hz)	28.5
		(4000 Hz)	32.5

these variables influence the measured value. With respect to the utility of the dB nHL scale, Picton (2011) has presented an intriguing idea to replace the confusing multistep-derived dB nHL scale with a physiologic threshold level (PTL). The PTL represents the mean stimulus specific threshold for detecting a physiologic response in a group of young adults. This measure would negate the need for determining the nHL level using behavioral thresholds and determining the difference between the behavioral and electrophysiologic measures. This novel idea warrants further consideration.

Finally, dB SL is the stimulus level above an individual's threshold. This measure, while useful in some suprathreshold perceptual measures, is not commonly used, in part because equal sensation levels across individuals with different audiometric thresholds (dB HL) are not the same SPL and therefore would be stimulating the system at different points along the dynamic range.

II. ANALOG SIGNAL CONDITIONING AND PREPROCESSING SECTION

The magnitude of the signal (stimulus-evoked response) being measured is very small (in the submicrovolt to nanovolt range) compared to the noise (ongoing brain activity, myogenic components, and artifacts) it is embedded in. This noise is several orders of magnitude larger (between 50 and 100 microvolts) and poses a challenge to extract the small signal. To optimally extract the signal, every step in the data acquisition process is aimed at increasing the signal magnitude and decreasing the noise magnitude—that is, increasing the signal-to-noise ratio (SNR). So, the *mantra for the data acquisition section is, "do whatever it takes to increase the SNR."* Let us first consider the initial preprocessing steps of the analog inputs, which includes a description of the electrodes and the basic principles of differential amplification (gain) and filtering. These preprocessing conditioning steps are essential to obtain as clean a signal as possible to optimize digital processing in the next stage.

Electrodes: This is the first and a very important step in data acquisition since the electrodes are the sensors that detect the brain's electrical activity from the scalp. Therefore, the choice of electrode type and the nature of the functional coupling between the electrode and the scalp can make the difference between a robust interpretable response and a noisy uninterpretable response. There are a variety of disposable and reusable EEG surface disc electrode types (made of plated gold, silver, or tin) that conduct low voltages readily with good SNR (Figure 3–8). The prewired sintered silver/silver chloride (Ag/AgCl) electrode is particularly desirable because of its high quality (low contact potential since the electrode itself does not touch the skin, and the Ag/AgCl coating reduces the noise, thus yielding a high SNR), durability, and ease of application with its ring-shaped adhesive sleeve. Noise associated with electrode contact is

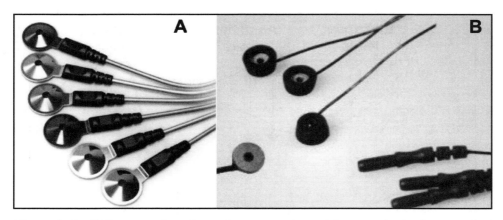

Figure 3–8. EEG-type surface electrodes commonly used for recording auditory evoked potentials. **A.** Electrodes made of different metals. **B.** Sintered Ag/AgCl-type electrode. Both reusable and disposable electrodes are used.

an issue primarily for a very low setting of the low-cutoff frequency of the analog filter. Since the aim is to improve SNR, the functional coupling between the surface of the electrode and scalp should yield contact electrical impedances below about 3000 ohms—the lower the better. Care should be taken to prep the skin at the electrode locations to achieve this. Indeed, it is important to ensure that the impedances are similar and balanced across all electrodes to optimize SNR (more on this under "Differential amplification"). It is also advisable to braid the electrode cables to facilitate the cancellation of stray fields picked up by the electrodes, particularly in an electrically noisy recording environment. In the end, it is worth spending the required time to apply the electrodes optimally to obtain low and balanced interelectrode impedances.

Figure 3–9 shows the commonly used electrode locations for a single channel recording for stimulation of each ear (in this case the left ear) and requires three electrodes. One electrode on the vertex (Cz) location or a more commonly used location now, the midline high-forehead at the hairline location (HFH) serves as the positive or more accurately the noninverting input to the differential amplifier; one electrode on the left mastoid (M1) serves as the negative or the inverting input, and a midline electrode on the mid-forehead (MFH) serves as the common ground input. Inadvertent switching of the inverting and noninverting inputs yields a polarity reversal of the acquired evoked potential waveform. It should be noted here that simultaneous multichannel recordings, using different electrode configurations or montages (the electrode locations serving as the inputs to the differential amplifier), are also utilized to enhance amplitude and/or improve the clarity of certain response components to aid in the accuracy of response detection (more on this in Chapter 4). Finally, we have used the more descriptive labels HFH and MFH to more accurately reflect the scalp locations of these electrodes, since they do not exactly represent the 10–20 system labels Fz (HFH) and Fpz (MFH).

Differential Amplification: As indicated in the previous paragraph, the electrical activity is picked up by the scalp electrode leads that are connected to the noninverting (NI), inverting (I), and common ground (GND) input of a differential amplifier as shown in Figure 3–9 (top row). A differential amplifier may be operationally defined as an electronic amplifier that amplifies (by a selectable gain factor) the difference between two input voltages but suppresses voltages that are common at the two inputs. Thus, in principle, the noise (the much larger ongoing EEG and other myogenic signals and artifacts) arriving at the two inputs (inverting and noninverting) is *the same (may not be identical so we still have residual noise that is amplified) and therefore is suppressed* substantially if not eliminated. On the other hand, the evoked responses elicited by the stimulus are *temporally different* at the two inputs and are therefore amplified. The result is an improvement in SNR. As the name implies, noninverting means the signal polarity is preserved at

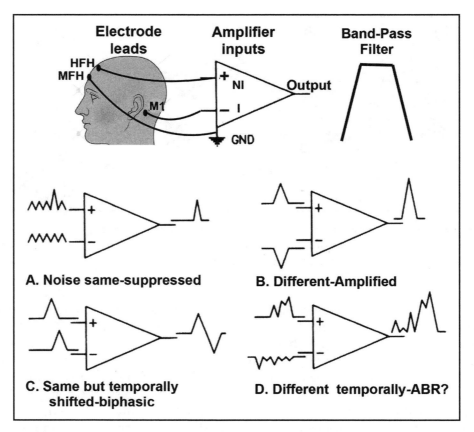

Figure 3–9. Operational principles of a differential amplifier. The top row shows the noninverting (NI), inverting (I), and ground (GND) inputs to the differential amplifier from scalp electrodes on HFH, M1, and MFH followed by analog band-pass filtering. Differential conditions and the resulting outputs are shown in panels A–D to illustrate the main principle of operation of the differential amplifier: amplify different signals and attenuate/eliminate common signals at the inputs.

this input, and inverting means that the signal at this input is inverted—this is how the differential amplification is achieved. This principle of differential amplification is illustrated in Figure 3–9; inputs that are the same (noise) are suppressed (A), and the signal (stimulus-evoked response) that is different at the two electrodes is amplified. Identical signals but opposite in polarity at the inputs are amplified (B); same signals but temporally shifted to produce a biphasic output are amplified (C); and finally, signals that are different at the two inputs over time (similar to the ABR signals picked up by electrodes at the forehead [NI input] and the ipsilateral mastoid [M1]) will result in a composite output that reflects all the temporal components (D). One important determinant of the effectiveness of a differential amplifier in improving SNR is its ability to reject the common mode signal (signals that are similar at the two inputs) and amplify the differential signal. The common mode rejection ratio (CMRR) is a measure of this ability and is given by the ratio, differential gain (Ad)/common mode gain (Acm), where Ad is the output gain measured when the amplifier is set to operate in the differential mode, and Acm is the output gain when the amplifier is set to the common mode, that is when the same signal is applied to both inputs. Typically, differential amplifiers with CMRR greater than 80 dB are considered effective. In the section on electrodes, we emphasized the importance of balance between electrical impedances across electrodes for achieving good SNR. If the impedances are different, then electrodes with higher impedances will be noisier (lower CMRR) than ones with lower impedances (higher CMRR), resulting in the noise being amplified and effectively reducing the SNR of the response. SNR may also be reduced by differential noise inputs resulting from the pickup of stray electrical fields by loosely routed electrode cables. It is advisable to keep the electrode length short and braided. The advent of evoked potential systems with considerable initial processing proximal to the electrodes and the transmission of this output via fiber-optic cables makes these systems less susceptible to these problems. Typically, differential amplifiers also have high input impedance to keep signal distortion well outside the frequency range of interest.

Filtering: Continuing with the mantra of increasing SNR, the output of the differential amplifier is next band-pass filtered (only the frequency components within a narrow range of frequencies are selectively passed through, while other frequency components are attenuated appreciably). This analog filter is a combination of a high-pass and a low-pass filter with different cutoff frequencies (Figure 3–10). The efficiency with which the frequencies beyond the passband are rejected depends on the decibel attenuation rate/octave (*slope of the filter skirt*) of spectral components outside the passband. Analog filtering for ABR recording typically uses a 3 to 6 dB/octave slope. The rationale for filtering is that frequency components outside the filter bandwidth largely contribute to the noise, and attenuating them improves the SNR. While narrowing the filter bandwidth in an attempt to isolate the signal from the noise improves the SNR, too much filtering will distort the recorded evoked potential, with the distortion manifesting as amplitude and latency changes. Most commonly, ABR recordings in a sound booth for threshold estimation are made with a high-pass cutoff frequency set at 30 Hz and a low-pass cutoff frequency set at 3000 Hz. If possible, it is advisable to set the analog filters open for data acquisition and subsequently utilize digital filtering (which overcomes the problem of waveform distortion and phase shifts). In addition to improving SNR, low- and high-pass filtering also helps in keeping the signal within the analog-to-digital converter's operating range and eliminating aliasing (the appearance of spurious low frequencies not in the original signal) during digitization. Aliasing in signal processing refers to the distortion or artifact that results when a signal reconstructed from samples is different from the original continuous signal.

III. DIGITAL SIGNAL PROCESSING SECTION

The preprocessed signal in the analog section is well conditioned and ready for digitization through a process called analog-to-digital conversion using an analog-to-digital converter (ADC). The optimally digitized representation of the analog signal is then converted back to its analog version using a digital-to-analog converter (DAC). The resulting analog signal is finally filtered to have a representation that closely matches the original analog signal. The sequence of steps for this processing is shown in Figure 3–11.

Analog-to-Digital Conversion: Since later manipulation of the signal for averaging will be on the digital representation of the input analog signal, the ADC converts the analog signal into a series of numbers (binary representation) representing the amplitude of the signal over its duration. This conversion is carried out by taking discrete-time samples of the amplitude of the analog signal at specified

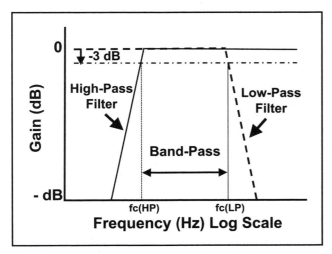

Figure 3–10. The combination of a high-pass and a low-pass filter to form a band-pass filter. The high-pass (fc[HP]); and low-pass (fc[LP]) cutoff frequencies, and the band-pass bandwidth (effective bandwidth) using the 3-dB down point are identified.

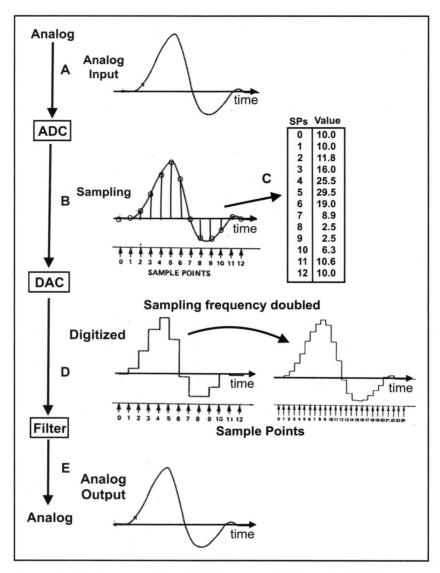

Figure 3-11. Analog-to-digital (ADC) and digital-to-analog (DAC) conversion. Analog waveform to be digitized (A); digitization (B) where discrete samples of the analog waveform are taken at regular intervals (sampling period); and assigned amplitude values (C). As the sampling frequency is doubled, the temporal resolution of the digitized signal increases (D: *left to right*). After completion of digitization, the waveform is plotted after reconverting to an analog signal (E). Note that the digitized signal looks almost identical to the input analog signal.

time intervals (*sampling period*) (Figure 3–11, B and C). The rate at which these samples are taken is known as the *sampling frequency*. Thus, Sampling frequency = 1/Sampling period. The accuracy with which this process digitally represents the analog signal is determined by two factors. One is the temporal resolution (Figure 3–11, D), which is determined by the sampling frequency (the rate at which discrete samples are taken), and the other is amplitude resolution, which is determined by the number of discrete binary steps (bits) available to represent the amplitude step size between sampled values. For complex signals like the EEG and the embedded auditory evoked potentials, the requirement of the minimum sampling rate needed to reproduce a signal with precision is informed by the Nyquist theorem of sampling. According to the Nyquist theorem, an analog waveform can be reconstructed digitally by taking samples at equal time intervals, if the sampling rate is ≥ twice the highest frequency component in the analog signal. The spectrum of the input arriving from the analog preprocessing stage is broad given the gradual slope characteristics of the analog filter (3–6 dB/octave). Thus, the Nyquist sampling rate must be set appropriately higher based on the highest frequency present in this input signal to avoid a distorted representation of the original analog signal and to prevent aliasing. More commonly, sampling rates higher than required by the Nyquist theorem rate are used to also minimize the distorting effects of sampling error and noise. In terms of the amplitude resolution, the greater the number of bits available (larger dynamic range) to represent amplitude, the better is the signal quality without distortion and the better is the ability to capture smaller signals. This is particularly the case when recording ABRs because the tiny ABR components are only a small portion of the overall input signal (at the lowest 10%–15% of the dynamic range). However, the number of bits in the ADC alone does not determine the precision of the measure. Increasing the number of sweeps during averaging also significantly improves precision by effectively increasing the number of available bits. So, the precision of the final measurement is determined by the combination of the number of ADC bits available and the number of sweeps averaged. For a more detailed treatise, readers are referred to the technical review on analog-to-digital conversion provided by Thornton (2007). Finally, care should be taken that the input stays within the ADC limits to avoid amplitude peak clipping and signal distortion.

Signal Averaging: This is the final and most powerful step in our quest to continually improve the SNR at each step of data acquisition. Recall that we started with the problem of extracting a small evoked response embedded in a large "noise." Even after applying all the necessary steps we described so far, we are not able to visually see the evoked response elicited by the auditory stimulus. Response averaging is required to accomplish this. The time-domain averaging of evoked potentials works on a very basic and effective principle —when like events repeat, they tend to add and grow in magnitude; when random events repeat, they tend to subtract and diminish in magnitude. Specifically, the stimulus-unrelated ongoing brain activity is random and therefore tends to diminish in magnitude with repeated stimulus presentations, but the stimulus-evoked response is nearly identical and grows in magnitude upon stimulus repetition.

Operation of Time-Domain Averaging: Shown at the bottom of Figure 3–12 are the essential elements of time-domain averaging. A preset number of sweeps of the stimulus with a fixed repetition rate (therefore a fixed interstimulus interval) is selected. The stimulus elicited evoked response components will occur in a fixed time window post stimulus onset (middle row of Figure 3–12). This temporal window used to average the response is called the *analysis time or epoch*. For example, for typical ABR recordings, this analysis epoch is about 12 to 20 ms. The onset location of this analysis epoch can be placed so that it is either synchronous with the onset of the stimulus or occurs 100 to 200 ms before the onset of the stimulus (thus providing an average of the *prestimulus baseline*). For the former, the stimulus trigger used to onset averaging will be synchronous with stimulus onset; for the latter, the stimulus trigger will occur 100 to 200 ms before stimulus onset. The prestimulus onset analysis epoch provides the prestimulus baseline activity that can be used to measure baseline to peak amplitude. Care is taken to ensure that slow enough repetition rates are used so that two successive stimuli do not occur within the same analysis window. Each sweep is sampled by the ADC and the value stored in memory. This memory keeps a running sum of the values measured in each sweep, which is averaged after a preset number of sweeps until data acquisition are completed. As the number of sweeps increases, the signal response grows linearly with the number of sweeps; since the noise is not time-locked to the stimulus, it overall begins to decrease (top of Figure 3–12 shows averaged ABR traces using three different sweep numbers). Averaging enhances the SNR by a factor equal to the square root of the number of sweeps. (***This holds only if the response is constant with little latency variability and the noise is truly random.***) This

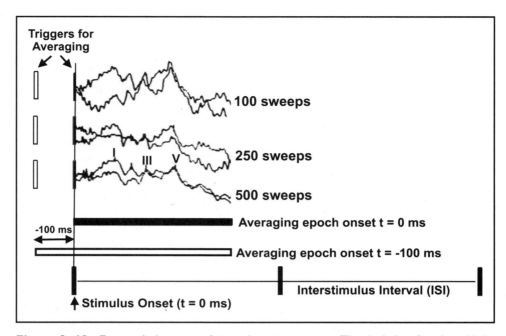

Figure 3–12. Essential elements of time-domain averaging. The dark (*t* = 0 ms) and light vertical bars (*t* = −100 ms) show the temporal location of the trigger pulses to start digitization. The dark and the light horizontal bars below the waveforms represent the analysis epoch or window. The stimulus-interstimulus interval is plotted at the bottom of the figure showing the temporal location of the stimulus. Note that only one stimulus occurs in each analysis epoch. Response averages show the response components increasing in amplitude, repeatability, and detectability as the number of averages is increased from 100 to 500 sweeps.

also means that the *gain in SNR* with increasing sweeps decreases, so continuing to average several thousands of sweeps is not necessarily beneficial and might simply use up valuable test time that is usually at a premium when recording from infants and young children.

Several different strategies, primarily aimed at minimizing the influence of noise, are utilized to estimate the quality of the response and/or to improve the SNR during averaging. The simplest and most commonly used online (while averaging) method is *artifact rejection* enabled over a specific portion of the acquisition window. Artifact rejection simply rejects sweeps that exceed a criterion amplitude in that window from consideration for averaging. Care should be taken that this amplitude criterion for rejection is not set too low (more samples are rejected, which appreciably increases the acquisition time) or too high (more noisy trials are included, resulting in a noisy recording). This same method could be more effective when acquired single trials are more carefully examined offline for artifacts and more selectively rejected. However, this takes considerably more time and therefore is seldom used in the clinic for brainstem evoked response assessment. A different and more sophisticated approach to reduce the influence of noisy sweeps in the average is the use of the *weighted average* (Elberling & Wahlgreen, 1985). Essentially, there is no rejection of any sweeps from the average, but rather the quieter sweeps are weighted more than the noisier sweeps so that the latter contribute minimally to the final average. The amount of weighting relies on the estimate(s) of the variance of the background noise distribution. Most of the difficulty in averaging a combination of signal plus noise arises from the assumption that the background noise is stationary, which may not be the case in every recording condition.

Another consideration for interpretation and transportability of results is some measure of the quality of the recorded waveform. The commonly used approach of averaging with a fixed number of sweeps does not necessarily yield the same SNR across test conditions. A measure of the noise variance and how it affects the SNR of the averaged response would be a useful index of response quality. Most current systems provide a residual noise estimate by subtracting averaged responses stored in split buffers. Split-buffered averaging stores half the total number of sweeps in buffer A and the other half in buffer B. Thus, A-B cancels the response, leaving only the noise. This noise estimate is then used to measure the SNR of each averaged response by measuring the ratio of the normal average (Signal + Noise) to the residual noise (A–B) estimate (Wong & Bickford, 1980). Operationally, the larger the signal component, the larger is the measured ratio. A more refined method of a quality estimate of the averaged ABR was proposed by Elberling and Don (1984) in which, unlike the previous method, the variance of the noise is calculated using the sweep-to-sweep values at a single fixed time (therefore, the name F_{sp}). Based on this ratio, the SNR criterion for the presence of response is determined. For example, if the F_{sp} ratio is equal to or greater than 3.1 after a minimum of 250 sweeps, a response was detected with 99% confidence. What this implies is that averaging can be automatically stopped once the criterion F_{sp} ratio is attained—an important time-saver in the clinic.

IV. SUMMARY

- The choice of stimuli for recording the auditory brainstem evoked response is an important consideration as it determines how robust the responses are and how narrow or broad the cochlear regions of primary activity contributing to the responses are. Broadband clicks and chirps with their abrupt onsets are ideal to elicit synchronized neural activity in the onset-sensitive neurons, but they activate a wide range of cochlear frequency regions. Chirps, compensating for traveling wave delay, elicit synchronous and more robust responses compared to clicks. Frequency-specific tone bursts and narrowband chirps, obtained by using more gradual rise-fall times and longer stimulus durations, on the other hand, engage restricted cochlear regions and are more suitable for obtaining audiogram-like information.

- It is important to precisely know the output and frequency-response characteristics of the transducer used to record the response, since responses can vary depending on both the transducer type and methods (e.g., use of different acoustic couplers) used to measure the evoked response. It is recommended that the output of brief stimuli (clicks and tone bursts) used to record evoked potentials be specified in terms of dB peSPL (ISO 389-6). This standard also provides the recommended peRETSPLs for clicks and tone bursts.

- Every sequential step in the data acquisition process (from electrode application, differential amplification, filtering, analog-to-digital conversion, and the different averaging methods to minimize noise) is aimed at improving the SNR to optimally extract the submicrovolt amplitude response at the scalp. For example, low and balanced electrode electrical impedances improve the CMRR and therefore increase the SNR; differential amplification effectively increases the SNR by suppressing signals that are the same (background EEG and noise) at the inputs and amplifying signals that are different (stimulus elicited neural activity relevant to the auditory evoked potential) at the inputs; filtering gets rid of the noise that is not part of the signal; and averaging works on the principle that like events time-locked to the stimulus grow when the stimulus is repeated, while random events, like the noise, tend to diminish with stimulus repetition. A clearly defined robust response is essential for accurate interpretation of the functional integrity of auditory nerve and brainstem pathways.

- While learning to use commercially available user-friendly evoked potential systems is relatively easy and does not require technical expertise, obtaining optimal responses and troubleshooting issues during recording requires a good understanding of the signal generation and data acquisition principles presented in this chapter.

V. RECOMMENDED READINGS

Excellent Chapters With More Details

Durrant, J. D., & Boston, J. B. (2007). Stimuli for auditory evoked potential assessment. In R. F. Burkard, M. Don, & J. J. Eggermont (Eds.), *Auditory evoked potentials: Basic principles and clinical applications* (pp. 65–69). Baltimore, MD: Lippincott Williams & Wilkins.

Picton, T. W. (2011). Acoustic stimuli: Sounds to charm the brain. In T. W. Picton, *Human auditory evoked potentials* (pp. 125–133). San Diego, CA: Plural Publishing.

Thornton, A. R. D. (2007). Instrumentation and recording parameters. In R. F. Burkard, M. Don, & J. J. Eggermont (Eds.), *Auditory evoked potentials: Basic principles and clinical applications* (pp. 73–102). Baltimore, MD: Lippincott Williams & Wilkins.

REFERENCES

Burkard, R. (1984). Sound pressure level measurement and spectral analysis of brief acoustic transients. *Electroencephalography and Clinical Neurophysiology, 57,* 83–91.

Dau, T., Wagner, O., Mellert, V., & Kollmeier, B. (2000). Auditory brainstem responses with optimized chirp signals compensating basilar-membrane dispersion. *Journal of the Acoustical Society of America, 107*(3), 1530–1540.

Durrant, J. D., & Boston, J. B. (2007). Stimuli for auditory evoked potential assessment. In R. F. Burkard, M. Don, & J. J. Eggermont (Eds.), *Auditory evoked potentials: Basic principles and clinical applications* (pp. 65–69). Baltimore, MD: Lippincott Williams & Wilkins.

Elberling, C., Callo, J., & Don, M. (2010). Evaluating auditory brainstem responses to different chirp stimuli at three levels of stimulation. *Journal of the Acoustical Society of America, 128,* 215–223.

Elberling, C., & Don, M. (1984). Quality estimation of averaged auditory brainstem evoked responses. *Scandinavian Audiology, 13,* 187–197.

Elberling, C., & Don, M. (2008). Auditory brainstem responses to a chirp stimulus designed from derived-band latencies in normal hearing subjects. *Journal of the Acoustical Society of America, 124,* 3022–3077.

Elberling, C., Kristensen, S. G. B., & Don, M. (2012). Auditory brainstem responses to chirps delivered by different insert earphones. *Journal of the Acoustical Society of America, 131*(3), 2091–2100.

Elberling, C., & Wahlgreen, O. (1985). Estimation of auditory brainstem response, ABR, by means of Bayesian inference. *Scandinavian Journal of Audiology, 14,* 89–96.

Fobel, O., & Dau, T. (2004). Searching for the optimal stimulus eliciting auditory brainstem responses in humans. *Journal of the Acoustical Society of America, 116*(4), 2213–2222.

Jansson, K-J. F., Hakansson, B., Johannsen, L., & Tengstrand, T. (2015). Electro-acoustic performance of the new bone vibrator RadioEar B81: A comparison with the conventional RadioEar B71. *International Journal of Audiology, 54*(5), 334–340.

Picton, T. W. (2011). Acoustic stimuli: Sounds to charm the brain. In T. W. Picton (Ed.), *Human auditory evoked potentials* (pp. 125–133). San Diego, CA: Plural Publishing.

Richter, U., & Fedtke, T. (2005). Reference zero for the calibration of audiometric equipment using 'clicks' as test signals. *International Journal of Audiology, 44,* 478–487.

Thornton, A. R. D. (2007). Instrumentation and recording parameters. In R. F. Burkard, M. Don, & J. J. Eggermont (Eds.), *Auditory evoked potentials: Basic principles and clinical applications* (pp. 73–102). Baltimore, MD: Lippincott Williams & Wilkins.

Wong, P. J. H., & Bickford, R. G. (1980). Brainstem auditory evoked potentials: The use of noise estimates. *Electroencephalography and Clinical Neurophysiology, 50,* 25–34.

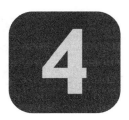

Normative Aspects of the Auditory Evoked Responses From the Brainstem

SCOPE

This chapter focuses on describing the characteristics and normative aspects of the ABR. The ABR represents transient neural activity synchronized to only the onset of brief stimuli. Before we consider the various clinical applications of these auditory brainstem evoked potentials (in Chapter 5), it is essential to first understand the normative aspects of these responses in terms of the overall response morphology, the response indices used to characterize them, their anatomical generator site(s), and how these response indices are predictably changed by stimulus factors, recording factors, and subject factors. This knowledge is a prerequisite to set up the normative database required to interpret these responses as normal or abnormal in clinical diagnosis.

I. AUDITORY BRAINSTEM RESPONSES (ABRS)

ABR Components and Response Morphology

The scalp-recorded ABR from normal-hearing individuals appear as a series of biphasic (positive and negative peak) components (waves) after onset of a high-intensity brief stimulus like a click. By convention (Jewett & Williston, 1971), the series of positive peaks, separated by approximately 1 ms, are identified using Roman numerals I–VII (Figure 4–1). At higher intensities (Figure 4–1 is an idealized response to an 80 dB nHL [decibels normal hearing level] click), all the ABR components are present, with wave V, the largest component, occurring 5.4 to 5.6 ms after stimulus onset. Waves I (presumably reflecting the whole nerve action potential from the auditory nerve and occurring about 4 ms earlier, 1.4–1.6 ms absolute latency) and III (occurring about 2 ms later than wave I and 2 ms earlier than wave V, about 3.4–3.6 ms absolute latency) are smaller but prominent. The other components (waves II, IV, VI, VII) are typically smaller, quite variable, and not always discernible in all individuals, thus limiting their clinical utility (Chiappa, Gladstone, & Young, 1979). One salient feature of these responses is their remarkable repeatability over a range of intensities. Add to this the ease with which these responses can be recorded, and it makes ABR assessment an ideal clinical tool to assess the functional integrity of auditory nerve and brainstem structures and to estimate audiogram-like hearing levels. For clinical diagnosis of site of lesion (more appropriately, level of the lesion along the auditory pathway in the brainstem), only waves I, III, and V are considered given that they are robust and repeatable at higher sound intensities. As we see later, only wave V is discernible and detectable near

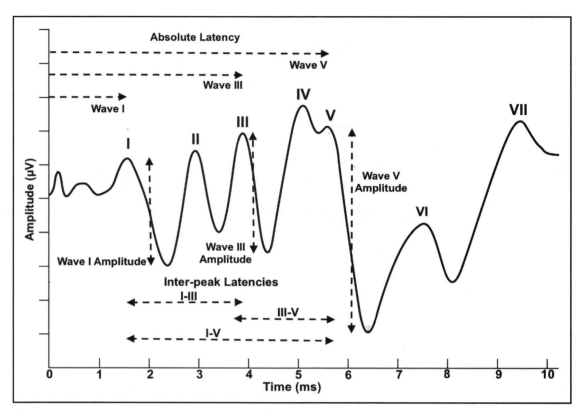

Figure 4–1. Idealized normal auditory brainstem response (ABR) waveform illustrating the characteristic morphology with several distinct biphasic components occurring post-stimulus onset with positive peaks labeled sequentially using Roman numerals I through VII by convention. The response indices of latency (both absolute and interpeak latencies) and amplitude are also depicted.

the threshold of the electrophysiologic response (about 10–15 dB nHL). The overall characteristic temporal signature of the ABR waveform (as shown in Figure 4–1) is referred to as its *waveform morphology*, which taken along with other quantitative response indices of the ABR, could serve as a soft qualitative indicator of functional integrity. While the overall waveform morphology is similar, normal individual variations in morphology are observed across individuals (Figure 4–2). Chiappa et al. (1979) identified six different patterns of the wave IV–V complex in 86% of a total of 52 individuals they tested. Variations are seen for other ABR components as well as shown in Figure 4–2. These normal individual variations in ABR morphology likely reflect differences in the algebraic sum at the electrode site(s) due to individual contributions of multiple sources to the ABR and/or differences in orientation of the dipole generators across individuals. Thus, it is important to be aware of these normal variations in response morphology to establish baseline criteria that could be used to identify abnormalities. Since clinical application of these responses includes assessment of the functional integrity of auditory nerve and brainstem structures to confirm or rule out structural and/or pathway abnormalities that may affect specific ABR components, *it is critical to know their anatomical generator sources to arrive at an accurate diagnosis of the site or level of the lesion.* Therefore, we next consider the neural generators of ABR components and then move to the description of the normative aspects of the ABR.

Neural Generators of the ABR Components

At the outset, it should be noted that although the research literature on the search for the neu-

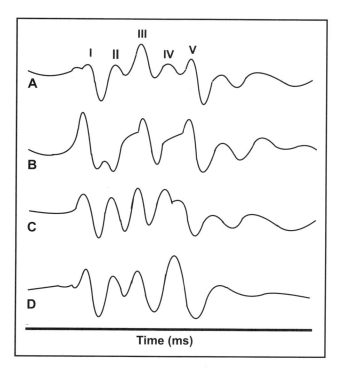

Figure 4–2. Auditory brainstem response (ABR) waveforms (A–D) showing normal individual variations in response morphology. (A) Both waves I and V show bifid peaks, particularly the clear separation of peaks IV and V. (B) Waves III and V show broad peaks that appear to be bifid. (C) Wave V shoulder is much smaller than the more prominent wave IV. (D) The wave IV–V complex is fused into a single peak.

ral generators of the ABR is extant, there is still a lack of closure on specific generator sites for most of the ABR components except for the certainty that wave I is generated in the distal portion of the auditory nerve. Because of the sequential temporal unfolding of the ABR components, initial formulations of successive activation of distinct nuclei and tracts consistent with the anatomical organization led to the simple formulation of the one peak, one anatomical generator notion (life would have been a lot easier this way) (Buchwald & Huang, 1975; Jewett, 1970; Lev & Sohmer, 1972). While it is generally agreed that the ABR generators are largely confined to the brainstem's classic lemniscal pathways (including the midbrain inferior colliculus), the difficulty in isolating the specific generator sources of each ABR component is complicated by the fact that the later components of scalp-recorded far-field potentials likely represent algebraically summed activity from several distinct but overlapping generator sites. There is evidence that multiple generators may contribute to the ABR components (Achor & Starr, 1980a, 1980b). Also, the increasing complexity of the bilateral structures and pathways (and the modulatory influence of descending pathways on these response components) along the ascending pathways starting with the cochlear nucleus (CN) makes it difficult to establish clear-cut associations between an ABR component and its anatomical source. Lastly, differences in the methods used in different investigations also add to the problem. Several different experimental approaches have been employed to address the issue of neural generators of the ABR. These include drawing inferences about the ABR component generator(s) by associating the changes in specific ABR components with discrete lesions of structures and pathways along the brainstem (animal studies), examining the latency correspondence between intracranial recordings directly from the auditory nerve and brainstem structures and simultaneously scalp-recorded ABR components (main method in human experiments), and by comparing the ABRs in normal individuals with the ABRs of individuals with confirmed auditory nerve and brainstem lesions (in humans, but hard to find individuals with confirmed isolated focal lesions). However, all these methods have limitations. For example, transection of the pathways may produce large alterations in the physiology of structures remote from the lesion. Also, a large-amplitude voltage field in a brainstem nucleus does not necessarily mean that the scalp recordings will reflect this field (Wada & Starr, 1983). Finally, a latency correspondence between the intracranial recording and a specific component of the scalp-recorded ABR does not necessarily mean that the intracranial site is the generator of the scalp-recorded component. Consistent with the scope of this chapter, we deliberately focus on the human studies related to the ABR generators. The intent here is to help maintain focus on the neural generators of the ABR in humans rather than be distracted by the difficulties applying animal ABR generator experimental data to humans. These difficulties primarily relate to differences in the auditory systems (e.g., differences in the length of the auditory nerve and brainstem tracts) and the resulting differences in morphologies of the ABR.

Latency Correspondence Between Intracranial and Scalp-Recorded ABR Components

The first study reported using this method in humans was by Hashimoto, Ishiyama, Yoshimoto, and Nemoto (1981), who recorded ABRs from the scalp and several brainstem structures including the auditory nerve, medulla, pons, and midbrain in patients undergoing neurosurgery. Based on the latency correspondence between the compound action potential directly recorded from the distal portion of the auditory nerve and ABR wave I, and the latency correspondence between a later response recorded near the cerebellopontine angle (where the auditory nerve enters the CN) and ABR wave II, these authors concluded that wave I was generated exclusively in the distal portion of the auditory nerve and wave II in the proximal portion of the auditory nerve. Essentially similar findings for waves I and II were reported by several other subsequent studies (Moller, 1981a; Moller & Jannetta, 1981; Moller, Jannetta, & Moller, 1981; Spire, Dohrmann, & Prieto, 1982) comparing intracranial recordings from the distal and proximal portions of the auditory nerve with scalp-recorded ABRs. These results suggest that the auditory nerve appears to generate two components—*waves I and II of the ABR from the distal and proximal portions of the auditory nerve, respectively* (Figure 4–3A–B). Responses recorded using short tone bursts from the vicinity of the CN revealed a robust negative peak that matched in latency with wave III of the scalp-recorded ABR when the stimulus was in the ipsilateral ear (Moller & Jannetta, 1983). This CN response was smaller in amplitude and had longer latency when the stimulus was in the contralateral ear. Based on these results, the authors concluded that the *ipsilateral CN was the main contributor for wave III generation and that it could also contribute to the negative peak that follows wave III* (Figure 4–3C). While it is likely that the CN may contribute to later ABR components, it is unlikely that structures above the CN in the brainstem contribute to the CN response. The responses recorded from the lateral brainstem proximal to the superior olivary complex (SOC) (Moller & Jannetta, 1984) and dorsal CN (Moller, Jannetta, & Jho, 1994) revealed several peaks that occurred later than the CN response, including a *negative peak that*

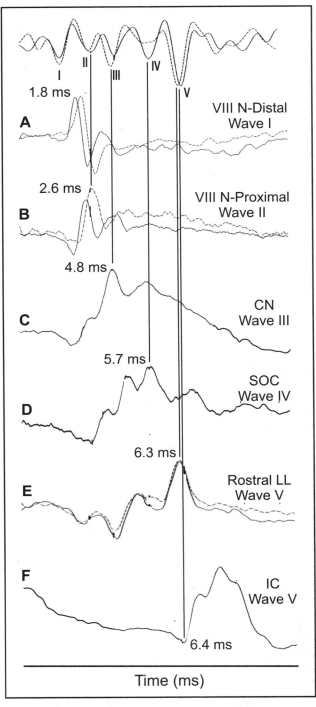

Figure 4–3. Idealized auditory brainstem response (ABR) waveform showing components I–V (*top*) and the intracranial recordings from distal VIIIN (A), proximal VIIIN (B), CN (C), SOC (D), rostral LL (E), and surface of IC (F). The presumed generator site(s) and the correspondence with each ABR component are identified to the right of each trace. While latency values for each intracranial component are accurate, the time axis for the composite figure is not. From data used with permission from Aage Moller.

approximately aligned with wave IV of the ABR, suggesting a SOC generator source (Figure 4–3D). Intracranial recordings from the dorsal CN on both sides and the midline over the dorsal acoustic stria (proximal to the lateral lemniscus [LL]) revealed a large negative peak that aligned with ABR wave V (Moller, Jannetta. & Jho, 1994), leading the authors to infer that *wave V of the ABR is generated in the rostral part of the contralateral LL proximal to its termination in the inferior colliculus (IC)* (Figure 4–3E). Finally, recordings from the surface of the IC showed a negative peak (Figure 4–3F) that (followed by a slow positive peak) aligned with *ABR wave V, which was interpreted to suggest LL inputs to the contralateral IC* (Moller & Jannetta, 1983). Hashimoto et al. (1981) also showed that the IC recorded component aligned with ABR wave V, but they inferred the wave V source to be the IC and not the LL inputs. While these results taken together (except for the more certain wave I generator source) appear to suggest a predominant single source for each component and possible contributions from several other sources, caution should be exercised in utilizing this information about the anatomical generator(s) of the ABR components for clinical decision-making about the site(s) of a lesion in the brainstem. In almost all the intracranial recordings from each structure along the brainstem, multiple peaks were observed. It is not clear how the volume-conducted multicomponent responses from different sources combine at the electrode site to form the multicomponent ABR that is recorded at the scalp. Nevertheless, based on these results, the putative auditory nerve and brainstem generator sites for the scalp-recorded ABR are illustrated in Figure 4–4.

Identification of ABR Generators in Individuals With Confirmed Focal Brainstem Lesions

The rationale for this experimental approach is quite simple. Since the components forming the scalp-recorded ABR waveform reflect neural activity originating in distinct anatomical locations along the ascending auditory pathway, any lesion that compromises the generation of a particular component will appear altered or will be absent in the scalp recording, thus leading to the inference that the functional integrity of the affected structure is essential for the presence of a normal component at the scalp recording site. Stockard and Rossiter (1977) correlated abnormalities of ABR

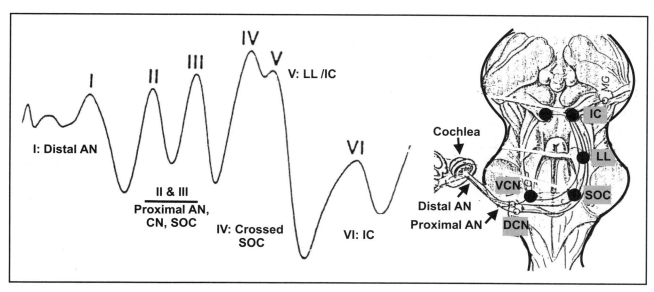

Figure 4–4. *Left:* Auditory brainstem response (ABR) waveforms with components (I–VI) identified. *Right:* A schematic dorsal view of the brainstem shows the generator sites of the ABR components from the distal and proximal portions (distal AN, proxima AN) of the auditory nerve, dorsal and ventral cochlear nucleus (DCN, VCN), superior olivary complex (SOC), lateral lemniscus (LL), and the inferior colliculus (IC). The neural generator(s) of each ABR wave is shown at the bottom of each peak of the ABR.

components with postmortem or radiologic locations of different brainstem lesions in over 100 patients. The results of their correlational analyses revealed that the auditory nerve generated wave I, cochlear nucleus wave II, caudal pons wave III, rostral pons or midbrain wave IV, IC wave V, and MGB wave VI. Essentially similar conclusions were drawn by Starr and Achor (1975) when they evaluated ABRs in individuals with neurological disease involving the auditory nerve and brainstem structures. Consistent with these findings, based on correlations between CT lesion sites and the selective absence of the ABR IV–V complex or wave V in individuals with discrete midbrain-pontine hemorrhages or tumors, Chu (1989) concluded that the intact dorsolateral area of the upper pons was essential for the presence of waves IV and V. These authors also observed that the ABRs were affected when stimulation was ipsilateral to the lesion. This ipsilateral laterality of the later generators, also reported by others (Brown, Chiappa, & Brooks, 1981; Chiappa, Harrison, Brooks, & Young., 1980; Markand, Farlow, Stevens, & Edwards, 1989; Oh et al., 1981; York, 1986), is at odds with the intracranial experimental data that suggest a contralateral location of generators for the later ABR components. However, characteristic clinical findings of ipsilateral ABR abnormalities for most auditory nerve and lower brainstem lesions and bilateral abnormalities for upper brainstem lesions are more consistent with intracranial findings that suggest ipsilateral generators for the earlier waves and contralateral generators for the later waves. In clinical testing situations in humans, a useful guideline that appears to work is to think that wave I originates from the VIIIth nerve, wave III from the pons (trapezoid body, superior olive), and wave V from the midbrain (LL, IC), while the generators of waves II, IV, VI, and VII are still uncertain (Starr & Hamilton, 1976). Given the uncertainty about the precise generator sites of most ABR components, it would be even better to continue to consider the common clinically used dichotomy of auditory nerve and lower brainstem lesions (using the I–III and I–V interpeak latency [IPL] metric) and upper brainstem lesions (using the III–V IPL metric and the V/I amplitude ratio), which focuses on the level of the lesion rather than on the specific anatomical site.

In summary, based on both experimental approaches (albeit leaning more toward the intracranial approach), we can draw the following conclusions about the ABR generators in humans (see Figure 4–3A–F):

1. Waves I and II of the ABR reflect activity from the distal and proximal portions of the auditory nerve, respectively.

2. Wave III is generated mainly by the ipsilateral CN, with the CN contributing to the negative peak that follows wave III and to some later components.

3. Wave IV of the ABR is generated by SOC bilaterally with a stronger contralateral component.

4. Wave V of the ABR is generated in the rostral part of the contralateral LL proximal to its termination in the IC.

5. The results of intracranial to surface recording comparison studies to determine ABR generators are to a first-degree approximation comparable with the ipsilateral site of generators, particularly for the earlier waves. Results of lesion studies are generally more difficult to interpret.

6. Given that multiple generators can contribute to each ABR component (with the possible exception of wave I), the notion of one wave one generator is not tenable.

ABR Indices

It is typical to quantify evoked potentials in terms of their latency and amplitude. The absolute latency (defined as the time interval between stimulus onset and response peak of interest) of waves I, III, and V is shown by the horizontal dotted line in Figure 4–1. Unlike the cortical evoked potentials where **peak amplitude** of a given response component is measured relative to a prestimulus baseline, the **peak-to-peak** (more correctly the peak-to-trough—that is, from a positive peak to the following negative peak or trough) amplitude measure is utilized for the ABR components as shown for waves I, III, and

V by the vertical dotted lines in Figure 4–1. Derived from these "absolute" measures of amplitude and latency are relative measures that include *amplitude ratio V/I (amplitude of wave V relative to wave I)*, and relative latency measures that include the interpeak latencies (IPLs) I–V, I–III, and III–V (shown below the waveform in Figure 4–1), which are a measure of the time interval between each of the three pairs of response peaks. There is also an additional relative measure called the *interaural latency difference (ILD)*, which evaluates the difference in latency for a given ABR component elicited by stimulation of each ear. For example, the most commonly used ILD_V measures the difference in wave V latency between the two ears.

What Are the Physiological Determinants of ABR Latency and Amplitude?

Absolute Latency: Absolute latency of the ABR components is determined by a combination of factors that include the frequency-dependent cochlear place of primary activity (the lower the frequency of the stimulus, the more apical is the activity, the longer is the traveling wave delay, and thus, the longer is the absolute latency of all ABR components); the intensity-dependent threshold of the cochlear excitatory process (the higher the stimulus intensity, the shorter is the latency of the presynaptic graded hair cell receptor or generator potential, which is the effective stimulus for action potential generation); the frequency-independent synaptic integration time (at each synapse from the hair cell through the brainstem pathways, delays are introduced due to the time taken to integrate information from multiple synapses); the neural conduction velocity (the faster the neural conduction, the shorter is the time for neural transmission along fiber tracts—recall from Chapter 1 that faster neural conduction occurs in myelinated and larger-diameter fibers); and the time to the generator site (the higher in the brainstem the generator for a given ABR component is, the longer will be its absolute latency). For example, the wave V generator is farther along the brainstem than the wave I generator, so wave I latency will be shorter than wave V latency. However, it should be noted here that cochlear contributions to each component could be different, particularly waves I and V.

Relative Latency—IPLs: Information about neural conduction time (often referred to as the central conduction time) between structures eliciting the ABR components is reflected in the IPL measures. There are three IPL temporal windows (I–V, I–III, and III–V) that are used to evaluate the neural conduction time between structures in the caudal brainstem (I–III), between structures in the rostral brainstem (III–V), and the overall integrity of the entire brainstem (I–V). This scheme is consistent with the site of generation of waves I (distal auditory nerve), III (caudal brainstem), and V (rostral brainstem) described earlier. To the extent that *IPL is a true measure of neural conduction time independent of cochlear events*, then it provides for a robust metric to assess the integrity of the transmission of neural activity in both the caudal and rostral brainstem and allows the clinician to draw inferences about the *level* of the lesion-caudal versus rostral brainstem. Again, both frequency-independent factors of neural conduction velocity and delays caused by integration across multiple synapses along the brainstem will determine each IPL measure.

Relative Latency—ILD: As defined earlier, ILD refers to the difference in latency between specific ABR components elicited by monaural stimulation of the right and left ear using the same stimulus and recording parameters. The rationale for this metric is that in a system with normal functional integrity of peripheral and brainstem structures, there should not be a significant ILD—that is, the latencies of a given component elicited by stimulation of either ear should be similar, producing a near-zero ILD. Thus, a significantly large ILD (corrected for peripheral asymmetries in hearing sensitivity) would point to a brainstem lesion.

Response Amplitude

Two factors contribute to the amplitude of the population neural response. One is the temporal synchrony and coherence of neural activity in the responding elements (the lower the synchrony, the smaller is the amplitude and the broader is the response waveform), and two is the number of neural elements contributing to the response (the greater the number of contributing neurons, the larger is the amplitude). The derived V/I amplitude ratio measure is used in clinical diagnosis because peak-to-peak amplitudes of ABR components show large intersubject variability (primarily due to the varying amount of residual noise during averaging) and therefore are not clinically useful. Since wave V is typically larger than wave I, any low ratio that would suggest the opposite may be indicative of a pathology. Relative ABR metrics, in general, are more sensitive in differentiating pathologies since they subtract the effects of electrode montage, head size, and sex as factors contributing to amplitude variability (King & Sininger, 1992; Mitchell, Phillips, & Trune, 1989; Trune, Mitchell, & Phillips, 1988; Verhulst, Jagadeesh, Mauermann, & Ernst, 2016).

Effects of Stimulus Factors

Intensity

Stimulus intensity is an important and robust determinant of changes in the amplitude and latency of the ABR components. For ABR measurements using clicks or brief tone bursts, stimulus intensity is expressed in decibels normal hearing level (dB nHL). (See the preceding chapter for more details on this measure.) Stimulus intensity is manipulated to either measure threshold or characterize how latency of the ABR components changes. In this section, the description of effects of intensity is limited to ABRs obtained in young normal-hearing adults using click stimuli. ABR waveforms to click stimuli are plotted in Figure 4–5 as a function of decreasing stimulus intensity. Several changes in the ABR components easily observable with the decrease in intensity include a systematic prolongation of the absolute latency of all components. (wave V is the largest component and is reliably detectable down to a threshold level of about 5–10 dB nHL). Also, there is a progressive reduction in response amplitude of all components with the detectability of the relatively smaller earlier components (waves I, II, and III) becoming increasingly difficult for levels below about 40 dB nHL. Only wave V is detectable near threshold making it the best candidate for threshold estimation. Plotting the latency as a function of intensity (latency-inten-

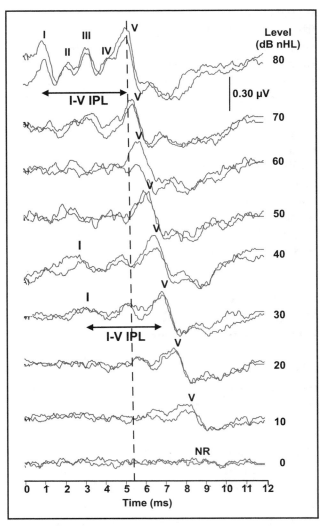

Figure 4–5. Grand averaged replicated click-elicited auditory brainstem response (ABR) waveforms from normal hearing adults plotted as a function of stimulus level in dB nHL. The ABR components and the stimulus levels are identified. The horizontal double-arrow lines below the waveforms for the 80 and 30 dB nHL conditions illustrates the decrease I–V IPL as stimulus intensity is decreased.

sity function [LIF]) provides a more complete characterization of how latency changes with intensity. The LIF for wave V (Figure 4–6) may be described as curvilinear with intensities above about 50 dB nHL showing a shallower slope of about a 0.1 to 0.2 ms latency change/10 dB change in intensity, and intensities below 50 dB nHL showing a relatively steeper slope of 0.5 to 0.6 ms latency change/10 change in intensity (Gorga, Worthington, Reiland, Beauchine, & Goldgar, 1985; Pratt & Sohmer, 1976). The differential latency changes for waves I, III, and

V in different intensity regions are seen in Table 4–1, re-created using data from Stockard and Stockard (1983). For click stimuli, the mean wave V latency at threshold (15–20 dB nHL) in normal-hearing individuals is around 7.8 to 8.2 ms and about 5.3 to 5.5 ms at 80 dB nHL (Hecox & Galambos, 1974; Picton, Woods, Baribeau-Braun, & Healey, 1977; Starr & Achor, 1975). Thus, wave V latency shifts about 2.6 ms between these two levels. Wave V latencies are more variable (SD = ±0.3–0.4 ms) at lower levels compared to latencies at higher levels (at 80 dB nHL SD = ±0.1–0.15 ms).

At 80 dB nHL, the absolute latency of wave I is around 1.4 to 1.5 ms, wave III is about 3.5 to 3.6 ms, and wave V is about 5.4 to 5.6 ms, thus yielding I–III and III–V IPLs of about 2 ms and I–V IPL of about 4 ms. IPLs are thought to reflect neural conduction times and therefore are not expected to change with intensity. However, there is evidence suggesting that IPLs I–III, and particularly I–V, decrease with intensity (Pratt & Sohmer, 1976; Starr & Achor, 1975; Stockard, Stockard, Westmoreland, & Corfits, 1979). This decrease in IPL is clear from the width of the bidirectional arrows in the waveform data in Figure 4–5. This trend toward decreasing I–III, III–V, and I–V IPL as intensity is decreased is clear in Table 4–2 with IPL I–V showing the greatest change.

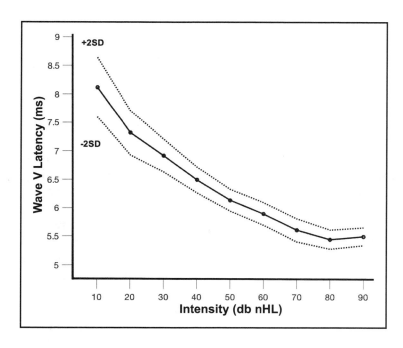

Figure 4–6. Wave V latency-intensity function. Note the steeper slope of the function below about 50 dB and relatively shallower slope at higher intensities. The dotted lines indicate the ±2 SD.

Table 4–1. Wave V Absolute Latency Changes (ms) per 10-dB Change in Intensity in Normal Young Adults

	Intensity Region (dB nHL)			
ABR Component	30–40	40–50	50–60	60–70
Wave	0.44 (0.19)	0.49 (0.24)	0.29 (0.13)	0.23 (0.11)
Wave III	0.37 (0.24)	0.49 (0.19)	0.23 (0.12)	0.18 (0.10)
Wave V	0.33 (0.15)	0.34 (0.16)	0.20 (0.10)	0.21 (0.09)

Source: Recreated from "Recording and Analyzing," by J. E. Stockard and J. J. Stockard. In *Bases of Auditory Brain-Stem Evoked Responses*, by E. J. Moore (Ed.), 1983, pp. 255–286. Copyright 1983 by Grune & Stratton, New York. Adapted by permission.

Table 4–2. Interpeak Latency (IPL) (I–III, III–V, I–V) Changes (ms) as a Function of Intensity in Normal Young Adults

IPL	\multicolumn{5}{c}{Stimulus Intensity (dB nHL)}
	30	40	50	60	70
I-III	1.95 (0.15)	2.02 (0.14)	2.03 (0.17)	2.09 (0.18)	2.14 (0.15)
III-V	1.73 (0.20)	1.74 (0.17)	1.89 (0.17)	1.92 (0.14)	1.89 (0.16)
I-V	3.68 (0.22)	3.76 (0.20)	3.91 (0.27)	4.00 (0.27)	4.02 (0.25)

Source: Recreated from "Recording and Analyzing," by J. E. Stockard and J. J. Stockard. In *Bases of Auditory Brain-Stem Evoked Responses*, by E. J. Moore (Ed.), 1983, pp. 255–286. Copyright 1983 by Grune & Stratton, New York. Adapted by permission.

As seen in Figure 4–5, the response amplitude of all ABR components decreases with a decrease in intensity. Since response amplitude is quite variable (Hecox & Galambos, 1974; Jewett & Williston, 1971; Lasky, 1984), few studies have tried to characterize the amplitude change of ABR components. While some report nonlinear behavior (Hecox & Galambos, 1974; Jewett & Williston, 1971), others report a linear growth function for wave V (Starr & Achor, 1975; Wolfe, Skinner, & Burns, 1978). The difficulty in accurately characterizing the ABR amplitude in general, and particularly at lower intensities, is due to the large variability resulting from both the small magnitude of the signal measured (submicrovolt range—even at high intensity, wave V amplitude is about 500 nanovolts [nV]) and the residual noise it is competing with.

Physiological Bases of the Intensity-Induced Absolute Latency and Amplitude Change

We need to invoke some of the physiological mechanisms we described earlier (under the section, What Are the Physiological Determinants of ABR Latency and Amplitude?) to explain the latency and amplitude changes produced by changing stimulus intensity. At high intensities, the ABRs to the broadband click are basally biased due to the higher traveling wave velocity near the base. That is, although a broad range of cochlear regions contributes to the response, particularly for wave V (Don & Eggermont, 1978; Eggermont & Don, 1980), the gradient of effective contribution reflected in the modal value of the latency distributions of cochlear regions contributing to the response is located more basally (consistent with the cochlear mechanics property of upward spread of excitation with increasing intensity); therefore, the response has a shorter latency. As intensity decreases, the modal value of the latency distribution shifts more apically due to a reduction in the basal bias, and thus response latency gets longer. This mechanism likely moves the modal value from around 4000 Hz at high intensities to about 1000 to 2000 Hz near the ABR threshold for clicks. While this across-place mechanism may account for the latency shift, Burkard and Don (2007) make a convincing argument that within-place mechanisms are probably the dominant contributor for intensity-dependent latency shifts observed for click ABR, since derived band responses do not show a substantial shift in cochlear regions contributing to the response across levels. Nevertheless, the fact that wave V is still present near threshold with a long latency does suggest the operation of an across-place mechanism. Additional experiments specifically designed to address this issue are needed to resolve this issue of the relative contributions of across-place and within-place mechanisms to level-dependent changes in latency. Additional intensity-dependent mechanisms have to be brought into play to realize the entire 2.5 to 3.0 ms shift in latency from high intensity to the threshold level ABR. It is likely that intensity-dependent changes associated with the cochlear excitatory process, which leads to the generator potential and the excitatory postsynaptic potential (EPSPs), may also contribute to the intensity-dependent latency change observed for the ABR components. Specifically, at high intensities, these processes are presumed to have shorter latency (i.e., both the generator potential and the EPSPs arise more quickly); as intensity is decreased, their generation takes longer (Moller, 1981b). The decrease in IPLs with decreasing intensity is largely due to the apparently greater intensity-induced latency shift for wave I compared to wave V. Specifically, wave I has both a short latency, high intensity component and a longer latency, low intensity component (N1, N2, respectively). At high intensities, the dominant short latency component determines wave I latency, thus providing the normal longer I–V IPL. At low intensities, only the longer latency wave I component is present, thus producing the relatively shorter I–V IPL.

The mechanism accounting for intensity-dependent amplitude change is relatively more straightforward. As intensity increases, the cochlear regions contributing to the ABR increase; therefore, more neurons contribute to the response, and because of the increasing basal (higher traveling wave velocity) bias, the synchrony of neural activity also increase. Thus, these two amplitude determinants combine effectively to produce a larger amplitude response. Conversely, at lower intensities, there is a reduction in the number of neural elements (reduced upward spread), and a more distributed cochlear regional contribution that disrupts the synchrony as well, thus resulting in a response that is smaller in amplitude and appears broader. The inability to detect the earlier components at lower levels suggests that synchronous activity with greater synchrony (i.e., from more basal regions) is essential to detect the evoked activity representing waves I and III at the scalp electrodes.

Frequency

Here we focus on the ABRs elicited by brief frequency-specific tone bursts that are used to estimate thresholds. As discussed in Chapter 3, limiting the dominant spectral energy of the stimulus to a narrow band around the nominal frequency of the tone burst is essential to obtain audiogram-like threshold information by restricting the cochlear place(s) contributing to the response to correspond as closely as possible to the nominal frequency of the stimulus. The assumption is that if the tone bursts are frequency specific, then they should elicit place-specific responses, at least near threshold levels. Consistent with this, the absolute latency of the ABR components should decrease as the frequency is increased. As expected, waveform data in Figure 4–7 show a systematic increase in latency of all ABR components as tone burst frequency is decreased from 4000 Hz to 500 Hz in octave steps. While wave V is easily identifiable at all four frequencies, waves I and III are discernible for only 4000 and 2000 Hz. Also, note that wave V is robust and sharper at 4000 and 2000 Hz, while wave V is smaller in amplitude and shows a broader waveform at 1000 and 500 Hz. This difference in wave V waveform morphology even at higher intensities suggests that wave V for these low frequencies would be more difficult to detect near the threshold. Gorga, Kaminski, and Beauchaine (1988) reported that the low-frequency responses were less reproducible and more variable. Similar to the click responses, absolute latency of wave V elicited by different frequency

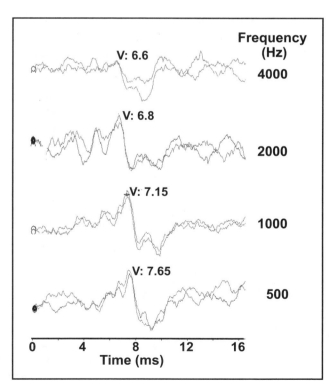

Figure 4–7. Auditory brainstem response (ABR) waveforms plotted as a function of decreasing frequency of tone bursts. Wave latency identified in each trace shows a progressive delay as frequency is decreased. The early components (I and III) are not discernible for the 1000 and 500 Hz stimulus. Also, wave V shows amplitude decrement and broadened waveform at 1000 and 500 Hz.

tone bursts also decreases with an increase in intensity, showing a similar nonlinear function although the slope of the function (Figure 4–8) is steeper for low frequencies compared to high frequencies (Gorga et al., 1988). It can also be seen in this figure that at any given level, latency decreases as the frequency is increased (see a downward-pointing line indicating movement from longer to shorter latency), and the latency spread across frequency decreases as intensity increases (indicated by the shorter arrow to the right of the figure)—that is, the widely separated functions at lower levels appear to converge as intensity increases. It should be noted here that similar frequency-related effects on latency and amplitude of the ABR may be observed using transducers with very different frequency response characteristics.

Physiological Bases of the Frequency-Induced Absolute Latency and Amplitude Change

The most straightforward interpretation of the latency change with frequency (with level fixed) can be made by invoking the cochlear place of primary activity contributing to the ABR. As tone burst frequency is decreased, the primary cochlear activity contributing to the ABR shifts progressively to more apical locations producing increasingly longer latency responses. This explanation assumes frequency-specific tone bursts of moderate intensity or lower. Since the rise-fall time used also varies, differences in rise-fall time could also affect the latency (longer latency responses for slower rise-fall times used with low-frequency tone burst). For example, the change in latency shown in our waveform data in Figure 4–7 for our stimuli is similar to that reported by Gorga et al. (1998). Place specificity is not guaranteed even for frequency-specific tone burst elicited responses at higher levels due to increasing excitatory spread that, in turn, increases the contributions from increasingly higher-frequency cochlear regions and thereby shortens the latency. The trend toward convergence of the latency intensity functions at higher levels seen in Figure 4–8 is likely due to the relatively steeper latency intensity slopes for low frequencies compared to high frequencies. The steeper slopes for the low frequencies could also be interpreted

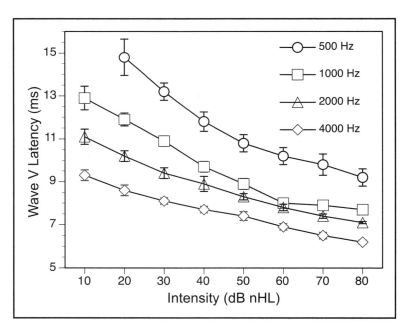

Figure 4–8. Wave V latency plotted as a function of intensity for tone bursts of different frequency. For each frequency, wave V latency decreases with an increase in intensity with greater separation in latency across frequency at low frequencies with a tendency to converge at high intensities. Also, at each level there is a progressive decrease in wave latency as frequency is changed from low to high frequencies.

to suggest a relatively greater excitatory spread for low-frequency stimuli.

With respect to response amplitude, since the ABR is sensitive to stimulus onset, the more rapid the rise times, the greater should be the synchrony of the generated neural activity and therefore the larger the amplitude of the response. The sharper and greater amplitude responses observed for the higher frequencies may be due to a combination of factors that increased synchrony and/or the number of neural elements, including the use of more rapid rise times at high frequencies, a larger neural population response consistent with the greater innervation density in the basal end of the cochlea relative to the apical regions (Spoendlin, 1972), and greater traveling wave velocity near the base (high frequencies). In addition to not having these advantages, low frequencies are more susceptible to phase effects (as when using an alternating polarity stimulus) on latency, which smear averaged responses to low-frequency stimuli producing low amplitude and broad responses (Moller, 1986).

Repetition Rate

Repetition rate, as the name implies, is simply the rate at which stimuli are presented in a unit of time (typically clicks or tone bursts per second). The reciprocal of repetition rate gives the measure of interstimulus interval (ISI). Thus, ISI is the time interval between the onset of one stimulus and the onset of the next stimulus (more appropriately referred to as stimulus onset asynchrony). Thus, the relationship Repetition rate = 1/ISI is illustrated in Figure 4–9. Manipulation of rate is used to evaluate the nature of neural adaptation (decreased responsiveness with sustained or rapidly repeating stimuli), which may be different in normal-hearing individuals and individuals with auditory nerve or brainstem pathology, and therefore could serve as a useful diagnostic metric. The literature evaluating stimulus repetition rate effects on the ABR is vast (selected references include Chiappa, Gladstone, & Young, 1979; Don, Allen, & Starr, 1977; Fowler & Noffsinger, 1983; Hyde, Stephens, & Thornton, 1976; Picton, Stapells, & Campbell, 1981; Pratt & Sohmer, 1976; Sininger & Don, 1989; Suresh & Krishnan, 2021; Thornton & Coleman, 1975; Weber & Fijikawa, 1977). Across studies, there is general agreement that increasing click rates above about 26/sec progressively increases the latency and reduces the amplitude of all components as shown in Figure 4–10. The amplitudes of the earlier components (waves I and III) appear to be more susceptible to the desynchronization effects of increasing stimulus rate (going from 10/sec to about 90/sec), while wave V appears to be more resilient with relatively smaller changes in amplitude (Chiappa et al.,

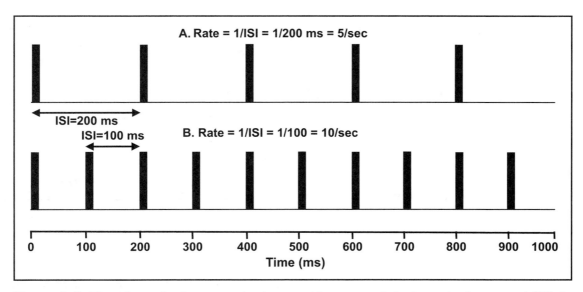

Figure 4–9. The relationship between stimulus repetition rate and the interstimulus interval (ISI). As the rate increases from 5/sec (*top trace*) to 10/sec, the ISI decreases from 200 to 100 ms. The faster the stimulus repetition rate, the shorter is the ISI.

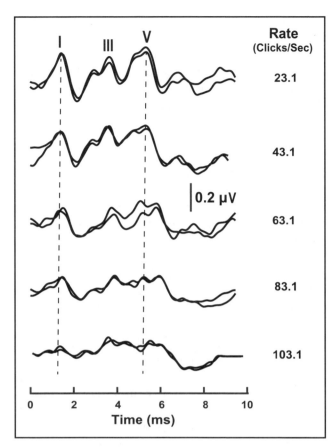

Figure 4–10. Auditory brainstem response (ABR) waveforms plotted as a function of increasing click rate. The vertical dotted line for wave I shows very little latency change as click rate is increased. In contrast, the vertical dotted line for wave V shows a progressive increase in latency as repetition rate is increased. While wave I shows a progressive decrease in amplitude, wave V amplitude appears to be more resilient to increase in rate.

1979; Hyde et al., 1976; Jewett & Williston, 1971; Picton et al., 1981: Pratt & Sohmer, 1976; Suzuki, Kobayashi, & Takaoi, 1986; Terkildsen, Osterhammel, & Huis in't Veld, 1975; Thornton & Coleman, 1975; Yagi & Kaga, 1979). Picton et al. (1981) reported a 50% reduction in amplitude (compared to the slowest rate of 10/sec) for the earlier components with only a 10% reduction in wave V amplitude. This resilience of wave V amplitude to faster rates allows consideration of using faster rates for threshold estimation to reduce test time, particularly while testing infants and young children. The amount of the intensity-independent (Don et al., 1977) latency shift from a slow rate (about 10–11/sec) to a rate of 90/sec is about 0.28 ms for wave I, 0.46 ms for wave III, and 0.61 ms for wave V for a stimulus level of 55 dB nHL (Suzuki et al., 1986). Several of these studies have reported this progressively increasing magnitude of latency shift (Figure 4–11) for the later waves compared to the relatively smaller latency changes for wave I, resulting in prolongation of the I–III and I–V IPL.

Physiological Bases of the Stimulus Rate Induced Absolute Latency and Amplitude Change

While adaptation is common in sensory systems, the specific mechanism(s) and their loci producing the latency prolongation and amplitude reduction of the ABR components is not well understood. The substantial rate effects observed at ISIs (between 10 and 35 ms) comfortably exceeding the rapid time course of neural refractoriness (1–2 ms) make it an unlikely mechanism to account for the observed changes in latency and amplitude. It is likely that rate-related changes in ABR reflect synaptic short-term adaptation and poststimulus recovery from this adaptation (Don, Allen, & Starr, 1977; Thornton & Coleman, 1975). This latter description is consistent with the neural basis of forward masking (wherein the response to the stimulus is adapted by a preceding masker) observed for auditory nerve fiber responses (Harris & Dallos, 1979). One likely

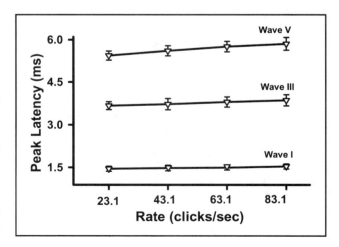

Figure 4–11. Mean latency shift for waves I, III, and V plotted as a function of stimulus repetition rate. Note the relatively steeper slope of the function for wave V compared to waves I and III. Thus, the I–V interval increases with an increase in stimulus repetition rate.

locus for this synaptic adaptation is the hair cell–nerve junction. While the specific sequence and dynamics of presynaptic and postsynaptic events associated with this synaptic adaptation are not clear, both the cochlear excitatory process (producing the generator potential) and the subsequent generation of excitatory postsynaptic potentials may be disrupted. The consequence is the prolongation of latency and reduction in amplitude of the ABR components. Rate studies cited earlier have also indicated that the amplitude of the earlier components is reduced more compared to wave V. Terkildsen et al. (1975) have interpreted this differential amplitude effect of the rate as reflecting greater susceptibility of the earlier components to neural desynchronization associated with adaptation. It is tempting to speculate here that the greater resilience of wave V amplitude to rate effects may, at least in part, relate to the triggering of central compensatory gain mechanisms when peripheral output is degraded by adaptation. Finally, the progressively larger latency shifts for the later waves are consistent with the notion of synaptic adaptation, wherein the latency shift is cumulative across the multiple synapses traversed by the neural activity. That is, a delay is added at each synapse from the auditory nerve (wave I), CN (wave III), SOC (wave IV), and LL/IC (wave V). It should be noted that the rapid rate paradigm to evaluate synaptic adaptation does have a potential confound caused by the overlap of the ABR components with later middle latency evoked responses for short ISIs, thereby obscuring the real rate effects associated with adaptation.

Onset Polarity

Onset polarity refers to the phase of the stimulus at onset, usually expressed as condensation (where the initial deflection of the stimulus voltage is in the positive direction), rarefaction (where the initial deflection of the stimulus voltage is in the negative direction), or alternating (alternating between condensation and rarefaction). Since neural activity occurs about half a period earlier for stimuli with a rarefaction onset phase compared to those with a condensation onset phase (see Physiological Bases of the Onset Polarity-Induced Latency Differences section for more details), response latency of the ABR components should be shorter for the rarefaction phase compared to the condensation phase, at least theoretically. However, the results across studies are equivocal with the lack of a consistent demonstration of predictable effects. Some studies suggest that the rarefaction onset phase produces more robust and shorter latency response components, as expected, thereby presumably increasing the sensitivity of the measure in clinical diagnosis (Kevanishvili & Aphonchenko, 1981; Rosenhamer, Lindstrom, & Lundborg, 1978; Schwartz et al., 1990; Stockard, Sharbrough, & Tinker, 1978). However, several studies have shown the opposite effect—earlier responses for condensation compared to the rarefaction onset polarity (Kevanishvili & Aphonchenko, 1981; Maurer, Schaefer, & Leitner, 1980; Rosenhamer et al., 1978; Ruth, Hildebrand, & Cantrell, 1982; Terkildsen et al., 1975). To further confuse the issue, several studies have failed to see any measurable difference in the responses elicited by these two onset polarities (Beattie, 1988; Kevanishvili & Aphonchenko, 1981; Maurer et al., 1980; Ruth et al., 1982; Terkildsen et al., 1975). In contrast to clicks, frequency-specific tone bursts that are lower in frequency (therefore have longer periods so that polarity differences are more clearly discernible) produce differences (Figure 4–12) in morphology and latency of the ABR (Fowler, 1992) that shows a predictable inverse relationship with frequency (Table 4–3). The latency differences do not quite approach the predicted theoretical half period (shown in the last column) probably due to the relative phase insensitivity of the higher-frequency contributions to the ABR resulting from the excitatory spread.

Physiological Bases of the Onset Polarity-Induced Latency Differences

Hair cell excitation and the subsequent activation of auditory nerve fibers occurs only during the rarefaction onset phase (Brugge, Anderson, Hind, & Rose, 1969; Zwislocki, 1975) because the hair cell stereocilia are sheared in the preferred direction (toward the outer cochlear wall radially) to depolarize hair cells (Peake & Kiang, 1962; Salomon & Elberling, 1971). The sequence of events leading to hair cell excitation and subsequent activation of the auditory nerve fibers includes movement of the stapes footplate toward the middle ear, which results in the basilar membrane being displaced

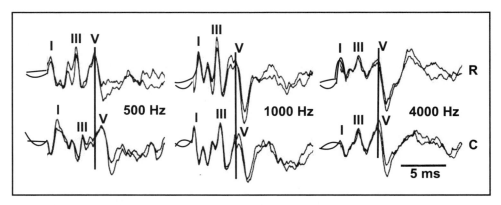

Figure 4–12. Auditory brainstem response (ABR) waveforms elicited by frequency tone bursts using rarefaction (R) and condensation (C) onset polarities. Frequencies of the tone burst are identified for each panel. The vertical solid line aligned with wave V in each panel serves to illustrate the wave V latency difference for the ABRs elicited using rarefaction, and condensation onset polarities. Note that the wave V latencies for the two polarities are larger and clearer at 500 Hz. Data from Fowler (1992).

Table 4–3. Mean Absolute Latency Differences (C-R) for ABR Waves I, III, and V Elicited by Tone Bursts Using Rarefaction and Condensation Onset Polarities

Frequency (Hz)	ABR Components			
	Wave I	Wave III	Wave V	Half Period
500	0.52	0.55	0.67	1.0 ms
1000	0.53	0.41	0.45	0.5 ms
2000	0.02	0.01	0.08	0.25 ms

Source: Created with permission using data from "Effects of Stimulus Phase on the Normal Auditory Brainstem Response," by C. Fowler, 1992, *Journal of Speech and Hearing Research*, 35, Table 2, p. 171.

upward toward the scala vestibuli and subsequently the shearing of the hair cell in the preferred direction for depolarization. Therefore, an acoustic click with condensation polarity can excite the hair cells only during the rarefaction phase, which occurs about half a period later for the condensation stimulus. Thus, the response latency will be half a period earlier for the rarefaction onset polarity stimulus, theoretically.

Several factors could account for the considerable variability of polarity effects reported in the literature using click stimuli. Since the ABR in response to broadband clicks represents summed activity across different cochlear regions, the extent and temporal differences in the cochlear regional contributions for the two polarities could significantly influence the response morphology and latency within and across individuals (Don, Vermiglio, Ponton, Eggermont, & Masuda, 1996). This means that the evaluation of polarity effects on the click-evoked responses has limited utility in clinical diagnosis. Because the click responses are dominated by high-frequency contributions (Don & Eggermont, 1978), polarity effects would be smaller than the standard deviation of the response latency and therefore not detectable.

Finally, the common practice of using alternating polarity in clinical testing (primarily to reduce or eliminate stimulus artifacts at high stimulus levels) is not advisable, particularly in individuals with high-frequency hearing loss where the click-evoked ABR may be largely determined by lower-frequency contributions. Consequently, the appreciable difference in the latency of the ABR for the two polarities will add to produce a smeared small-amplitude response with broad or bifid peaks. In such cases, it would be better to record the response to each polarity separately to obtain cleaner data. Stimulation with both rarefaction and condensation clicks separately has been suggested as a means to obtain more meaningful clinical data (Fowler, 1992; Gorga, Kaminski, Beauchaine, Jesteadt, & Neely, 1991).

Rise-Fall Time

Since the ABR represents neural activity synchronized to the onset of the stimulus, it is important to understand how the latency and amplitude of the ABR components are altered by changes in the stimulus rise time to make an informed choice about the optimal rise time to use for both clinical and research applications. We learned in Chapter 3 that the choice of a particular rise time is a trade-off between ensuring frequency specificity (therefore place-specific responses) of the stimulus using a longer rise time, and a rise time fast enough to elicit a robust onset response (Stapells & Picton, 1981). Several studies using either tone bursts (Beattie, Moretti, & Warren, 1984; Cobb, Skinner, & Burns, 1978; Kodera, Yamane, Yamada, & Suzuki, 1977; Stapells & Picton, 1981; Suzuki & Horiuchi, 1981; Suzuki, Yasuhito, & Horiuchi, 1981) or noise bursts (Barth & Burkard, 1993; Hecox & Deegan, 1983; Hecox, Squires, & Galambos, 1976) have consistently shown that response amplitude and absolute latency of all components decrease as rise-fall time is increased, with wave V barely discernible at a rise time of 10 ms (Figure 4–13). Beattie et al. (1984) reported that the detectability of the response components was high and unaltered for rise times as long as 4 ms. Also, Barth and Burkard (1993) noted that the slope of the latency/rise time function increased with a decrease in noise burst level.

Physiological Bases of the Rise Time Induced Latency and Amplitude Changes

The latency prolongation and amplitude reduction observed with increases in the rise time of the stim-

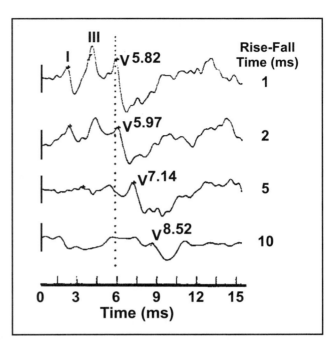

Figure 4–13. Auditory brainstem response (ABR) waveforms plotted as a function of increasing rise times. All ABR components are identified for the 1-ms rise time condition. For each condition the absolute latency of the wave is shown. As rise-fall time is increased all ABR components show a systematic increase in latency and decrease in amplitude with waves I and III becoming difficult to identify for rise-fall times of 5 and 10 ms.

ulus can be explained by a spectral splatter effect at fast rise times and a specific rise time effect associated with the stimulus cycle involved in the generation of the response at longer rise times. Tone burst spectra change with stimulus rise-fall times up to about 3 to 4 ms with shorter rise-fall times producing broader spectra (with significant energy in the sidebands well beyond the nominal frequency) because of spectral splatter associated with gating a brief stimulus on and off abruptly (Durrant & Boston, 2007; Picton, 2011). A longer rise-fall time will appreciably reduce this spectral spread and limit the prominent energy to the nominal frequency creating a frequency-specific stimulus (Figure 4–14, left panel). Thus, the shorter latency at the fast rise-fall time is due to greater contribution to the ABR from more basal regions, which moves the mode of the latency distribution more basally. This basal bias is reduced (modal value of the latency distribution begins to shift more apically) as rise

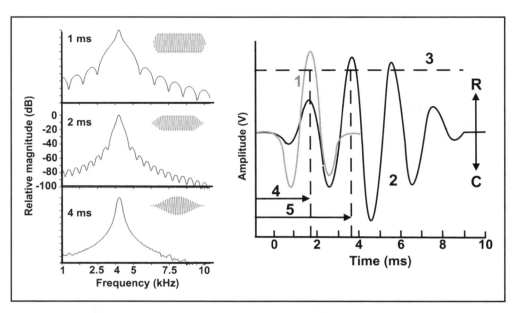

Figure 4–14. *Left:* The narrowing of the spectrum of a 2000 Hz tone burst as rise-fall time is increased. Note the sharp reduction in spectral splatter and side band energy. *Right:* The effective cycle reaching criterion amplitude to elicit a response (indicated by the dashed line 3) earlier (arrow 4) for a tone-pip with 1-ms rise time (1) and later (arrow 5) for a 500 Hz tone pip with a 4 ms rise time (2). Bidirectional arrow on the right indicates the onset polarity rarefaction (R) condensation (C).

time is decreased, and the latency begins to get longer. However, since there is no further appreciable change in stimulus spectrum with further increases in rise time, the continued latency prolongation and amplitude reduction at longer rise times therefore requires another explanation. For the spectral independent effects of rise time on the ABR, we need to invoke the effective cycle in the stimulus waveform that has sufficient amplitude to generate the neural activity underlying the ABR. The right panel in Figure 4–14 is a schematic illustration showing that for the faster rise time, the effective cycle reaches criterion amplitude (shown by dashed line 3) to generate the ABR *earlier in time* (arrow 4), thus producing an ABR with shorter latency. For the longer rise time, the response latency is longer because the stimulus amplitude growth takes a relatively *longer time* to reach criterion amplitude to generate the ABR. It should be noted here that this explanation will hold for shorter rise times as well but is confounded by the changes in the spectral width at the shorter rise times. In terms of cochlear place contributions to the rise time effects, Hecox and Deegan (1983) showed that rise-time effects did not depend on derived-band frequency, suggesting that place mechanisms cannot account for the ABR rise-fall time effects. Finally, for clinical applications, Stapells and Picton (1981) recommend the use of tone bursts with rise-fall times of 5 ms or less since longer rise-fall times showed a substantial reduction in response amplitude. The reduction in response amplitude could reflect both a reduction in the number of neural elements (faster rise-fall times may recruit more neurons because of spectral spread) and neural synchrony.

Effects of Recording Factors

Electrode Configuration/Montage

Since volume-conducted potentials are propagated in all directions toward the scalp from deep generators located within the brainstem, they can be recorded by electrodes placed on multiple locations of the head. However, the voltages and morphology of the recorded ABRs vary depending on the orientation of the dipole generator(s) and the configuration of the recording electrodes (Starr & Squires, 1982; Terkildsen & Osterhammel, 1981). Therefore, it is important to place the electrodes using the proper electrode configuration to optimally record the multiple components of the ABR. To standardize recordings and facilitate transportability of results, and to facilitate scientific replication of studies, the 10-10 electrode placement system (a higher-density extension of the International 10-20 system, adopted by the American Electroencephalographic Society in 1991, and as the International Federation 10-10 system guideline in 1998) is used. In the 10-20 system (Figure 4–15), each electrode has a letter label (sagittal [front-to-back] scalp locations identified as **F**rontal, **C**entral, **T**emporal, **P**arietal, and **O**ccipital) and a number (location from side-to-side). The numbers, even over the right hemisphere and odd over the left hemisphere, increase from the midline electrodes to the lateral electrodes. The main front-back axis measure is the midline nasion (NZ—dip between the top of the nose and the forehead) to inion (IZ—a small dent in the back of the skull above the neck). All midline electrodes along this axis are identified by a subscript Z (zero). As implied by the name, the electrodes closest to nasion and inion, and the mastoids are placed at 10% of the total distance of the electrode layout axis. For example, the first electrode from nasion, and inion is placed at 10% of the total length of this axis with subsequent electrodes along this axis at 20% intervals. The currently accepted 10-10 system places all electrodes at equal intervals. Cz, one of the common electrode sites serving as a noninverting input for ABR recordings, is halfway along the nasion to inion axis. Electrode locations for the right and left mastoid (used as inverting inputs for ABR recordings) are labeled as A2 (M2) and A1 (M1), respectively. It is generally good practice to identify both electrode locations using the correct labels and the electrode placement system (10-20, 10-10, or caps) being used.

Recall from Chapter 4, that ABRs are recorded using differential recording consisting of a noninverting input, inverting input, and common ground. An electrode configuration commonly employed in clinical assessment to capture all ABR components optimally can be characterized as a *vertical-ipsilateral* recording configuration with a noninverting electrode placed on the vertex (Cz) or high forehead at the hairline (HFH), the inverting electrode on the ipsilateral mastoid (A2 or A1, ipsilateral to the stimulus ear), and the common ground electrode on the mid-forehead (FPz) or the contralateral mastoid (A1 or A2). ABRs recorded simultaneously from three different electrode configurations (commonly used in clinical applications to improve the accuracy of ABR wave identification) are shown in Figure 4–16. The top ABR trace using the *vertical-ipsilateral* configuration (HFH-A1) shows the classic ABR morphology with a clear definition of all ABR components.

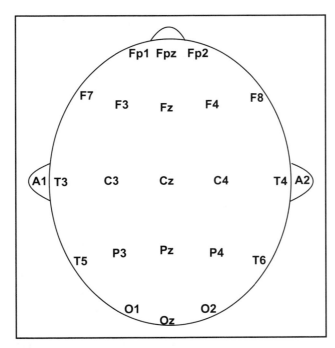

Figure 4–15. The 10-20 system of electrode placement. The electrode location identifier indicates the scalp region (e.g., F = Frontal, C = Central, T = Temporal, P = Parietal, and O = Occipital), the subscript z indicates midline electrodes, even numbers indicate electrodes on the right side of the head, and odd numbers are used for electrode locations on the left side of the head. A1/M1 and A2/M2 indicate left and right mastoids, respectively.

Comparison of Vertical-Ipsilateral and Vertical-Contralateral Recordings

The ABR in the middle trace of Figure 4–16, recorded using a *vertical-contralateral* (HFH-A2) electrode configuration, is characterized by an absent wave I positive peak (expected since the reference

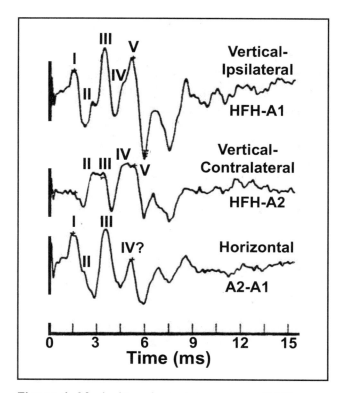

Figure 4–16. Auditory brainstem response (ABR) waveforms plotted for three (vertical-ipsilateral [HFH-A1]; vertical-contralateral [HFH-A2]; and horizontal [A2-A1]) different electrode configurations using clicks presented to the left ear at 80 dB nHL. All ABR components are robust for the vertical-ipsilateral configuration; as expected wave I is absent, waves II and III are almost fused; and waves IV and V shows a bifid peak for the vertical-contralateral configuration. Waves I and III are robust with an earlier smaller peak closer to the latency of wave IV in the horizontal configuration. Thus, the electrode configuration alters the morphology of the ABR.

electrode is far away from the left auditory nerve), the presence of a negative trough of wave I, bifid waves II and III, and better separation of the wave IV/V complex. Comparing the *vertical-ipsilateral and vertical-contralateral* recordings improves the clinician's accuracy in identifying the response components in the *vertical-ipsilateral recordings*. For example, wave I can be confirmed if it peaks before the negative trough of wave I in the contralateral recordings, and since there is better separation of the IV–V complex in the contralateral recordings, wave V latency can be more accurately measured (Hughes, Fino, & Gagnon, 1981; Starr & Squires, 1982; Stockard, Stockard, & Sharbrough, 1978). This accuracy is needed in determining the site of lesion where absolute latencies are used to derive the IPLs, which in turn are used to determine if there is an abnormality. The utility of these comparisons is limited in newborns since the contralateral configuration does not show any discernible response components (Katbamma, Metz, Adelman, & Thodi, 1993).

Comparison of Horizontal and Vertical Recordings

The bottom trace in Figure 4–16 shows ABR traces recorded using a *horizontal* electrode configuration wherein the noninverting and inverting electrodes were placed on the contralateral (A2) and the ipsilateral mastoid (A1), respectively. Comparing the three traces in Figure 4–16, it can be seen that waves I and III are very prominent in the *horizontal* recording with a much smaller amplitude and earlier latency wave for V. Since the latency of this component is more proximal to wave IV, it is tempting to suggest that this is more likely an unmasked wave IV rather than wave V, which may not be detectable in this electrode configuration (Ruth, Hildebrand, & Cantrell, 1982; Starr & Squires, 1982). Also, Krishnan and Durrant (1991) reported a significantly shorter latency for wave II in the horizontal configuration compared to wave II in the vertical-ipsilateral configuration, suggesting the possibility that these two response components may reflect activity from distinct generators.

In summary, the HFH placement is preferred to Cz placement since the preparation and placement of the electrode are much easier, the stability of the electrode during recording is better, wave V amplitude is only slightly smaller compared to the Cz location, wave I is bigger in amplitude compared to Cz, and the responses are more robust in infants using noninverting electrode on the HFH (Starr & Squires, 1982). These authors also found that the amplitude of waves II–V is optimal at Cz or HFH but diminishes dramatically at the mastoid as we saw in the horizontal recording. Increasingly, there is a move toward using a recording configuration using HFH as the noninverting input and an electrode placed on the seventh cervical vertebra (C7) as the inverting electrode. This configuration is particularly useful for threshold estimates since wave V is larger and reliably identifiable down to

10 above the threshold for clicks (King & Sininger, 1992; Sininger & Don, 1989). Finally, since volume conduction occurs in a purely resistive medium, changes in recording electrode configuration should only produce changes in amplitude of specific components and overall morphology due to differences in the orientation of the ABR generators (and consequently, how the different electrode configurations line up with the flow of the electrical field). Therefore, if consistent and significant latency differences are observed (like we reported for waves IV and II), then these latency differences may suggest neural activity from different generators (Krishnan & Durrant, 1991). While a multichannel recording is useful in older children and adults, its utility is limited in infants because only the vertex-ipsilateral configuration produces a clear ABR with a normal response morphology.

Analog Filter Settings

As we reviewed in Chapter 3, analog filtering is performed on the input signal before analog-to-digital conversion to remove frequency components that are not part of the signal of interest (the auditory evoked potential). Typical analog filters used in this stage of processing have a relatively gradual rejection rate (3–6 dB/octave) with several high-pass and low-pass filter cutoff settings available. For suprathreshold measures, a band-pass setting of 100 to 3000 Hz is commonly used. For measures near threshold, a more open band-pass setting of 30 or 50 Hz to 3000 Hz is used to optimally capture the broad, lower-frequency wave V near threshold. However, certain challenging test environments, like an electrically noisy patient room or intraoperative monitoring, force one to use restricted filter settings that allow recording but have the undesired consequence of altered response morphology, including appreciable latency changes. Increasingly, clinicians are beginning to realize the merits of using open analog filter settings to minimize waveform distortions associated with too much filtering. Since analog filter settings can distort the recorded ABR, it is important to know the types of changes in latency and amplitude associated with specific low-pass and high-pass filter settings to be able to interpret the data accurately. Fortunately, most clinical systems can perform zero phase shift digital filtering on the recorded responses that overcome the distortion problems associated with analog filtering. So, the strategy should be more open filter settings (e.g., 30–5000 Hz) for data acquisition followed by digital filtering using the desired bandwidth to capture all components optimally. However, opening the filter bandwidth allows higher-amplitude (usually low-frequency "noise") to come through that may trigger preset artifact rejection and increase data acquisition time because more sweeps are rejected. The solution is to adjust the artifact reject threshold so that no more than 10% of the total sweeps are rejected (e.g., 100 sweeps out of a total of 1,000 sweeps).

The effects of analog filter settings on the ABR components have been systematically investigated (Boston & Ainslie, 1980; Doyle & Hyde, 1981a; Elberling, 1979; Kevanishvili & Aphochenko, 1979; Laukli & Mair, 1981; Osterhammel, 1981). Let us first consider the effects of changes in the low-frequency cutoff of the band-pass filter (i.e., the high-pass filter cutoff frequency) followed by a description of the effects of changes in the high-frequency cutoff.

Effects of Changing the Low-Frequency Cutoff of the Band-Pass Filter

The effects of changing the low-frequency cutoff of the band-pass filter from 5 to 200 Hz (with the high-frequency cutoff of the band-pass filter held constant at 3000 Hz) on the ABR waveform morphology are shown in Figure 4–17. At the lowest setting, the ABR components appear to be riding on a slow wave with all components robust and easily identifiable. As the cutoff is increased, the ABR waveform morphology becomes flatter (due to the filtering of the slow wave component), but the components are still clearly present, absolute latencies of all components decrease, and amplitudes (particularly for wave V) decrease appreciably for the 200-Hz condition. The changes described here are consistent with results in the literature (Chiappa et al., 1979; Laukli & Mair, 1981; Stockard et al., 1978). Since the latency and amplitude of the slower, broader waveforms elicited by low-frequency tone bursts are more susceptible to changes in the lower cutoff of band-pass filters, care should be taken to use a more open filter setting (e.g., a low-pass cutoff for the band-pass filter of 30 Hz is desirable).

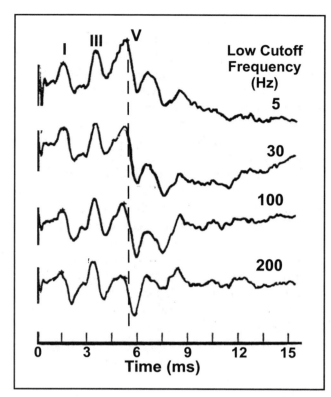

Figure 4–17. Auditory brainstem response (ABR) waveforms plotted as a function of increasing low frequency cutoff of band-pass filter. The vertical dotted line aligned with wave V peak for the 5 Hz cutoff condition shows the decrease in latency of wave V as cutoff frequency is increased. The filtering effects on latency appear to be more pronounced for wave V with little change for the earlier components. Also, note that the waveform loses the slow wave and becomes flatter as the cutoff frequency is increased.

Effects of Changing the High-Frequency Cutoff of the Band-Pass Filter

The effects of changing the high-frequency cutoff of the band-pass filter from 1000 to 8000 Hz (with the low-frequency cutoff of the band-pass filter held constant at 100 Hz) on the ABR waveform morphology are shown in Figure 4–18. At the 1000 and 2000-Hz high-frequency cutoff of the band-pass filter, the ABR waveform appears smooth, with the former showing appreciably smaller amplitudes and longer latencies for all components. The latency continues to shorten as the cutoff frequency increases. Wave V is largest for the commonly used 100 to 3000 Hz band-pass condition. For the 8000-

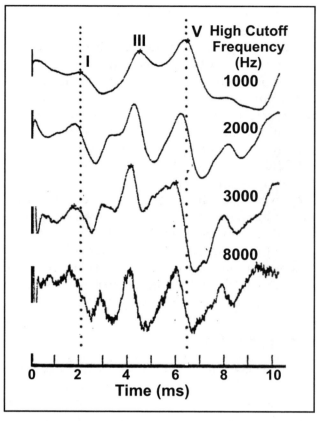

Figure 4–18. Auditory brainstem response (ABR) waveforms plotted as a function of increasing high-frequency cutoff of band-pass filter. The vertical dotted lines aligned with waves I and V peak latency for the 1000 Hz low-pass filter condition show the decrease in latency for wave V only as cutoff frequency is increased. The filtering effects on latency appear to be more pronounced for wave V with little change for the earlier components. Also, note the addition of high-frequency noise for the 8000 Hz low-pass filter condition.

Hz high-frequency cutoff, the ABR waveform appears noisier. Most of the changes are prominent when the cutoff frequency is 2000 Hz or less.

Digital Filtering to the Rescue

All the changes in latency and amplitude associated with analog filtering described earlier are due to phase shifts (manifesting as latency and amplitude changes of frequency components) [Doyle & Hyde, 1981a]). These artifactual changes in latency have the potential for clinical misinterpretation and misdiagnosis. There is widespread approval for the use of post–data acquisition digital filtering (as indicated earlier, it is better to use as open an analog filter setting as possible during ABR acquisition) to improve detection and analysis of waveforms, since they do not produce phase shifts that appear as latency and amplitude changes. Most current clinical systems have implemented a user-friendly application of digital filtering. Figure 4–19 shows a comparison of the effects of analog and digital filtering on the latency (left panels) and amplitude (right panels) of the ABR (data from Boston & Ainslie, 1980). For both the high-pass filter cutoff (top pair) and low-pass filter cutoff (bottom pair), the latency remains unchanged with digital filtering, while the latency decreases with increasing cutoff frequency for analog filtering. Similarly, for both high cutoff (top right) and low cutoff (bottom right), the amplitude remains essentially unchanged as the frequency is increased using digital filtering, but amplitude decreases with increasing low-frequency cutoff (particularly above 200 Hz) and

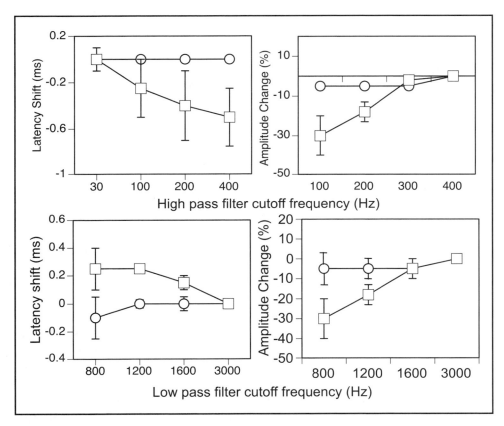

Figure 4–19. Effects of analog and digital filtering on the latency (*left panels*) and amplitude (*right panels*) of the auditory brainstem response. For both the high-pass cutoff (*top pair*) and the low-pass cutoff conditions (*bottom pair*), the latency decreases for analog filtering (*open squares*) with little or no appreciable latency change observed with digital filtering (*open circles*). Similarly, response amplitude with analog filtering decrease at high cutoff frequencies for the high-pass filter (*top right*), and for the low low-pass cutoff frequencies of the low-pass filter (*bottom right*). In contrast, digital filtering does not alter the response amplitude appreciably (*top and bottom right panels*). Figures created using data from "Effects of Analog and Digital Filtering on Brainstem Auditory Evoked Potentials," by J. R. Boston and P. J. Ainslie, 1980, *Electroencephalography Clinical Neurophysiology, 48*, pp. 361–364. Copyright 1980 by Elsevier Scientific Publishers.

decreases for high-frequency cutoff below 1200 Hz using analog filtering.

In summary, the recommended filter settings for suprathreshold ABR measures using clicks is 100 to 3000 Hz. However, for threshold estimation, newborn screening, and responses elicited by low-frequency tone bursts, a setting of 30–50 Hz to 3000 Hz is preferable (Elberling, 1979; Kavanagh, Harker, & Tyler, 1985; Schwartz & Berry, 1985) to optimally detect wave V near threshold. Digital filtering can be subsequently utilized to improve ABR detection. It should be noted that too much filtering, analog or digital, will lose information and therefore should be avoided.

Effects of Background Noise in the Test Environment

Just as behavioral thresholds are elevated when measurements are made outside a sound-treated booth due to the masking effects of background noise, ABRs obtained outside a test booth (e.g., in a busy practice, neonatal intensive care units, or during surgery) also show prolongation in latency and reduction in amplitude. Burkard and Hecox (1983) showed latency prolongation and amplitude reduction of click-evoked ABRs (for a range of intensity levels) in the presence of broadband noise greater than 30 dB SPL. The prolongation of the I–III and I–V IPL with increasing noise level argues against a within-place mechanism contributing to the noise-induced latency shifts. On the contrary, the increase in IPL with noise level appears to be more consistent with synaptic adaptation invoked to explain rate effects (Burkard & Hecox, 1987). The clinical implication of these ABR changes in the presence of background noise is that care should be taken to minimize noise levels in the test environment failing which proper adjustments should be made to mitigate these noise effects while establishing normative data for the test environment.

Effects of Subject Factors

Factors like *age, sex, and body temperature* of an individual can dramatically affect at least one or several ABR indices including response morphology, absolute latencies, IPLs, and response amplitude. Therefore, the clinician needs to consider the effects of these factors and rule them out while interpreting unexpected "abnormal" ABR results.

Age: It is convenient to describe the effects of age on the ABR under two separate categories given that these represent two distinct and well-separated points along the age spectrum. The first, development, describes the maturation of ABR indices from birth to about 2 years of age when the ABR morphology and other response indices attain adult values. The second describes the consequences of age-related structural and functional changes past about 55 years of age. This assumes that ABRs are quite stable between the age of 2 and 55 years.

Neural Maturation of the ABR From Birth to Three Years of Age

The general principle of neural maturation in the central nervous system is that the time course of development proceeds from peripheral to cortical structures. This caudal to rostral temporal course of maturation means that the auditory nerve matures before the caudal brainstem, the caudal brainstem before the rostral brainstem, the rostral brainstem before the thalamus, and the thalamus before the primary auditory cortex. The ABR provides a robust metric to evaluate the time course of this neural maturation at least up to the midbrain and implications for the development of auditory function and its clinical assessment. Therefore, it is not surprising that the literature is replete with studies trying to characterize the time course of ABR maturation. (Just a few examples are listed here: Salamy, 1984; Eggermont, Brown, Ponton, & Kimberley, 1996; Eggermont & Salamy, 1988; Fria & Doyle, 1984; Gorga, Kaminski, & Beauchaine, 1988; Gorga et al., 1989; Gorga, Reiland, Beauchaine, Worthington, & Jesteadt, 1987; Jiang, Brosi, & Wilkinson, 1998; Lauter, Oyler, & Lord-Maes, 1993; Zimmerman, Morgan, & Dubno, 1987). Remarkably, the ABR can be recorded as early as 27 to 28 weeks of *conceptional age* (Galambos & Hecox, 1978; Stockard & Westmoreland, 1981). Conceptional age is the estimated gestational age relative to actual time of conception (which is at least 14 days after the first day of the last menstrual period). The newborn ABR morphology is characterized by three prominent, almost equal amplitude peaks (waves I, III, and V) as early as 32 weeks' conceptional age (Figure 4–20A) and begins to show the emergence of the other components by about 3 months of age. The absolute latencies, particularly of waves III and V, continue to decrease with little change in the absolute latency of wave V after 40 weeks conceptional age (Figure 4–20A–F). Consequently, the IPLs (I–III and I–V) progressively decrease (indicated by the bidirectional arrows below waveforms A and F in Figure 4–20). Absolute latencies of waves I and V are about 1.8 ms, and 6.8 to 7 ms at term with a mean I–V IPL of about 5.5 ms. Figure 4–21, left panels show the latency change for wave V (top left) and wave I (bottom left). Wave I latency reaches adult values as early as 3 months of age (Gorga et al., 1989), while wave V latency and the IPLs (I–III and I–V) continue to decrease and reach adult values by age 18–24 months (Figure 4–21, top left, and right panels). However, more recently, Skoe, Krizman, Anderson, and Kraus (2015) and Spitzer, White-Schwoch, Carr, Skoe, and Kraus (2015) have reported that the ABR latencies continue to decrease through early childhood before they stabilize and then begin to increase with aging.

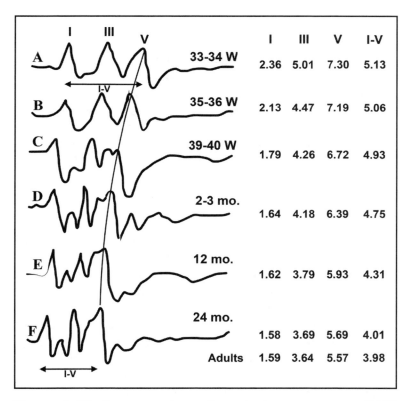

Figure 4–20. Representative auditory brainstem response (ABR) waveforms from birth to 2 years (age identified to the right of each trace) illustrating the neural maturation of the ABR components. Both the absolute latency of all components and the interpeak latencies decrease (see values to the right of each trace) with increasing age. The horizontal bidirectional arrows below the top and the bottom traces indicate the reduction in the I–V interval with age. The solid sloping line aligned to wave V illustrates the exponential change in wave V latency with increasing age. Note that by age 24 months (2 years), the absolute and IPLs have attained adult values (values on the right).

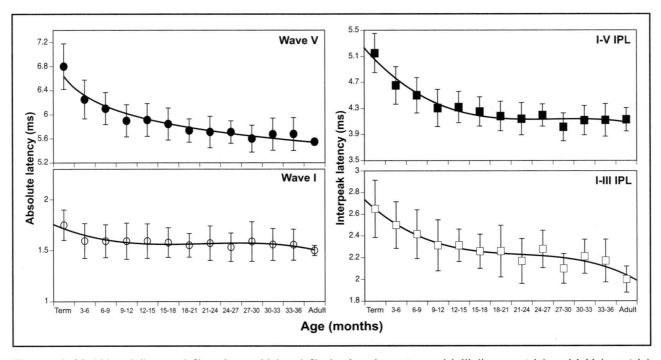

Figure 4–21. Wave I (*bottom left*) and wave V (*top left*) absolute latencies, and I–III (*bottom right*) and I–V (*top right*) IPL changes plotted as a function of age (months) from term (T) to adult (A) with age (from term [T] to adult [A]). Wave V latency changes with age can be best characterized by an exponential decrease including a rapid initial change and a more gradual later change after about 10 to 12 months. Note the relatively smaller change in latency for wave I and the much earlier attainment of the adult latency value (*bottom left*). Figures created using mean data from Gorga et al. (1989).

The temporal course of this neural maturation of the ABR components, particularly wave V, is best characterized by a decaying exponential function with two distinct time constants. A rapid change in latency from birth to about 12 months, followed by a more gradual change in latency from about 12 to 24 months of age (see inset in Figure 4–21, top left). This developmental time course is the same for both I–III and III–V IPLs (Figure 4-21, top right and bottom panels) suggesting that I–V IPL also follows the same developmental time course. Further, the level independence of these changes suggests that central neural (rather than cochlear mechanism) changes are driving the neural maturation of the ABR components. Neural maturation of several physiological determinants of latency and amplitude of ABR are invoked in trying to explain these developmental changes. These include incomplete myelinization and smaller fiber diameter that reduce neural conduction velocity causing the observed IPL delays and poor synaptic efficiency, which can also account for latency delay and disruption in neural synchrony (Eggermont & Salamy, 1988; Fria & Doyle, 1984; Hecox & Burkard, 1982). It is likely that the two distinct time constants may reflect the same underlying process that changes from rapid to slow change over the first two years. Alternatively, it is tempting to speculate that these processes reflect a more rapid peripheral process and a more gradual central process. Eggermont and Salamy (1988) reported that all time constants (absolute latency of all ABR components) were longer for prematurely born infants compared to full-term infants. However, the absence of differences in the I–V IPL between the two groups suggests a peripheral conductive loss given the higher incidence of otitis media in the prematurely born group.

The observation of robust responses that can be seen with fewer averages in a term baby may be because of a smaller head size that results in smaller amplitude reduction during volume conduction. In summary, with these dynamic changes in the ABR during the first two years, it is important to utilize age-appropriate latency norms in the assessment of the functional integrity of auditory nerve and brainstem structures in children. Also, since the maturing neural processes underlying ABR generation are more susceptible to stimulus rate–induced adaptation (Cox, 1985; Despland & Galambos, 1980; Jiang et al., 1998; Lasky, 1984; Pratt & Sohmer, 1976; Stockard et al., 1979), clinicians should ensure that appropriately slower stimulus rates are used to minimize the effects of more pronounced adaptation of the ABRs in children below 2 years of age.

Normal Aging-Related ABR Changes in Older Adults

Purely aging-related changes in ABR are difficult to disentangle because of their interaction with gender effects and the accompanying cochlear hearing loss due to aging (Jerger & Johnson, 1988; Rupa & Dayal, 1993). Thus, it is not surprising that the results presented in the literature on the effects of aging on the ABR have been equivocal, with some studies showing a small but significant increase in both the absolute latencies (about a 0.1–0.2 ms latency increase/decade above age 50 years) and IPLs, and a decrease in amplitude of all ABR components (Allison, Hume, Wood, & Goff, 1984; Allison, Wood, & Goff, 1983; Chu, 1985; Don and Eggermont, 1978; Eggermont & Don, 1980; Harkins, 1981; Houston & McClelland, 1985; Jerger & Hall, 1980; Oku & Hasegewa, 1997; Rowe, 1978; Trune et al., 1988), while others show no significant latency changes with aging (Beagley & Sheldrake, 1978; Rosenhall, Bjorkman, Pedersen, & Kall, 1985; Rosenhamer, Lindstrom, & Lundborg, 1980). The amplitude of wave I has been reported to decrease with age and hearing loss (Don & Eggermont, 1978; Eggermont & Don, 1980; Harkins, 1981; Kjaer, 1980; Stockard et al., 1978). It is generally thought that the IPLs I–III and I–V remain stable and do not change appreciably. Even in the studies that show these "age-related" changes, it is difficult to rule out the role of sex, and particularly hearing loss that invariably accompanies aging. To our knowledge, there are no reported findings to date that convincingly isolate specific aging-related changes in the ABR. The lack of compelling evidence for age-related changes in the ABR is rather surprising given the pervasive nature of age-related changes in the central nervous system that include loss of neurons, demyelination, and decrease in synaptic efficiency. Taking these small and equivocal age-related findings together, the need does not arise for separate age-appropriate norms for the older adult population.

Sex

Unlike the equivocal age effects, there is a small but significant effect of sex on the latency and amplitude of adult ABRs (Elberling & Pabro, 1987; Jerger & Hall, 1980; Lopez-Escamez, Salguero, & Salinero, 1999; Rosenhall et al., 1985; Rupa & Dayal, 1993; Watson, 1996). Females consistently show shorter absolute latencies (waves III and V shorter by about 0.15–0.3 ms with no difference for wave I, thus shortening the I–III and I–V IPLs) and larger response amplitudes than males for waves III through V. Although these sex differences are not much bigger than the normal latency variability, it is important to establish norms using an equal number of male and female participants to reduce the risk of misinterpretation of the ABR data if the norms largely reflected the latency values of only one group. For example, if normal limits are set using only the shorter latencies from females, then there is a risk of interpreting ABR data from older male individuals as being abnormal. The sex differences in infants and young children are quite small and not consistently observed across studies, with some studies showing differences similar to those seen in adults and others showing no difference.

Several less than convincing explanations are provided for the sex differences, including hearing sensitivity and body temperature, smaller head size and brainstem distances between nuclei, and hormonal differences. Females tend to have better hearing sensitivity in the higher frequencies and on average a higher body temperature (Watson, 1996) that could account for both their shorter absolute and interpeak latencies. However, no significant sex difference in body temperature was found in a well-controlled study (McGann, Marion, Camp, & Spangler, 1993). The next explanation suggests that the smaller head size in women means that the brainstem will also be smaller and the distances between nuclei will be shorter and thus will produce shorter absolute and interpeak latencies and larger response amplitudes because the electrodes are closer to the ABR generators (Allison et al., 1983; Haug, 1977; Stockard et al., 1978). However, the fact that sex differences in the ABR persist even when ABRs from head-size-matched males and females are compared suggests that head size alone cannot account for the sex differences in the ABR (Durrant, Sabo, & Hyre, 1990). Finally, there is no clear direct evidence to suggest that specific hormonal differences between males and females can account for the shorter absolute and IPLs in the females compared to the males. A more intriguing possibility is that the shorter length of the cochlea in women (Sato, Sando, & Takahashi, 1991) may be associated with a greater traveling-wave velocity. Don, Ponton, Eggermont, and Masuda (1993) provided evidence in support of this notion by showing a shorter latency shift across derived narrowband responses (from about 11 to 0.7 kHz) for women (about 1 ms shorter than that for males with a total latency shift of 2.4 ms for women versus 3.4 ms for men across the range of narrowbands examined). These findings can account for both the larger amplitude (greater traveling wave velocity in women could increase synchrony and thereby increase amplitude) and the shorter IPLs that may represent a greater basal bias of wave V (meaning shorter wave V latency). Importantly, these findings also suggest that the location of the cochlear initiation site of primary activity generating the ABR could also contribute to the IPL.

Body Temperature

Small changes in body temperature (as little as 1°C–3°C), associated with either the normal circadian variations or other conditions producing hypothermia or hyperthermia, can significantly impact neural activity by influencing events leading to action potential generation, neurotransmitter release, synaptic transmission, and neural conduction velocity. There is evidence from human and animal studies showing latency prolongation and amplitude reduction for the later components of the ABR (thus resulting in increased I–III and I–V IPLs) with a decrease in body temperature (Doyle & Fria, 1985; Hall, Bull, & Cronau, 1998; Jones, Stockard, & Weidner, 1980; Marsh, Yamane, & Potsic, 1984; Marshall & Donchin, 1981; Stockard et al., 1978). Stockard et al. (1978) observed abnormal IPL prolongations compared to an age-matched control group when body temperature dropped to 32°C. The IPLs returned to normal upon rewarming to normal body temperature of 37°C. Marsh et al. (1984) showed a linear decrease in guinea pig ABR I–V latency and a more variable amplitude reduction as body temperature was increased from 25°C to 40°C. These authors inferred that the decrease in latency for the later waves reflected a temperature-related increase in the rate of chemical processes underlying the events involved in the neural activity generating the ABR. To the extent that the I–V IPL reflects neural conduction time, these results suggest an increase in neural conduction speed with increasing temperature presumably mediated by temperature-sensitive synaptic plasticity and larger axonal depolarizations to increase conduction velocity.

While body temperature fluctuation is not a real concern in the routine clinical use of the ABR, it is an important factor to consider while testing and interpreting ABR results from individuals undergoing treatment that could appreciably change body temperature (e.g., hypothermia during serial monitoring of comatose patients or individuals with alcohol intoxication, and increased body temperature in individuals undergoing hyperthermic therapy).

II. SUMMARY

- The normal morphology of the ABR waveform elicited by brief auditory stimuli consists of a series of six to seven biphasic waves in the first 10 to 15 ms after stimulus onset, identified by roman numerals I–VII. Peaks I through V are consistently observed with the peaks occurring about 1 ms apart and wave V exhibiting the largest amplitude.

- The ABR is characterized by several measures including absolute and interpeak latencies and peak-to-peak amplitude. Latency measures provide information about the cochlear place of activity contributing to the response, synaptic processing time, neural conduction time, and the time taken to activate a particular structure or neural tract along the auditory pathway in the brainstem. Response amplitude provides information about the number of neural elements contributing to the response and the degree of neural synchrony in the activated population of neurons. Thus, both measures can be used to assess the structural and functional integrity of cochlear and brainstem structures.

- The different experimental approaches used to localize the anatomical generators of the ABR components have not precisely identified the anatomical generator site(s) for the components of the ABR. It is known that the auditory nerve and several different nuclei and tracts along the brainstem contribute to ABR components. Based on latency correlations between surface-recorded ABR components and intracranially recorded responses from specific auditory structures along the brainstem, it is inferred that wave I is from the distal portion of the auditory nerve exclusively; wave II is from the proximal portion of the auditory nerve as it enters the cochlear nucleus; wave III is from the ipsilateral cochlear nucleus; wave IV is from the superior olivary complex contralaterally; and wave V is from the rostral lateral lemniscus proximal to the IC and its inputs to the IC. However, caution should be exercised about the specificity of these generator sites, as multiple generators likely contribute to a single component beyond wave I.

- Stimulus, recording, and subject factors substantially affect the latency and amplitude of the ABR components. Thus, it is important to understand the nature and size of these effects and adopt appropriate adjustments to the normative data to be able to correctly interpret ABR results with minimal errors. Given that ABRs are recorded in various test environments, it cannot be emphasized enough that all these factors affecting the ABR indices should be seriously considered and incorporated into the normative database used in interpreting the ABR results to minimize incorrect diagnoses.

REFERENCES

Achor, L. J., & Starr, A. (1980a). Auditory brain stem responses in the cat. I. Intracranial and extracranial recordings. *Electroencephalography and Clinical Neurophysiology, 48*, 154–173.

Achor, L. J., & Starr, A. (1980b). Auditory brain stem responses in the cat. II. Effects of lesions. *Electroencephalography and Clinical Neurophysiology, 48*, 174–190.

Allison, T., Hume, A. L., Wood, C. C., & Goff, W. R. (1984). Developmental and aging changes in somatosensory, auditory and visual evoked potentials. *Electroencephalography and Clinical Neurophysiology, 58*, 14–24.

Allison, T., Wood, C. C., & Goff, W. R. (1983). Brain stem auditory, pattern-reversal visual, and short-latency somatosensory evoked potentials: Latencies in relation to age, sex, and brain and body size. *Electroencephalography and Clinical Neurophysiology, 55*, 619–636.

Barth, C. D., & Burkard, R. F. (1993). Effects of noise burst rise time and level on the human brainstem auditory evoked response. *Audiology, 32*(4), 225–233.

Beagley, H. A., & Sheldrake, J. B. (1978). Differences in brainstem response latency with age and sex. *British Journal of Audiology, 12*, 69–77.

Beattie, R. C. (1988). Interaction of click polarity, stimulus level, and repetition rate on the auditory brainstem response. *Scandinavian Audiology, 17*, 99–109.

Beattie, R. C., Moretti, M., & Warren, V. (1984). Effects of rise-fall time, frequency, and intensity on the early/middle evoked response. *Journal of Speech and Hearing Disorders, 49*(2), 114–127.

Boston, J. R., & Ainslie, P. J. (1980). Effects of analog and digital filtering on brainstem auditory evoked potentials. *Electroencephalography and Clinical Neurophysiology, 48,* 361–364.

Brown, R. H., Chiappa, K. H., & Brooks, E. B. (1981). Brainstem auditory evoked responses in 22 patients with intrinsic brainstem lesions: Implications for clinical interpretations. *Electroencephalography and Clinical Neurophysiology, 51,* 38P.

Brugge, J. F., Anderson, D. J., Hind, J. E., & Rose, J. E. (1969). Time structure of discharges in single auditory nerve fibers of the squirrel monkey in response to complex periodic sounds. *Journal of Neurophysiology, 32,* 386–340.

Buchwald, J. S., & Huang, C. -M. (1975). Far-field acoustic responses: Origins in the cat. *Science, 189,* 382–384.

Burkard, R. F., & Don, M. (2007). The auditory brainstem response. In R. F. Burkhard, M. Don, & J. J. Eggermont (Eds.), *Auditory evoked potentials, basic principles and clinical applications* (pp. 248–249). Baltimore, MD: Lippincott Williams & Wilkins.

Burkard, R., & Hecox, K. (1983). The effect of broadband noise on the human brainstem auditory evoked responses. I. Rate and intensity effects. *Journal of the Acoustical Society of America, 74,* 1204–1213.

Burkard, R., & Hecox, K. (1987). The effect of broadband noise on the human brainstem auditory evoked responses. III. Anatomic locus. *Journal of the Acoustical Society of America, 81,* 1050–1063.

Chiappa, K. H., Gladstone, K. J., & Young, R. R. (1979). Brain stem auditory evoked responses studies of waveform variations in 50 normal human subjects. *Archives of Neurology, 36*(2), 81–87.

Chiappa, K. H., Harrison, J. L., Brooks, E. B., & Young, R. R. (1980). Brainstem auditory evoked responses in 200 patients with multiple sclerosis. *Annals of Neurology, 7,* 135–143.

Chu, N. S. (1985). Age-related latency changes in the brain-stem auditory evoked potentials. *Electroencephalography and Clinical Neurophysiology, 62,* 431–436.

Chu, N. S. (1989). Brainstem auditory evoked potentials' correlation between CT midbrain-pontine lesion sites and abolition of wave V or the IV-V complex. *Journal of the Neurological Sciences, 91,* 165–177.

Cobb, J., Skinner, P., & Burns, J. (1978). Effects of signal rise time and frequency on the brainstem auditory evoked response. *Journal of Speech and Hearing Research, 21,* 408–416.

Cox, L. C. (1985). Infant assessment: Development and age-related considerations. In J. T. Jacobson (Ed.), *The auditory brainstem response* (pp. 297–316). San Diego, CA: College-Hill Press.

Despland, P. A., & Galambos, R. (1980). The auditory brainstem response (ABR) is a useful diagnostic tool in the intensive care nursery. *Pediatric Research, 14,* 154–158.

Don, M., Allen, A. R., & Starr, A. (1977). Effect of click rate on the latency of auditory brainstem responses in humans. *Annals of Otology, Rhinology, and Laryngology, 86,* 186–195.

Don, M., & Eggermont, J. J. (1978). Analysis of the click-evoked brainstem potentials in man using high-pass noise masking. *Journal of the Acoustical Society of America, 63,* 1084–1092.

Don, M., Ponton, C. W., Eggermont, J. J., & Masuda, A. (1993). Gender differences in cochlear response time: An explanation for gender amplitude differences in the unmasked auditory brain-stem response. *The Journal of the Acoustical Society of America, 94*(4), 2135-2148.

Don, M., Vermiglio, A. J., Ponton, C. W., Eggermont, J. J., & Masuda, A. (1996). Variable effects of click polarity on auditory brain-stem response latencies: Analysis of narrow-band ABRs suggest possible explanations. *Journal of the Acoustical Society of America, 100,* 458–472.

Doyle, D. J., & Hyde, M. L. (1981a). Analogue and digital filtering of auditory brainstem responses. *Scandinavian Audiology, 10,* 81–89.

Doyle, W. J., & Fria, T. (1985). The effects of hypothermia on the latencies of the auditory brain-stem response (ABR) in the rhesus monkey. *Electroencephalography and Clinical Neurophysiology, 60*(3), 258–266.

Durrant, J. D., & Boston, J. R. (2007). Stimuli for auditory evoked potential assessment. In R. F. Burkard, M. Don, & J. J. Eggermont (Eds.), *Auditory evoked potentials: Basic principles and clinical applications* (pp. 42–65). Baltimore, MD: Lippincott Williams & Wilkins.

Durrant, J. D., Sabo, D. L., & Hyre, R. J. (1990). Gender, head size and ABRs examined in a large clinical sample. *Ear and Hearing, 11,* 210–214.

Eggermont, J. J., Brown, D., Ponton, C., & Kimberley, B. (1996). Comparison of distortion product otoacoustic emissions (DPOAE) and auditory brainstem response (ABR) traveling wave delay measurements suggest frequency-specific synapse maturation. *Ear and Hearing, 17,* 386–394.

Eggermont, J. J., & Don, M. (1980). Analysis of the click-evoked brainstem potentials in man using high-pass masking. II. Effects of click intensity. *Journal of the Acoustical Society of America, 68,* 1671–1675.

Eggermont, J. J., & Salamy, A. (1988). Maturational time course for the ABR in preterm, and full-term infants. *Hearing Research, 33,* 35–47.

Elberling, C. (1979). Auditory electrophysiology: Spectral analysis of cochlear and brainstem evoked potentials. *Scandinavian Audiology, 8,* 57–64.

Fowler, C. (1992). Effects of stimulus phase on the normal auditory brainstem response. *Journal of Speech and Hearing Research, 35,* 167–174.

Fowler, C., & Noffsinger, D. (1983). Effects of stimulus repetition rate and frequency on the auditory brainstem response in normal, cochlear-impaired and VII nerve/brainstem impaired subjects. *Journal of Speech and Hearing Research, 26,* 560–567.

Fria, T. J., & Doyle, W. J. (1984). Maturation of the auditory brain stem response (ABR): Additional perspectives. *Ear and Hearing, 5,* 361–365.

Galambos, R., & Hecox, K. E. (1978). Clinical application of the auditory brainstem response. *Otolaryngology Clinics of North America, 11,* 709–722.

Gorga, M. P., Kaminski, J. R., & Beauchaine, K. A. (1988). Auditory brainstem responses from graduates of an intensive care nursery using an insert earphone. *Ear and Hearing, 9,* 144–147.

Gorga, M. P., Kaminski, J. R., & Beauchaine, K. L. (1991). Effects of stimulus phase on the latency of the auditory brainstem response. *Journal of the American Academy of Audiology, 2,* 1–6.

Gorga, M. P., Kaminski, J. R., Beauchaine, K. L., Jesteadt, W., & Neely, S. (1989). Auditory brainstem responses from children three months to three years of age: Normal patterns of responses II. *Journal of Speech and Hearing Research, 32,* 281–288.

Gorga, M. P., Reiland, J. K., Beauchaine, K. A., Worthington, D. W., & Jesteadt, W. (1987). Auditory brainstem responses from graduates of an intensive care nursery: Normal patterns of response. *Journal of Speech and Hearing Research, 30,* 311–318.

Gorga, M. P., Worthington, D. W., Reiland, J. K., Beauchaine, K. A., & Goldgar, D. E. (1985). Some comparisons between auditory brainstem response threshold, latencies, and the pure-tone audiogram. *Ear and Hearing, 6,* 105–112.

Hall, J. W., Bull, J., & Cronau, L. (1998). The effect of hypo- versus hyperthermia on auditory brainstem response: Two cases. *Ear and Hearing, 9,* 137–143.

Harkins, S. W. (1981). Effects of age and interstimulus interval on the brainstem auditory evoked potential. *International Journal of Neuroscience, 15,* 107–118.

Harris, D. M., & Dallos, P. (1979). Forward masking of auditory nerve fiber responses. *Journal of Neurophysiology, 42*(4), 1083–1107.

Hashimoto, I., Ishiyama, Y., Yoshimoto, T., & Nemoto, S. (1981). Brainstem auditory evoked potentials recorded directly from human brainstem and thalamus. *Brain, 104,* 841–859.

Haug G. (1977). Age and sex dependence of the size of normal ventricles on computed tomography. *Neuro-radiology, 14,* 201–204.

Hecox, K., & Burkard, R. (1982). Development dependencies of the human brainstem auditory evoked response. *Annals of the New York Academy of Sciences, 388*(1), 538–556.

Hecox, K., & Deegan, D. (1983). Rise-fall time effects on the brainstem auditory evoked response: Mechanisms. *Journal of the Acoustical Society of America, 73*(6), 2109–2016.

Hecox, K., & Galambos, R. (1974). Brainstem evoked responses in human infants and adults. *Archives of Otolaryngology, 99,* 30–33.

Hecox, K. E., Squires, N. K., & Galambos, R. (1976). Brainstem auditory evoked responses in man. I. Effect of stimulus rise-fall time and duration. *Journal of the Acoustical Society of America, 60*(5), 1187–1192.

Houston, H. G., & McClelland, R. J. (1985). Age and gender contributions to intersubject variability of the auditory brainstem potentials. *Biological Psychiatry, 20,* 419–430.

Hughes, J. R., Fino, J., & Gagnon, L. (1981). The importance of phase stimulus and reference recording electrode in brainstem auditory evoked potentials. *Electroencephalography and Clinical Neurophysiology, 51,* 611–623.

Hyde, M. L., Stephens, S. D. G., & Thornton, A. R. D. (1976). Stimulus repetition rate and early brainstem responses. *British Journal of Audiology, 10,* 41–50.

Jerger, J., & Hall, J. (1980). Effects of age and sex on auditory brainstem response. *Archives of Otolaryngology, 106,* 387–391.

Jerger, J. J., & Johnson, K. (1988). Interactions of age, gender, and sensorineural hearing loss on ABR latency. *Ear and Hearing, 9,* 168–176.

Jewett, D. L. (1970). Volume-conducted potentials in response to auditory stimuli as detected by averaging in the cat. *Electroencephalography and Clinical Neurophysiology, 28,* 609–618.

Jewett, D. L., & Williston, J. S. (1971). Auditory-evoked far fields averaged from the scalp of humans. *Brain, 94,* 681–696.

Jiang, Z., Brosi, D., & Wilkinson, A. (1998). Immaturity of electrophysiological responses of the neonatal auditory brainstem to high repetition rates of click stimulation. *Early Human Development, 52,* 133–143.

Jones, T. A., Stockard, J. J., & Weidner, W. J. (1980). The effects of temperature and acute alcohol intoxication on brain stem auditory evoked potentials in the cat. *Electroencephalography and Clinical Neurophysiology, 49,* 23–30.

Katbamma, B., Metz, D., Adelman, C., & Thodi, C. (1993). Auditory evoked responses in chronic alcohol and drug abusers. *Biological Psychiatry, 33,* 750–752.

Kavanagh, K. T., Harker, L. A., & Tyler, R. S. (1984). Auditory brainstem and middle latency responses: I. Effects of response filtering and waveform identification; II. Threshold responses to a 500 Hz tonepip. *Acta Otolaryngologica (Stockholm), 108,* 1–12.

Kevanishvili, Z., & Aphochenko, V. (1979). Frequency composition of the brainstem auditory evoked potentials. *Scandinavian Audiology, 8,* 51–55.

Kevanishvili, Z., & Aphonchenko, V. (1981). Click polarity inversion effects upon the human brainstem auditory evoked potential. *Scandinavian Audiology, 10,* 141–147.

King, A. J., & Sininger, Y. S. (1992). Electrode configuration for auditory brainstem response audiometry. *American Journal of Audiology, 1*(2), 63–67.

Kodera, K., Yamane, H., Yamada, O., & Suzuki, I. J. (1977). The effect of onset offset and rise-decay times of tone bursts on brain stern response. *Scandinavian Audiology, 6,* 205–210.

Krishnan, A., & Durrant, J. J. (1991). On the origin of wave II of the auditory brainstem responses. *Ear and Hearing, 12*(3), 174–179.

Lasky, R. E. (1984). A developmental study on the effect of stimulus rate on the auditory evoked brain-stem response. *Electroencephalography and Clinical Neurophysiology, 59,* 411–419.

Laukli, E., & Mair, I. W. S. (1981). Early auditory-evoked responses: Spectral content. *Audiology, 20,* 453–464.

Lauter, J., Oyler, R., & Lord-Maes, J. (1993). Amplitude stability of auditory brainstem responses in two groups of children compared with adults. *British Journal of Audiology, 27,* 263–271.

Lev, A., & Sohmer, H. (1972). Sources of averaged neural responses recorded in animal and human subjects during cochlear audiometry (electrocochleography). *Archiv für klinische und experimentelle Ohren- Nasen- und Kehlkopfheilkunde, 201,* 79–90.

López-Escámez, J. A., Salguero, G., & Salinero, J. (1999). Age and sex differences in latencies of waves I, III and V in auditory brainstem response of normal hearing subjects. *Acta oto-rhino-laryngologica belgica, 53*(2), 109-115.

Markand, O. N., Farlow, M. R., Stevens, J. C., & Edwards, M. K. (1989). Brain stem auditory evoked potential abnormalities with unilateral brainstem lesions demonstrated by magnetic resonance imaging. *Archives of Neurology, 46,* 295–299.

Marsh, R. R., Yamane, H. Y., & Potsic, W. P. (1984). Auditory brain-stem response and temperature: Relationship in the guinea pig. *Electroencephalography and Clinical Neurophysiology, 57,* 289–293.

Marshall, N. K., & Donchin, E. (1981). Circadian variation in the latency of brainstem responses and its relation to body temperature. *Science, 212*(4492), 356–358.

Maurer, K., Schaefer, E., & Leitner, H. (1980). The effect of varying stimulus polarity rarefaction vs condensation of early auditory evoked potentials. *Electroencephalography and Clinical Neurophysiology, 50,* 332–334.

McGann, K. P., Marion, G. S., Camp, L., & Spangler, J. G. (1993). The influence of gender and race on mean body temperature in a population of healthy older adults. *Archives of Family Medicine, 2*(12), 1265–1267.

Mitchell, C., Phillips, D. S., & Trune, D. R. (1989). Variables affecting the auditory brainstem response: Audiogram, age, gender and head size. *Hearing Research, 40*(1), 75–85.

Moller, A. R. (1981a). Neural delay in the ascending auditory pathway. *Experimental Brain Research, 43,* 93–100.

Moller, A. R. (1981b). Latency in the ascending auditory pathway determined using continuous sounds: Comparison between transient and envelope latency. *Brain Research, 207,* 184–188.

Moller, A. R. (1986). Effect of click spectrum and polarity on round window N1N2 response in the rat. *Audiology, 25,* 29–43.

Moller, A. R., & Jannetta, P. J. (1981). Compound action potentials recorded intracranially from the auditory nerve in man. *Experimental Neurology, 74,* 862–874.

Moller, A. R., & Jannetta, P. J. (1983). Auditory evoked potentials recorded from the cochlear nucleus and its vicinity in man. *Journal of Neurosurgery, 59,* 1013–1018.

Møller, A. R., Jannetta, P. J., & Jho, H. D. (1994). Click-evoked responses from the cochlear nucleus: a study in human. *Electroencephalography and Clinical Neurophysiology/Evoked Potentials Section, 92*(3), 215–224.

Moller, A. R., Jannetta, P. J., & Moller, M. B. (1981). Neural generators of brainstem evoked potentials. Results from human intracranial recordings. *Annals of Otology Rhinology and Laryngology, 90,* 591–596.

Oh, S. J., Kuba, T., Soyer, A., Choi, S., Bonikowski, F. P., & Vitek, J. (1981). Lateralization of brainstem lesions by brainstem auditory evoked potentials. *Neurology, 31,* 14–18.

Oku, T., & Hasegewa, M. (1997). The influence of aging on auditory brainstem response and electrocochleography in the elderly. *ORL Journal for Otorhinolaryngology and Its Related Specialties, 59,* 141–146.

Osterhammel, P. (1981). The unsolved problems in analog filtering on the auditor brainstem responses. *Scandinavian Audiology, Supplementum, 13,* 69–74.

Peake, W., & Kiang, N. Y. S. (1962). Cochlear responses to condensation and rarefaction clicks. *Biophysics Journal, 2,* 23–34.

Picton, T. W. (2011). Acoustic stimuli: Sounds to charm the brain. In T. W. Picton (Ed.), *Human auditory evoked potentials* (pp. 131–132). San Diego, CA: Plural Publishing.

Picton, T. W., Stapells, D. R., & Campbell, K. B. (1981). Auditory evoked potentials from the human cochlea and brainstem. *Journal of Otolaryngology (Toronto), 9,* 1–41.

Picton, T. W., Woods, D. L., Baribeau-Braun, J., & Healey, T. M. G. (1977). Evoked potential audiometry. *Journal of Otolaryngology (Toronto), 6,* 90–119.

Pratt, H., & Sohmer, H. (1976). Intensity and rate functions of cochlear and brainstem evoked response to click stimuli in man. *Archives of Otorhinolaryngology, 212,* 85–92.

Rosenhall, U., Bjorkman, G., Pedersen, K., & Kall, A. (1985). Brain-stem auditory evoked potentials in different age groups. *Electroencephalography and Clinical Neurophysiology, 62,* 426–430.

Rosenhamer, H. J., Lindstrom, B., & Lundborg, T. (1978). On the use of click-evoked electric brainstem responses in audiological diagnosis. I. The variability of the normal response. *Scandinavian Audiology, 7,* 193–205.

Rosenhamer, H. J., Lindstrom, B., & Lundborg, T. (1980). On the use of click-evoked electric brainstem responses in audiological diagnosis. II. The influence of sex and age upon the normal response. *Scandinavian Audiology, 9,* 93–100.

Rowe, M. J. (1978). Normal variability of the brainstem auditory evoked response in young and old adult subjects. *Electroencephalography and Clinical Neurophysiology, 44,* 459–470.

Rupa, V., & Dayal, A. (1993). Wave V latency shifts with age and sex in normals and patients with cochlear hearing loss: Development of a predictive model. *British Journal of Audiology, 27,* 273–279.

Ruth, R. A., Hildebrand, D. L., & Cantrell, R. W. (1982). A study of methods used to enhance Wave I in the auditory brainstem response. *Archives of Otolaryngology-Head and Neck Surgery, 90,* 635–640.

Salamy, A. (1984). Maturation of the auditory brainstem response from birth through early childhood. *Journal of Clinical Neurophysiology, 1*(3), 293–329.

Salomon, G., & Elberling, C. (1971). Cochlear nerve potentials recorded from the ear canal in man. *Acta Otolaryngology (Stockholm), 71,* 319–325.

Sato, H., Sando, I., & Takahashi, H. (1991). Sexual dimorphism and the development of the human cochlea. Computer 3-D measurement. *Acta Otolaryngologica (Stockholm), 111,* 1037–1040.

Schwartz, D. M., & Berry, G. A. (1985). Normative aspects of the ABR. In J. T. Jacobson (Ed.), *The auditory brainstem response* (pp. 66–93). San Diego, CA: College-Hill Press.

Schwartz, D. M., Morris, M. D., Spydell, J. D., Brink, C. T., Grim, M. A., & Schwartz, J. A. (1990). Influence of click polarity on the brain-stem auditory evoked response (BAER) revisited. *Electroencephalography and Clinical Neurophysiology, 77,* 445–457.

Sininger, Y. S., & Don, M. (1989). Effects of click rate and electrode orientation on threshold of the auditory brainstem response. *Journal of Speech and Hearing Research, 32,* 880–886.

Skoe, E., Krizman, J., Anderson, S., & Kraus, N. (2015). Stability and plasticity of auditory brainstem function across the lifespan. *Cerebral Cortex, 25,* 1415–1426.

Spire J. P., Dohrmann, G. J., & Prieto, P. S. (1982). Correlation of brainstem evoked responses with direct acoustic nerve potential. *Advances in Neurology, 32,* 159–167.

Spitzer, E., White-Schwoch, T., Carr, K. W., Skoe, E., & Kraus, N. (2015). Continued maturation of the click-evoked auditory brainstem response in preschoolers. *Journal of the American Academy of Audiology, 26,* 30–35.

Spoendlin, H. (1972). Innervation densities of the cochlea. *Acta Otolaryngologica, 73*, 235–248.

Stapells, D. R., & Picton, T. W. (1981). Technical aspects of brainstem evoked potential audiometry using tones. *Ear and Hearing, 2*, 20–29.

Starr, A., & Achor, L. (1975). Auditory brainstem responses in neurological disease. *Archives of Neurology, 32*, 761–768.

Starr, A., & Hamilton, A. E. (1976). Correlation between confirmed sites of neurological lesions and abnormalities of far-field auditory brainstem responses. *Electroencephalography and Clinical Neurophysiology, 41*, 595–608.

Starr, A., & Squires, K. (1982). Distribution of auditory brainstem potentials over the scalp and nasopharynx in humans. *Annals of the New York Academy of Sciences, 388*, 427–442.

Stockard, J. E., & Stockard, J. J. (1983). Recording and analyzing. In E. J. Moore (Ed.), *Bases of auditory brain-stem evoked responses* (pp. 255–286). New York, NY: Grune & Stratton.

Stockard, J. E., Stockard, J. J., Westmoreland, B. F., & Corfits, J. L. (1979). Brainstem auditory-evoked responses: Normal variation as a function of stimulus and subject characteristics. *Archives of Neurology, 36*, 823–831.

Stockard, J. J., & Rossiter, V. S. (1977). Clinical and pathologic correlates of brain stem auditory response abnormalities. *Neurology, 27*(4), 316–325.

Stockard, J. J., Sharbrough, F. W., & Tinker, J. A. (1978). Effects of hypothermia on the human brainstem auditory response. *Annals of Neurology, 3*(4), 368–370.

Stockard, J. J., Stockard, J. E., & Sharbrough, F. W. (1978). Nonpathologic factors influencing brainstem auditory evoked potentials. *American Journal of EEG Technology, 18*, 177–209.

Stockard, J. J., & Westmoreland, B. F. (1981). Technical considerations in the recording and interpretation of the brainstem auditory evoked potential for neonatal diagnosis. *American Journal of EEG Technology, 21*, 31–54.

Suresh, C. H., & Krishnan, A. (2021). Search for electrophysiological indices of hidden hearing loss in humans: Click auditory brainstem response across sound levels and in background noise. *Ear and Hearing, 42*(1), 53–67.

Suzuki, T., & Horiuchi, K. (1981). Rise time of pure-tone stimuli in brain stem response audiometry. *Audiology, 20*, 101–112.

Suzuki, T., Kobayashi, K., & Takaoi, N. (1986). Effects of stimulus repetition rate on the slow and fast components of auditory brainstem responses. *Electroencephalography and Clinical Neurophysiology, 65*, 150–156.

Suzuki, T., Yasuhito, H., & Horiuchi, K. (1981). Simultaneous recording of early and middle components of auditory electric responses. *Ear and Hearing, 2*, 276–282.

Terkildsen, K., & Osterhammel, P. (1981). The influence of reference electrode position on recordings of the auditory brainstem responses. *Ear and Hearing, 2*, 9–14.

Terkildsen, K., Osterhammel, P., & Huis in't Veld, F. (1975). Farfield electrocochleography: Frequency specificity of the response. *Scandinavian Audiology, 4*, 167–172.

Thornton, A. R. D., & Coleman, M. J. (1975). The adaptation of cochlear and brainstem evoked potentials in humans. *Electroencephalography and Clinical Neurophysiology, 39*, 399–406.

Trune, D. R., Mitchell, C., & Phillips, D. S. (1988). The relative importance of head size, gender and age on the auditory brainstem response. *Hearing Research, 32*(2), 165–174.

Verhulst, S., Jagadeesh, A., Mauermann, M., & Ernst, F. (2016). Individual differences in auditory brainstem response wave characteristics relations to different aspects of peripheral hearing loss. *Trends in Hearing*. https://doi.org/10.1177/23312165166721863

Wada S-I., & Starr, A. (1983). Generation of auditory brainstem responses (ABRs). I. Effects of injection of a local anesthetic (Procaine HCL) into the trapezoid body of guinea pigs. *Electroencephalography and Clinical Neurophysiology, 56*, 326–339.

Watson, D. R. (1996). The effects of cochlear hearing loss, age and sex on the auditory brainstem response. *Audiology, 35*(5), 246–258.

Weber, B. A., & Fijikawa, S. M. (1977). Brainstem evoked responses (BER) audiometry at various stimulus presentation rates. *Journal of the American Audiology Society, 3*, 59–62.

Wolfe, J. A., Skinner, P., & Burns, J. (1978). Relationship between the sound intensity and latency the latency and amplitude of the brainstem auditory evoked response. *Journal of Speech and Hearing Research, 21*, 387–400.

Yagi, T., & Kaga, K. (1979). The effect of the click repetition rate on the latency of the auditory evoked brain stem response and its clinical use for a neurological diagnosis. *Archives of Otorhinolaryngology, 222*, 91–97.

York, D. H. (1986). Correlation between a unilateral midbrain-pontine lesion and abnormalities of the brain-stem auditory evoked potential. *Electroencephalography and Clinical Neurophysiology, 65,* 282–288.

Zimmerman, M. C., Morgan, D. E., & Dubno, J. R. (1987). Auditory brainstem evoked response characteristics in developing infants. *Annals of Otology, Rhinology, and Laryngology, 96,* 291–299.

Zwislocki, J. J. (1975). Phase opposition between inner and outer hair cells and auditory sound analysis. *Audiology, 14,* 443–455.

5

Clinical Applications of the Auditory Brainstem Responses: Audiologic Applications for Hearing Screening and Threshold Estimation

SCOPE

It is well established that the auditory brainstem response (ABR) has proven to be a relatively rapid and reliable objective clinical measure to assess the functional integrity of auditory peripheral and brainstem structures. In this chapter, we consider the clinical applications of the ABR and auditory steady-state response (ASSR) in hearing screening and threshold estimation. Since ABR is the more commonly used (with a still persistent reluctance to utilize ASSR in clinical practice) clinical objective measure, we first focus on the description of clinical applications of the ABR. We then try to make the case for incorporating ASSR measures, as a complementary accurate and rapid supplement in threshold estimation. The clinical applications of the ABR can be described under three main categories: *hearing screening* for early identification of hearing loss; *estimation of hearing thresholds* or minimum hearing levels to develop management strategies in the event of a hearing loss (both applications are crucial to providing adequate auditory stimulation through the critical period of speech and language development); and a range of *neuro-otologic applications*, including determination of site/level of lesion, serial monitoring of comatose patients, and intraoperative monitoring. The neuro-otologic applications are addressed in Chapter 7. While there is no single standard protocol for each application across clinics to date, the aim here is to present the latest developments relevant to hearing screening and threshold estimation to move toward the development of effective and efficient protocols that utilize next-generation technology to both increase accuracy and reduce test time—the essential tenets of the recent recommendations of the Joint Committee on Infant Hearing (JCIH, 2019). The goal is to move toward the much-needed standardization of stimuli and automated response detection algorithms for both hearing screening and threshold estimation.

I. HEARING SCREENING

Hearing Screening: Factors Determining Optimal Implementation

One important goal in clinical audiology is the identification, characterization, and appropriate intervention of hearing loss as early as possible to minimize the potential negative impact of auditory sensory deprivation on the acquisition of speech and language, academic achievement, and social and emotional development. Since behavioral measures do not permit accurate determination of the status of hearing in infants, young children, and adults incapable of reliably performing the tasks required by behavioral hearing tests, an objective reliable measure like the ABR is essential for early identification of any abnormalities in auditory function in these individuals. Although ABRs have been used for hearing screening since the mid-1980s, a major push for universal hearing screening for all infants gained momentum following the 1993 National Institutes of Health (NIH) consensus statement (NIH, 1993) on the importance of early identification of hearing loss in infants and young children. Before this, there were only a handful of hospitals performing newborn hearing screening. This momentum for early identification and intervention of hearing impairment grew rapidly following the recommendations of the American Academy of Pediatrics (1999, 2007), and the Joint Committee on Infant Hearing position statements (JCIH, 2000, 2007). With the help of these sustained efforts, we now have a mandatory universal newborn hearing screening program (hearing screening performed before the baby is discharged from the hospital) using electrophysiologic measures (ABRs and/or otoacoustic emissions [OAEs], with a follow-up complete threshold evaluation for infants who do not pass the screening) implemented in all U.S. states. The main stated goal of the JCIH's revised guidelines (2007 and reinforced in 2019) on early hearing detection and intervention (EHDI) is to maximize linguistic and communicative competence and literacy development. Every U.S. state has established an EHDI program. The EHDI program strives to identify every child born with a permanent hearing loss before the age of 3 months and provide timely and appropriate intervention services before 6 months of age, provide culturally competent family support, create a "medical home" (a patient-centered, team-based health care delivery concept to provide comprehensive and sustained medical care to obtain maximal health outcomes) for all newborns, and have effective newborn hearing screening tracking and data management systems that are linked with other relevant public health information systems. Also, the JCIH sets benchmarks and quality indicators to ensure high-quality hearing screening with low postscreening referral rates (4%) and a 95% or better follow-up rate. *A review of these well-principled and thorough documents should be required reading for all audiology students and practicing audiologists.*

Justification for a Hearing Screening Program

To warrant a screening program for any disorder, there are several general criteria (related to the importance of the disorder, prevalence, diagnosis, treatment resources, responsiveness to treatment, and advantages of early intervention) that have to be met, and these also apply to justify universal newborn hearing screening (UNHS). Ruth, Dey-Sigman, and Mills (1985) have provided a concise description of how each of these requirements can be specifically applied to justify newborn hearing screening. To warrant screening, the disorder must be ***sufficiently serious and prevalent:*** Hearing impairment in infants has a high enough prevalence (4%–5% of high-risk infants; about 1.5–2.75 cases/1,000 for a permanent bilateral sensorineural hearing loss of 40 dB HL, respectively) (Bamford et al., 2007)) and can produce significant deficits in speech and language, academic achievement, and social and emotional development. ***The disorder can be diagnosed:*** Newborn otologic pathology and auditory deficits are well defined and can be clinically assessed and diagnosed. ***Effective treatment/ therapy should be available:*** Effective medical and/or audiologic management of hearing impairment is available and accessible. ***The disorder should be responsive to treatment:*** Some auditory pathologies can be treated medically while other irreversible impairments can be managed effectively by hearing prosthetic devices (hearing aids or cochlear implants) that provide the necessary auditory input to the auditory system to minimize the impact of hearing impairment on speech and language acquisition and communicative skills. ***Screening warranted only if there is an advantage to early identification:*** Early identification of hearing impairment and timely and appropriate intervention are critical to minimize the negative impact of hearing impairment on speech and language acquisition, and its ripple effects on academic achievement and social and emotional development of the individual. Children whose hearing impairments are identified earlier (before the age of 6–9 months) and receive effective auditory stimulation are more likely to acquire speech and language and show better language scores later in childhood compared to children for whom identification and intervention occurred much later (Moeller, 2000; Nelson, Bougatsos, & Nygren, 2008; Watkin et al., 2007; Yoshinaga-Itano, Sedey, Coulter, & Mehl, 1998). Early detection promotes early intervention that, in turn, results in better communication skills outcomes (Sininger, Grimes, & Christensen, 2010).

Hearing Screening: Measures to Be Used

While there is a multitude of factors (related to type and degree of hearing loss, measures to be used, their sensitivity and specificity, cost) to consider when implementing a hearing screening protocol, it is important to focus on the main objective of hearing screening—early identification of hearing impairment in all infants who need further evaluation to determine the type and degree of loss to facilitate timely, appropriate, and effective intervention. The JCIH (2007, 2019) guidelines recommend the use of automated *OAEs* and/or *automated auditory brainstem response (A-ABR)* screening technology as acceptable methods for initial and rescreening of newborns. These are noninvasive measures that can be easily administered by trained nursery staff. Since they are objective measures with automated interpretation, errors due to subjective bias are ruled out. OAE provides information about the functional integrity of the outer hair cell (OHC) subsystem that presumably is dysfunctional in cochlear hearing losses. OAE protocols use either the broadband transient evoked otoacoustic emissions (TEOAEs) or the frequency-specific distortion product otoacoustic emissions (DPOAEs). In contrast, the ABR measure assesses the functional integrity of both peripheral structures (outer ear, middle ear, and cochlear hair cells) and auditory nerve and brainstem structures. Given these differences in the measures, infants with auditory neuropathy will likely fail the ABR and pass the OAE screening. Therefore, ABR screening is recommended for babies needing care in the neonatal intensive care unit (NICU) for more than 5 days, who may be at risk for not only late-onset or progressive hearing loss but also auditory neuropathy spectrum disorders (ANSDs) (disorders of the afferent auditory system involving the inner hair cell [IHC] and the auditory nerve). The use of ABR in this high-risk group ensures that this neural disorder is not missed. Well babies and babies in the NICU for less than 5 days (with no risk indicators for late-onset or progressive hearing loss) can be screened initially with OAE.

Over 90% of all newborns in the United States are screened for hearing loss before their discharge from the hospital. Many hospitals use a two-stage protocol for newborn hearing screening in which all infants are screened first with OAEs. No additional testing is done with infants who pass the OAE, but infants who fail the OAE are next screened with A-ABR. Infants who fail the A-ABR screening are referred for diagnostic evaluation to determine whether they have permanent hearing loss (PHL). Those who pass the A-ABR are considered at low risk for hearing loss and are not tested further.

While it is generally acknowledged that these measures are very effective for early detection of hearing impairment, certain limitations have to be kept in mind while administering and interpreting the results. Both measures, OAE in particular (higher failure rates have been reported for OAE [van Dyk, Swanepoel, & Hall, 2015]), are influenced by outer and middle ear problems that could, in turn, produce a fail in the automated screening, even when the inner ear and brainstem are functionally normal. Both measures also are not sufficiently sensitive to detect slight or mild hearing losses of about 25 to 40 dB HL. Levit, Himmelfarb, and Dollberg (2015) reported that 42% of children who failed TEOAE screening but passed an A-ABR screening were later found to have a mild to moderate hearing loss.

What Is the Appropriate Time to Screen?

While hearing screening of well babies can be performed as early as 6 hours after birth, it is better to perform the screening closer to discharge time (allowing sufficient time to minimize the possibility of a transient threshold elevation due to debris [vernix] in the ear canal) to improve both efficiency and accuracy of screening and to reduce referrals. Based on screening results from low-risk term and late-preterm newborns, Johnson et al. (2018) reported that false-positive rates for congenital sensorineural hearing loss diagnosis decreased with increasing age at test time in the first 48 hours of life, thereby reducing the referral rate for audiologic evaluation.

The JCIH (2007, 2019) also recommends that a single repeat screening be performed if the infant does not pass the initial screening before discharge. Only a single repeat screen, preferably several hours after the first one, is recommended because multiple repeated screenings will increase the probability of obtaining a PASS by chance alone (type I error). The JCIH report (2019) further reinforces the recommendation that only two high-quality screenings be performed before discharge and only one postdischarge screening before referral to a pediatric audiologist. "High quality" here refers to recordings while the baby is asleep or resting quietly with minimal movements and with a patent ear canal.

For babies in the NICU, hearing screening should be performed just before the infant's discharge from the hospital. For babies born at home or in a birthing facility, the recommendation is to perform the hearing screening within the first 2 weeks of the infant's life or to conform to a more stringent guideline of the state EHDI program. Finally, infants with congenital aural atresia of one or both ears or other visible deformities of the pinna or ear canal (e.g., stenosis) should be referred for a complete audiologic evaluation, instead of screening, in the NICU or inpatient hospital if possible or immediately after discharge.

Location of Screening

Most environments for screening are outside a sound-treated booth, in less than ideal conditions both in terms of electrical interference and background noise levels (well-baby nursery, NICU, or a relatively quiet office room). Thus, care should be taken to select the most optimal environment possible to minimize the confounding effects of both electrical and acoustic noise on the recorded responses.

Loss to Follow-Up a Serious Concern

One of the major limitations of hearing screening is the loss of patients to follow-up for various reasons. The loss to follow-up rates for UNHS are highly variable across states, from less than 5% in some states to greater than 75% in others (CDC, 2012; Liu, Farrell, MacNeil, Stone, & Barfield, 2008). Although the loss to follow-up continues to improve through the diligent work of EHDI programs, close to 33% of newborns who do not pass the initial screening do not receive timely follow-up, thereby limiting the effectiveness of the screening and realization of the goal of early intervention following appropriate diagnosis with follow-up testing (CDC, 2012; Hunter et al., 2016; Russ, Hanna, DesGeorges, & Forsman, 2010). However, it is encouraging to note that a review of 53 published reports (between 2005 and 2015) on loss to follow-up rates showed a rate of 20% (Rohit et al., 2016).

Hearing Screening Protocols

Consistent with JCIH recommendations, both OAEs and A-ABR, in somewhat varying combinations, are currently used for hearing screening. We provide below a brief overview of OAE screening, but the major focus is on the description of the use of the A-ABR.

Hearing Screening Using Otoacoustic Emissions (OAEs)

OAEs are small acoustic signals, presumably reflecting functional integrity of the OHC subsystem, that are backpropagated through the middle ear and recordable in the ear canal. Thus, the presence of OAEs at a moderate intensity level is taken to reflect the normal function of the OHC subsystem, and by extension, normal-hearing thresholds (30 dB nHL or less). This, of course, assumes normal functional integrity of the IHCs, auditory nerve, and the central auditory system. It should be noted here that the absence of OAEs does not always mean OHC dysfunction because a middle ear pathology with a functionally intact OHC subsystem can also account for its absence. Two types of OAEs are commonly used. The **TEOAE** reflects broadband responses elicited by clicks, and the **DPOAE** reflects a frequency-specific cubic difference tone (2f1-f2) resulting from nonlinear processing of a pair of tones presented simultaneously. Both responses are more robust in the high frequencies (in part due to the reduced noise floor, less effective transmission of the low frequencies through the middle ear, and their basal bias) and less reliable at frequencies below about 1000 Hz. They are difficult to record in the presence of a middle ear problem due to attenuation of the backpropagated OAEs, therefore limiting their clinical utility. Also, OAEs do not provide any information about the functional status of the afferent IHC nerve synapse or of the auditory nerve itself. However, OAE measurement lends itself well as a newborn hearing screening tool because data acquisition is easy and quick, and it is affordable. Therefore, it has been commonly used as an initial hearing screening method in the dual OAE/A-ABR protocol. However, there are concerns about the OAEs' high referral and false-positive rates. Recall that the JCIH has set a 4% tolerance for referral rate. To determine the factors contributing to the high referral and false-positive rates associated with OAE newborn hearing screening, Akinpelu, Peleva, Funnell, and Daniel (2014) reviewed 10 published reports between 1990 and 2012 that met their specific inclusion criteria. Results, reflecting a large pool of newborn participants, revealed significantly lower referral rate (RR) and false positive (FP) rate when initial screening age was increased from less than 2 days to more than 2 days (RR: 13.8% versus 4.7%; FP: 13.1% versus 4.4%); pass criterion was set at 6 dB signal-to-noise ratio (SNR) instead of 3 dB (RR: 3.2% versus 9.4%; FP: 2.96% versus 9.1%); and screening higher (2–4 or 2–5 kHz) compared to lower (1–4 kHz) frequencies (RR: 1.6% versus 6.08%; FP: 1.28% versus 5.8%). Thus, to improve the sensitivity and viability of OAE as an initial newborn screening test, these factors have to be optimized (that is, later screening age, use of high frequencies, and a 6 dB SNR pass criterion) in the OAE protocol. However, due to the possibility that later testing might have the unintended consequence of increasing the loss to follow-up rate, this strategy does not appear practical. Based on these results, it would be worthwhile to utilize the ability to repeat the OAE measures at several close time points after the initial screening to increase the sensitivity (the ability of the test to correctly identify infants with hearing impairment when they do have a hearing impairment) and specificity (the ability of the test to correctly identify infants with normal hearing when they do have normal hearing). Several screening programs practice this strategy to reduce RRs to under the 4% JCIH benchmark. Most of these hearing screening tests have a high sensitivity as well as a high specificity (usually between 95% and 100%). In recent times, OAE devices have become smaller, use improved technology for processing OAEs in background noise, and use automated algorithms. Also, early screening has moved from TEOAE to the use of DPOAE.

Hearing Screening Using the ABR

The ABR has been time tested and is the gold standard screening and threshold estimation tool. It enjoys this privilege because it is a very reliable and easy to administer test, and importantly, it has been proven to be a reliable frequency-specific predictor of hearing sensitivity in normal and hearing-impaired infants, children, and adults. Also, it is well established that the ABR measure is superior to OAE in terms of sensitivity, lower susceptibility to middle ear pathology, and ability to detect retrocochlear hearing impairments, such as auditory neuropathy, which has an estimated prevalence of about 5% to 10% in newborns at risk for hearing loss (Foerst et al., 2002; Rance et al., 1999). Finally, with the advent of A-ABR devices and algorithms, it has become a very efficient, cost-effective (does not require an audiologist) screening tool that can achieve standardization across facilities easily. Ideally, newborn hearing screenings should be least disruptive to personnel resources, fast, and have high sensitivity (low false negatives) and high specificity (low false positives, which reduces unnecessary over-referrals).

Earlier ABR screening used the conventional approach where responses were recorded to clicks using a repetition rate of about 23 to 37 clicks/s at stimulus levels of 35 dB nHL (to confirm normal hearing or a mild hearing loss) and 70 dB nHL (to determine greater hearing loss) if babies failed the screening at the 30 dB nHL level. Pass criteria were based on either the presence of wave V (PASS) or its absence (REFER) upon visual examination or more stringent wave V latency-based pass/fail criteria (Figure 5–1). Sensitivity and specificity were high for these measures, particularly upon rescreening 2 weeks after the initial screening.

A-ABR screening devices were introduced in the late 1980s after successful validation trials in nursery settings using ALGO1 (Hermann, Thornton, & Joseph, 1995; Jacobson, Jacobson, & Spahr, 1990; Kileny, 1987). ALGO1 uses a binary template matching algorithm to objectively arrive at a statistically based decision about the presence (PASS) or absence (REFER) of a response by comparing the sampled amplitude values of discrete temporal points on the template, corresponding to prominent response regions, with the averaged response. To increase its sensitivity to selectively detect wave V, the template places more weight on the time points corresponding to wave V latency and the following slow negative trough (the SN10—slow negativity around 10 ms). The algorithm also allows a time window shift of ±1.5 ms in this region to ensure detection of wave Vs that differ in latency across infants due to maturational differences and/or transient middle ear problems. This also serves to minimize a false REFER decision. The ABR temporal waveform template represents the composite response from a group of infants with normal hearing that were simultaneously obtained with the A-ABR. Before we consider the newer generation of automated screeners and their hearing screening performance, a brief introduction to the fundamentals of operation of the A-ABR detection and decision-making algorithm would be helpful.

An Overview of a Time-Domain Approach to Automatic Detection in A-ABR

Recall from Chapter 3 that response averaging involves cancellation/reduction of random noise and addition of the constantly repeating time-locked ABR neural activity (the signal) detected by the electrodes that form the noninverting and inverting inputs to the differential amplifier. Essentially, the automated algorithm has to reliably distinguish between the two distributions (noise and signal + noise distributions) by determining the proportion of activity due to noise, and that due to the signal in the averaged response in the temporal window (where wave V and the following trough occur) of interest. We also know that response detection gets better with an increasing number of averages, so the algorithm has to decide the presence of a reliable response before averaging is terminated using a stop criterion. The decision-making component of the algorithm uses a combination of the basic principles of signal detection and statistical theory to detect the response by using estimates of the signal and the noise variance in an SNR-like measure (similar to the automated algorithms for response detection described in more detail by Sininger, 2007). Most current A-ABR detection algorithms use time-domain methods that start with a precise temporal template of the ABR elicited by a 35 dB nHL alternating polarity click. Using this template, five to nine discrete time points in the response area are

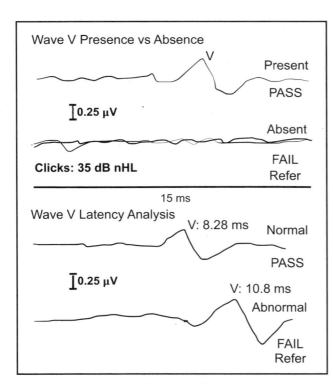

Figure 5–1. The pass-refer criteria for auditory brainstem response screening. *Top:* A "pass" is based on the presence of the response; a "refer" is when the response is absent. *Bottom:* For a pass, the response must be present and occur with normal latency, while the presence of a delayed wave V is considered abnormal and generates a referral.

assigned a value of one (if the amplitude is greater than 0) or zero (if the amplitude is negative) for each sweep of the stimulus (Figure 5–2). Amplitude values for the time points in the template falling in the region of wave V and the following trough are weighted more to increase the sensitivity of detection. That is, the specific location of these temporal sampling points serves to optimize the variance of the target waveform for faster detection. If there is no response present, then the weighted sum should be zero (equivalent to a noise distribution alone); if a response is present, the weighted sum will continue to grow with each sweep in the averaging process, thus improving the SNR estimates. For each sweep, the ratio of the summed estimate of the signal and an estimate of noise (similar to the F_{SP}, but algorithms in recent automated devices estimate variance using multiple points in the ABR waveform) are compared using the z-statistic (which essentially compares the variance of the signal with that of the noise) to determine if the signal variance is significantly greater than the noise variance. Averaging is continued until a clear response is detected, or it is stopped after a fixed number of sweeps. Another important aspect of this automated algorithm is the use of a sliding template that keeps the relationship between sampled points in the response temporal region the same but shifts in time to allow optimal detection of responses with different latencies. That is, the time window for response detection is moved over a range of latencies to ensure responses with delayed latencies are also detected. The sliding template range of 1.5 ms used easily covers the 0.5-ms standard deviation in latency of wave V observed for infants at 30 dB nHL (Sininger et al., 2000). In terms of the number of sweeps used, most automated systems have a stop criterion based on reaching a statistically significant SNR-type measure. For example, Norton et al. (2000a, 2000b) reported that a criterion F_{SP} value of 3.1 is sufficient to make a PASS versus REFER decision.

Later models of ALGO (ALGO2, 3, and now 5) have progressively incorporated several improvements in earphone coupling and electrode adhesion (that improve ambient noise attenuation and electrode stability), enhancements in the screening algorithm to improve signal acquisition and data processing using separate ambient and myogenic noise rejection algorithms (that serve to reduce screening time and initial referral rates while keeping sensitivity high), and the addition of database

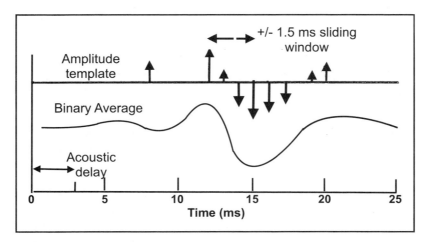

Figure 5–2. The temporal template used for the automated wave V detection in the ALGO1 automated auditory brainstem response device. The detection algorithm tests to see if amplitude values in a sliding temporal window (latency region for wave V and the following negative trough region with some tolerance) significantly exceed the residual noise levels. Created using data from "Automated and Conventional ABR Screening Techniques in High-Risk Infants," by J. T. Jacobson, C. A. Jacobson, and R. C. Spahr, 1990, *Journal of the American Academy of Audiology*, 1(4), pp. 187–195.

management capability in the recent ALGO 5. ALGO 3, for example, has been shown to complete screening in an average time of about 71 seconds with relatively low REFER results of about 5.7% (Murray et al., 2004). All ALGO screening systems have multiple components, including disposable earphones and electrodes, that are critical for performance and accuracy. ALGO devices screen for hearing loss in both ears simultaneously using alternating clicks presented at 30 to 35 dB nHL using a click rate of about 37 click/s. The choice of the level appears to aim at detecting a mild to moderate hearing loss. Remember that the click threshold correlates best with pure-tone thresholds in the 2000 to 4000 Hz region (Baldwin & Watkin, 2013; Gorga, Worthington, Reiland, Beauchaine, & Goldgar, 1985; Lu, Wu, Chang, & Lin, 2017; Van der Drift, Brocaar, & Van Zanten, 1987). The faster rate is used to make the test time shorter. The faster rate might produce some neural adaptation of the ABR because of the greater susceptibility of the maturing system to the faster stimulus rate in term and preterm infants. However, since the goal is to detect wave V and/or the following negative trough [SN10], this should not be a serious concern. The most recent models of ALGO screeners have been shown to have 100% clinical sensitivity and 97% to 100% clinical specificity (Stewart et al., 2000; van Straaten, Groote, & Oudesluys-Murphy, 1996). The automatic algorithm-driven decision of PASS means that the probability of the infant having normal hearing is 99.96%. The REFER decision occurs when the PASS criteria are not met.

An Overview of a Frequency Domain Statistical Approach to Automatic Response Detection

Here we describe another method that employs statistical analysis of the phase and spectral information contained in the response. Only a sustained response that is periodic or quasiperiodic like the ASSR or the envelope following response (EFR) will be amenable to a spectrum analysis using fast Fourier transform (FFT). The spectra of these sustained responses will contain a large peak at the fundamental frequency (corresponding to the inverse of the envelope periodicity) and five to six peaks, with increasingly smaller amplitudes, at integer multiples of the fundamental frequency. Stimuli with envelopes containing more rapid changes will produce more robust responses as they engage a broader cochlear region (John, Dimitrijevic, & Picton, 2002; Stürzebecher, Cebulla, & Pschirrer, 2001). Since the envelope of these stimuli deviates from being a simple sine wave, appreciable energy is introduced into the higher harmonics, thereby producing higher-amplitude response components at the higher harmonics. Once the FFT analysis is completed, both the phase information and the weighted spectral amplitudes (at the fundamental and the harmonics below 800 Hz) are subjected to a statistical analysis (modified Q-sample test) to detect the presence (PASS) of a response (Cebulla, Stürzebecher, & Elberling, 2006; Cebulla, Stürzebecher, Elberling, & Müller, 2007; Cebulla, Stürzebecher, & Wernecke, 2000; Stürzebecher, Cebulla, & Wernecke, 1999) above the noise floor (similar to finding a significant SNR to indicate the presence of response) or a response indistinguishable from the noise (REFER). The weighting of the spectral amplitudes by the mean amplitude of the spectral noise components in the adjacent bands (noise was estimated as the average of the noise estimates for 30 components below and 30 components above each response peak in the spectrum) improves detection, reduces the time of detection, and enhances the performance index (Cebulla et al., 2006). These authors also report that the inclusion of spectral information of multiple harmonics in addition to the fundamental frequency improves performance with respect to test time and reliability.

Hearing Screening Using Frequency-Domain Algorithms for A-ABR

This type of frequency-domain approach to automated response detection has been implemented in some A-ABR devices. MAICO, MB11 BERAphone (MAICO Diagnostics GmbH, Germany) uses the CE-chirp stimulus (with an option to choose the conventional click stimulus) presented at 35 dB nHL using a very rapid rate (92 clicks/s) thus achieving a faster test time (maximum test time 3 minutes). The use of this rapid rate generates a sustained periodic response (similar to the envelope following a response) that lends itself well to a frequency domain spectral analysis followed by a response detection statistical analysis (modified Q-sample test) that uses the phase and weighted spectral components of the response at the fundamental periodicity (92 Hz) and its harmonics below 800 Hz as described in the preceding paragraph (Cebulla et al., 2006, 2007; Stürzebecher et al., 1999). The MB11 BERAphone utilizes three steel reusable electrodes (adjustable noninverting vertex, inverting mastoid, and a ground electrode located between the two positioned closer to the temple) to record the electroencephalograph (EEG; no disposable adhesive electrodes are required), a soft earmuff, and a preamplifier, which are all incorporated into a compact device. Like the ALGO, test results are shown as "PASS" or "REFER." Unlike the ALGO devices where simultaneous binaural screening can be performed, the BERAphone is only capable of monaural testing. As described in Chapter 3, chirp stimuli (Figure 5–3), unlike clicks, elicit more robust responses due to greater neural synchrony resulting from the removal of cochlear delays associated with contributions from different cochlear regions to the click-elicited ABR (Cebulla & Elberling, 2010; Dau, Wegner, Mellert, & Kollmeier, 2000; Elberling, Don, Cebulla, & Stürzebecher, 2007).

Cebulla and Shehata-Deiler (2012) analyzed pre- and postdischarge screening results obtained from a large population (6,866 babies) of well babies screened over 5 years using the MB11 BERAphone. The results showed a predischarge pass rate of 96.2% (RR of 3.8%), with a median test time/ear of 28 s (range = 15–112 s). Of the 259 infants who failed the predischarge screening, 27.4% (71) passed the postdischarge screening bilaterally, and 72.6% (188) failed this screening in one or both ears. Thus, the overall pass rate was 97.3% with a referral rate of 2.8%. Subsequent diagnostic evaluation of all the referred babies (188) showed that 75% (141) had normal hearing (specificity of 97.9%), and 25% (47) had a hearing loss. None of the babies who passed screening had a hearing loss later, suggesting a sensitivity of 100%. Consistent with these findings, the authors concluded that this device provides a very effective and fast screening option. Importantly, they also report a mean age of hearing impairment identification of 2.15 months, a follow-up diagnostic evaluation starting at a mean age of 2.9 months, and intervention occurring at a mean age of 6.74 months. While a few other studies have reported similar results using this device, differences in methods used prevent direct comparisons.

An effective method to determine the sensitivity of screening devices is to investigate children who pass newborn screening and go on to develop a hearing loss much later or children with known hearing loss. Cebulla, Hofmann, and Shehata-Dieler (2014) did a follow-up analysis of results (targeted for 2 years postscreening) from questionnaires sent to parents of such children who passed newborn hearing screening using the MB11, BERAphone and showed that none of the children had permanent hearing loss 2 years after screening, suggesting 100% sensitivity of the

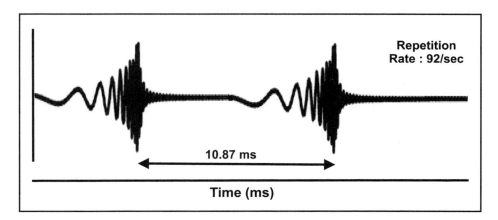

Figure 5–3. Broadband-optimized chirp stimuli presented at 92/s rate. The horizontal double arrow line represents the envelope periodicity of the stimulus (1/92 chirps/s = 10.87 ms).

measure. Kunze, Nickisch, Fuchs, and von Voss (2004), using the same screening device in children with known hearing impairment, did not find any hearing-impaired child in their subject group who passed the hearing screening, again suggesting that the screening test had 100% sensitivity. Similar high sensitivity using the MB11, BERAphone has been reported by Melagrana, Casale, Calevo, and Tarantino (2007), and van den Berg, Deiman, and van Straaten (2010). However, Stuart and Cobb (2014) noted that chirps might show a tendency to produce false-negative results (passing when a hearing loss is actually present) and affect threshold estimation in individuals with low- or high-frequency hearing loss due to the enhanced synchronization in other areas of the cochlea. Also, click correction factors to estimate effective hearing levels cannot be used with chirps. These authors suggest the need for further research to address these potential limitations of using chirp stimuli.

The efficiency of any automated response detection algorithm that is trying to reliably detect a very small response near threshold depends on the amount of background noise in the recorded EEG. Thus, to improve reliable response detection near threshold, care should be taken to record when the infant is relaxed and lying still or preferably asleep.

Is There an Advantage to the Integration of OAE and A-ABR Screening?

Recall that the OAE tests the functional integrity of the OHC subsystem, while the ABR provides a more complete assessment of the functional integrity of the outer and middle ear, cochlea (OHCs and IHCs), auditory nerve, and the brainstem including the midbrain.

Thus, these measures could provide complementary information if used strategically. The JCIH recommends that in the well-baby nursery, A-ABR screening should follow failure on an initial OAE screening. Since there is a concern about the greater risk of the A-ABR to miss mild hearing losses, this two-stage process presumably ensures that babies with mild to moderate hearing loss and auditory neuropathy are not missed when OAE is combined with A-ABR. It would be ideal if both steps are completed before discharge on all babies. However, the higher incidence of transient middle problems in NICU babies (Hunter, Prieve, Kei, & Sanford, 2013) might increase the referral rate for diagnostic evaluation. Also, the use of two different measures would add cost to resources and increase screening time. Several commercially available devices permit a combined automated OAE/A-ABR screening test. The advantage of the A-ABR, particularly in the high-risk group (cytomegalovirus, hyperbilirubinemia, sepsis, and gentamycin exposure) will be the ability to detect auditory neuropathy which has been reported to be the case in about 8% to 10% of infants and young children with permanent hearing (Foerst et al., 2006; Rance, 2005).

Hall (2006) reasons that the use of the combined approach provides more information about the nature of the hearing problem and increases test efficiency (faster and more accurate screening). Hall, Smith, and Popelka (2004) using a combined approach (DPOAE at 2000, 3000, 4000, and 5000 Hz elicited at moderate levels, and click ABRs at 35 dB nHL with a stimulus rate of 37/s obtained 13–42 hours after birth in the well-baby nursery) and an F_{SP} detection criterion of 3.2 or greater for PASS and less than 3.2 for REFER, found higher sensitivity and "acceptable" specificity for this approach. These authors also report that the pattern of the OAE and ABR results can differentiate between normal (both measures normal), mild conductive (OAE abnormal, ABR normal), cochlear (both abnormal), and neural (e.g., auditory neuropathy), where OAE is normal and ABR is abnormal. They also suggest that the low REFER rate using the combined approach reduces the need for follow-up diagnostic evaluation, thereby decreasing cost and reducing parental anxiety. However, the higher rates of OAE failures when babies are screened earlier, compared with A-ABRs, is still a serious limitation. Based on referral rates, cost analysis, and learning curves to improve the efficiency of both measures, Lemons et al. (2002) concluded that A-ABR is the preferred method for newborn hearing screening since its costs were lower, it had lower referral rates at discharge, and it was quicker to learn to administer it efficiently.

However, more recent reports evaluating the efficacy of the most commonly used two-stage OAE/A-ABR screening procedure raise *real and unexpected* concerns about the A-ABR's sensitivity to detect mild-to-moderate hearing losses. The practice of not performing the A-ABR when the baby in the well-baby nursery passes the OAE appears to be justified since it does not miss babies profiled for auditory neuropathy—less than 1% in the well-baby nursery show the pattern of A-ABR-Refer/OAE-Pass (Berg, Prieve, Serpanos, & Wheaton, 2011).

Does the A-ABR Fail to Identify Babies With Hearing Loss?

Since OAE screening can detect milder hearing losses (30–35 dB HL) compared to A-ABR screening (40–45 dB HL), it is possible that A-ABR may miss milder hearing losses in the 25 to 40 dB range. While most recent studies have reported high sensitivity, specificity, and the failure to see babies identified with a hearing loss later after initially passing A-ABR screening, there are a few published reports that suggest the presence of a later identified hearing loss in infants who failed the OAE and passed the A-ABR. Young, Reilly, and Burke (2011) found that about 33% of their pediatric cochlear implant recipients passed the newborn hearing screening. White et al. (2005) and Johnson et al. (2005) in a multisite study examined the efficacy of the OAE/A-ABR screening protocol. They evaluated a very large data set (86,634 infants) obtained from a two-stage OAE/A-ABR protocol. Of the total number, 1,524 infants who failed the OAE but passed the A-ABR were enrolled in the study. A diagnostic evaluation was performed on 64% (973 infants, 1,432 ears) of these infants at age 8 to 12 months. Twenty infants who passed the newborn A-ABR were found to have a permanent hearing loss (about 71% of these had a mild loss). They concluded that a typical two-stage OAE/A-ABR would pass nearly 23% of those with permanent hearing loss at age 8 to 12 months. A similar evaluation of the efficacy of the OAE and A-ABR screening results showed an even higher percentage (42%) of infants, who were later confirmed to have a hearing loss of 45 dB HL or greater, passed the 45 dB HL A-ABR screening after initial failure on OAE (Levit et al., 2015). Based on these results, Levit et al. (2015) suggest that an audiologic follow-up referral be made for all babies who have a Refer OAE/Pass A-ABR pattern on screening. They also suggest that a repeat of the TEOAE test at the age of 10 to 30 days may be a good alternative for second-stage screening to minimize this problem. Given the stability and reliability of the ABR, these findings may be more consistent with a delayed-onset permanent hearing loss. Unfortunately, it may not be possible for a differential diagnosis of neonatal and late-onset hearing loss (Minami et al., 2013; Norris et al., 2006). Levit et al. (2015), in trying to explain these unexpected findings, considered the possibility that their population may have had a greater number of babies with mild hearing loss that may have been missed by their use of a higher level (45 dB HL) for screening rather than the more commonly used level of 35 dB HL. Also, recall that the broadband stimuli used for A-ABR correlate best with pure-tone hearing thresholds in the 2000 to 4000 Hz region, so theoretically all infants with fragmentary normal hearing in this region could go undetected.

As we stated earlier, these results support the notion that most A-ABR devices are not designed to reliably identify responses at levels consistent with normal hearing levels. Thus, it is clear there is a need to improve the detection algorithms in these A-ABR devices, considering the use of multiple-channel recordings (e.g., the standard mastoid placement of the inverting electrode, plus another channel with an inverting electrode on the nape, which has been shown to provide larger wave V amplitude responses, therefore potentially improving detection of the response at levels closer to normal hearing levels) to improve the reliable detection of responses near normal levels. Cebulla et al (2014), using a frequency domain analysis of sustained periodic brainstem responses implemented in the BERAphone, reported that none of the babies who passed the screening had a hearing loss later, suggesting a sensitivity of 100%. These results could, at least in part, be due to the greater sensitivity of their detection algorithm. Given that this frequency-domain detection algorithm for sustained responses elicited by chirps is already implemented in several devices and appears to be performing well, it may be appropriate to consider the possibility of using multiple narrowband chirps to obtain frequency-specific information simultaneously for both ears (similar to the multifrequency ASSR). In the interim, these results suggest the need for continued monitoring of hearing status during early childhood. Collectively, the judicial use of a combined approach with an optimized time of testing before discharge using a two-stage screening program appears to be more beneficial, in terms of both sensitivity and specificity, compared to relying on just one measure alone. It may also be prudent to chart out a follow-up serial monitoring of hearing status, at least for high-risk babies, at some feasible periodicity postdischarge.

Stimulus Intensity Calibration Issues in Screening

The challenges associated with the calibration of brief stimuli described in Chapter 3 clearly apply to both screening and diagnostic electrophysiologic ABR measures. While the International Organization for Standardization (ISO) standard specifies reference threshold sound pressure levels (SPLs) and stimulus temporal characteristics, there is, unfortunately, no recognized calibration standard for stimuli used in the screening devices we have described. The problem is complicated by a lack of a reliable method to apply adult threshold values to infants, and a lack of standardization of stimuli, stimulus parameters, transducer type, and coupler type. Thus, effectively different stimulus spectra and levels may be presented across studies. Also, there is appreciable variability in the accuracy of using ABR to predict individual behavioral thresholds (McCreery et al., 2015). Given the lack of a standard, it is imperative that manufacturers of these devices provide reliable calibration information (that closely aligns with the ISO standard) and expected PASS/REFER rates for normal and hearing-impaired infants in the interim. Fortunately, there are several commercially available devices capable of performing in-the-ear calibration of stimulus intensity, which would then allow a more accurate specification of stimulus intensity in each ear screened.

JCIH Recommended Hearing Screening Protocol

Based on the very low prevalence of auditory neuropathy and the persistence of high loss to follow-up for babies in the well-baby nursery, the JCIH (2019) recommends a two-stage screening and rescreening with either OAE or A-ABR before discharge from hospital. If the baby does not pass the initial A-ABR screening, then rescreening should be done using A-ABR again because persistent transient middle ear problems may decrease the sensitivity of the OAE. Given the higher prevalence of elevated thresholds in babies in the NICU (Robertson, Howarth, Bork, & Dinu, 2009; Vohr et al., 2000) and their higher risk for auditory neuropathy, particularly for infants with hyperbilirubinemia and exposure to mycin-class antibiotics (Berg, Spitzer, Towers, Bartosiewicz, & Diamond, 2005), use of only A-ABR is recommended for screening and rescreening of NICU infants. The reasoning is that babies who do not pass the A-ABR can be immediately referred to an audiologist for rescreening, and if warranted, a complete diagnostic ABR can be performed. However, Wood, Davis, and Sutton (2013) pointed out that one pattern of results in NICU babies that has a strong association with delayed-onset hearing loss is the pattern of OAE failure and A-ABR PASS in both ears. Berg et al. (2005) recommended the use of an initial A-ABR followed by OAE screening. They believe that screening with both measures will ensure detection of both auditory neuropathy and a mild/moderate hearing loss. However, the JCIH's new recommendation takes into consideration the higher transient middle problem among high-risk infants in the NICU (Hunter et al., 2013), higher costs to implement and run a multiple test program, and increased screening time. Furthermore, they recommend continued surveillance of both hearing skills and language development in all individuals (with particular attention to high-risk individuals) through early childhood and up until entrance to kindergarten to identify mild progressive and late-onset hearing loss.

Postdischarge screening upon initial failure, for both groups, should be a single screening performed as soon as possible or within a month. Failure on this rescreening in one or both ears should immediately trigger a complete diagnostic ABR evaluation. Multiple screenings should be avoided as this delays prompt diagnosis and intervention (White, Nelson, & Munoz, 2016). An example of a protocol mostly consistent with the JCIH's new recommendation but with the addition of an OAE rescreen is shown in Figure 5–4.

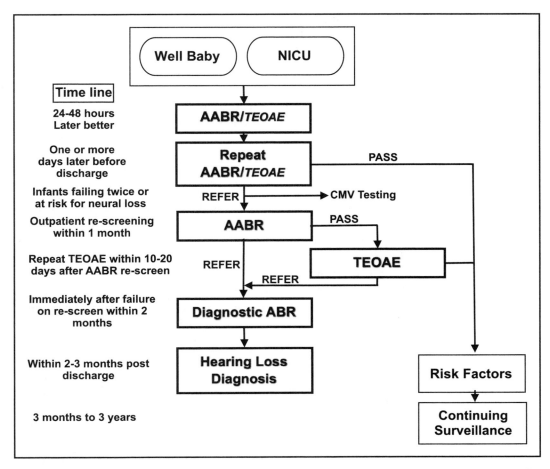

Figure 5–4. Example of a flowchart for a two-stage newborn hearing screening program for infants in both well-baby nursery and neonatal intensive care unit. The conditional decisions and time lines are shown.

II. FREQUENCY-SPECIFIC THRESHOLD ESTIMATION USING AUDITORY BRAINSTEM RESPONSES

As a logical follow-up to hearing screening, the JCIH recommends a diagnostic evaluation to confirm the presence and degree of hearing loss for babies who do not pass the two stages of newborn hearing screening. This diagnostic evaluation entails the use of an appropriate electrophysiologic measure (since behavioral measures are not possible) such as the ABR (or ASSR—description follows after consideration of the ABR first) using frequency-specific stimuli to accurately estimate hearing threshold before the baby is 2 to 3 months old. Since babies in this age range are likely to sleep longer, the ABR protocol can be completed during natural sleep. While every effort should be made to reduce delays, it may be necessary to delay evaluation in some babies who need other time-sensitive urgent care for medical problems.

Every effort should be made to begin intervention between the ages of 3 and 6 months. Information about frequency-specific hearing levels (type, degree, and configuration of hearing loss) is essential for optimal selection of hearing aids or to determine alternative management strategies (like consideration of cochlear implants for profound hearing losses). The ABR measure using frequency-specific stimuli is considered the gold standard for testing children under 6 months of age (Gorga et al., 2006). However, it should be noted here that the ABR is not a perceptual hearing test; therefore, any inferences about hearing ability should await results of behavioral tests that may be possible only when the child is older than 4 to 5 months of age. Since the use of frequency-specific stimului is recommended, we first provide an overview of the concepts of frequency and place specificity and how they are ensured while recording the ABR.

Frequency and Place Specificity

The specification for use of frequency-specific stimuli to elicit ABRs for threshold estimation is to ensure that the ABR thresholds reflect, like the pure-tone audiogram, the primary activity in the cochlea restricted to a place corresponding to the nominal frequency of the stimulus. The rationale is that a frequency-specific stimulus generates a place-specific response. Thus, frequency specificity (as described in Chapter 3) in this context refers to the narrowband spectrum of the stimulus; place specificity refers to the restricted cochlear place of primary activity contributing to the ABR in response to this stimulus. While broadband stimuli like clicks and chirps are optimal to generate the onset synchronized neural activity underlying the ABR due to their fast rise-fall times, they reflect activity along a broad portion of the cochlear partition and therefore are not place specific. However, there are effective methods to break down this broadband activity into frequency specific parts by *deriving narrowband contributions* (that reflect place-specific activation) using *high-pass masking* or *restricting activity contributing to the ABR to a narrow region around the stimulus frequency* by selectively removing contributions to the ABR from adjacent regions using *notched noise (NN) masking.*

Derived Narrowband Responses Using High-Pass Masking Noise on Click-Evoked ABRs

It has been well established that the auditory filter asymmetry favoring upward spread of excitation accounts for the observation that low-frequencies are better maskers of high frequencies (with the reverse not being true). Given that ABR responses to moderate intensity clicks represent a sum of contributions from different regions along the cochlear partition from base to apex (albeit the responses from the base are more synchronous and therefore have larger amplitudes), it should be possible to selectively eliminate high-frequency contributions in a systematic way using high-pass masking with successively lower high-pass cutoff frequency. That is, as the cutoff frequency of the masker is systematically lowered, more and more high-frequency contributions are progressively eliminated and increasingly only the cochlear apical regions contribute to the ABR. Consequently, the latency of the response also increases as the activity contributing to the response is increasingly restricted to the apical regions. This technique, first developed by Teas, Eldridge, and Davis (1962) to evaluate regional contributions to the click-evoked whole nerve action potential, was subsequently applied effectively to scalp-recorded click-elicited ABR by Don and Eggermont (1978) to derive narrowband contributions to the ABR— an attempt at obtaining place-specific responses. The high-pass masking technique (section A), its effects on the ABRs (section B), narrowband derivation (section C), and derived narrowband responses (section D) are illustrated in Figure 5–5. The procedure essentially consists of several steps: (a) ABRs are elicited by clicks presented alone at moderate intensity (the top box in section A shows that all cochlear regions contribute to the unmasked response shown at the top of section B); (b) subsequently, ABRs for the same clicks are obtained in the presence of broadband noise with noise level adjusted to produce both perceptual and electrophysiologic masking of the ABR so that no discernible response is present; (c) keeping the spectrum level of the noise the same, responses to clicks are obtained with the broadband noise high-pass filtered using steep filter rejection rates (at least 96 dB/octave) at successively lower cutoff frequencies (section B shows the cutoff frequencies of 8, 4, 2, 1, and 0.5 kHz). Note the spread of the masked region (in black) to the right, leaving increasingly smaller apical regions to contribute to the ABR. Thus, for each high-pass condition, the neuronal contribution from regions above the cutoff is eliminated from contributing to the response (remember the spread of masking is toward the higher frequencies). For example, the use of a 4-kHz HP noise would eliminate the

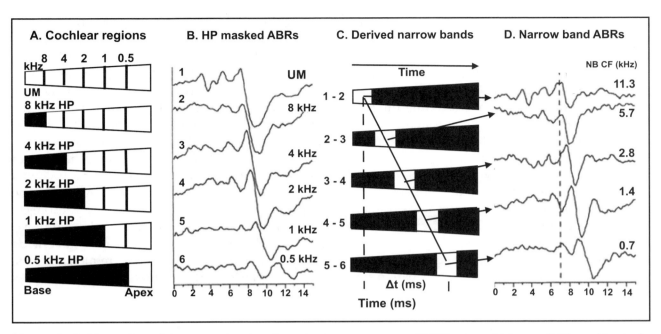

Figure 5–5. Derivation of the narrowband auditory brainstem response (ABR) using a high-pass (HP) masking technique. **A.** Top box depicts the cochlear regions contributing to the click ABR in the unmasked and in HP masking conditions with cutoff frequencies of 8, 4, 2, 1, and 0.5 kHz. Note that as the HP masking cutoff is decreased, the ABR responses are progressively restricted to increasingly more apical cochlear regions. **B.** Consistent with this, the HP masked ABRs showing the progressive delay in wave V latency prolongation, amplitude decrement, and loss of early components as the cochlear contributions are increasingly restricted to the apical cochlear region. **C.** The narrowband-derived regions obtained by pairwise subtraction of ABRs obtained in successive HP conditions. Also shown (C, *bottom*) is the amount of latency change in the response (Δt in ms) from a derived narrowband of 11.3 kHz to a derived narrowband of 0.7 kHz. **D.** The derived narrowband responses, which also exhibit latency prolongation as the center frequency of the derived band decreases from 11.3 to 0.7 kHz. Re-created using data from "Analysis of the Click-Evoked Brainstem Potentials in Humans Using High-Pass Noise Masking," by M. Don and J. J. Eggermont, 1978, *Journal of the Acoustical Society of America*, 63, pp. 1–20.

contribution to the ABR of cochlear regions 4 kHz and above. Consequently, the recorded ABR in this condition only represents summed activity from cochlear regions below about 4 kHz and therefore would have a longer latency compared to the 8-kHz HP masking condition, since the response region has shifted apically (see Figure 5–5, section B); and (d) once the HP masking step is completed, narrowband responses are derived by subtracting response pairs of ABRs from successive HP conditions as shown in section C of Figure 5–5. That is, 8 kHz HP ABR minus 4 kHz HP ABR, 4 kHz HP ABR minus 2 kHz HP ABR, 2 kHz HP ABR minus 1 kHz; and 1 kHz HP ABR minus 0.5 kHz HP ABR. The rationale is that this successive subtraction will yield a narrow band (between the two cutoff frequencies) of neural activity contributing to the ABR that is presumably unaffected by the noise. Thus, with subtractions of the paired conditions identified earlier, a series of derived narrowbands contributing to the ABR moving from base to apex can be realized as shown in section C. The resulting ABR waveforms from these derived narrowbands are shown in section D of the same figure. As expected, the latency of the derived ABR increases as the narrowband center frequency decreases. The narrowband center frequency is taken as the geometric mean of the two cutoff frequencies used for subtraction (that is, multiplying the two cutoff frequencies used for subtraction and then taking the square root, e.g., for 8- and 4-kHz cutoff, 8 × 4 = 32, square root of 32 = 5.7 kHz).

As shown in Figure 5–5, wave V latency shifts about 3 to 4 ms (due to both a traveling wave delay and receptor filtering delay) in going from a narrow band centered at 11.3 to 0.7 kHz. The broader distribution of latencies in the apical cochlear region likely accounts for the smaller amplitude and broader waveforms for the low-frequency narrowband-derived responses. While the validity of this method has been confirmed (Parker & Thornton, 1978b) and has been used to accurately estimate pure-tone thresholds (Don, Eggermont, & Brackmann, 1979; Oates & Stapells, 1997a, 1997b; Parker & Thornton, 1978a), it does not enjoy widespread clinical use to predict thresholds primarily because of longer acquisition and analysis time, and the successful use of frequency-specific tone bursts to accurately estimate hearing thresholds without any masking or response derivation steps.

Notched Noise Masking to Ensure Place Specificity of the ABR

Another simpler and more direct method of ensuring place specificity of the ABR is NN masking. The concern about the spread of spectral energy beyond the nominal frequency of the tone bursts (thus rendering the response less place-specific) prompted the consideration of recording tone burst ABRs in NN to ensure place specificity and therefore more accurate prediction of the behavioral threshold (Stapells et al., 1995). Although Stapells et al. (1995) have reported correlations ≥0.94 between the two measures at 500, 2000, and 4000 Hz using the NN technique, it is not in widespread clinical use. Unlike HP masking described in the previous section, the NN method does not require the use of multiple high-pass masking conditions followed by a narrowband derivation step. As the name implies, the NN masker is created by band-reject filtering (where the low-pass and the high-pass filter cutoff are the same) using a 1-octave-wide notch centered on the nominal frequency of the tone (see Figure 5–6) with high-pass and low-pass rejection slopes of 48 dB per octave and the noise level set to 20 dB below that of the tone at the center of the notch (Stapells, Picton, Durieux-Smith, Edwards, & Moran, 1990). Thus, as the frequency of the stimulus is changed, so is the notch location, which is always centered on the stimulus frequency. The rationale for this method is to prevent the signal energy in the sidebands (off-frequencies where hearing may be normal, e.g., low frequencies in the case of a sloping high-frequency loss) that

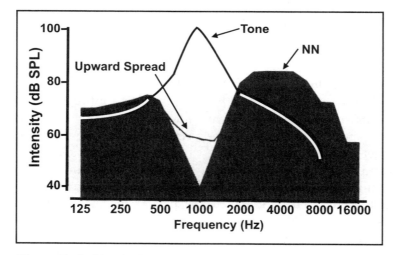

Figure 5–6. Notched noise masking. The notched noise spectrum (in solid black) and the 1000-Hz tone centered on the notch are identified. The upward spread of masking from the lower side of the notch into the notch area, effectively reducing the notch depth, is also identified. Re-created using template from "Brainstem Evoked Potentials to Tonepips in Notched Noise," by T. W. Picton, J. Ouellette, G. Hamel, and A. D. Smith, 1979, *Journal of Otolaryngology, 8*(4), pp. 289–314.

exceeds the hearing threshold to contribute to the ABR, thereby affecting threshold estimation at the test frequency (Picton, Ouellette, Hamel, & Smith, 1979; Stapells, Picton, & Durieux-Smith, 1994; Stapells, Picton, Perez-Abalo, Read, & Smith 1985). In other words, the masker energy outside the notch prevents off-frequency contribution to the ABR and ensures that the primary cochlear activity contributing to the ABR is limited to the place corresponding to the nominal frequency of the stimulus. Thus, using NN masking may improve the frequency specificity (and therefore the place specificity) of the tone burst ABR (Stapells & Oates, 1997). Using NN masking with varying NN center frequency, Oates and Purdy (2001) demonstrated that ABR wave V amplitude was greatest when the NN center frequency matched the nominal frequency of either a 500- or 2000-Hz tone burst evoked ABR at 90 dB peak-to-peak equivalent SPL, suggesting place specificity within an octave (Figure 5–7).

Several studies have shown that using this masking paradigm gives reliable threshold estimates (within 10–20 dB of behavioral thresholds) from 500 to 4000 Hz in most infants/young children, and adults with normal hearing and with hearing loss (Munnerley, Greville, Purdy, & Keith, 1991; Picton et al., 1979; Stapells, Gravel, & Martin, 1995; Stapells et al., 1985, 1990, 1994).

Notched noise masking has also been used with broadband clicks to isolate place-specific contributions to the ABR by placing the notch at different frequencies, like the derived narrowband responses using HP masking. Results from the few studies using this procedure have been equivocal (Pratt & Bleich, 1982; Stapells et al., 1985; van Zanten & Brocaar, 1984), with van Zanten and Brocaar (1984) reporting expected latency changes as the notch frequency was changed, while Pratt and Bleich (1982) and Pratt, Ben-Yitzhak, and Attias (1984) did not report any latency change. These

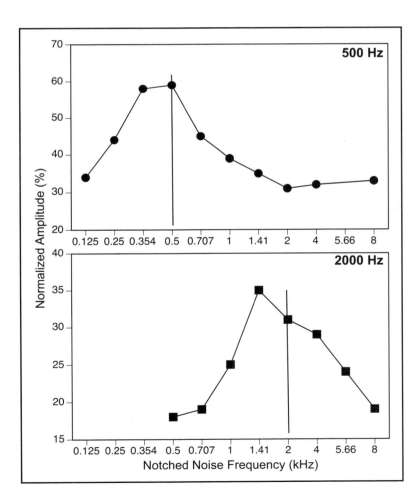

Figure 5–7. Mean auditory brainstem response wave V amplitude plotted as a function of notched noise center frequency for a 500-Hz tone burst (*top*) and a 2000-Hz tone burst (*bottom*) presented at 90 dB p-p peak equivalent SPL. Amplitude SD profile is plotted at the bottom of each mean amplitude profile. The vertical solid line is aligned at the tone burst frequencies of 500 and 2000 Hz. Note that for each frequency, maximal amplitude was proximal to the nominal frequency of the tone bursts. Data from "Frequency Specificity of Human Auditory Brainstem and Middle Latency Responses Using Notched Noise Masking," by P. Oates and S. Purdy, 2001, *Journal of the Acoustical Society of America*, *110*(2), Figures 4 and 5.

results led Pratt et al. (1984) to conclude that clicks in NN are not effective in estimating frequency-specific hearing thresholds. Also, Stapells et al. (1985) suggested that the amplitude of the ABRs elicited by clicks in NN were too small for reliable detection.

The clinical utility of the NN method with clicks or tone bursts is limited because both the poor response morphology (particularly at low frequencies) and the degraded response SNR (presumably due to the upward spread of masking into the notch region) make visual response detection more difficult unless automatic detection can be implemented to enhance response detection. Since the masking level is close to the click level in the click in NN method, the degradation of the response (due to upward spread of masking from the low side of the notch into the notch containing the stimulus) is greater compared to tone in NN because the noise is presented 20 dB SPL below the peak intensity of the tone. This tone to masker level difference allows for a discernible place-specific response since the potential for off-frequency contribution to the ABR is eliminated.

Estimation of the Air-Conduction Threshold Using ABRs Elicited by Frequency-Specific Tone Bursts

The JCIH (2019) recommends the use of frequency-specific stimuli to elicit ABRs or ASSRs. While the use of frequency-specific tone bursts to elicit ABRs would be the preferred method, it is not clear if just frequency-specific tone bursts (as opposed to a combination of clicks and low-frequency tone bursts) to estimate behavioral threshold are in widespread clinical use. Until recently, the more common approach was the combined use of clicks to represent the behavioral thresholds in the 2000 to 4000 Hz region (e.g., Gorga et al., 1985, 2006; van der Drift et al., 1987) and low-frequency tone bursts to estimate behavioral thresholds in the 250 to 500 Hz region. The use of the ABR measure using frequency-specific tone bursts is at present considered the gold standard, since it can provide accurate information about the type, degree, and configuration of hearing loss (Gorga et al., 2006; McCreery et al., 2015; Stapells, 2000; Purdy & Abbas, 2002).

Below, we present reasons why click-elicited ABR is still an indispensable part of the assessment. Emerging newer stimuli and measures are considered later in this chapter.

Several studies evaluating the relationship between tone burst elicited ABR and behavioral threshold for infants, children, and adults have confirmed that ABR thresholds accurately predict behavioral thresholds in children with normal hearing and children with hearing loss (Gorga et al., 2006; Lee, Jaw, Pan, Hsieh, & Hsu, 2008; McCreery et al., 2015; Sininger, Abdala, & Cone-Wesson, 1997; Stapells, 2000; Vander Werff, Prieve, & Georgantas, 2009). Earlier studies have also shown agreement between tone burst elicited ABR thresholds and behavioral thresholds (Kodera, Yamane, Yamada, & Suzuki, 1977; Munnerly et al., 1991; Suzuki, Hirai, & Horiuchi, 1977; Purdy & Abbas, 2002), suggesting that frequency-specific tone burst evoked ABR thresholds can be used to predict the magnitude and configuration of hearing loss.

Stapells' (2000) detailed meta-analysis of tone burst ABR results from 32 studies that included adults and children with normal hearing and sensorineural hearing loss revealed that ABR thresholds at 500, 1000, 2000, and 4000 Hz predicted behavioral thresholds to within 5 to 10 dB in approximately 95% of cases. They also showed that adults and infants with normal hearing showed similar thresholds; ABR threshold at 500 Hz was about 19 to 20 dB above the behavioral threshold at that frequency and this difference decreased with increasing frequency to about 11 to 15 dB at 4000 Hz. Sininger, Abdala, and Cone-Wesson (1997) showed similar trends but with smaller differences between ABR and behavioral thresholds (11 dB for adults, and 16.5 dB for infants/children at 500 Hz decreasing to 5 dB for adults and 6 dB for infants/children at 4000 Hz. Gorga et al. (2006) and McCreery et al. (2015) found an excellent correlation (>0.87) between ABR threshold (obtained under the age of 5 days) and behavioral thresholds (obtained about 6 months after the ABR) at 250, 1000, 2000, and 4000 Hz in normal-hearing and hearing-impaired young children and young adults (Figure 5–8). They found the difference between the ABR thresholds and pure-tone thresholds to be less than 20 dB for all frequencies tested. Besides, they reported a tendency for the ABR thresholds to overestimate

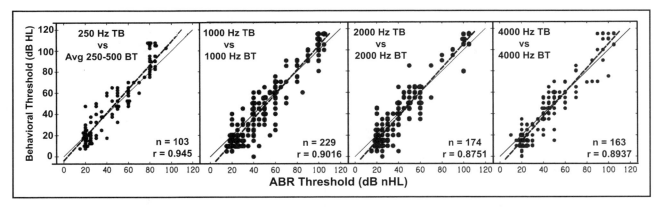

Figure 5–8. Behavioral thresholds (BTs) plotted against auditory brainstem response thresholds for frequencies 250, 1000, 2000, and 4000 Hz. The specific comparisons, number of observations (n), and correlations are provided within each panel. The solid thin line is a reference with a slope of 1. The dashed line represents a best-fit line to the data in each panel and has a slope greater than 1. From "The Impact of Degree of Hearing Loss on Auditory Brainstem Response Predictions of Behavioral Thresholds," by R. W. McCreery, J. Kaminski, K. Beauchaine, N. Lenzen, K. Simms, and M. P. Gorga, 2015, *Ear and Hearing, 36*(3), pp. 309–319.

behavioral thresholds (suggesting elevated threshold when hearing is normal) in normal-hearing individuals and underestimate (suggesting better hearing than behavioral threshold) behavioral thresholds in individuals with hearing loss. This discrepancy is likely caused by the differential effects of stimulus duration on primarily the behavioral threshold (presumably due to reduced temporal integration in hearing-impaired individuals), since the ABR is determined by onset synchronization. Thus, the application of the same correction factors for individuals with normal hearing and hearing loss may produce spurious threshold estimates. Gorga et al. (2006) suggest the use of a linear regression equation to more accurately predict behavioral thresholds.

The results from the above studies taken together suggest that ABRs elicited by frequency-specific tone bursts provide an accurate estimate of pure-tone thresholds across the typical audiometric frequency range. However, Gorga et al. (2006) observed that the differences between ABR and behavioral threshold depended on the degree of hearing loss as measured by behavioral thresholds. Specifically, ABR thresholds overestimate behavioral threshold in cases of normal hearing and underestimate behavioral threshold in cases of hearing loss. Since ABR estimates of behavioral thresholds are the primary information used to select hearing aids (Bagatto et al., 2010) in infants and young children, it is even more important that this estimate be accurate. Underestimation of the behavioral threshold may reduce the much-needed audibility of amplified speech, and overestimation could lead to an even more serious consequence of overamplification and possible noise-induced hearing damage (Macrae, 1994, 1995). To address this problem associated with the use of correction factors without regard to the degree of hearing loss, McCreery et al. (2015) evaluated the relationship between ABR and behavioral threshold as a function of the degree of hearing loss in infants and young children. As suspected, they observed that the difference between the ABR threshold and behavioral threshold varied with the degree of hearing loss (Figure 5–9). Similar to the observations in the Gorga et al. (2006) study, the ABR underestimated hearing loss in individuals with moderate or greater degrees of hearing loss. These authors demonstrated more accurate ABR prediction of behavioral thresholds using frequency-specific correction factors (see Table 5–1) that were based on the linear relationship between the ABR and behavioral threshold differences (i.e., taking into account the effects of degree of hearing loss on the ABR-behavioral threshold differences). Also, they found that the improvements in accuracy of predicted thresholds are greater for the more variable low-frequency responses and for greater degrees of hearing loss. As stated earlier, improvement in

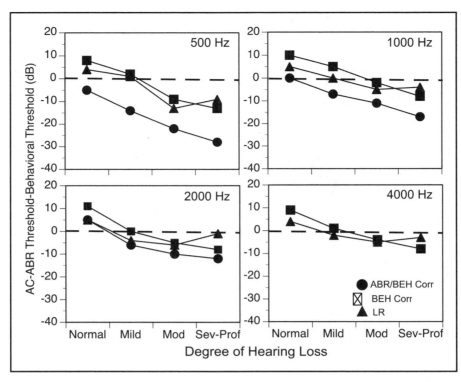

Figure 5–9. Mean air conduction auditory brainstem response (AC-ABR) behavioral threshold correction factors using three methods (ABR-behavioral correction [circles], behavioral correction [BEH, squares], and linear regression [LR, triangles]) plotted as a function of hearing loss category (normal, mild, moderate, severe-profound) for 500, 1000, 2000, and 4000 Hz. For all frequencies, the ABR-BEH threshold difference correction changed as the degree of loss increased, suggesting the need for hearing loss dependent correction factors. Data from "The Impact of Degree of Hearing Loss on Auditory Brainstem Response Predictions of Behavioral Thresholds," by R. W. McCreery, J. Kaminski, K. Beauchaine, N. Lenzen, K. Simms, and M. P. Gorga, 2015, *Ear and Hearing, 36*(3), pp. 309–319.

Table 5–1. Frequency-Dependent ABR t = Threshold Correction Factors as a Function of the Degree of Hearing Loss

Frequency (Hz)	Correction/Hearing Loss			
	20	40	60	80
500	5	−3	−7	−12
1000	5	3	0	−2
2000	5	2	−1	−4
4000	6	3	0	−3

Note: Correction factors to be subtracted from ABR threshold to predict behavioral threshold.

Source: Data from "The Impact of Degree of Hearing Loss on Auditory Brainstem Response Predictions of Behavioral Thresholds," by R. W. McCreery, J. Kaminski, K. Beauchaine, N. Lenzen, K. Simms, and M. P. Gorga, 2015, *Ear and Hearing, 36*(3), pp. 309–319, Table 4.

accuracy of estimating behavioral thresholds will improve hearing aid selection, particularly for children with moderate or greater severity of hearing loss. This approach also negates the underestimation of hearing thresholds (as much as 25 dB) that may lead to a lower gain selection. It should be noted here that the correction values shown in Table 5–1 for 500 Hz are estimates using the 250-Hz tone burst data from Gorga et al. (2006) and likely underestimate the needed correction factor at 500 Hz.

Overall, there is compelling evidence to support the clinical utility of tone burst elicited ABR in the estimation of hearing sensitivity in infants and young children with normal hearing and with hearing loss. For infants and young children displaying sensorineural hearing loss, tone burst ABR hearing threshold estimates range from 5 dB better to 5 dB poorer than the stimulus presentation level, depending on the stimulus presentation intensity and frequency.

Estimation of the Bone-Conduction Threshold Using ABRs Elicited by Frequency-Specific Tone Bursts

As in pure-tone audiometry, the difference in ABR air-conduction (AC-ABR) threshold and the ABR bone-conduction (BC-ABR) threshold (the air-bone gap, ABG) can be used to accurately quantify the magnitude of the conductive component and to differentiate normal versus impaired cochlear sensitivity in infants with conductive, mixed, or sensorineural hearing loss. Specifically, if the AC-ABR threshold is elevated in the presence of normal BC-ABR thresholds, then it points to a conductive hearing loss. If both AC-ABR and BC-ABR thresholds are elevated, it points to a sensorineural hearing loss. If ABR thresholds to bone-conduction stimuli are elevated, a sensorineural component is present. Given that elevated AC-ABR thresholds in young infants referred for diagnostic ABR are commonly due to a conductive hearing loss (Gravel, 2002), it is imperative that diagnostic ABR protocols include BC-ABR to determine if a conductive component is present. In addition to medical management of a detected conductive component, BC thresholds are essential to estimate additional hearing aid gain and output in the presence of a conductive component. While the inclusion of BC-ABR testing is not uniform in clinical practice, and likely underutilized, there is a considerable body of work over nearly three decades that validates its effective complementary role in objective threshold estimation (Campbell, Harris, Hendricks, & Sirimanna, 2004; Cobb & Stuart, 2016; Cone-Wesson, 1995; Cone-Wesson & Ramirez, 1997; Elsayed et al., 2015; Gorga, Kaminski, Beauchaine, & Bergman, 1993; Hatton, Janssen, & Stapells, 2012; Nousak & Stapells, 1992; Stapells & Ruben, 1989; Stuart & Yang, 1994; Vander Werff, Prieve, & Georgantas, 2009). The reliance on acoustic immittance tests alone is not sufficient to estimate the degree of hearing loss or to rule out a sensorineural hearing loss in the presence of a flat tympanogram. The JCIH (2007, 2019) guidelines also emphasize the need for BC-ABR testing to differentiate between conductive and sensorineural hearing loss.

Like AC-ABR, the same frequency-specific tone bursts are used to elicit BC-ABR to obtain place-specific responses. However, most published studies to date have been in infants with normal hearing and conductive hearing loss with testing limited to 500 and 2000 Hz. While there are no clearly established estimated hearing levels for BC-ABR to date, most clinicians continue to use 30 and 20 dB nHL as "normal" levels for 500- and 2000-Hz elicited BC-ABR, respectively—levels first suggested by Stapells and Ruben (1989) based on their results in infants with normal hearing and conductive hearing loss. Vander Werff, Prieve, and Georgantos (2009) reported similar mean thresholds at these two frequencies in their normal-hearing control group of infants. Also, they found that the absolute ABR threshold and the magnitude of the ABR-ABG could be used to accurately classify the type of hearing loss (conductive, mixed, or sensorineural); BC-ABR latencies were similar for the two groups, and AC-ABR latencies were longer for the conductive loss infants compared to the normal-hearing infants; and correlations between ABR and behavioral thresholds, were strong at all three test frequencies (500 Hz, $r = 0.86$; 2000 Hz, $r = 0.90$; and 4000 Hz, $r = 0.91$). These findings led them to conclude that it is clinically feasible to develop protocols for AC-ABR, BC-ABR, and behavioral thresholds that meet the guidelines for early intervention. More recently, Elsayed et al. (2015) evaluated normative thresholds and wave V latencies for click and tone burst elicited AC-ABR and BC-ABR in normal-hearing infants using tone bursts at frequencies between 500 and 4000 Hz. Median air-conduction hearing thresholds using tone burst ABR ranged from 0 to 20 dB nHL, depending on stimulus frequency. Median bone-conduction thresholds were 10 dB nHL across all frequencies, and median air-bone gaps were 0 dB across all frequencies. While these levels appear to be somewhat lower, they are well within the range of other earlier studies reviewed here.

Despite almost three decades of collective clinical experience in the use of BC-ABR in testing infants (albeit with somewhat sporadic application across clinics), to our knowledge, there is only one published report of a complete (as opposed to anecdotal report on clinical cases) study specifically evaluating the test performance of tone-elicited BC-ABR in infants in terms of its ability not only to identify conductive and sensorineural hearing loss but to accurately categorize them. Hatton, Janssen, and Stapells (2012) compared 500- and 2000-Hz tone burst elicited BC-ABR thresholds with follow-up behavioral thresholds in 108 infants with conductive or sensorineural hearing to determine if BC-ABR was sensitive enough to differentiate infants with conductive and sensorineural hearing loss and to determine if BC-ABR thresholds correlated well with the subsequently measured severity of sensorineural hearing loss behaviorally (Figure 5–10). They reported that for most infants, the BC-ABR obtained at normal levels of 20 dB nHL for 500 Hz and 30 dB nHL were sufficient to accurately differentiate normal-hearing infants from infants with conductive loss (normal BC-ABR, elevated AC-ABR) and sensorineural hearing loss (elevated BC-ABR and AC-ABR), with a sensitivity of 97% and a specificity of 100% at both 500 and 2000 Hz. Comparison of the BC-ABR responses at maximum BC outputs (50 dB nHL for 500 Hz, and 60 dB nHL for 2000 Hz) with behavioral follow-up thresholds in a subset of these infants with elevated BC-ABR indicated that the BC-ABR correctly categorized the functional status of the cochlea at 2000 Hz (with 92.8% accuracy) into normal 20 to 30 dB HL, mild-moderate 30–50 dB HL, and severe sensorineural hearing loss >50 dB HL). That is, if no BC-ABR is present at 60 dB nHL, then behavioral thresholds are greater than 65 dB HL. If BC-ABR is elevated but present between 35 and 50 dB nHL, then behavioral thresholds are 30 to 50 dB HL. The authors reported a similar accuracy (94.7%) for a limited data set at 500 Hz. Based on the observation of essentially no difference between the BC-ABR and the BC-behavioral threshold (and about 6.2 dB better BC-ABR than AC-behavioral) for the 2000-Hz stimulus, these authors propose a preliminary correction factor of 0 dB for the 2000-Hz BC-ABR (i.e., 40 dB nHL BC-ABR = 40 dB eHL BC-behavioral). Although their limited data at 500 Hz did not permit the determination of a reliable correction factor, a larger correction at this frequency will likely be required since BC-ABR threshold is 10 to 20 dB better than BC-behavioral thresholds in infants. It should be noted here that BC-ABR, typically obtained only when the AC thresholds are elevated, is limited to 500 and 2000 Hz, since normative data or normal levels are not available for 1000 and 4000 Hz.

While frequency-specific tone bursts are used successfully in research and clinical practice to estimate the behavioral thresholds in infants and young children, there is no real uniformity in the specification of the tone burst stimuli in terms of the temporal characteristics of the stimulus waveform, windowing function (linear, cosine squared, Blackman) used to achieve frequency specificity, calibration methods used to specify the stimulus output (dB pSPL versus dB peSPL) in dB nHL, and the reference equivalent threshold sound pressure levels (RETSPL). In fairness, major research/clinical institutions and national early hearing/infant hearing programs have developed their own sound methods using compelling clinical data that support their specific methods. Also, only recently has ISO provided recommendations for the RETSPL for tone bursts and clicks for insert earphones (and the B71 bone-conduction vibrator) using peak-to-peak equivalent SPL measurements (Table 5–2). With respect to the choice of different windowing functions being used, it may be argued that there is no convincing evidence that these different windowing functions produce different degrees of place specificity in the ABR (Oates & Stapells, 1997a, 1997b).

5. Clinical Applications of the ABR: Audiologic Applications for Hearing Screening and Threshold Estimation   105

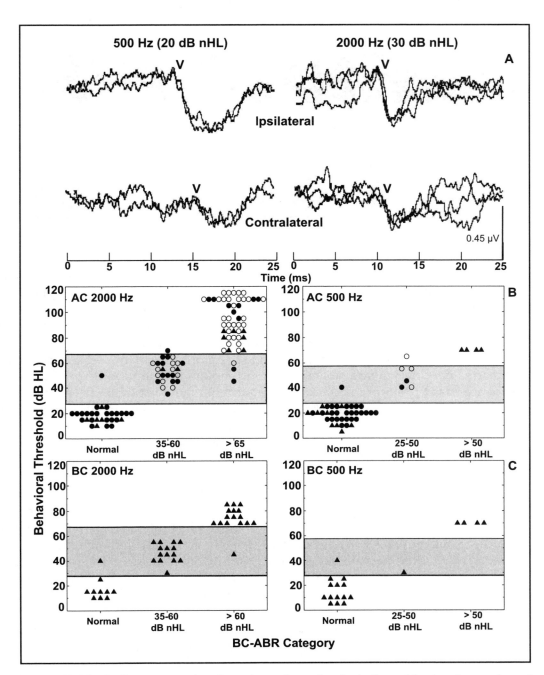

Figure 5–10. A. Superimposed replicated waveforms for the ipsilateral (*top*) and contralateral (*bottom*) montage using 500-Hz (*left*) and 2000-Hz bone-conducted stimuli. Note the shorter latency for the ipsilateral response, more readily apparent at 500 Hz, suggesting ipsilateral cochlear activity. **B** and **C.** The ways auditory brainstem response (ABR) is able to categorize degree of loss accurately for air conduction ABR and bone conduction ABR, respectively. Data from "Auditory Brainstem Responses to Bone-Conducted Brief Tones in Young Children With Conductive or Sensorineural Hearing Loss," by J. L. Hatton, R. M. Janssen, and D. R. Stapells, 2012, *International Journal of Otolaryngology, 2012*, pp. 1–12.

Table 5–2. Peak Equivalent Reference Equivalent Threshold Sound Pressure Levels (peRETSPL) for Tone Bursts and Clicks (ER3-A Tubal Insert Earphone) and RadioEar B71 Bone Oscillator (Tone Bursts and Clicks)

Transducer Type	Frequency (Hz)				
	500	1000	2000	4000	Clicks
ER3-A TIP					
ISO-389-6 (2007)	24	22	29	33	36
Stapells (2011)	25	23	28	30	38
RADIOEAR B71W					
Stapells (2011)	62	49	47	39	47

Note: Insert earphones: re 20 µPa; BC Oscillator: re 1 µN. RETSPL adjustment for 0 dB nHL.

However, the question does arise about the validity of simply relying on manufacturer-provided calibration values to perform clinical assessment since the accuracy of the threshold estimates depends on the specific stimulation and data acquisition methods used in each clinic. Thus, it is important to use in-house normative data, where available, to develop an evidence-based protocol to accurately estimate hearing thresholds that is transportable.

AC-ABR and BC-ABR Protocols for Threshold Estimation

In the clinic, ABRs in newborns or infants can be recorded to estimate AC and BC thresholds during their natural sleep (and at times when they are quiet and relaxed). This would be the ideal situation to record responses with optimal SNR (not contaminated by noise and artifact) and complete the test protocol in the short time window of about 35 to 50 minutes. The average sleep time for 80% of infants below the age of 4 months is about 49 minutes, allowing estimation of only four thresholds, and is only 33 minutes in the remaining 20% (Janssen, Usher, & Stapells, 2010). Thus, it is not surprising that a more complete ABR evaluation takes longer to complete than the natural sleep time.

Given the relatively short time window available, the development of ABR protocols for diagnostic evaluation should factor in data acquisition time and develop a protocol that is efficient and has the flexibility to make conditional decisions concerning the choice of stimulus and ear tested.

Sedation or anesthesia may be required to test some older infants to buy sufficient time to not only get clean responses but to be able to complete all planned diagnostic measures. However, sedation requires additional on-site medical resources and therefore adds to the cost and may still not last long enough to complete the protocol. Ideally, the protocol(s) should optimize the ability to detect the type and degree of hearing loss or obtain as much information as possible about the characteristics of the hearing loss. In the interest of promoting the development of a standard protocol and uniformity across clinics, we attempt here to present protocols for AC-ABR and BC-ABR that incorporate the combined clinical and research wisdom of recognized institutions (e.g., Boys Town National Research Hospital) and national organizations (Ontario Infant Hearing Program's [OIHP] ABR protocol; British Columbia Early Hearing Program's [BCEHP] ABR protocol) that developed and confirmed the clinical utility and validity of protocols for estimating minimum hearing levels in infants and young children. The specific protocol described next is a summary of the salient elements of the recently revised version (2018.01) of the rather comprehensive ABR threshold estimation protocol developed by the OIHP (2018).

Preliminary Considerations

Subject: To ensure that the child sleeps through or at least is in a relaxed state during testing, advise the parents to bring in a tired and hungry baby who can soon be put to sleep after feeding upon arrival in the clinic. A cursory otoscopic examination is recommended to determine if there is debris in the ear canal or any other abnormality that could invalidate the planned test. It is better to feed the child to induce sleep after placement of the electrodes. Ideally, testing should be done in a sound-treated booth or, in its absence, in a quiet room where ambient octave band noise levels are below 22 dB SPL at 500 Hz, 30 dB SPL at 1000 Hz, 35 dB SPL at 2000 Hz, and 45 dB SPL at 4000 Hz (BCEHP, 2012).

Electrode Placement and Recording Montage: Before placement, each electrode site should be gently scrubbed with an alcohol pad and cotton gauze strip to cleanse the skin of debris to reduce electrode impedance. A two-channel recording is recommended using electrodes placed as follows: midline on the high forehead at the hairline (noninverting electrode); one each on the lower portion of the ipsilateral and contralateral mastoid (inverting), and another electrode on the lateral forehead, about 2 to 3 centimeters from the noninverting electrode, to serve as the common ground. Electrode impedance at each electrode site should be less than 3 kilo-ohms and evenly balanced to optimize common-mode rejection that provides for better SNR. While a single high forehead to ipsilateral channel electrode configuration is sufficient for recording and analyzing AC-ABR, the recommendation for two channels is primarily required to compare the ipsilateral and contralateral BC-ABRs to infer the cochlea producing the response (wave V amplitude is greater and latency is shorter on the side ipsilateral to the stimulus compared to the contralateral side, particularly near threshold levels (Stapells, 2011). The theoretical basis for the inference of the responding cochlea based on latency and amplitude differences between ipsilateral and contralateral recordings is still not clear and not very convincing. One plausible explanation is that the bone oscillator imparts an effectively greater stimulus level to the cochlea on the ipsilateral cochlea compared to the contralateral cochlea, and/or the vibrational force is restricted to a segmental vibration proximal to the ipsilateral mastoid since the skull bones are not fused to optimally transfer the stimulus-elicited vibrations across the skull. In our opinion, the optimal method would be to isolate each ear using contralateral masking.

Stimuli: For AC-ABR, frequency-specific tone bursts using either a linear exact Blackman windowing function with a 2-1-2 cycle (two cycles of rise—one cycle plateau—two cycles of fall time) are recommended. For both AC-ABR and BC-ABR, testing at 2000 and 500 Hz is mandatory (when elevated AC thresholds mandate BC testing) with testing using 1000 and 4000 Hz conditional (see specific ABR protocol, later, for more details). Calibration of stimulus intensity should use the ISO-recommended decibel peak-to-peak equivalent (ppe) SPL to dB nHL to establish 0 dB nHL. These values are shown in Table 5–2. Both the BCEIP and the OIHP programs use this measurement based on Stapells' (2011) data. For AC-ABR, all stimuli are presented through insert earphones (Etymōtic, ER-3A), and for BC-ABR all stimuli are presented using the RadioEar, B70/71 bone oscillator. All stimuli are presented at a repetition rate of 39.1/s using alternating onset polarity. For BC-ABR, the bone oscillator should be placed on the mastoid process more superior and posterior to the canal opening and firmly held in place by a Velcro band or handheld with firm pressure (Small, Hatton, & Stapells, 2007). Binaural placement of the inserts is recommended while testing, as there is no real concern about the influence of the occlusion effect (Small et al., 2007), and it would be less disruptive in running the protocol. While the handheld approach provides flexibility, it also assumes some degree of training to achieve stable placement within and across tests. In our view, it would be preferable to adopt a standard repeatable procedure that uses a Velcro band.

Filter and Amplifier Gain Settings: For both AC-ABR and BC-ABR using tone bursts, the high-pass filter setting should be 30 Hz, and the low-pass filter setting should be 1500 Hz. For click ABR (described later), the low-pass filter setting should be increased to 3000 Hz to capture the cochlear microphonic. Amplifier gain of 100,000 or 150,000 is recommended. The artifact reject system and amplifier gain should be set so that approximately 5% to 10% of the sweeps are rejected during averaging. Some systems utilizing weighted averaging methods to improve SNR do not require artifact rejection.

Averaging: Responses are averaged over an analysis epoch of 25 to 26 ms for the tone burst and about 12 to 15 ms for clicks to be able to capture the delayed, slow and long duration response, particularly for the 500-Hz tone burst. Typically, split buffer averaging is utilized in most current systems that enable an online measure of residual noise (RN—subtraction of responses in each buffer [A-B]), response SNR, and the correlation between the responses in the two buffers. It is recommended that any split-buffer averaging be not less than 2,000 sweeps (so that there are 1,000 sweeps to each buffer) and not more than 4,000 sweeps. At least one replication of each response is recommended to evaluate repeatability. The recent application of automated response detection and average stop once a preset SNR is attained (Sininger, Hunter, Hayes, Roush, & Uhler, 2018) may reduce the number of averages required in the search stage, and thereby reduce test time.

ABR-AC and ABR-BC Threshold Estimation Procedure

Start With AC Threshold Estimates: Threshold estimation consists of both mandatory and conditional steps incorporated into a procedure that consists of search (using 20–30 dB steps) followed by bracketing (using 10-dB steps) to estimate threshold. Since 2000 Hz is considered the most important frequency in psychoacoustic measures and its proximity to speech frequencies, the threshold search is begun in the referred ear using the 2000-Hz tone burst and replicated using a starting level equal to the minimal level of 30 dB nHL (because most babies tested have normal hearing). If a clear, repeatable response well above the noise floor is present (RP), then this is taken as the threshold (TH), which will be ≤30 dB, that is a threshold within normal limits. The practice of obtaining responses at 10 dB above the minimum level, even when a clear response is present at the minimum level, to validate the minimum-level response (using amplitude and latency change) takes up valuable time and is not considered necessary. If the response is not clear at the minimum level, and therefore taken as inconclusive (INC), then two responses are obtained at a level 10 dB above the minimum level. If a response is present, then the 10-dB level is the upper bracket for threshold, and the threshold is between 30 and 40 dB nHL. Once you have the 2000-Hz threshold for one ear, the protocol calls for a switch to the opposite ear and repeat threshold search and bracketing at 2000 Hz to establish threshold in the other ear. This switching is to ensure that the most important information is obtained for both ears given the time constraints. If this ear also shows an RP at the minimum level at 2000 Hz, immediately test 4000 Hz at the minimum level (25 dB nHL). This is because 4000-Hz responses are robust and clear, so the threshold can be estimated rather quickly. This strategy is warranted to check for progressive high-frequency hearing losses that may be more common than previously thought. Once the testing is completed at 4000 Hz, switch to the opposite ear and complete threshold estimation for 4000 Hz. Now that there are threshold estimates at 2000 and 4000 Hz for both ears, testing can proceed to complete threshold estimation at 500 Hz for both ears. Ear switching typically occurs when RP is observed at the minimum level for each frequency (see example threshold level ABR waveforms for both ears in Figure 5–11).

Elevated AC Thresholds Trigger BC-ABR Threshold Estimates: If AC-ABR shows no response (NR) at the minimum level (30 dB nHL), obtain a response at 60 dB nHL and continue to 80 dB nHL. If there is still NR, obtain responses at the maximum output of the equipment. Since we are now beginning to suspect a significant hearing loss, it is important at this stage to determine the type of hearing loss. Therefore, the BC-ABR threshold estimate using the same steps described earlier for AC should be completed at 2 kHz starting at the minimum level (30 dB nHL). Remember that the BC maximum output is lower than the AC output. As mentioned earlier, there is no need to remove inserts while obtaining BC-ABR data, since the occlusion effect for this measure is negligible in young infants. If both AC-ABR and BC-ABR at 2000 Hz show elevated thresholds, switch to BC-ABR search and bracketing at 500 Hz (minimum level is 25 dB nHL) before shifting to 4000 Hz. If a conductive component is found at 2 kHz, it may not be necessary to obtain an accurate estimate of BC-ABR threshold at 500 Hz. If the BC-ABR threshold estimates at 2000 Hz reveals a conductive component, it is reasonable to expect the presence of a conductive component at 500 Hz; thus, confirmation by the BC-ABR threshold at 500 Hz may be redundant. However, the presence of a conductive component at 500 Hz cannot rule

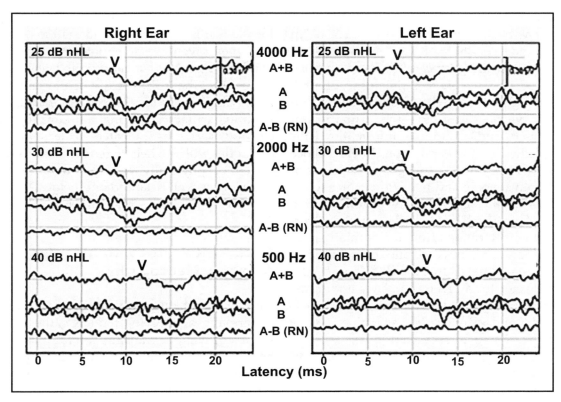

Figure 5–11. Auditory brainstem response waveforms for right ear (*left*) and left ear (*right*) at minimum levels at 4000, 2000, and 500 Hz. For each frequency and ear, the top is the average (A + B), the middle pair A and B, and the bottom trace (A − B) is used to estimate the residual noise. Adapted with permission from the Ministry of Children, Community and Social Services, Ontario Infant Hearing Program (OIHP), Protocol for Auditory Brainstem Response-Based Audiological Assessment (ABRA), Version 2018.01, 2018.

out a sensorineural component at 2000 Hz. If AC-ABR at 4000 Hz is the only frequency showing elevated thresholds, then BC-ABR threshold estimates for this frequency have to be obtained. ABR threshold estimates at 1000 Hz are only required if the difference between AC-ABR thresholds in dB nHL is 25 dB. Finally, a 5-dB final bracketing step size is recommended for ABR threshold estimates greater than 70-dB estimated hearing level (eHL). While this may satisfy the hearing loss–dependent changes in correction factors for estimating behavioral thresholds (McCreery et al., 2015) for thresholds above 70 dB eHL, the benefit-to-time cost ratio is minimal for threshold estimates below 70 dB eHL, since 5 dB steps may not produce changes that can be reliably detected. Therefore, bracketing using a 5-dB step to estimate the AC-ABR threshold above 70 dB nHL at 2000 and 4000 Hz should only be attempted if time permits upon completion of all other mandatory elements of the protocol.

Response Detection Criteria: The ABR protocol used by OHIP categorizes the outcome of the ABR test as ABR bracketed threshold (TH); response-positive (RP), no response (NR), and inconclusive response (INC). When RP and NR are separated by 10 dB, RP is considered the TH. An RP decision occurs when a clear negative deflection in the 6 to 20-ms time window, at least 50 nV in peak-trough amplitude of wave V is observed for a replicated 2,000 sweeps average. For an NR decision, needed are an RP at a 10-dB higher level as a reference and essentially flat replicated tracings of at least 1,000 sweeps at a level 10 dB below RP. Additionally, the residual noise (RN), derived from the A-B waveforms, should be no greater than half the amplitude of the smallest RP—that is, 25 nV. An

INC response falls between NR and RP where the response may be discernible but less than 50 nV in amplitude and closer to the RN.

Estimated Hearing Level (eHL): Once the tone burst evoked ABR threshold estimates in dB nHL are obtained, they have to be related to the audiometric behavioral threshold—the primary aim being to obtain "audiogram-like" information. This is accomplished by the expression dB eHL. Since there are differences in the threshold SPL between the electrophysiologic and behavioral thresholds, we need correction factors to convert from dB nHL to dB eHL. The dB eHL is derived by applying correction factors determined from the normative statistical relationships between tone burst ABR and VRA-based behavioral thresholds. The specific correction factor for a given frequency and transducer is based on the median difference in decibels between ABR and VRA thresholds obtained from a large group of young infants (Table 5–3).

Limitations of BC-ABR: While the BC-ABR is very useful in differentiating conductive and cochlear hearing loss, there are a few limitations that have to be pointed out. The main limitation of BC stimulation is the reduced output available (maximum 50 dB nHL at 500 Hz, and 60 dB nHL at 2000 and 4000 Hz) and the higher energy needed to elicit threshold level BC-ABR, which effectively reduces the range of intensities available for testing to about 25 to 30 dB. This, in turn, limits the degree of cochlear hearing loss that may be estimated with the BC-ABR. Stimulus artifacts are also observed at levels above 40 dB nHL and are particularly large for the 500 Hz longer duration (10 ms) stimulus. However, given the much later response latency window, this should not appreciably affect the ability to detect the ABR. The use of alternating polarity for threshold estimation can significantly reduce stimulus artifact. Also, making sure to keep the electrode leads (as indicated earlier, braiding the electrodes will also help to reduce artifacts) and the transducer physically well separated, and electrode impedances well balanced and below 3 kilo-ohms will help to minimize this problem.

Click ABR Protocol to Identify Auditory Neuropathy

Auditory neuropathy (AN) is a disorder that reflects abnormalities involving the IHCs, the IHC-nerve synapses, synaptic transmission to spiral ganglion neurons, and/or the temporal neural encoding of auditory information in the auditory nerve (therefore affecting the neural responses), without altering the sensory transduction and active gain mechanisms of the OHC subsystem; therefore, OAEs should be present (Moser & Starr, 2016; Rance & Starr, 2015). Given the loci and nature of the functional changes associated with AN, a more accurate nomenclature would be ***IHC/auditory nerve dysfunction or impairment***. The typical absence of any discernible neural response component likely reflects either a reduction in the number of neural

Table 5–3. Minimum Normal Threshold Levels, Correction Factors, and Effective Normal Hearing Levels for Tone Burst Elicited AC-ABR and BC-ABR

	AC-ABR				BC-ABR			
	Frequency (Hz)				Frequency (Hz)			
Measure	500	1000	2000	4000	500	1000	2000	4000
Minimum Hearing Level (db nHL)	40	35	30	25	25	30	25	25
Correction Factor (dB)	−15	−10	−5	0	0	0	−5	0
Effective Hearing Level (EHL)	25	25	25	25	25	30	20	25

Note: All values are drawn from ABR protocols developed by the Ontario Infant Hearing Program (OIHP, 2018).

elements and/or of poor temporal synchrony in the responding neural elements (unfortunately, the coinage auditory neuropathy is not consistent with either the description of the underlying pathology or the changes in the neuronal function observed). Since the incidence of AN is substantially higher in infants with permanent hearing loss, it is well justified to include in the protocol a measure to identify AN early. Evaluation to identify AN is mandatory if (after the tone burst threshold estimates have been completed) the 2000-Hz ABRs are absent or abnormal at high levels. It is likely that a second session may be needed to complete the AN assessment. Both the OAE (to assess OHC functional integrity) and a high-intensity click ABR (to assess the functional integrity of the auditory nerve and the brainstem) are currently the measures of choice for assessment of AN.

OAE tests have to be performed to confirm the presence of OAEs. Failing this, absence of ABRs alone does not automatically indicate AN. Then, ABRs should be obtained separately for rarefaction and condensation onset polarity at 90 dB nHL using a repetition rate of 21.1/s with the filter set to band-pass 100 to 3000 Hz. Note that with ABRs recorded with alternating polarity using systems with split-buffer averaging, responses to each polarity are saved in the split buffers (A and B) that can be accessed for evaluation. ABRs to each click polarity should be averaged using 2,000 sweeps. If no response is observed at 90 dB nHL, recording should be repeated at the maximum output of the system.

The aim is to show the presence of receptor potentials (cochlear microphonic [CM] and summating potential [SP], both presumably from the OHCs, although there is the possibility that IHC could also produce receptor potentials) and the absence of any discernible neural components in the ABR response elicited by the click. Click is the stimulus of choice because of its ability to produce robust synchronized responses from activation of a broad cochlear region. Although chirps have not been used to identify AN, they may be potentially useful since they have been shown to produce more synchronous and robust ABRs.

To determine the presence/absence of CM, the response to each onset polarity should be compared. To determine whether the observed response is a true biologic response and not a stimulus artifact (which overlaps the CM and follows the time course of the stimulus and inverts with the change in polarity), the response for each polarity is compared with responses obtained with the insert earphone tubing clamped. If the initially recorded response is a true biologic CM, it should be absent when the tubing is clamped. If the response persists with the tube clamped, then it is not a biologic response and instead is a stimulus artifact. This method is the only recognized and verified method for identifying AN (Starr, Picton, Sininger, Hood, & Berlin, 1996). It is possible to see a delayed wave V occasionally in some children at 90 dB nHL, which would be more consistent with a retrocochlear pathology distinct from ANSD. If there is an asymmetry in the threshold between the ears, the use of contralateral masking would be prudent to rule out a contralateralized response from the better ear.

Emergence of Narrowband Chirp Stimuli to Estimate AC-ABR and BC-ABR Thresholds

As described earlier, broadband chirp stimuli have been shown to elicit larger-amplitude wave V response compared to traditional click stimuli by optimizing the temporal synchronization of contributions from different portions of the cochlea through the elimination of the different delays associated with neural contributions from different cochlear locations (Cebulla & Elberling, 2010; Cebulla, Stürzebecher, Elberling & Muller, 2007; Dau et al., 2000; Stürzebecher, Cebulla, Elberling, & Berger, 2006). Recently, a few published studies comparing ABRs elicited by narrowband (NB) frequency-specific versions of chirp stimuli and tone burst stimuli have also observed larger-amplitude wave V responses to NB chirps compared to tone bursts (Cobb & Stuart, 2016; Dzulkarnain et al., 2018; Ferm, Lightfoot, & Stevens, 2013; Rodrigues, Ramos, & Lewis, 2013). For example, Rodrigues et al. (2013) and Ferm et al. (2013) reported that wave V amplitude to narrowband chirps was 26% to 74% larger compared to their tone burst counterparts. Cobb and Stuart (2016) found, in general, larger wave V amplitudes for the NB chirp stimuli for both AC-ABR and BC-ABR at 1000 and 4000 Hz (similar to Ferm et al., 2013) but not at 500 Hz (Ferm et al., 2013, did not test at 500 Hz). The authors speculate that the absence of the amplitude advantage for the NB chirp stimulus at 500 Hz may be due to a reduced number of active neurons resulting from the relatively narrow spectrum of the 500-Hz NB chirp. Also, for high intensities, Rodrigues et al. (2013) did not observe any amplitude advantage for the chirp stimuli presumably due to smearing resulting from the upward spread of excitation (Figure 5–12). Finally, Cobb and Stuart (2013) observed that the wave V amplitude advantage at 1000, 2000, and 4000 Hz for both AC-ABR, and BC-ABR persisted at levels near threshold (30 dB nHL), suggesting that NB chirp ABR hold promise for threshold estimation.

Given this wave V amplitude advantage, there is growing interest to evaluate whether NB chirp ABRs could provide a faster, more sensitive, and more accurate estimate of AC and BC thresholds in normal-hearing infants and infants with hearing loss (Cobb & Stuart, 2016; Eder et al., 2020; Ferm et al., 2013; Rodrigues, Ramos, & Lewis, 2013; Sininger et al., 2018; Xu, Cheng, & Yao, 2014; Zirn et al., 2014). There is growing evidence to suggest that NB chirp ABR can successfully be used to estimate auditory thresholds in normal-hearing infants and infants with hearing loss (Eder et al., 2020; Ferm et al., 2013; Rodrigues & Lewis, 2014; Sininger et al., 2018 [see the section on ASSR/ABR later in this chapter for more details); Xu et al., 2014; Zirn et al., 2014). Ferm et al. (2013) reported that the ABR threshold to NB chirp stimuli was 10 dB nHL better than the threshold estimated using tone burst ABR, and they proposed a 5 dB nHL correction factor for infants with normal hearing. The utility of NB chirp ABR to estimate hearing thresholds in infants is further reinforced by the findings of Xu et al. (2014) who reported that NB chirp ABR thresholds were within 3 to 5 dB of behavioral thresholds in infants with moderate hearing loss across the frequency range. Recently, Eder et al. (2020) reported that while initial reports look promising, further studies are needed to validate the frequency specificity of these NB chirp stimuli, the nature of the level and frequency dependence of the wave V amplitude advantage, and the sensitivity and specificity of the threshold estimates in infants with normal hearing and hearing loss. To replace the well-established current gold standard of using frequency-specific tone bursts to estimate hearing threshold, any new procedure should show unequivocally clear and substantial advantages in accuracy and shorter test time.

III. FREQUENCY-SPECIFIC THRESHOLD ESTIMATION USING THE BRAINSTEM AUDITORY STEADY-STATE RESPONSE (ASSR)

Unlike the ABR that represents neural activity synchronized to the abrupt onset of a brief stimulus, ASSR represents a sustained neural activity that is phase locked to either the envelope periodicity of an amplitude-modulated tone or the repetition frequency of a complex stimulus. Unlike the typical ABR recording protocol, ASSRs can be recorded simultaneously for multiple frequency-specific stimuli binaurally, and with automated frequency domain analysis followed by an optimal statistically based response detection method, making the test time significantly shorter compared to ABR. While the ABR is still considered the gold standard for estimating hearing thresholds in infants, the test time to complete a full ABR assessment exceeds the natural sleep time of a large majority of infants, thereby limiting clinical information gathered in a single session. There is growing evidence in support of the clinical utility of the sustained ASSR using improved stimuli and automatic detection algorithms (applied to both ASSR and ABR) that suggests that ASSR provides accurate frequency-specific estimates of hearing threshold in normal-hearing infants and infants with hearing loss in a significantly shorter time compared to the ABR (Cebulla & Stürzebecher, 2015; Cebulla, Lurz, & Shehata-Dieler, 2014; Eder et al., 2020; Rodrigues, Fichino, & Lewis (2010); Rodrigues & Lewis, 2014; Sininger et al., 2018; Venail, Artaud, Blanchet, Uziel, & Mondain, 2015).

ASSR studies, particularly the more recent ones that have utilized improved stimuli and response detection algorithms, have consistently reported short test times (as short as 19–25 minutes—less than the natural sleep time) to complete simultaneous binaural four frequency threshold estimates in infants/adults with normal hearing and

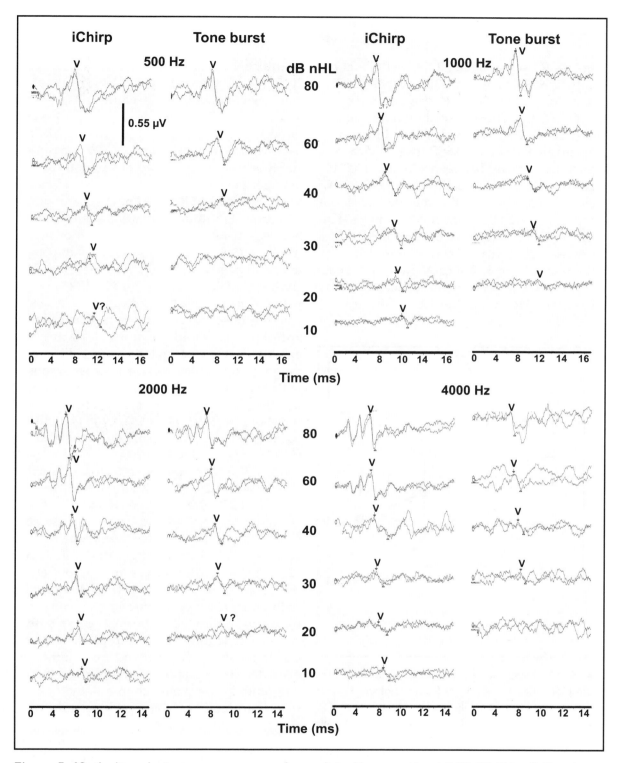

Figure 5–12. Auditory brainstem response waveforms elicited by narrowband (NB) CE-Chirp (*left*) and tone bursts (*right*) at 500 Hz (*top*) and 4000 Hz (*bottom*) at 80, 60, 40, and 20 dB nHL. The response latencies tend to be paradoxically shorter for the low-frequency narrowband chirps compared to the high-frequency narrowband chirps. This is artifactual in the sense that the 0-time reference here corresponds to the estimated arrival time of the 8000-Hz component at the tympanic membrane. Thus, the shorter latency for the low frequencies reflects their earlier arrival time. The consistently observed greater amplitude for the chirp stimuli (compared to clicks and tone bursts) is clearly evident upon comparison, particularly for the 4000-Hz stimuli. Data reprinted with permission from Dr. Delgado, Intelligent Hearing Systems.

hearing loss (Casey & Small, 2014; Cebulla et al., 2014; Cebulla & Stürzebecher, 2015; Eder et al., 2020; Michel & Jørgensen, 2017; Rodrigues & Lewis, 2014; Sininger et al., 2018). Also, it is promising that these newer studies, although fewer in number, report equivalent or better ASSR thresholds across the octave frequencies between 500 and 4000 Hz compared to ABR. This recent evidence is in sharp contrast to previous studies that reported questionable accuracy of the ASSR threshold estimates (Figure 5–13) and much higher ASSR threshold values (Cone-Wesson et al., 2002; Levi, Folsom, & Dobie, 1995; Lins et al., 1996; Rance & Rickards, 2002; Rance et al., 2005; Rance, Tomlin & Rickards, 2006; Rickards et al., 1994; Savio, Cárdenas, Pérez Abalo, González, & Valdés, 2001; Swanepoel & Ebrahim, 2009; Van Maanen & Stapells, 2009) relative to ABR and behavioral thresholds (Figure 5–14). Rodrigues and Lewis (2010) using tone-pips presented at a rapid rate and Michel and Jørgensen (2017) using narrowband chirps found closer agreement of ASSR with both ABR and behavioral thresholds. Sininger et al. (2018), used narrowband chirps for both ASSR and ABR and a "next-generation" ASSR detection algorithm (similar to Cebulla et al., 2006; Stürzebecher et al., 1999). This detection algorithm used F_{MP} (instead of F_{SP}) wherein multiple spaced temporal points were used to estimate the SNR. For clinical decision-making, an F_{MP} likelihood ratio value of 2.25 is used to indicate the presence of a true response. These authors reported that ASSR and ABR thresholds in normal-hearing infants exhibited strong correlations (see Figure 5–14) ranging from 0.769 to 0.963 across frequencies, with ASSR thresholds significantly better than ABR thresholds. Their observed average ASSR/ABR thresholds were 25 (SD = 6.9)/20.19 (4.8) dB nHL at 500 Hz; 16.0 (7.3)/13.1 (3.3) dB nHL at 1000 Hz; 7.8 (5.7)/10.1 (1.5) dB nHL at 2000 Hz; and 6.3 (6.8)/10 (0) dB nHL at 4000 Hz. The corrected ABR–ASSR difference was 14.39 dB at 500 Hz, 10.12 dB at 1000 Hz, 3.73 dB at 2000 Hz, and 3.67 dB at 4000 Hz, which is similar to the threshold values reported by one other study using the same technology (Rodrigues & Lewis, 2014). Their average test time for ABR was 32.15 (SD = 18.23) minutes and 19.93 (SD = 8.73) minutes for the ASSR, which tended to increase with an increase in hearing loss. Finally, this significantly improved performance for both measures in general, and ASSR in particular, is likely due to the use of narrowband chirp stimuli which elicit detectable responses at lower levels, and the substantial improvements in automatic response detection algorithms that enable accurate response detection at lower levels.

Several other studies have also shown better threshold estimates for ASSR compared to ABR (Eder et al., 2020; Han, Mo, Liu, Chen, & Huang, 2006; Michel & Jørgensen, 2017; Rodrigues, Lewis, & Fichino, 2010). Comparing NB chirp ABR and ASSR threshold estimates in children with severe or profound hearing loss, Eder et al. (2020) reported correlations ranging from 0.69 to 0.711 between the two measures at 1000, 2000, and 4000 Hz (correla-

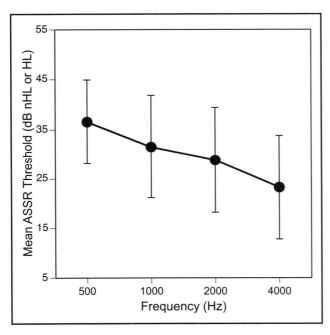

Figure 5–13. Mean auditory steady-state response threshold plotted as a function of frequency from several studies. Note the large variability in the mean thresholds. The newer studies using similar stimuli and intensity calibration show less variability. In addition, recent reports using newer detection algorithms and NB chirp stimuli show thresholds that are equal to or better than auditory brainstem response thresholds. Mean plot created with data presented in "Evaluation of Speed and Accuracy of Next-Generation Auditory Steady State Response and Auditory Brainstem Response Audiometry in Children With Normal Hearing and Hearing Loss," by Y. S. Sininger, L. L. Hunter, D. Hayes, P. A. Roush, and K. M. Uhler, 2018, *Ear and Hearing, 39*(6), pp. 1207–1223, Figure 11.

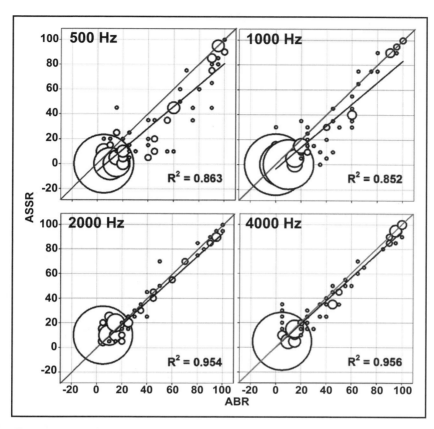

Figure 5–14. Bubble plots of the correlation between auditory brainstem response (ABR; x-axis) and auditory steady-state response (ASSR; y-axis) thresholds in dB eHL for 500, 1000 (*top*), 2000, and 4000 Hz (*bottom*). Scaled symbol size represents the number of subjects at a given intersection. The perfect fit diagonal is shown in gray, and the regression line fit to the data is shown in black. Overall, the plots show that the ABR thresholds are higher (poorer) than ASSR thresholds. The strength of correlation, R2 is shown in the lower right of each panel. The modified version of "Evaluation of Speed and Accuracy of Next-Generation Auditory Steady State Response and Auditory Brainstem Response Audiometry in Children With Normal Hearing and Hearing Loss," by Y. S. Sininger, L. L. Hunter, D. Hayes, P. A. Roush, and K. M. Uhler, 2018, *Ear and Hearing*, *39*(6), pp. 1207–1223, Figure 5.

tion was only 0.49 at 500 Hz). These correlations are much lower than the excellent correlations reported by several other studies in hearing-impaired children (Han et al., 2006; Michel & Jørgensen, 2017; Rodrigues & Lewis, 2010). Eder et al. (2020) also reported better thresholds for ASSR compared to ABR, in their group of 55 participants, with 22% of this group showing differences greater than 15 dB. Also, several studies have reported that ASSR was able to estimate threshold when ABR was unable to estimate threshold in children with profound hearing loss (Eder et al. 2020; Luts et al., 2004; Rodrigues & Lewis, 2010; Stueve & O'Rourke, 2003; Vander Werff, Brown, Gienapp, & Schmidt Clay, 2002), suggesting that ASSR may allow measurement of a greater degree of hearing loss and therefore residual hearing.

In summary, comparative evaluation of both ABR and ASSR using narrowband chirps and the newer more optimal automated signal detection algorithms suggests that both measures are excellent for accuracy of threshold prediction and test time for behavioral threshold prediction, which is reduced for both measures, but significantly shorter and well within the natural sleep window for the ASSR. The ASSR also has the potential to determine more accurately the magnitude of residual hearing in infants with severe to profound hearing loss, which might be useful for determining hearing aid prescription more accurately. More studies providing validation of these findings for the ASSR in both normal-hearing infants and infants with hearing loss are needed before widespread clinical use of ASSR. Any new measure and analysis technique considered to supplement or replace ABR for clinical objective estimation of frequency-specific hearing thresholds should be rigorously evaluated and independently validated for its ability to accurately predict behavioral hearing thresholds in a time-efficient manner in normal-hearing and hearing-impaired infants and young children across age groups. Although both ABR and ASSR show good correlation with behavioral thresholds, it is important to use behavioral testing to validate the electrophysiologic estimates of hearing as soon as possible given individual variability. It is equally important to have ongoing evaluations to monitor for progressive hearing loss in children with high risk for hearing loss and those using amplification devices.

IV. SUMMARY

- The primary purpose of hearing screening is the early identification of hearing loss. This allows for early audiologic evaluation to be completed to characterize the type and degree of hearing loss and enable appropriate intervention as early as possible to minimize the potential negative impact of auditory sensory deprivation on the acquisition of speech and language, academic achievement, and social and emotional development.

- The JCIH's revised guidelines (2007, 2019) on early hearing detection and intervention (EHDI) are focused to maximize linguistic and communicative competence and literacy development. Every U.S. state has established an EHDI program. The EHDI program strives to identify every child born with a permanent hearing loss before the age of 3 months and to provide timely and appropriate intervention services before 6 months of age. One major concern that affects hearing screening efficiency is the loss to follow-up.

- The need for hearing screening is amply justified because hearing impairment in infants and young children meets the criteria of sufficient *prevalence* and the possibility of producing *significant deficits* in speech, language, academic and emotional development; it is diagnosable, treatable, and/or effectively manageable; and there is a clear advantage to *early identification*.

- The JCIH (2007, 2019) guidelines recommend the use of either automated ***otoacoustic emissions (OAEs)*** and/or ***automated ABR (A-ABR)*** screening technology as acceptable methods for initial and rescreening of newborns. The best time for screening is closer to the time of discharge to minimize over-referrals due to transient hearing loss. Also, a single repeat screening is recommended if the infant does not pass initial screening before discharge.

- To improve the sensitivity of OAE screenings (to keep referral rates to below 4%), screening time should be later, use high frequencies (or DPOAEs), and use a 6 dB SNR pass criterion.

- Highly accurate time-domain, and more recently, frequency-domain response detection algorithms are utilized. However, it might still miss mild hearing loss. There is a need to improve response detection algorithms.

- Judicial use of a combined screening approach (OAE/A-ABR) with an optimized time of testing before discharge using a two-stage screening program appears to be more beneficial, in terms of both sensitivity and specificity.

- See Figure 5–4 for the hearing screening protocol.

- Diagnostic follow-up evaluation for infants not passing the screening should be completed before 2 to 3 months of age using ABRs elicited by frequency-specific tone burst (narrowband chirp is an emerging effective stimulus), and intervention should begin within 3 to 6 months—the earlier the better. There is growing evidence that ASSR could be an accurate, faster measure than ABR and has the potential of providing a more accurate estimate of residual hearing in infants and young children with profound hearing loss. Both of these measures provide an accurate estimate of behavioral threshold (to within 10–15 dB), and the correlation between the threshold estimates provided by these two measures is strong, with ASSR showing better thresholds than ABR in more recent studies that utilize more advanced automatic response detection algorithms.

- Both AC-ABR and BC-ABR should be used to estimate threshold, with BC only recommended if AC-ABR thresholds are elevated. It is recommended that providers use the threshold estimation strategy with the described preliminary considerations developed by OIHP and BCEHP. The protocol calls for a threshold search starting at the minimum hearing level at 2000 Hz with 20-dB increments if NR is present and a bracketing stage where levels are changed in 10-dB steps to approximate threshold. The sequence would be to switch to the other ear after determining the threshold in one ear and determine the threshold for the same frequency. The sequence of frequencies recommended is 2000, 4000, and then 500 Hz. A protocol including click-evoked ABR at high intensity using both rarefaction and condensation onset polarity and OAEs should be recorded in infants/young children identified with permanent hearing loss to confirm/rule out auditory neuropathy.

- Once the tone burst evoked ABR threshold estimates in dB nHL are obtained, they have to be related to the audiometric behavioral threshold. This is accomplished by the decibel estimated hearing level (dB eHL). See Table 5–3 for the correction factor at each frequency for this conversion.

- Comparative evaluation of both ABR and ASSR using narrowband chirps and the newer-generation automated signal detection algorithms suggests that both measures are excellent for the accuracy of threshold prediction and the test time for behavioral threshold prediction, which is reduced for both measures, but significantly shorter and well within the natural sleep window for the ASSR. The ASSR also has the potential to determine more accurately the magnitude of residual hearing in infants with severe to profound hearing loss, which might be useful for determining hearing aid prescription. More studies providing validation of these findings for the ASSR in both normal-hearing infants and infants with hearing loss are needed before widespread clinical use of ASSR.

REFERENCES

Akinpelu, O. V., Peleva, E., Funnell, W. R. J., & Daniel, S. J. (2014). Otoacoustic emissions in newborn hearing screening: A systematic review of the effects of different protocols on test outcomes. *International Journal of Pediatric Otorhinolaryngology, 78*, 711–717.

American Academy of Pediatrics, Joint Committee on Infant Hearing. (2007). Position statement: Principles and guidelines for early hearing detection and intervention programs. *Pediatrics, 12*(4), 898–921.

American Academy of Pediatrics Task Force on Newborn and Infant Hearing. (1999). Newborn and infant hearing loss: Detection and intervention (RE9846). *Pediatrics, 103*, 527–530.

Bagatto, M., Scollie, S. D., Hyde, M., & Seewald, R. (2010). Protocol for the provision of amplification within the Ontario infant hearing program. *International Journal of Audiology, 49*(Suppl. 1), S70–S79.

Baldwin, M., & Watkin, P. (2013). Predicting the degree of hearing loss using click auditory brainstem response in babies referred from newborn hearing screening. *Ear and Hearing, 34*(3), 361–369.

Bamford, J., Fortnum, H., Bristow, K., Smith, J., Vamvakas, G., Davies, L., . . . Hind, S. (2007). Current practice, accuracy, effectiveness, and cost-effectiveness of the school entry hearing screen. *Health Technology Assessment, 11* (32), 1–168.

Berg, A. L., Prieve, B. A., Serpanos, Y. C., & Wheaton, M. A. (2011). Hearing screening in a well-infant nursery: Profile of automated ABR-fail/OAE-pass. *Pediatrics, 127*(2), 269–275.

Berg, A. L., Spitzer, J. B., Towers, H. M., Bartosiewicz, C., & Diamond B. E. (2005). Newborn hearing screening in the NICU: Profile of failed auditory brainstem response/passed otoacoustic emission. *Pediatrics, 116*(4), 933–938.

British Columbia Early Hearing Program. (2012). *Audiology Assessment Protocol. v 4.1*. Retrieved from http://www.phsa.ca/Documents/bcehpaudiology assessmentprotocol.pdf

Campbell, P. E., Harris, C. M., Hendricks, S., & Sirimanna, T. (2004). Bone conduction auditory brainstem responses in infants. *Journal of Laryngology and Otology, 118*(2), 117–122.

Casey, K. A., & Small, S. A. (2014). Comparisons of auditory steady state response and behavioral air conduction and bone conduction thresholds for infants and adults with normal hearing. *Ear and Hearing, 35*, 423–439.

Cebulla, M., & Elberling, C. (2010). Auditory brain stem responses evoked by different chirps based on different delay models. *Journal of the American Academy of Audiology, 21*(7), 452–460.

Cebulla, M., Hofmann, S., & Shehata-Dieler, W. (2014). Sensitivity of ABR based newborn screening with the MB11 BERAphone. *International Journal of Pediatric Otorhinolaryngology, 78*(5), 756–761.

Cebulla, M., Lurz, H., & Shehata-Dieler, W. (2014). Evaluation of waveform, latency and amplitude values of chirp ABR in newborns. *International Journal of Pediatric Otorhinolaryngology, 78*(4), 631–636.

Cebulla, M., & Shehata-Dieler, W. (2012). ABR-based newborn hearing screening with MB11 BERAphone using an optimized chirp for acoustical stimulation. *International Journal of Pediatric Otorhinolaryngology, 76*, 536–543.

Cebulla, M., & Stürzebecher, E. (2015). Automated auditory response detection: Further improvement of the statistical test strategy by using progressive test steps of iteration. *International Journal of Audiology, 54*, 568–572.

Cebulla, M., Stürzebecher, E., & Elberling, C. (2006). Objective detection of auditory steady state responses: Comparison of one-sample and q-sample tests. *Journal of the American Academy of Audiology, 17*, 93–103.

Cebulla, M., Stürzebecher, E., Elberling, C., & Müller, J. (2007). New click-like stimuli for hearing testing. *Journal of the American Academy of Audiology, 18*(9), 725–738.

Cebulla, M., Stürzebecher, E., & Wernecke, K. D. (2000). Objective detection of auditory brainstem potentials: Comparison of statistical tests in the time and frequency domains. *Scandinavian Audiology, 29*(1), 44–51.

Centers for Disease Control and Prevention. *Summary of 2012 National CDC EHDI data*. Retrieved from https://www.cdc.gov/ncbddd/hearingloss/2012-data/2012_ehdi_hsfs_summary_b.pdf

Cobb, K. M., & Stuart, A. (2016). Neonate auditory brainstem responses to CE-chirp and CE-chirp octave band stimuli I: Versus click and tone burst stimuli. *Ear and Hearing, 37*(6), 710–723.

Cone-Wesson, B. (1995). Bone-conduction ABR tests. *American Journal of Audiology, 4*, 14–19.

Cone-Wesson, B., & Ramirez, G. M. (1997). Hearing sensitivity in newborns estimated from ABRs to bone-conducted sounds. *Journal of the American Academy of Audiology, 8*(5), 299–307.

Cone-Wesson, B., Rickards, F., Poulis, C., Parker, J., Tan, L., & Pollard, J. (2002). The auditory steady-state response: Clinical observations and applications in infants and children. *Journal of American Academy of Audiology, 13*, 270–282.

Dau, T., Wegner, O., Mellert, V, & Kollmeier, B. (2000). Auditory brainstem responses with optimized chirp signals compensating basilar-membrane dispersion. *Journal of the Acoustical Society of America, 107*(3), 1530–1540.

Don, M., & Eggermont, J. J. (1978). Analysis of the click-evoked brainstem potentials in humans using high-pass noise masking. *Journal of the Acoustical Society of America, 63*, 1–20.

Don, M., Eggermont, J. J., & Brackmann, D. E. (1979). Reconstruction of the audiogram using brainstem responses and high-pass noise masking. *Annals of Otology, Rhinology, and Laryngology, Supplement, 88*(3), 1–20.

Dzulkarnain, A. A. A., Abdullah, S. A., Ruzai, M. A. M., Ibrahim, S. H. M. N., Anuar, N. F. A., & Rahim, A. E. A. (2018). Effects of different electrode configurations on the narrow band level-specific CE-chirp and tone burst auditory brainstem response at multiple intensity levels and frequencies in subjects with normal hearing. *American Journal of Audiology, 27*(3), 294–305.

Eder, K., Schuster, M. E., Polterauer, D., Neuling, M., Hoster, E., Hempel, J-M., & Semmelbauer, S. (2020). Comparison of ABR and ASSR using NB-chirp-stimuli in children with severe and profound hearing loss. *International Journal of Pediatric Otorhinolaryngology, 131*, 109864.

Elberling, C., Don, M., Cebulla, M., & Stürzebecher, E. (2007). Auditory steady-state responses to chirp stimuli based on cochlear traveling wave delay. *Journal of the Acoustical Society of America, 122*, 2772–2785.

Elsayed, A. M., Hunter, L. L., Keefe, D. H., Feeney, P. M., Brown, D. K., Meinzen-Derr, J. K., . . . Schaid, L. G. (2015). Air and bone conduction click and toneburst auditory brainstem thresholds using Kalman adaptive processing in nonsedated normal-hearing infants. *Ear and Hearing, 36*(4), 471–481.

Ferm, I., Lightfoot, G., & Stevens, J. (2013). Comparison of ABR response amplitude, test time, and estimation of hearing threshold using frequency specific chirp and tone pip stimuli in newborns. *International Journal of Audiology, 52*(6), 419–423.

Foerst, A., Beutner, D., Lang-Roth, R., Huttenbrink, K. B., von Wedel, H., & Walger, M. (2006). Prevalence of auditory neuropathy/synaptopathy in a population of children with profound hearing loss. *International Journal of Pediatric Otorhinolaryngology, 71*, 1415–1422.

Gorga, M. P., Johnson, T. A., Kaminski, J. R., Beauchaine, K. L., Garner, C. A., & Neely, S. T. (2006). Using a combination of click- and tone burst-evoked auditory brain stem response measurements to estimate pure-tone thresholds. *Ear and Hearing, 27*(1), 60–74.

Gorga, M., Kaminski, J., Beauchaine, E. K., & Bergman, B. (1993). A comparison of auditory brain stem response thresholds and latencies elicited by air- and bone-conducted stimuli. *Ear and Hearing, 14*(2), 85–94.

Gorga, M. P., Worthington, D. W., Reiland, J. K., Beauchaine, K. A., & Goldgar, D. E. (1985). Some comparisons between auditory brain stem response thresholds, latencies, and the pure-tone audiogram. *Ear and Hearing, 6*, 105–112.

Gravel, J. S. (2002). Potential pitfalls in the audiological assessment of infants and young children. In R. C. Seewald & J. S. Gravel (Eds.), *Foundation through early amplification and proceedings of the second international conference* (pp. 85–101). Stafa, Switzerland: Phonak AG.

Hall, J. W. (2006). ABR: Pediatric clinical applications and populations. In J. W. Hall III (Ed.), *New handbook of auditory evoked potentials* (pp. 313–365). Boston, MA: Allyn & Bacon.

Hall, J. W. III., Smith, S. D., & Popelka, G. R. (2004). Newborn hearing screening with combined otoacoustic emissions and auditory brainstem responses. *Journal of the American Academy of Audiology, 15*, 414–425.

Han, D., Mo, L., Liu, H., Chen, J., & Huang, L. (2006). Threshold estimation in children using auditory steady-state responses to multiple simultaneous stimuli. *ORL: Journal for Otorhinolaryngology and Its Related Specialties, 68*(2), 64–68.

Hatton, J. L., Janssen, R. M., & Stapells, D. R. (2012). Auditory brainstem responses to bone-conducted brief tones in young children with conductive or sensorineural hearing loss. *International Journal of Otolaryngology, 2012*, 1–12. https://doi.org/10.1155/2012/284864

Hermann, B. S., Thornton, A. R., & Joseph, J. M. (1995). Automated infant hearing screening using the ABR: Development and validation. *American Journal of Audiology, 4*, 6–14.

Hunter, L. L., Meinzen-Derr, J., Wiley, S., Horvath, C. L., Kothari, R., & Wexelblatt, S. (2016). Influence of the WIC program on loss to follow-up for newborn hearing screening. *Pediatrics, 138*, 1–8.

Hunter, L. L., Prieve, B. A., Kei, J., & Sanford, C. A. (2013). Pediatric applications of wideband acoustic immittance measures. *Ear and Hearing, 34*(Suppl. 1), 36S–42S.

Jacobson, J. T., Jacobson, C. A., & Spahr, R. C. (1990). Automated and conventional ABR screening techniques in high-risk infants. *Journal of the American Academy of Audiology, 1*(4), 187–195.

Janssen, R. M., Usher, L., & Stapells, D. R. (2010). The British Columbia's Children's Hospital tone-evoked auditory brainstem response protocol: How long do infants sleep and how much information can be obtained in one appointment? *Ear and Hearing, 31*, 722–724.

John, M. S., Dimitrijevic, A., & Picton, T. W. (2002). Auditory steady-state responses to exponential modulation envelopes. *Ear and Hearing, 23*, 106–117.

Johnson, J. L., White, K. R., Widen, J. E., Gravel, J. S., James, M., Kennalley, T., . . . Holstrum, J. (2005). A multicenter evaluation of how many infants with permanent hearing loss pass a two-stage otoacoustic emissions/automated auditory brainstem response newborn hearing screening protocol. *Pediatrics, 116*(3), 663–672.

Johnson, L. C., Toro, M., Vishnja, E., Berish, A., Mills, B., Lu, Z., & Lieberman, E. (2018). Age and other factors affecting the outcome of A-ABR screening in neonates. *Hospital Pediatrics, 8*(3), 141–147.

Joint Committee on Infant Hearing. (2000). Year 2000 position statement: Principles and guidelines for early hearing detection and intervention programs. *American Journal of Audiology, 9*, 9–29.

Joint Committee on Infant Hearing. (2007). Year 2007 position statement: Principles and guidelines for early hearing detection and intervention programs. *Pediatrics, 120*(4), 898–921.

Joint Committee on Infant Hearing. (2019). Year 2019 position statement: Principles and guidelines for early hearing detection and intervention programs. *Journal of Early Hearing Detection and Intervention, 4*(2), 1–44.

Kileny, P. R. (1987). ALGO-1 automated infant screener: Preliminary results. *Seminars in Hearing, 8*, 125–131.

Kodera, K., Yamane, H., Yamada, O., & Suzuki, J. I. (1977). Brain stem response audiometry at speech frequencies. *Audiology, 16,* 469–479.

Kunze, A., Nickisch, A., Fuchs, M., & von Voss, H. (2004). Bestimmung der Sensitivitäteines Horscreeninggerats (BERAphon1 MB 11) an einer Gruppe hörgeschädigter Kinder. In *International Conference on Newborn Hearing Screening, Diagnosis and Intervention,* Italy.

Lee, C.-Y., Jaw, F.-S., Pan, S.-L., Hsieh, T. H., & Hsu, C.-J. (2008). Effects of age and degree of hearing loss on the agreement and correlation between sound field audiometric thresholds and tone burst auditory brainstem response thresholds in infants and young children. *Journal of Formosa Medical Association, 107*(11), 869–875.

Lemons, J., Fanarhoff, A., Stewart, E., Bantkover, J., Murray, G., & Diefendorf, A. (2002). Newborn hearing screening: Cost of establishing a program. *Journal of Perinatology, 22,* 120–124.

Levi, E. C., Folsom, R. C., & Dobie, R. A. (1995). Coherence analysis of envelope-following responses (EFRs) and frequency-following responses (FFRs) in infants and adults. *Hearing Research, 89,* 21–27.

Levit, Y., Himmelfarb, M., & Dollberg, S. (2015). Sensitivity of the automated auditory brainstem response in neonatal hearing screening. *Pediatrics, 136*(3), e641–e647.

Lins, O. G., Picton, T. W., Boucher, B. L., Durieux-Smith, A., Champagne, S. C., Moran, L. M., . . . Savio, G. (1996). Frequency-specific audiometry using steady-state responses. *Ear and Hearing, 17,* 81–96.

Liu, C. L., Farrell, J., MacNeil, J. R., Stone, S., & Barfield, W. (2008). Evaluating loss to follow-up in Massachusetts. *Pediatrics, 121*(2), e335.

Lu, T.-M., Wu, F.-W., Chang, H., & Lin, H.-C. (2017). Using click-evoked auditory brainstem response thresholds in infants to estimate the corresponding pure-tone audiometry thresholds in children referred from UNHS. *International Journal of Pediatric Otorhinolaryngology, 95,* 57–62.

Luts, H., Desloovere, C., Kumar, A., Vandermeersch, E., & Wouters, J. (2004). Objective assessment of frequency-specific hearing thresholds in babies. *International Journal of Pediatric Otorhinolaryngology, 68*(7), 915–926.

Macrae, J. H. (1994). An investigation of temporary threshold shift caused by hearing aid use. *Journal of Speech and Hearing Research, 37,* 227–237.

Macrae, J. H. (1995). Temporary and permanent threshold shift caused by hearing aid use. *Journal of Speech, Language, and Hearing Research, 38*(4), 949–959.

McCreery, R. W., Kaminski, J., Beauchaine, K., Lenzen, N., Simms, K., & Gorga, M. P. (2015). The impact of degree of hearing loss on auditory brainstem response predictions of behavioral thresholds. *Ear and Hearing, 36*(3), 309–319.

Melagrana, A., Casale, S., Calevo, M. G., & Tarantino, B. (2007). MB11 BERAphone and auditory brainstem response in newborns at audiologic risk: Comparison of results. *International Journal of Pediatric Otorhinolaryngology, 71,* 1175–1180.

Michel, F., & Jørgensen, K. F. (2017). Comparison of threshold estimation in infants with hearing loss or normal hearing using auditory steady state response evoked by narrow band CE-chirps and auditory brainstem response evoked by tone pips. *International Journal of Audiology, 56,* 99–105.

Minami, S. B., Mutai, H., Nakano, A., Arimoto, Y., Taiji, H., Morimoto, N., . . . Matsunaga, T. (2013). GJB2-associated hearing loss undetected by hearing screening of newborns. *Genetics, 532*(1), 41–45.

Moeller, M. P. (2000). Early intervention and language development in children who are deaf and hard of hearing. *Pediatrics, 106*(3), e43.

Moser, T., & Starr, A. (2016). Auditory neuropathy—Neural and synaptic mechanisms. *Nature Reviews/Neurology, 12*(3), 135–149.

Munnerley, G. M., Greville, K. A., Purdy, S. C., & Keith, W. J. (1991). Frequency-specific auditory brainstem responses relationship to behavioral thresholds in cochlear-impaired adults. *Audiology, 30,* 25–32.

Murray, G., Ormson, M. C., Loh, M. H. L., Ninan, B., Ninan, D., Dockery, L., & Fanaroff, A. A. (2004). Evaluation of the Natus ALGO 3 Newborn Hearing Screener. *Journal of Obstetric, Gynecologic, and Neonatal Nursing, 22*(2), 183–190.

National Institutes of Health. (1993). Early identification of hearing impairment in infants and young children. *NIH Consensus Statement, 11*(1), 1–24.

Nelson, H. D., Bougatsos, C., & Nygren, P. (2008). Universal newborn hearing screening: Systematic review to update the 2001 U.S. Preventative Service Task Force Recommendation. *Pediatrics, 122,* e266–e277.

Norris, V. W., Arnos, K. S., Hanks, W. D., Xia, X., Nance, W. E., & Pandya, A. (2006). Does universal newborn hearing screening identify all children with GJB2 (Connexin 26) deafness? Penetrance of GJB2 deafness. *Ear and Hearing, 27*(6), 732–741.

Norton, S. J., Gorga, M. P., Widen, J. E., Folsom, R., Sininger, Y., Cone-Wesson, B., . . . Fletcher, K. A. (2000a). Identification of neonatal hearing impairment: evaluation of transient otoacoustic emission, distortion product otoacoustic emission, and auditory brainstem response test performance. *Ear and Hearing, 21,* 5, 508–528.

Norton, S. J., Gorga, M. P., Widen, J. E., Folsom, R., Sininger, Y., Cone-Wesson, B., . . . Fletcher, K. A. (2000b). Identification of neonatal hearing impairment: Summary and recommendations. *Ear and Hearing, 21,* 529–535.

Nousak, J. M. K., & Stapells, D. R. (1992). Frequency specificity of the auditory brain stem response to bone-conducted tones in infants and adults. *Ear and Hearing, 13*(2), 87–95.

Oates, P., & Purdy, S. (2001). Frequency specificity of human auditory brainstem and middle latency responses using notched noise masking, *Journal of the Acoustical Society of America, 110*(2), 995–1009.

Oates, P., & Stapells, D. R. (1997a). Frequency specificity of the human auditory brainstem and middle latency responses to brief tones. I. High pass noise masking. *Journal of the Acoustical Society of America, 102,* 3597–3608.

Oates, P., & Stapells, D. R. (1997b). Frequency specificity of the human auditory brainstem and middle latency responses to brief tones. II. Derived response analyses. *Journal of the Acoustical Society of America, 102,* 3609–3619.

Ontario Infant Hearing Program (OIHP). (2018). Protocol for auditory brainstem response-based audiological assessment (ABRA). Version 2018.01. Retrieved from https://www.uwo.ca/nca/pdfs/clinical_protocols/2018.01%20ABRA%20Protocol_Oct%2031.pdf

Parker, D. J., & Thornton, A. R. (1978a). Frequency specific components of the cochlear nerve and brainstem evoked responses of the human auditory system. *Scandinavian Audiology, 7*(1), 53–60.

Parker, D. J., & Thornton, A. R. (1978b). The validity of the derived cochlear nerve and brainstem evoked responses of the human auditory system. *Scandinavian Audiology, 7*(1), 45–52.

Picton, T. W., Ouellette, J., Hamel, G., & Smith, A. D. (1979). Brainstem evoked potentials to tonepips in notched noise. *Journal of Otolaryngology, 8,* 289–314.

Pratt, H., Ben-Yitzhak, E., & Attias, J. (1984). Auditory brainstem potentials evoked by clicks in notch-filtered masking noise: Audiological relevance. *Audiology, 23,* 380–387.

Pratt, H., & Bleich, N. (1982). Auditory brain stem potentials evoked by clicks in notch-filtered masking noise. *Electroencephalography and Clinical Neurophysiology, 53,* 417–426.

Purdy, S. C., & Abbas, P. J. (2002). ABR thresholds to tone bursts gated with Blackman and linear windows in adults with high-frequency sensorineural hearing loss. *Ear and Hearing, 23,* 358–368.

Rance, G. (2005). Auditory neuropathy/dys-synchrony and its perceptual consequences. *Trends in Amplification, 9,* 1–43.

Rance, G., Beer, D. E., Cone-Wesson, B., Shepherd, R. K., Dowell, R. C., King, A. M., Rickards, F. W., & Clark, G. M. (1999). Clinical findings for a group of infants and young children with auditory neuropathy, *Ear and Hearing, 20,* 238–252.

Rance, G., & Rickards, F. (2002). Prediction of hearing threshold in infants using auditory steady-state evoked potentials. *Journal of the American Academy of Audiology, 13,* 236–245.

Rance, G., Roper, R., Symons, L., Moody, L.-J., Poulis, C., Dourlay, M., & Kelly, T. (2005). Hearing threshold estimation in infants using auditory steady-state responses. *Journal of the American Academy of Audiology, 16,* 291–300.

Rance, G., & Starr, A. (2015). Pathophysiological mechanisms and functional hearing consequences of auditory neuropathy. *Brain, 139,* 3141–3158.

Rance, G., Tomlin, D., & Rickards, F. W. (2006). Comparison of auditory steady-state responses and tone-burst auditory brainstem responses in normal babies. *Ear and Hearing, 27,* 751–762.

Rickards, F. W., Tan, L. E., Cohen, L. T., Wilson, O. J., Drew, J. H., & Clark, G. M. (1994). Auditory steady-state evoked potential in newborns. *British Journal of Audiology, 28,* 327–337.

Robertson, C. M. T., Howarth, T. M., Bork, D. L. R., & Dinu, I. A. (2009). Permanent bilateral sensory and neural hearing loss of children after neonatal intensive care because of extreme prematurity: A thirty-year study. *Pediatrics, 123*(5), e797–e807.

Rodrigues, G. R. I., Lewis, D.R., & Fichino, S. N. (2010). Auditory steady state responses in diagnostic audiological child: Comparisons with the auditory brainstem responses. *Brazilian. Journal of Otorhinolaryngology, 76*(1), 96–101.

Rodrigues, G. R. I., & Lewis, D. R. (2010). Threshold prediction in children with sensorineural hearing loss using the auditory steady-state responses and tone-evoked auditory brain stem response. *International Journal of Pediatric Otorhinolaryngology, 74,* 540–546.

Rodrigues, G. R. I., & Lewis, D. R. (2014). Establishing auditory steady-state response thresholds to narrow band CE-chirps in full-term neonates. *International Journal of Pediatric Otorhinolaryngology, 78,* 238–243.

Rodrigues, G. R. I., Ramos, N., & Lewis, D. R. (2013). Comparing auditory brainstem responses (ABRs)

to tone burst and narrow band CE-chirp in young infants. *International Journal of Pediatric Otorhinolaryngology, 77*(9), 1555–1560.

Rohit, R., Dhanshree, R. G., Krishna, Y., Lewis, L. E., Driscoll, C., & Rajashekar, B. (2016). Follow-up in newborn hearing screening—A systematic review. *International Journal of Pediatric Otorhinolaryngology, 90*, 29–36.

Russ, S. A., Hanna, D., DesGeorges, J., & Forsman, I. (2010). Improving follow-up to newborn hearing screening: A learning collaborative experience. *Pediatrics, 126*, S59–S69.

Ruth, R. A., Dey-Sigman, S., & Mills, J. A. (1985). Neonatal ABR hearing screening. *Hearing Journal*, 39–40.

Savio, G., Cárdenas, J., Pérez Abalo, M., González, A., & Valdés, J. (2001). The low and high frequency auditory steady responses mature at different rates. *Audiology and Neuro-otology, 6*, 279–287.

Sininger, Y. S. (2007). The use of auditory brainstem response in screening for hearing loss and audiometric threshold prediction. In R. F. Burkard, M. Don, & J. J. Eggermont (Eds.), *Auditory evoked potentials: Basic principles and clinical applications* (pp. 254–274). Baltimore, MD: Lippincott Williams & Wilkins.

Sininger, Y. S., Abdala, C., & Cone-Wesson, B. (1997). Auditory threshold sensitivity of the human neonate as measured by the auditory brainstem response. *Hearing Research, 104*, 27–38.

Sininger, Y. S., Cone-Wesson, B., Folsom, R. C., Gorga, M. P., Vohr, B. R., Widen, J. E., . . . Norton, S. J. (2000). Identification of neonatal hearing impairment: Auditory brainstem responses in the perinatal period. *Ear and Hearing, 21*, 383–399.

Sininger, Y. S., Grimes, A., & Christensen, E. (2010). Auditory development in early amplified children: Factors influencing auditory-based communication outcomes in children with hearing loss. *Ear and Hearing, 31*, 166–185.

Sininger, Y. S., Hunter, L. L., Hayes, D., Roush, P. A., & Uhler, K. M. (2018). Evaluation of speed and accuracy of next-generation auditory steady state response and auditory brainstem response audiometry in children with normal hearing and hearing loss. *Ear and Hearing, 39*(6), 1207–1223.

Small, S. A., Hatton, J. L., & Stapells, D. R. (2007). Effects of bone oscillator coupling method, placement location, and occlusion on bone-conduction auditory steady-state responses in Infants. *Ear and Hearing, 28*(1), 83–98.

Stapells, D. R. (2000). Threshold estimation by the tone-evoked auditory brainstem response: A literature meta-analysis. *Journal of Speech Language Pathology and Audiology, 24*, 74–83.

Stapells, D. R. (2011). Frequency-specific threshold assessment in young infants using the transient ABR and the brainstem ASSR. In R. Seewald & A. M. Tharpe (Eds.), *Comprehensive handbook of pediatric audiology* (pp. 409–448). San Diego, CA: Plural Publishing.

Stapells, D. R., Gravel, J. S., & Martin, B. A. (1995). Thresholds for auditory brain stem responses to tones in notched noise from infants and young children with normal hearing or sensorineural hearing loss. *Ear and Hearing, 16*, 361–371.

Stapells, D. R., & Oates, P. (1997). Estimation of the pure tone audiogram by the auditory brainstem response: A review. *Audiology and Neuro-otology, 2*, 257–280.

Stapells, D. R., Picton, T. W., Durieux-Smith, A., Edwards, C. G., & Moran, L. M. (1990). Thresholds for short-latency auditory-evoked potentials to tones in notched noise in normal hearing and hearing-impaired subjects. *Audiology, 29*, 262–274.

Stapells, D. R., Picton, T. W., & Durieux-Smith, A. (1994). Electrophysiologic measures of frequency-specific auditory function. In J. T. Jacobson (Ed.), *Principles and applications in auditory evoked potentials* (pp. 251–283). Boston, MA: Allyn & Bacon.

Stapells, D. R., Picton, T. W., Perez-Abalo, M., Read, D., & Smith, A. (1985). Frequency specificity in evoked potential audiometry. In J. T. Jacobson (Ed.), *The auditory brainstem response* (pp. 147–177). San Diego, CA: College-Hill Press.

Stapells, D. R., & Ruben, R. J. (1989). Auditory brain stem responses to bone-conducted tones in infants. *Annals of Otology, Rhinology, and Laryngology, 98*(12, Pt. I), 941–949.

Starr, A., Picton, T. W., Sininger, Y., Hood, L. J., & Berlin, C. I. (1996). Auditory neuropathy. *Brain, 119*, 741–743.

Stewart, D., Mehl, A., Hall, J. W. III., Thompson, V., Carroll, M., & Hamlett, J. (2000). Universal newborn hearing screening with automated auditory brainstem response: A multisite investigation. *Journal of Perinatology, 20*, S128–S131.

Stuart, A., & Cobb, K. M. (2014). Effect of stimulus and number of sweeps on the neonate auditory brainstem response. *Ear and Hearing, 35*, 585–588.

Stuart, A., & Yang, E. Y. (1994). Effect of high-pass filtering on the neonatal auditory brainstem response to air- and bone-conducted clicks. *Journal of Speech and Hearing Research, 37*, 475–479.

Stueve, M. P., & O'Rourke, C. (2003). Estimation of hearing loss in children: Comparison of auditory steady-state response, auditory brainstem response, and behavioral test methods. *American Journal of Audiology, 12*(2), 125–136.

Stürzebecher, E., Cebulla, M., Elberling. C., & Berger, T. (2006). New efficient stimuli for evoking frequency-specific auditory steady-state responses. *Journal of the American Academy of Audiology, 17,* 448–461.

Stürzebecher, E., Cebulla, M., & Pschirrer, U. (2001). Efficient stimuli for recording of the amplitude-modulation following response. *Audiology, 40,* 63–68.

Stürzebecher, E., Cebulla, M., & Wernecke, K. (1999). Objective response detection in the frequency domain: Comparison of several q-sample tests. *Audiology and Neuro-otology, 4*(1), 2–11.

Suzuki, T., Hirai, Y., & Horiuchi, K. (1977). Auditory brainstem responses to tone pips. *Scandinavian Audiology, 6,* 123–126.

Swanepoel, D., & Ebrahim, S. (2009). Auditory steady-state response and auditory brainstem response thresholds in children. *European Archives of Otorhinolaryngology, 266,* 213–219.

Teas, D. C., Eldredge, D. H., & Davis, H. (1962). Cochlear responses to acoustic transients: An interpretation of whole-nerve action potentials. *Journal of the Acoustical Society of America, 34,* 1438–1459.

van den Berg, E., Deiman, C., & van Straaten, H. L. (2010). MB11 BERAphone hearing screening compared to ALGO portable in a Dutch NICU: A pilot study. *International Journal of Pediatric Otorhinolaryngology, 74,* 1189–1192.

Van der Drift, J. F., Brocaar, M. P., & van Zanten, G. A. (1987). The relation between the pure-tone audiogram and the click auditory brainstem response threshold in cochlear hearing loss. *Audiology, 21*(1), 1–10.

Van Dyk, M., Swanepoel, D. W., & Hall, J. W. (2015). Outcomes with OAE and A-ABR screening in the first 48 h—Implications for newborn hearing screening in developing countries. *International Journal of Pediatric Otorhinolaryngology, 79*(7), 1034–1040.

Van Maanen, A., & Stapells, D. R. (2009). Normal multiple auditory steady state response thresholds to air-conducted stimuli in infants. *Journal of the American Academy of Audiology, 20,* 196–207.

Van Maanen, A., & Stapells, D. R. (2010). Multiple-ASSR thresholds in infants and young children with hearing loss. *Journal of the American Academy of Audiology, 21,* 535–545.

Van Stratten, H. L., Groote, M. E., & Oudesluys-Murphy, A. M. (1996). Evaluation of an automated auditory brainstem response infant hearing screening method in at risk patients. *European Journal of Pediatrics, 155,* 702–705.

van Zanten, G. A., & Brocaar, M. P. (1984). Frequency-specific auditory brainstem responses to clicks masked by notched noise. *Audiology, 23,* 253–264.

Vander Werff, K. R., Brown, C. J., Gienapp, B. A., & Schmidt Clay, K. M. (2002). Comparison of auditory steady-state response and auditory brainstem response thresholds in children. *Journal of the American Academy of Audiology, 13*(5), 227–235.

Vander Werff, K. R., Prieve, B., & Georgantas, L. M. (2009). Infant air and bone conduction tone burst auditory brain stem responses for classification of hearing loss and the relationship to behavioral thresholds. *Ear and Hearing, 30*(3), 350–368.

Venail, F., Artaud, J. P., Blanchet, C., Uziel, A., & Mondain, M. (2015). Refining the audiological assessment in children using narrow-band CE-Chirp-evoked auditory steady state responses. *International Journal of Audiology, 54,* 106–113.

Vohr, B. R., Widen, J. E., Cone-Wesson, B., Sininger, Y. S., Gorga, M. P., Folsom, R. C., & Norton, S. J. (2000). Identification of neonatal hearing impairment: Characteristics of infants in the neonatal intensive care unit and well-baby nursery. *Ear and Hearing, 21,* 373–382.

Watkin, P., McCann, D., Law, C., Mulle, M., Petrou, S., Stevenson, J., . . . Kennedy, C. (2007). Language abilities in children with permanent hearing impairment: The influence of early management and family participation. *Pediatrics, 120,* e631–e636.

White, K. R., Nelson, L. H., & Munoz, K. F. (2016). How many babies with hearing loss will be missed by repeated newborn hearing screening with otoacoustic emissions due to statistical artifact? *Journal of Early Hearing Detection and Intervention, 1*(2), 56–62.

White, K. R., Vohr, B. R., Meyer, S., Widen, J. E., Johnson, J. L., Gravel, J. S., . . . Weirather, Y. (2005). A multisite study to examine the efficacy of the otoacoustic emission/automated auditory brainstem response newborn hearing screening protocol: Research design and results of the study. *American Journal of Audiology, 14*(2), S186–S199.

Wood, S. A., Davis, A. C., & Sutton, G. J. (2013). Effectiveness of targeted surveillance to identify moderate to profound permanent childhood hearing impairment in babies with risk factors who pass newborn screening. *International Journal of Audiology, 52*(6), 394–399.

Xu, Z. M., Cheng, W. X., & Yao, Z. H. (2014). Prediction of frequency-specific hearing thresholds using chirp auditory brainstem response in infants with hearing losses. *International Journal of Pediatric Otorhinolaryngology, 78,* 812–816.

Yoshinaga-Itano, C., Sedey, A. L., Coulter, D. K., & Mehl, A. L. (1998). Language of early- and later-identified children with hearing loss. *Pediatrics, 102*(5), 1161–1171.

Young, N. M., Reilly, B. K., & Burke, L. (2011). Limitations of universal newborn hearing screening in early identification of pediatric cochlear implant candidates. *Archives of Otolaryngology-Head and Neck Surgery, 137*(3), 230–234.

Zirn, S., Louza, J., Reiman, V., Wittlinger, N., Hempel, J.-M., & Schuster, M. (2014). Comparison between ABR with click and narrow band chirp stimuli in children. *International Journal of Pediatric Otorhinolaryngology, 78*(8), 1352–1355.

6

Clinical Applications of the Auditory Brainstem Response: Differential Diagnosis

SCOPE

The auditory brainstem response's (ABR) ability to rapidly and accurately estimate hearing thresholds in both normal-hearing individuals and individuals with various degrees and configurations of hearing loss is well established. Most of the ABR applications related to threshold estimation are largely confined to children. ABR is rarely used in adults since behavioral measures can be easily accomplished. We have also established that there is a predictable relationship between certain stimulus factors (e.g., intensity and frequency) and absolute latency and amplitude of ABR components. Finally, we also know that the ABR indices (like absolute latency, interpeak latencies, and V/I amplitude ratio) provide information about the functional integrity of the auditory nerve and the brainstem. Given these attributes of the ABR, we examine here the clinical utility of the ABR to differentiate hearing losses resulting from structural abnormalities in the (a) conductive mechanism, (b) sensory-to-neural transduction in the cochlea, and (c) synaptic processing and neural transmission in the auditory nerve and brainstem. Specifically, do the patterns of changes in the ABR indices accurately identify the type, degree, configuration of hearing loss, and the level(s) of the lesion along the auditory pathway in the brainstem. Effective clinical application of ABR in the assessment of structural and functional integrity of peripheral (conductive mechanism and cochlear processing), auditory nerve, and auditory brainstem requires a clear understanding of the distinct ways in which type, degree, and configuration of hearing loss alter the response components. Remember, the application of ABR in differential diagnosis is indicated when the basic battery of audiologic tests cannot differentiate between a cochlear and a retrocochlear pathology. Unlike threshold testing, this neurodiagnostic application is more common in adults. We first consider the clinical utility of the ABR in the differential diagnosis of the "site of lesion" followed by the ABR's role in the monitoring of neural function (Chapters 6 and 7). The intent here is to provide information relevant to the optimal application of the ABR to distinguish between the different sites of pathologies producing a hearing loss.

I. ABR IN CONDUCTIVE HEARING LOSS (CHL)

Effects on ABR Characteristics

A CHL is characterized by elevated pure-tone air-conduction thresholds accompanied by normal bone-conduction threshold (the size of the air-bone gap [ABG] is an estimate of the magnitude of the conductive component), with acoustic immittance results confirming a middle ear disorder. Most CHLs exhibit a slightly rising (therefore greater loss in the low frequencies) or a flat configuration with a mild-to-moderate degree of hearing loss. Since air-conduction thresholds are elevated, it may be inferred that the stimulus reaching the cochlea is attenuated by the magnitude of the conductive component (McGee & Clemis, 1982). Since both absolute latency and the amplitude of the ABR components are inversely related to stimulus intensity (that is, a decrease in intensity produces a latency prolongation and an amplitude reduction), it follows that a similar change in ABR absolute latency and amplitude should be observed in individuals with CHL due to attenuation of the signal reaching the cochlea. To the extent that CHL is simply a signal attenuation problem that elevates the air-conduction threshold by the magnitude of the conductive component, then the wave V latency-intensity function should simply be shifted to the right by the amount of the conductive component with the slope of the function essentially unchanged compared to normal. McGee and Clemis (1982), evaluating wave V latency changes in individuals with CHLs due to ear canal occlusion or middle ear effusion, found that the parallel shift in wave V latency-intensity function correlated well with the ABG. Several other studies have also shown this characteristic parallel shift to the right of the wave V latency-intensity (LI) function in addition to an absolute latency shift for wave I (Borg & Löfqvist, 1982; Fria & Sabo, 1979; Mackersie & Stapells, 1994; Van der Drift, von Zanten, & Brocaar, 1989; Van der Drift, Brocaar, & von Zanten, 1988; Yamada, Yagi, Yamane, & Suzuki, 1975). Some of these studies were also interested in determining if the size of the ABG (and therefore the degree of CHL) could be predicted from the shifted wave V latency-intensity function. This would necessarily require that the normal and shifted functions are essentially parallel—that is, they exhibit the same slope.

Mackersie and Stapells (1994) used wave I latencies to predict the magnitude of the conductive component in infants and children with CHL due to otitis media or aural atresia. They used two prediction methods, one based on a 0.3 ms/10 dB slope value, and the other a regression analysis of wave I latency delays. Based on their prediction errors of 15 dB or greater in 33% of the subjects using either method, they questioned the validity of the clinical utility of wave I latencies to predict the magnitude of the conductive component and instead recommended the use of bone-conduction auditory brainstem response (BC-ABR) to assess cochlear status. Yamada et al. (1975) proposed a method to estimate the size of the ABG by comparing the right-shifted wave V LI functions in individuals with simulated conductive loss and confirmed conductive loss due to middle ear disorder with the normal wave V LI function. Their method was to quite simply determine the intensity correction required to move the shifted LI function to the left to overlay the normal function. Since they used clicks, their best CHL prediction, as expected, was at 4000 Hz and was within 15 dB of the actual loss in a majority of their subjects. Fria and Sabo (1979) found that ABR wave I and wave V latencies provided a sensitive index to not only identify otitis media with effusion (OME) but also to estimate the degree of CHL in infants and young children. However, they reported that wave I had much better specificity compared to wave V, which showed prolonged latencies even in children without OME. It is likely that the relatively longer maturational time course for wave V (18–24 months) compared to wave I (which attains adult values in the first 2 months) could be a confounding factor. These authors also found that they could predict CHL to within 15 dB using Yamada et al.'s intensity correction method. The 0.3 ms/10 dB slope value, also used by Fria and Sabo (1979), presumably reflects the relatively smaller change in latency for waves I and V at moderate intensities. For example, using this slope value, a 1-ms shift in wave V latency would predict a 33-dB conductive component. The slope and regression methods (Mackersie & Stappels, 1994; Yamada et al., 1975) used to predict the magnitude of the conductive component are illustrated in Figure 6–1. ABRs were recorded in a normal-hearing individual without and with the ears plugged with a foam earplug. With the ear plugged, an essentially flat loss with a high-frequency pure-tone average (HFPTA) of 42 dB HL was obtained. The replicated ABR waveforms to clicks plotted as a function of decreasing intensity (panel A) show responses down to 10

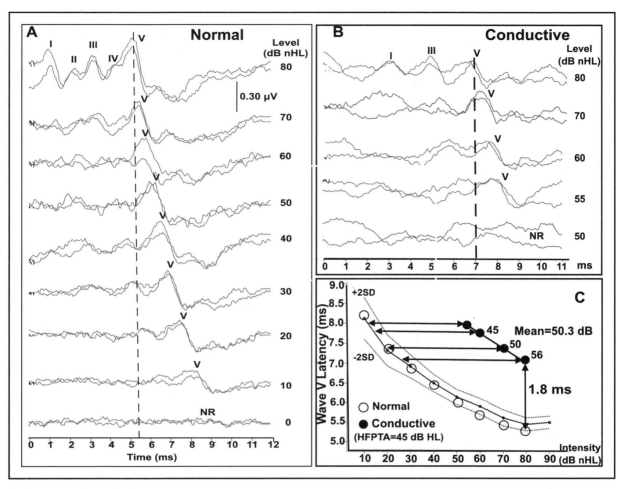

Figure 6–1. Auditory brainstem response waveforms from a normal-hearing young adult obtained with ears unplugged (**A**) and ears plugged (**B**). **C.** Wave V latency-intensity (LI) functions for normal (*open circles*) and simulated conductive loss (*shifted solid circles*) conditions are overlaid on the normal wave V LI function (*solid line*). The double-arrowed solid horizontal line from the shifted data pointing to the normal function depicts the decibel change needed to move the shifted LI function to the normal region. The decibel correction needed for this shift is shown to the right of each data point on the shifted LI function, with a mean of 50.3 dB (the estimated conductive component). The vertical double-arrowed line from the conductive loss LI function to the normal LI function indicates the magnitude of the latency shift (1.8 ms). Using a slope value of 0.4 ms/10 dB, the estimated conductive component is 45 dB.

dB nHL with normal wave V LI function (shown by open circles in panel C) consistent with normal hearing at least in the 2000–4000 Hz region. Replicated ABR waveforms obtained with the ear plugged are shown as a function of stimulus level in panel B. While all response components are present at 80 dB nHL, only wave V is easily discernible below this level, with no identifiable response component at 50 dB nHL. As expected, the simulated condition produces responses with longer latencies (see LI function plotted with black solid circles in panel C) and smaller amplitudes compared to the unplugged condition. The LI function for the "conductive" loss condition is shifted up and to the right and is essentially parallel to the "normal" LI function, showing similar slopes for both functions. In the first method, we calculated the intensity correction needed (shown by the length of the multiple horizontal lines straddling the normal and conductive LI functions) to move the conductive LI function to approximate the normal function using the mean of three data points (which yielded values of 56, 50, and 45 dB for intensities 80, 70, and 60 dB, respectively). The resulting estimate of the conductive component is 50.3 dB, which compares well with both the HFPTA and the ABR threshold estimate (remember electrophysiologic thresholds are typically 10 to 15 dB higher than behavioral thresholds). Applying the second method to our data to predict the magnitude of the conductive component, we calculated the intensity in decibels required to produce a latency shift of about 1.8 ms (see vertical bidirectional arrow in panel C) using a slope value of 0.3 ms/10 dB. The resulting estimate was 55 dB, again in agreement with the HFPTA and the ABR threshold. It should be noted here that these estimates depend on the number of data points across levels averaged; fewer data points will likely lead to prediction errors. For example, if the slope is changed from 0.3 ms/10 dB to 0.4 ms/10 dB, then the predicted value will be 45 dB, which underestimates the conductive component and the ABR threshold. Best estimates are obtained when the range of latency values considered has a slope closer to 0.3 ms/10 dB. Thus, the use of latency values from a small range of moderate-intensity sounds where the slope does not change appreciably might provide a better estimate of the size of the conductive component.

While these estimation methods seem reasonable if the assumption of identical wave V LI slopes for normal and conductive losses is, in fact, true, there are several drawbacks with these methods. When using click or tone burst stimuli, both methods may miss or underestimate hearing loss or may not meet the assumption of similar wave V LI slopes for normal and conductive loss for certain configurations of CHL (Eggermont; 1982; Gorga, Reiland, & Beauchaine, 1986; Stapells, 1989); therefore cautious application of these methods is suggested. First, the click response is basally biased and could miss hearing loss at frequencies below 2000 Hz and above 4000 Hz. Thus, it would be difficult to compare this response with different configurations of hearing loss except for a flat hearing loss similar to the one in our example. So, hearing losses in the low and higher frequencies may be missed or underestimated (Stapells, 1989). Second, since the normal variability of ABR latency is equivalent to an intensity change of about 20 to 30 dB, the estimation error could be as much as 30 dB (Eggermont, 1982). Third, CHLs are not always flat, so a high-frequency sloping conductive loss may exhibit a steeper slope (compared to a flat loss) similar to a cochlear hearing loss and therefore may not satisfy the requirement of slope equivalence essential for the estimation methods described earlier (Gorga, Reiland, & Beauchine, 1985). Gorga et al. (1985) measured ABR to clicks in an individual with a high-frequency mild CHL above 500 Hz (Figure 6–2, audiogram top right), presumably due to increased middle ear mass. Repeatable wave V was discernible down to 40 dB nHL with abnormally delayed latencies and essentially normal interpeak latencies (Figure 6–2, left panel). Unlike what is observed in most flat CHLs, their wave V LI function (Figure 6–2, bottom right panel) was abnormal and exhibited a steep slope (106 μs/dB) similar to what is commonly observed in a sloping cochlear hearing loss. However, it should be noted here that in a sloping high-frequency cochlear loss, wave V latency at high intensities is commonly normal or near-normal, unlike the prolonged latency observed in this CHL loss case presented here. Gorga et al. (1986) hypothesize that the slope of the LI function is largely determined by the intensity-dependent change in cochlear regions contributing to the response in CHL. In this case of high-frequency loss (albeit mild in degree), the more sensitive low-frequency contributions may likely be dominating the response, thus producing a latency prolongation. The steeper slope may reflect larger apical shifts in the modal value of the latency distribution with changes in intensity. Specifically, basal cochlear regions dominate the response at high intensities with the observed abnormally longer latency reflecting the attenuation effect of the conductive component. Apical cochlear regions increasingly begin to dominate the response as intensity is decreased, as indicated by the progressively increasing delay in response latency. This steeper wave V LI slope notwithstanding, estimation of the conductive component based on the first method (that is, intensity correction needed to move the LI function into the normal range) may still yield a reasonably good estimate of the magnitude of the conductive component. Taking together these observations, the reported variable effects of

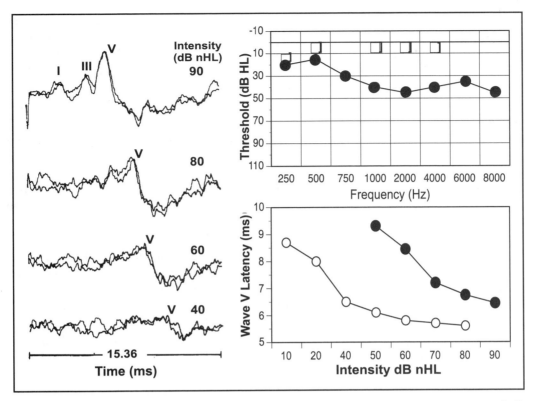

Figure 6–2. Auditory brainstem response waveforms plotted as a function of intensity (*left*); audiogram (*top right*) showing high-frequency mild conductive hearing loss, and wave V latency-intensity (*bottom right*) showing a steeper slope (*solid black circles*) compared to normal (*open circles*) more characteristic of a cochlear hearing loss. Waveform rendering based on data from "Auditory Brainstem Responses in a Case of High-Frequency Conductive Hearing Loss," by M. P. Gorga, J. K. Reiland, and K. A. Beauchaine, 1985, *Journal of Speech and Hearing Disorders, 50*, pp. 346–350.

OME on wave V latency, and the poor correlation between latency shift and thresholds in other middle ear disorders like stapedial fixation or ossicular discontinuity, caution should be exercised in interpreting ABR latency data to estimate the conductive component in individuals with certain degrees and configurations of CHL.

Effects of Chronic Middle Ear Infection on the Brainstem Response

Adequate and sustained auditory input to the central auditory system during development is critical for the normal development of central auditory structures and their function. Thus, reduced input to the auditory system during development could potentially disrupt and/or delay the normal development of speech and language and may lead to other auditory perceptual deficits. There is consistent evidence that recurring bouts of chronic middle ear infections in young children, which produce repeated periods of slight to mild hearing loss during early development, do alter the ABR, suggesting functional changes. Specifically, several studies have shown that compared to controls, children with OME or a history of recurrent OME consistently show significant ABR differences that persist even after resolution of the OME (Anteby, Hafner, Pratt, & Uri, 1986; Chambers, 1989; Folsom, Weber, & Thompson, 1983; Fria & Sabo, 1979; Gunnarson & Finitzo, 1991; Hall & Grose, 1993; Lenhardt, Shaia, & Abedi, 1985). However, the reported pattern of changes in IPLs varies across studies. For example, Chambers (1989) observed prolongation of only the I–III IPL; Gunnarson and Finitzo (1991) and Hall and Grose (1993) observed prolongation of both I–III and I–V IPL (Figure 6–3); Folsom, Weber, and Thompson (1983) observed prolongation of I–III and III–V; and Ferguson, Cook, Hall, Grose, and Pillsbury (1998) and Anteby et al. (1986) observed prolongation of I–V and III–V IPL. The prolongation in IPLs may suggest sensory deprivation–induced degradation of synaptic processing, neural conduction delays, or both resulting from weaker depolarizations affecting conduction velocity along fiber tracts.

Additionally, a behavioral measure of binaural function using the binaural masking level difference (BMLD) in children with a history of OME (Hall, Grose, & Pillsbury, 1995; Moore, Hutchings, & Meyer, 1991; Pillsbury, Grose, & Hall, 1991) and adults with acquired CHL (Ferguson et al., 1998; Hall & Derlacki, 1986; Hall & Grose, 1993; Hall, Grose, & Pillsbury, 1990; Magliulo, Gagliardi, Muscatello, & Natale, 1990) is significantly reduced. BMLD is a binaural phenomenon wherein there is an improvement in signal detection in dichotic antiphasic conditions (NoSπ: noise in phase and signal out of phase; or NπSo: noise out of phase and signal in phase) relative to a homophasic condition (NoSo; noise and signal in phase). Ferguson et al. (1998) also found a strong correlation between ABR IPL (I–III and I–V) and BMLD, suggesting that deprivation of optimal inputs to the binaural system in the brainstem may have altered binaural processes relevant to BMLD. Finally, the presence of ABR with delayed IPLs and reduced BMLD in adults (Ferguson et al., 1998) with acquired CHLs suggests that these brainstem changes are not necessarily the consequences of sensory deprivation during the critical period of development (that is, developmental plasticity). Rather the central changes in adults with acquired CHL likely reflect homeostatic adaptive plasticity due to reduced input.

CHL Causes Structural and Functional Changes in the Auditory Brainstem

Until recently, studies of structural and functional changes in the central auditory system consequent to CHL have largely focused on more central structures along the auditory pathway, with little attention paid to earlier stages of processing (e.g., brainstem). However, the earlier stages of processing also play an important role in the neural encoding of acoustic features essential for the perception of complex auditory stimuli and the processing of binaural cues important for localization and signal selection. Also, the optimal processing of sounds at later stages depends on the fine-grained representations from the early stages of processing. Zhuang, Sun, and Xu-Friedman (2017) examined the effects of CHL (produced by occlusion of the ear canal) on the structural and response properties of the large calyx of Held auditory nerve-bushy cells synapse in the mouse anteroventral cochlear nucleus. They found that CHL modified the properties of the synapses by decreasing their size and the number of

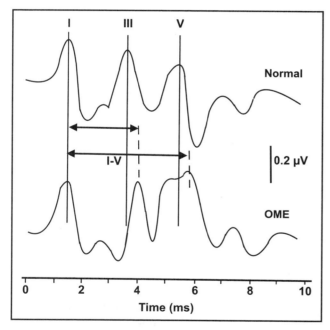

Figure 6–3. Representative auditory brainstem response waveforms from a normal-hearing child (*top*) and a child with a history of otitis media with effusion (OME) (*bottom*), but no conductive hearing loss at the time of testing. Both waves III and V are delayed for the child with OME with prolonged I–III and I–V interval indicated by the horizontal bidirectional arrows. Waveform rendering based on data from "The Effect of Otitis Media With Effusion on the Masking Level Difference and the Auditory Brainstem Response," by J. W. Hall and J. H. Grose, 1993, *Journal of Speech and Hearing Research, 36*, pp. 210–217.

synaptic vesicles and sites, and showed depressed activity that consequently resulted in the bushy cells firing fewer action potentials in response to evoked synaptic activity. The authors interpreted their results to suggest the operation of a homeostatic, adaptive response of the synapse to reduced activity. The consequences of these local changes might be reflected as reduced fidelity of neural representations at higher levels along the auditory pathway, which in turn might adversely affect the perception of sounds. Using a similar procedure, Clarkson, Antunes, and Rubio (2016) induced CHL in young adult rats and found that 10 days of monaural CHL produced an elevation of click and tone elicited ABR thresholds that persisted even after ears were unplugged (Figure 6–4A and B). In addition, cochlear nucleus neural output was reduced followed by enhancement of the response at the level of lateral lemniscus triggered by local compensatory gain mechanisms responding to reduced input (Figure 6–4C). Structural changes they observed at the auditory nerve-cochlear nucleus (calyx of Held) synapse that account for these physiologic changes included a decrease in transmitter expression in the presynaptic terminal, smaller synaptic vesicles, and an increase in postsynaptic density thickness and upregulation of the neurotransmitter. Ten days after removal of the plug, the density and size of the synaptic vesicles increased with the upregulation of the neurotransmitter still maintained. These results suggest that sound deprivation has a long-lasting change in the structural as well as presynaptic and postsynaptic dynamics at the auditory nerve-cochlear nucleus synapse that may degrade neural representation.

Several studies have also demonstrated that experimentally induced monaural CHL during critical periods of development leads to alterations in the symmetry of projections from the cochlear nucleus (CN) to the binaural neurons in the inferior colliculus (IC) and abnormalities in the development of binaural neurons (Clopton & Silverman, 1977, 1978; Moore, Hutchings, King, & Kowalchuk, 1989; Moore & Irvine, 1981). Examining the effects of sound deprivation (in ferrets reared with monaural plugging of the right ear canal) on the development of the auditory brainstem, Moore et al. (1989) showed that connectivity in the brainstem (evaluated by cell labeling) was altered, which could, in turn, alter binaural processing. Specifically, the symmetry of projections from each cochlear nucleus to the IC was changed, primarily by an increase of projections contralateral to the plugged side (that is more cells in CN ipsilateral to the IC were labeled). Clopton and Silverman (1978) evaluated the latency and spike duration in the IC in normally hearing rats and rats deprived of monaural auditory stimulation during early development using surgical blocking of the ear canal. Neurons in the contralateral IC with characteristic frequencies below 10 kHz showed response latencies similar to controls. However, most neurons above 10 kHz had two to three times longer latencies and shorter spike duration compared to the controls. Interestingly, rats that were sound deprived 60 days after birth also had changes in latencies and response durations, but much smaller than observed in the developmentally deprived rats. Also, their observation of no changes in the latencies of the auditory nerve response suggests a central origin of the early deprivation effect. Developmental auditory sensory deprivation via temporary and reversible CHL can also lead to distortion of tonotopic maps, degradation of neural representation from the affected ear, enhancement of representation in the opposite ear, and disruption of binaural cues important for localization (Polley, Thompson, & Guo, 2013; Popescu & Polley, 2010). Recently, Okada, Welling, Liberman, and Maison (2020) showed that patients with chronic conductive impairment and moderate to moderately severe hearing loss had lower word recognition scores on the affected side compared to the unaffected side. Liberman, Liberman, and Maison (2015) showed in mice that a chronic (1-year duration) CHL from eardrum resection in the mature animal led to a reduction in cochlear lateral efferent innervation to the inner hair cells (IHCs) and a loss of up to 30% of the afferent synapses between the cochlear nerve and sensory cells (cochlear synaptopathy). The authors suggest that the reduced auditory nerve drive consequent to cochlear synaptopathy (therefore still a peripheral dysfunction) may be a contributing factor to the reduced word recognition scores in individuals with chronic CHL of a moderate to a moderately severe degree.

Taken together, these findings suggest that a clear understanding of the structural and functional

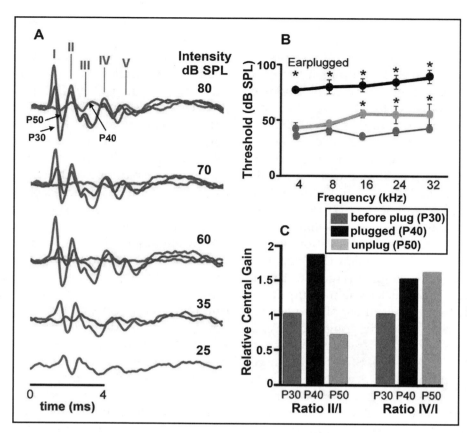

Figure 6–4. A. Auditory brainstem response (ABR) recorded from a young adult rat in a developmental deprivation study plotted as a function of decreasing intensity. The robust trace with the largest amplitude (P30) is the recording before ears were plugged (P30 days); trace with reduced amplitude of all components and response components barely discernible is recording obtained 10 days after the ear was plugged (arrow associated with label P40); and the trace with clear response peaks with smaller amplitudes is recording obtained 10 days (P50) after ear was unplugged. Note the persistence of delayed responses with appreciably reduced amplitude compared to the control condition. **B.** ABR thresholds plotted as a function of frequency. The plugged condition (P40: *black plot*) shows the expected threshold shift of about 40 dB with a slightly greater shift at higher frequencies. The thresholds improve after unplugging (P50, *light gray plot*) but are still significantly greater than the threshold in the control condition (*dark gray plot*) at higher frequencies. **C.** An appreciable central gain for the plugged condition (*black bar*) for both II/I and IV/I amplitude ratio with the unplugged condition showing a central gain for only the IV/I ratio. Adapted from "Conductive Hearing Loss Has Long-Lasting Structural and Molecular Effects on Presynaptic and Postsynaptic Structures of Auditory Nerve Synapses in the Cochlear Nucleus," by C. Clarkson, F. M. Antunes, and M. E. Rubio, 2016, *Journal of Neuroscience*, 36(39), pp. 10214–10227.

consequences of developmental auditory deprivation and their potential for reversibility is essential to develop optimal management strategies to reduce the negative impact of recurrent fluctuating CHL due to chronic OME on speech and language acquisition and to mitigate the perceptual auditory deficits that may follow. In terms of a test strategy to identify CHL, a full clinical battery approach including pure-tone audiometry and acoustic immittance tests should also be utilized in conjunction with air-conduction ABR (AC-ABR) and BC-ABR.

II. ABR IN COCHLEAR HEARING LOSS

Effects on ABR Characteristics

Unlike the primary problem of signal attenuation in CHL, cochlear hearing loss is more complicated since it involves dysfunction of sensory, neural, or both components. The sensory component includes cochlear regions available to contribute to the response (e.g., a significantly greater high-frequency loss would reduce or eliminate high-frequency contribution to the response), the functional integrity of the outer hair cell (OHC) subsystem (to provide gain and frequency selectivity via the active cochlear amplifier), and the functional integrity of the IHCs (role in neural transduction that provides the major drive of the auditory nerve). Thus, dysfunction of any of these components could produce distinct changes in the ABR. Given this possibility of a variable multicomponent problem across individuals, it could be challenging to establish a predictable relationship between a cochlear loss and specific changes in the ABR indices. We focus here on the commonly observed changes in ABR resulting from cochlear hearing loss that may help differentiate cochlear, conductive, and retrocochlear sites of pathology. There are two aspects of wave V latency behavior in a cochlear loss that would be useful to consider in the differential diagnosis. One is the relationship between the magnitude of latency increase and degree and configuration of hearing loss, and the second is the relationship between the slope of the wave V LI function and degree and configuration of hearing loss.

Relationship Between Magnitude of Latency Shift and Degree and Configuration of Cochlear Hearing Loss

While most earlier studies using clicks consistently report that wave V latency increases with about 50 dB or greater degree of cochlear hearing loss at 4000 Hz, the relationship between the latency shift and configuration of loss is not clear (Coats, 1978; Fowler & Mikami, 1993; Jerger & Johnson, 1988; Jerger & Mauldin, 1978; Moller & Blevgad, 1976; Rosenhammer, Lindstrom, & Lundborg, 1981; Yamada, Kodera, & Yagi, 1979). Jerger and Johnson (1988) reported wave V latency changes only for hearing losses greater than about 55 to 60 dB at 4000 Hz with no appreciable change below 55 dB. They observed a maximum latency shift of 0.4 ms at 90 dB nHL (approximately 0.1 ms for every 10-dB elevation in threshold at 4000 Hz). Some studies have also suggested that wave V latency increases were greater for high frequency sloping cochlear losses compared to cochlear losses with flatter configurations. Based on this relationship between wave V latency increase and audiogram slope, some investigators have proposed that a latency shift correction for cochlear hearing loss (e.g., 0.1 ms for every 10 dB of loss in the 2000–4000 Hz region) could be used to distinguish between cochlear and retrocochlear pathologies (Jerger & Mauldin, 1978; Prosser & Arslan, 1987; Selters & Brackmann, 1977). The rationale here is that if the latency increase exceeds the value predicted for cochlear loss, then it would point to a retrocochlear pathology (Selters & Brackmann, 1977). However, the use of a correction factor to account for the cochlear component has to be somewhat tempered, since some studies have failed to observe a predictable relationship between the configuration of hearing loss and magnitude of wave V latency shift (Jerger & Johnson, 1988; Rosenhammer, 1981).

An important issue not addressed in most of the earlier ABR studies in individuals with cochlear hearing loss is the selection of stimulus level(s) for ABR wave V latency comparisons between normal hearing and cochlear hearing loss. That is, the use of equal sound pressure level (SPL) or equal sensation level (SL) could produce different results because when using equal SPLs, comparisons are made with a lower SL for the hearing loss group; when equal SLs are used, comparisons are made with a higher SPL for the hearing loss group. Thus, it is difficult to discern if the observed ABR differences between the two groups are due to cochlear pathology or stimulus level-dependent changes in the cochlear-mechanics. To address this, Lewis et al. (2015) evaluated wave V latencies of ABRs elicited using tone-burst stimuli over a range of intensities in normal-hearing and hearing loss groups with mild-to-moderate cochlear hearing loss (Figure 6–5A). The range of intensities used

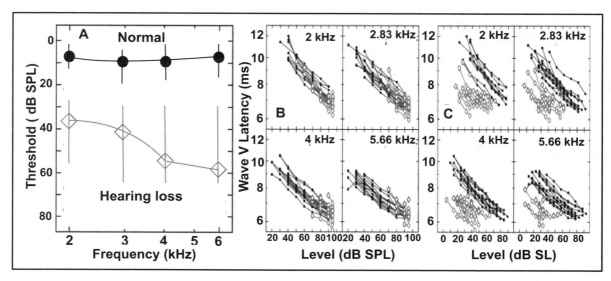

Figure 6–5. A. Hearing thresholds plotted as a function of frequency for normal hearing (*black*) and for individuals with a mild to moderate cochlear hearing loss (*light gray*). **B.** Wave V latency plotted as a function of intensity (*middle*, equal sound pressure level [SPL]; **C.** Wave V latency plotted as a function of intensity (right, equal sensation level [SL]) for the four frequencies. When plotted using equal SL, latencies are shorter for the hearing-impaired group. Reprinted with permission from "Tone-Burst Auditory Brainstem Response Wave V Latencies in Normal-Hearing and Hearing-Impaired Ears," by J. D. Lewis, J. Kopun, S. T. Neely, K. K. Schmid, and M. P. Gorga, 2015, *Journal of the Acoustical Society of America*, *138*(5), pp. 3210–3219. Copyright 2015, Acoustic Society of America.

allowed comparison of wave V latencies at equal SPL and equal SL. They found that when wave V latencies were compared using equal SLs, latencies were shorter in the hearing loss group for all frequencies, but wave V latencies were similar for the two groups when comparisons were made at equal SPLs (Figures 6–5C and 6–5B, respectively). Similar shortening of latency in individuals with mild-to-moderate cochlear hearing loss has been reported at high intensity levels for wave V (Don, Ponton, Eggermont, & Kwong, 1998; Strelcyk et al., 2009) and wave I (Eggermont, 1979; Henry, Kale, Scheidt, & Heinz, 2011; Strelcyk, Christoforidis, & Dau, 2009). However, Henry et al. (2011) used equal SPL comparisons and observed shorter latencies at all intensities and frequencies, based on chinchilla post–noise exposure data. They observed even shorter latencies for the postexposure animals when the comparison was made at equal SLs. Lewis et al. (2015) suggest that their observation of shorter latencies for equal SLs reflects a reduction of the active mechanism's filter build-up time (Don et al., 1998) due to a decrease in the gain of the cochlear amplifier consequent to OHC damage. As the active gain is reduced, the peak of the passive cochlear excitation pattern broadens, and the peak shifts basally accounting for the shorter latency, which shortens further with an increase in level and/or hearing loss. The absence of this latency shortening (i.e., similar wave V latencies for the two groups) when comparisons were made using equal SPLs suggests that stimulus level effects are similar for the two groups and that greater stimulus levels are required with increasing hearing loss to be able to elicit an ABR.

Finally, Lewis et al. (2015) reasoned that if cochlear hearing loss reduces the magnitude of the basilar membrane excitation, then it is likely that the IHC drive of the auditory nerve will also be reduced. Consequently, ABR will show a decrease in amplitude and an increase in wave V latency. Their data showed smaller amplitudes and shallower growth functions at frequencies above 2 kHz, suggesting a greater synaptic delay in cochlear hearing loss (Figure 6–6, see the light gray plots). The absence of shorter latencies in the cochlear loss group above 2 kHz may likely indicate that the decrease in latency with hearing loss was offset by the prolongation of latency by the synaptic delay due to reduced auditory nerve drive from the IHCs.

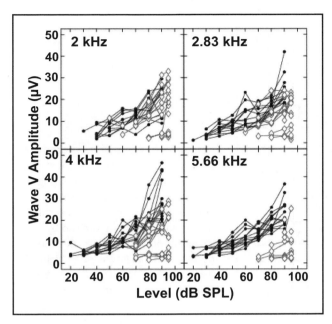

Figure 6–6. Wave V amplitude plotted as a function of stimulus level (dB SPL) for frequencies 2, 2.83, 4, and 5.66 kHz for the normal-hearing (*black*) and the hearing-impaired (*light gray*) groups. Plots show the smaller amplitude and shallower amplitude growth functions above 2 kHz for the hearing-impaired group suggesting synaptic delay. Reprinted with permission from "Tone-Burst Auditory Brainstem Response Wave V Latencies in Normal-Hearing and Hearing-Impaired Ears," by J. D. Lewis, J. Kopun, S. T. Neely, K. K. Schmid, and M. P. Gorga, 2015, *Journal of the Acoustical Society of America, 138*(5), pp. 3210–3219. Copyright 2015, Acoustic Society of America.

Relationship Between Slope of Wave V Latency-Intensity Function and Degree and Configuration of Cochlear Hearing Loss

There have been concerted efforts to determine if there is a predictable relationship between the slope of the wave V LI function and the degree and configuration of cochlear hearing loss (Coats, 1978; Gorga, Worthington, et al., 1985; Jerger & Maudin, 1978; Keith & Greville, 1987; Møller & Blegvad, 1976; Selters & Brackmann, 1977; Serpanos, O'Malley, & Gravel, 1997; Sohmer, Kinarti, & Gafni, 1981; Verhulst, Jagadeesh, Mauermann, & Ernst, 2016; Yamana, Kodera, & Yagi, 1979). While the findings are not consistent across studies, results from a majority of the studies (using click-elicited ABRs) report steeper slopes for wave V latency-intensity functions in sloping high-frequency cochlear hearing loss compared to hearing loss with a flat configuration (e.g., Coats, 1978; Gorga et al., 1985; Keith & Greville, 1987; Verhulst et al., 2016; Yamada, Kodera, & Yagi, 1979). The LI function in high-frequency sloping hearing loss is characterized by essentially normal latencies at high intensities (even in the presence of moderately severe high-frequency hearing loss) and abnormally long latencies at lower stimulus intensities (the so-called "recruiting" LI function). Coats (1978) observed that the slope of the wave V LI function increased as the magnitude of cochlear hearing loss in the 4000 to 8000 Hz region increased. Keith and Greville (1987) observed different patterns of wave V LI functions for high-frequency sloping, rising, flat, and notched audiograms with different degrees of hearing loss (Figure 6–7). Consistent with several other studies, they showed the characteristic recruiting LI function for high-frequency sloping loss. Mild hearing loss with a rising configuration in the 2000 to 8000 Hz region showed a normal LI function that tended to run along the lower limits of the confidence interval (meaning shorter latencies). It should be noted here that an audiogram with a rising and falling component with normal hearing in the 2000 to 4000 Hz region will produce a normal LI function for click-elicited ABRs, highlighting the click ABR's insensitivity to low- and high-frequency loss beyond the 2000 to 4000 Hz region. The flat, moderate hearing loss showed normal latencies at high intensities with latency prolongation near the ABR threshold. However, mild flat losses tend to show normal wave V LI functions. Notch-shaped hearing loss of moderate degree centered in the vicinity of 4000 Hz showed latency prolongation at high intensity and a latency delay near the ABR threshold with the truncated pattern not that different from the one observed for the high-frequency sloping loss. However, for a notch at 2000 Hz, wave V latency, although delayed compared to normal was essentially within normal limits. "Similar results were reported by both Gorga, Reiland, and Beuchaine (1985) and Yamada et al. (1979). In addition, Gorga, Reiland, et al. (1985) observed that wave V latency at high intensities in most high-frequency sloping losses converged to normal latency and was abnormal only when there was a significant loss in the 3000-Hz region. Taken

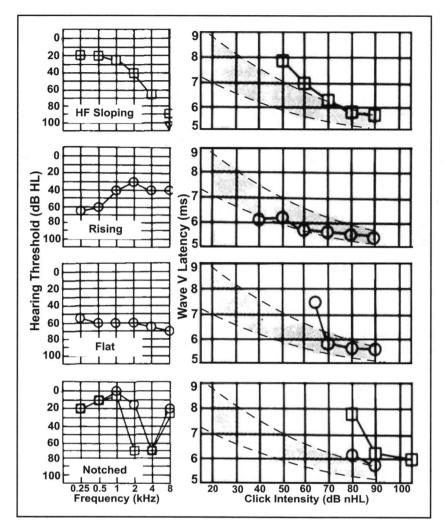

Figure 6–7. Wave latency-intensity (LI) function in different degrees and configurations of cochlear hearing loss. High-frequency sloping losses produce the characteristic "recruiting" LI function characterized by longer latencies at lower intensities and near-normal latencies at higher intensities. Flat configuration hearing losses tend to produce LI functions with a shallower slope. Created using data from "Effects of Audiometric Configuration on the Auditory Brain Stem Response," by W. J. Keith and K. A. Greville, 1987, *Ear and Hearing*, 8(1), pp. 49–55.

together, these results suggest that the pattern of the wave V LI function is largely determined by the degree and configuration of hearing loss above about 2000 Hz. Gorga, Worthington, et al. (1985) showed that the slope of the LI function depended largely on the slope of the loss, with sloping high-frequency losses showing a steeper slope than normal and flat hearing losses (Figure 6–8). For both mild and severe flat hearing losses, they found lower than normal slope values.

Differences in both the cochlear regions contributing to the response and the level of cochlear excitation could account for these different patterns of LI functions. In the case of the sloping high-frequency hearing loss, it is likely that the presence of a robust wave V with near normal latency at high intensity reflects the dominance of basally biased contributions to the ABR. However, given normal or near-normal hearing in the lower frequencies and the sloping high-frequency loss, the basal contribution is reduced considerably, and the activity contributing to the ABR from the apical regions increases at lower intensities resulting in a dramatic prolongation in latency (Coats, 1978; Don & Eggermont, 1978; Gorga, Worthington, et al., 1985). In the notched hearing loss, as in high-frequency sloping loss, high-frequency contributions to wave V are absent, and its latency is dominated by later occurring activity from more apical regions along the basilar membrane. For flat configurations, cochlear regions contributing to the response would likely be similar to the normal ABR once threshold is exceeded. In the case of the rising configuration, shorter latency basal contribution dominates the response, while the lon-

6. Clinical Applications of the Auditory Brainstem Response: Differential Diagnosis   137

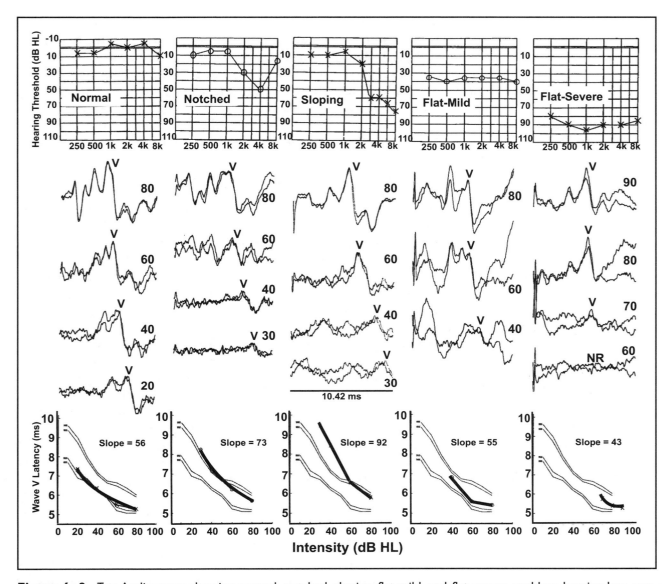

Figure 6-8. *Top:* Audiograms showing normal, notched, sloping, flat-mild, and flat-severe cochlear hearing loss configurations. Auditory brainstem response waveforms are plotted as a function of intensity. Clear wave V component is discernible down to the threshold level for each degree and configuration of loss. *Bottom:* Wave V latency-intensity (LI) functions. Only the high-frequency sloping loss exhibits a recruiting-like LI function. For the severe flat loss, unusually robust components are still present at 90 and 80 dB nHL, only 5 to 10 dB above the behavioral threshold consistent with recruitment. Flat losses tend to have shallower wave V LI function slope. Data from Gorga et al., 1985.

ger latency apical contributions to wave V latency are reduced in amplitude at low intensities.

Despite these qualitative relationships, empirical data are lacking to quantitatively characterize the relationship between wave V latency slope and the degree and configuration of hearing loss. Several factors that contribute to the difficulty in accurately determining this relationship include differences in cochlear excitation levels and cochlear regions contributing to responses across individuals with different degrees and configurations of hearing loss; differences in the etiology of the hearing loss that may produce distinct underlying cochlear structural changes; differential involvement of the OHC subsystem and the IHC subsystem; and combined cochlear and retrocochlear pathology. These factors may largely account for the considerable intersubject variability observed in the data across studies that preclude not only an accurate characterization of the relationship between the wave V LI function slope and the degree and configuration of hearing loss but also limit the clinical utility of this metric in differential diagnosis.

To address this issue of individual differences that limit the utility of the ABR's LI function metric to differentiate between cochlear losses due to OHC deficits and other peripheral hearing deficits such as cochlear synaptopathy, Verhulst et al. (2016) used a functional model for human ABRs (Verhulst, Bharadwaj, Mehraei, Shera, & Shinn-Cunningham, 2015) to simulate different combinations of hearing deficits (OHC, IHC, AN synapse, and auditory brainstem). They demonstrated that a reduction in high-frequency cochlear gain (OHC damage) steepened the slope of both the ABR wave V LI function and the amplitude intensity function. They confirmed the predicted relationship between the ABR LI function and the audiogram slope by comparing them with click-ABRs recorded from individuals with normal or high-frequency sloping hearing losses. Consistent with the other studies described earlier, they observed longer latencies at 70 dB peSPL for the hearing-impaired models than for the normal-hearing model, suggesting a more dominant contribution of low-frequency channels, and shorter latencies at 100 dB peSPL, reflecting increased high-frequency contributions due to broadening of the excitation pattern with an increase in stimulus level. Based on these results, they suggest that the individual ratio of ABR latency and amplitude growth may be used to differentiate between hearing losses due to AN fiber population deficits versus hearing loss from OHC-related deficits. While this novel approach shows excellent promise, their data from hearing-impaired individuals showed considerable variability. Therefore, further clinical validation is required to assess its clinical utility.

Effects of Cochlear Hearing Loss on ABR Interpeak Latencies

The ABR I–III, III–V, and I–V interpeak latencies (IPLs), thought to reflect neural conduction times between nuclei generating the ABR, have been successfully used by clinicians to differentiate cochlear and retrocochlear lesions at different levels along the auditory pathways in the brainstem. However, these IPLs may not be a pure measure of the neural conduction time, since data exist to show that the latencies of waves V and I are differentially altered by degree and configuration of hearing loss and therefore could produce I–V IPL changes (Coats, 1978; Coats & Martin, 1977; Don & Eggermont, 1978; Gorga, Worthington, et al., 1985; Eggermont, Don, & Brackmann, 1980; Keith & Greville, 1987; Klein, 1986; Rosenhamer et al., 1981; Sturzebecher, Kevanishvili, Werbs, Meyer, & Schmidt, 1985; Yamada et al., 1979) that have to be distinguished from IPL changes associated with auditory nerve and brainstem abnormalities. Don and Eggermont (1978), using high-pass masking to examine narrowband cochlear contributions to the click ABR, demonstrated that wave I is derived by synchronous cochlear activity largely restricted to basal cochlear regions above about 4000 Hz, while wave V receives contributions from a much broader cochlear region extending down to about 400 Hz. Eggermont, Don, and Brackmann (1980) showed that the wave I latency corresponds to the center frequency bands of 4000 and 8000 Hz, while wave V corresponds to about 1000 to 2000 Hz. That the wave I and wave V latencies are determined by intensity-dependent changes in cochlear regions contributing to the response (i.e., degree and configuration of hearing loss) rather than the type of the hearing loss is suggested by the results of Gorga, Worthington, et al. (1985), showing a delay of both waves I and V and a reduction of I–V IPL.

These results suggest that the I–V IPL could be altered differentially for low- and high-frequency hearing loss. Klein (1986), evaluating the effects of high-pass masking noise on ABRs elicited by a 4000-Hz tone burst, reported differential effects on the latency and amplitude of waves I and V consistent with the notion that different cochlear regions that contribute to waves I and V can also alter the I–V interval. Keith and Greville (1987) made several observations about changes in I–V intervals in individuals with different audiogram configurations. For low-frequency hearing losses, they observed shorter I–V intervals, more prominent at low intensities, because the basal regions contributing to waves I and V are unaffected, but the wave V latency is shorter because of a reduction of apical contributions. In notch-shaped hearing losses, they observed a longer I–V interval because of relatively greater prolongation of wave V due to the reduction of basal contributions. For high-frequency hearing losses, wave I is delayed more relative to wave V resulting in a reduced I–V IPL. This is because the high-frequency hearing loss affects the generation of wave I more than wave V since the latter can rely on contributions from a broader cochlear region. This shortening of the I–V IPL can be clearly distinguished from the abnormally increased IPLs typically observed in auditory nerve and brainstem lesions.

III. ABR IN AUDITORY NERVE AND BRAINSTEM LESIONS

Effects on ABR Characteristics

The ABR reflects synchronized neural activity in the auditory nerve and nuclei and tracts along the auditory brainstem including the midbrain IC. Thus, the components of the ABR provide a sensitive clinical index to evaluate the functional integrity of these structures. Specifically, pathologies at different levels along this pathway may produce distinct changes in the response components' latencies (including IPLs) and amplitudes that enable the clinician to determine the level of the lesion. ABR indices do not permit the identification of specific site(s) of lesion along the auditory pathway in the brainstem, with the exception of identifying acoustic neuroma. Therefore, a level-based classifier is most commonly used—auditory nerve and low (caudal) brainstem lesions versus upper (rostral) brainstem lesions. ABRs continue to be used in the clinic (despite an increased tendency to bypass ABR and perform magnetic resonance imaging [MRI]) to differentiate cochlear and retrocochlear pathologies, more precisely to rule out retrocochlear pathology. The use of ABR, a proven, sensitive, cost-effective measure in screening for auditory nerve and brainstem pathology (Selters & Brackmann, 1977), is desirable despite MRI becoming the gold standard for tumor detection. It should be noted that most referrals for MRI show negative results due to the low incidence of acoustic tumors in the population.

A quick overview of the ABR indices commonly used for identifying retrocochlear pathology would be useful here. The strategy is to use response indices that are particularly sensitive to pathologies beyond the conductive and cochlear mechanisms in the auditory periphery. These include the measurement of IPLs I–III, I–V, and III–V; ILDv; absolute latency of wave V; and the V/I amplitude ratio. IPLs provide a measure of the integrity of neural conduction in the auditory nerve, lower brainstem, and upper brainstem and permit the differentiation of the level of the lesion into auditory nerve and lower brainstem lesion, where IPLs I–III and I–V are characteristically abnormal with normal III–V IPL; or upper brainstem lesion where I–III is normal and III–V and I–V IPLs are typically abnormal. The interaural latency difference in the wave V (ILDv) measure assumes that a structurally intact and normal functioning brainstem should not produce a significant ILDv. Therefore, if a significant ILDv is present (after correcting for any latency difference due to asymmetry in peripheral hearing loss), then it may be consistent with a retrocochlear pathology. ILDv may be the only measure available if earlier components are absent, which is not uncommon. Absolute latency of wave V may also be a useful indicator of retrocochlear pathology but should be used with caution since both cochlear and CHL also produce a prolongation of wave V. Another measure that is useful, more for the identification of upper brainstem lesions affecting the neural generators of wave V, is the V/I amplitude ratio. Normally, wave V is about 1.55 to 1.7 bigger than wave I; however, in some upper brainstem lesions (e.g., a demyelinating disorder affecting the wave V generator), wave V is significantly smaller than wave I, yielding a V/I amplitude ratio of less than 0.75, pointing to a retrocochlear lesion. Finally, stimulus rate effects are also examined to determine if a particular pathology (e.g. multiple sclerosis) is more susceptible to rate-induced neural adaptation.

Effects of Auditory Nerve and Lower (Caudal) Brainstem Lesions on the ABR

This section focuses on lesions involving the auditory nerve (generator of wave I), the cerebellopontine angle (CPA), and the lower brainstem (medulla and caudal pons) that contribute to the generation of waves II and III. The most common auditory nerve mass lesion is acoustic neuroma (80%–90% of all CPA tumors), more appropriately vestibular schwannoma, since it arises from the Schwann cells (that form the myelin sheath around the nerve) in the vestibular portion of the VIIIth cranial nerve. In the posterior fossa region, tumors in the CPA are the most common and account for 5% to 10% of all intracranial tumors; and meningiomas are the most common (3%–13%) nonacoustic tumors in the CPA region (Hall, 2006; Rad, 2011; Shohet, 2012). These benign acoustic tumors start within the internal auditory canal (intracanalicular) and with progression extend into the CPA, are usually unilateral, slow-growing, and associated with a progressive high-frequency (presumably due to compression of the superficially located high-frequency fibers in the auditory nerve bundle) sensorineural hearing loss. Although the specific mechanisms producing a cochlear hearing loss in individuals with an acoustic neuroma are not clear, it is likely a consequence of mechanical injury to the cochlear nerve, vascular compromise, and increased intracanalicular pressure due to the tumor (Lapsiwala, Pyle, Kaemmerle, Sasse, & Badie, 2002). Large acoustic neuromas can displace the brainstem in a caudal-to-rostral direction toward the contralateral rostral brainstem. One common reason for referring a patient for ABR to rule out a retrocochlear pathology is asymmetric high-frequency sensorineural hearing loss, accompanied by disproportionally reduced word recognition score, or absent or elevated acoustic reflex when stimulating the affected side. These individuals may also exhibit tinnitus, vestibular symptoms of vertigo, and neurologic symptoms of facial numbness, tingling, and spasms. However, it should be pointed out that some small intracanalicular tumors (less than 1 cm in size) and posterior fossa tumors will show essentially normal audiograms and excellent word recognition scores.

The characteristic ABR findings in auditory nerve and lower brainstem lesions include the following: the I–III IPL (and I–V interval) may be abnormally prolonged; the ILDv may be significant; absolute latencies of all components may be abnormally prolonged; earlier response components or the entire ABR waveform may be absent.

Abnormalities are usually ipsilateral to the lesion unless the tumor is large and displacing the brainstem, resulting in both ipsilateral and contralateral ABR abnormalities (Figure 6–9). The contralateral

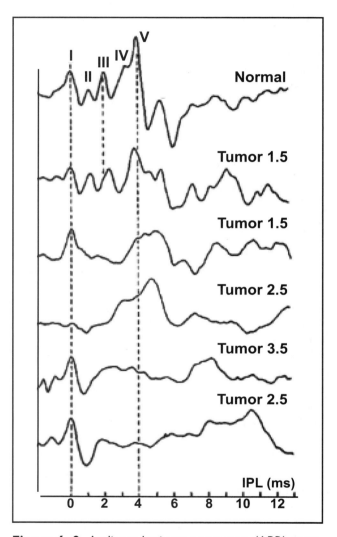

Figure 6–9. Auditory brainstem response (ABR) waveforms in auditory nerve and lower brainstem lesions plotted as a function of tumor size. Vestibular schwannoma size in centimeters is indicated to the right of each trace. ABR morphology ranges from normal to abnormal with only wave I present. The vertical dotted lines aligned with waves I and V show the progressively longer wave V latency and disruption of wave V morphology as tumor size increases. Adapted from "Electrocochleography and Auditory Brainstem Electric Responses in Patients With Pontine Angle Tumors," by J. J. Eggermont, M. Don, and D. E. Brackmann, 1980, *Annals of Otology, Rhinology, and Laryngology, 89*(6, Pt. 2), pp. 1–19. Reprinted by Permission of SAGE Publications, Inc.

abnormality is usually a prolongation in the I–V interval (primarily via III–V prolongation) or I–IV interval in cases where wave V is absent.

Abnormal Interpeak Latencies (IPL: I–III, I–V, and III–V)

The IPLs, particularly I–III and I–V, are abnormally prolonged (see examples of AN and low BS lesions in Figures 6–10 and 6–11) in over 90% of individuals with acoustic neuroma (Antonelli, Bellotto, & Grandori, 1987; Bauch, Olsen, & Pool, 1996; Moller & Moller, 1983; Musiek, Josey, & Glasscock 1986a; Musiek, McCormick, & Hurley, 1996) in contrast to the shortening of these IPLs observed in high-frequency sloping cochlear losses (Coats & Martin, 1977; Gorga, Reiland, & Beauchaine, 1985; Keith & Greville, 1987; Sturzebecher et al., 1985; Yamada, Kodera, & Yagi, 1979). The commonly used tolerance value for I–III IPL set at 2 SD units is about 2.4 ms (Musiek, Josey, & Glasscock, 1986a, 1986b; Rowe, 1978) and for I–V is about 4.5 ms (Eggermont, Don, & Brackmann, 1980). While I–V prolongation is also a strong indicator of a retrocochlear pathology, the prolongation of I–III IPL has to be considered to localize the lesion to the auditory nerve and or lower brainstem (Don & Brackman, 1980; Musiek, McCormick, & Hurley, 1996).

A relatively high percentage of individuals (32%–59%) with an VIIIth nerve tumor may not show any identifiable ABR components (Barrs, Brackmann, Olson, & House, 1985; Bauch & Olsen, 1989; Bauch, Olsen, & Harner, 1983; Eggermont et al., 1980) at all. In others, the only component that is repeatable is wave V; therefore, IPLs cannot be measured. Musiek, Josey, and Glasscock (1986a, 1986b) were able to measure all three ABR wave components and IPLs in only 27% of their subjects with acoustic neuroma. Cashman and Rossman (1983) were able to measure IPLs in only 15% of their subjects. Eggermont et al. (1980) could not identify wave I in 30% of their subjects with a CPA tumor. Thus, it appears that IPL information is available in only a small percentage of individuals with acoustic neuroma. The absence of wave I is somewhat surprising given that most tumors are medial to the site of wave I generation. It is

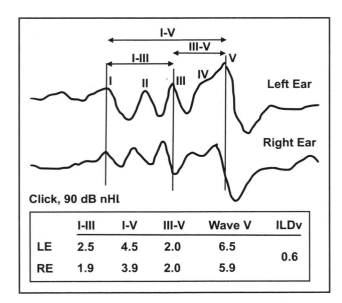

Figure 6–10. Auditory brainstem response (ABR) waveforms for the left ear (*top*) and right ear (*bottom*). Left ear response showing abnormal I–III and I–V IPL with normal III–V interval consistent with an auditory nerve or a lower brainstem lesion. All absolute and interpeak latencies are normal for the right ear.

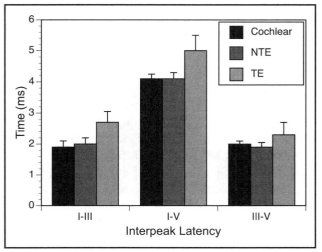

Figure 6–11. Mean interpeak latencies (IPL) for I–III, III–V, and I–V for the tumor ears (TE), nontumor ears (NTE), and cochlear lesion ears (Cochlear). Note that I–III and I–V are abnormally prolonged, for the tumor ear is prolonged with large variability. All IPLs are normal for the NTE and Cochlear ears. Data from "Auditory Brain Stem Response: Interwave Measurements in Acoustic Neuromas," F. E. Musiek, A. F. Josey, and M. E. Glasscock, 1986, *Ear and Hearing*, 7, Figure 1.

likely that a significant high-frequency loss could be contributing to the absence of wave I. There is also some suggestion that the III–V interval in addition to the I–III interval could be prolonged in individuals with acoustic neuromas or CPA tumors (Cashman & Rossman, 1983; Moller & Moller, 1983; Musiek, Josey, & Glasscock, 1986a). Musiek, Josey, and Glasscock (1986a) found that the III–V IPL was significantly longer on the tumor side compared to the nontumor side. However, they did report that abnormal I–III IPL was seen in about 88% of their tumor patients, while 43% of the patients showed an abnormal III–V prolongation. These authors speculated that unlike intracanalicular tumors, the larger-sized VIIIth nerve tract and CPA tumors may be more susceptible to brainstem displacement, compression, and stretching effects that could prolong both I–III and III–V IPLs.

Abnormal Interaural Latency Difference in Wave V (ILDv)

The rationale for the use of ILDv is that symmetrical normal hearing and asymmetrical purely cochlear hearing loss cannot solely account for the large ILDv that is typically suggestive of retrocochlear pathology. ILDv has also been shown to be a highly sensitive metric in detecting VIIIth nerve tumors when the absence of wave I (due to the difficulty in recording a clear wave I either due to a significant high-frequency loss and/or using conventional montage and electrodes) precludes IPL measurements (Bauch & Olsen, 1986, 1989; Bauch et al., 1983; Bauch, Rose, & Harner, 1982; Jerger & Johnson, 1988; Jerger & Mauldin, 1978; Prosser & Arslan, 1987; Selters & Brackmann, 1977). Use of ILDv, with a recommended tolerance of 0.4 ms without any correction for cochlear loss to differentiate cochlear and retrocochlear pathologies also has shown high sensitivity (exceeding 90%) in detecting VIIIth nerve tumors with false-positive rates below 10% (Bauch & Olsen, 1989; Bauch et al., 1996; Moller & Moller, 1983; Musiek, Johnson, Gollegly, Josey, & Glasscock, 1989; Prosser, Arslan, & Pastore, 1984; Selters & Brackmann, 1977; Sturzebecher et al., 1985; Terkildsen, Osterhammel, & Thomsen, 1981). Although we presented the use of a correction factor earlier in this chapter, there is no reliable method to accurately determine the amount of latency shift due to cochlear loss given the variability in latency in individuals with similar degrees of hearing loss, A potential limitation therefore is that ILDv can be confounded by latency shifts produced by the presence of cochlear hearing loss. That is, the ILDv in these cases could reflect a combination of cochlear and retrocochlear components, which may not be easily disentangled and could lead to false-positive results (Bauch & Olsen, 1989; Selters & Brackmann, 1977). Attempts at developing a metric to subtract out the wave V delay due to cochlear loss by applying a correction factor of 0.1 ms for every 10 dB loss greater than 50 dB in the 2000 to 4000 Hz region (Selters & Brackmann, 1977, 1979) have not reduced decision errors in tumor detection (Cashman & Rossman, 1983; Prosser & Arslan, 1987). Given that cochlear hearing loss and individuals with similar hearing loss show considerable variability, Fowler and Durrant (1994) rightly point out that categorization of hearing loss and development of an effective correction factor to fit all is not feasible. These potential drawbacks notwithstanding, the ILDv measure has high sensitivity in tumor detection. An ILDv tolerance value of 0.4 ms is more commonly used without using any correction factor for hearing loss (Cashman & Rossman, 1983; Eggermont et al., 1980; Musiek, Johnson, et al., 1989; Telian, Kileny, Niparko, Kemink, & Graham, 1989). In cases where wave V is the only component present in the affected ear, an absolute latency greater than 6 ms at the maximum output of the system also suggests a retrocochlear pathology. Musiek et al. (1989) have shown that the ILDv is sufficiently sensitive to differentiate between normal hearing, cochlear hearing loss, and auditory nerve and brainstem lesions as shown in the ILDv bar plot in Figure 6–12. However, note that ILDv values for auditory nerve and brainstem lesions essentially overlap. Since IPL I–V and ILDv are derived metrics using wave V latency, it is not surprising to see a strong positive correlation between the two (Figure 6–13), and combined use of both metrics, when available, will improve the accuracy of clinical decision-making regarding presence or absence of an auditory nerve tumor.

Musiek et al. (1996) compared the relative effectiveness of six different ABR indices (wave V latency; IPLs I–III, I–V, III–V); ILDv; and V/I amplitude ratio in 26 individuals with cochlear loss and 26 with confirmed vestibular schwannoma. They

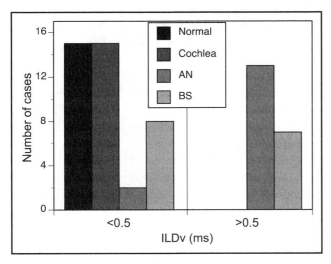

Figure 6–12. Bar plots of ILDv for normal, cochlear, auditory nerve, and brainstem lesions. While there is a clear differentiation between normal, cochlear, and retrocochlear lesions (auditory nerve [AN] and brainstem [BS] lesions), there is considerable overlap in ILDv values for auditory nerve and brainstem lesions. Note that normal and cochlear lesion ears showed ILDv less than 0.5 ms, whereas only the groups with auditory nerve and BS lesions showed ILDv greater than 0.5 ms. Data from "The Auditory Brain Stem Response Interaural Latency Difference (ILD) in Patients With Brainstem Lesions," by F. E. Musiek, G. D. Johnson, K. M. Gollegly, A. F. Josey, and M. E. Glasscock, 1989, *Ear and Hearing, 10*, pp. 131–134, Figure 1.

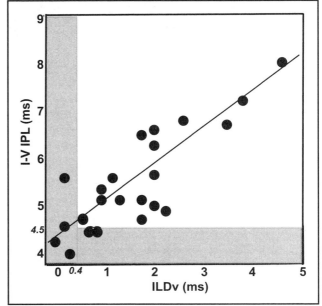

Figure 6–13. Scatterplot showing a strong positive relationship between interpeak latency (IPL) I–V and ILDv suggesting that as IPL I–V increases, so does the ILDv, as expected. The gray vertical and horizontal bars represent the normal limits of ILDv and I–V IPL, respectively. Data from "Electrocochleography and Auditory Brainstem Electric Responses in Patients With Pontine Angle Tumors," by J. J. Eggermont, M. Don, and D. E. Brackmann, 1980, *Annals of Otology, Rhinology, and Laryngology, 89*(6, Pt. 2), pp. 1–19.

found that the I–V interval showed the highest hit rate, lowest false alarms, and high efficiency (Table 6–1). Given that wave I is absent is as many as 40% of individuals with acoustic tumors, wave V latency and ILDv was found to have the highest clinical utility. They also showed that both I-V and ILDv were highly sensitive in differentiating individuals with acoustic neuroma from individuals with a cochlear hearing loss. Most individuals with cochlear hearing loss had an absolute latency of wave V less than 6 ms, I-V IPL less than 4.3 ms, and ILDv less than 0.4 ms

ABR Sensitivity Is Reduced in the Detection of Small Auditory Nerve Tumors

Table 6–2 shows the sensitivity of the ABR in detecting tumors smaller than 1 cm and tumors between 1 and 2 cm in size from several studies. Overall, the mean ABR tumor detection sensitivity is about 96% for larger tumors (>2 cm) and about 79% for tumors smaller than 1 cm, suggesting that standard ABR will likely miss detection of a substantial number of tumors smaller than 1 cm. However, Table 6–2 lists several individual studies that show higher sensitivity for small tumors as well. Also, Bauch et al. (1996) indicated that the sensitivity of the combined indices of I–V IPL and ILD$_V$ is higher (82% for tumors 1.0 cm or smaller, 93% for 1.1–2.0 cm tumors, and 100% for tumors larger than 2.0 cm). The higher sensitivity of the ABR to detect smaller tumors is desirable since early diagnosis of these tumors has been shown to improve the success rate of hearing preservation (Dornhoffer, Helms, & Hoehmann, 1995; Josey, Glasscock, & Jackson, 1988; Shelton, Brackmann, House, & Hitselberger, 1989). For example, Dornhoffer et al. (1995) were able to preserve hearing in 58% of their patients who underwent auditory neuroma resection (for tumors extending less than 1 cm into the CPA).

Table 6–1. Relative Effectiveness of ABR Indices Tolerance Values in Differentiating Cochlear Hearing Loss and Acoustic Neuroma

ABR Metric	Value (ms)	HR (%)	FA (%)	Performance	Efficiency (%)
Wave V					
Latency	>6.0	85	15	0.91	83
I–V	>4.3	87	8	0.94	92
ILDv	>0.3	80	12	0.91	88
I–III	>2.3	67	12	0.86	87
V/I	<0.75	43	0	0.83	97
III–V	>2.1	30	8	0.74	87

Note: Performance is a measure of area under the curve; Efficiency is the percentage overall correct responses.

Source: Created using data from "Effects of Stimulus Phase on the Normal Auditory Brainstem Response," by C. Fowler, 1992, *Journal of Speech and Hearing Research, 35,* p. 171, Table 2.

Table 6–2. ABR Sensitivity for Confirmed Small (<1 cm) and Big (1–2 cm) VIIIth Nerve Tumors Across Studies

	Smaller Tumors (<1 cm)	Larger Tumors (1–2 cm)
Selters & Brackmann, 1979		93%
Glasscock et al., 1979		98%
Eggermont et al., 1980		95%
Terkildsen et al., 1981		96%
Bauch et al., 1982		96%
Wilson et al., 1992	67%	96%
Dornhoffer et al., 1994	93%	100%
Chandrasekhar et al., 1995	83%	100%
Gordon & Cohen, 1995	69%	90%
Zappia et al., 1997	89%	98%
Chandrasekhar et al., 1997	93%	
Godfrey et al., 1998	77%	94%
Robinette et al., 2000	82%	94%
Schmidt et al., 2001	58%	94%
Kochanek et al., 2015		100%*
Mean:	79 (11.57)	96 (2.85)

Note: *Out of 29 patients, ABR correctly identified 13 tumors larger than 1 cm and missed 16 tumors smaller than 1 cm. Thus, overall sensitivity would be reduced to 48%. Means and standard deviations (within parentheses) are shown at the bottom.

Although others have reported similar results (Brooks & Woo, 1994; Josey et al., 1988), Kemink, LaRouere, Kileny, Telian, and Hoff (1990) found no correlation between ABR results and the ability to preserve hearing. Several of these authors have reported that chances for hearing preservation were better when ABR components were present preoperatively, even with delayed latencies as they can provide useful information to decide on a surgical approach.

Stacked ABR as a Method to Improve Detection of Small Acoustic Tumors

Current advanced otoneurologic surgical techniques are capable of removing small tumors with preservation of hearing (Bush, Shinn, Young, & Jones, 2008; Lasek et al., 2008; Timmer et al., 2009; Yamakami, Yoshinori, Saeki, Wada, & Oka, 2009). It is clear from the previous review that the standard ABR may not be adequately sensitive to detect small (less than 1 cm in size) intracanalicular tumors. Consequently, it is not surprising that the more expensive MRI with gadolinium contrast has essentially replaced the low-cost, easily accessible standard ABR, to become the gold standard for the diagnosis of acoustic tumors. However, considering that the ABR is easily accessible and cost-effective, some researchers believe that efforts should be made to improve the sensitivity of the ABR to detect small tumors so that a combination of ABR and MRI would be a better option (Fortnum et al., 2009; Murphy & Selesnick, 2002; Robinette et al., 2000). That is, a process wherein an initial ABR screening is done in all suspected tumor patients followed by an MRI if needed.

In an effort aimed at specifically increasing the sensitivity of the ABR to detect small acoustic tumors, Don, Masuda, Nelson, and Brackmann (1997) developed and validated a clever method called stacked derived narrowband ABR (SABR). In this technique, the broad-spectrum 60 dB nHL click response was high-pass masked at high-pass cutoff frequencies of 8, 4, 2, 1, and 0.5 kHz to derive narrowband cochlear regional contributions centered at 11.3, 5.7, 2.8, 1.4, and 0.7 kHz (Figure 6–14, two left panels). Subsequently, wave V amplitudes were summed by temporally aligning wave V of each derived band; therefore, the name SABR (Figure 6–14, two right panels). Using cumulative percentile curves of the SABR wave V amplitude derived from normal hearing nontumor individuals, they developed amplitude criteria for detecting small tumors. Specifically, if wave V amplitude fell in the lower 20% (corresponding to wave V amplitude of 780 nV or smaller) along the cumulative percentile distribution, then it would indicate the presence of a tumor (Figure 6–15, bottom panel). The top panel of Figure 6–15 shows both the standard ABR (top pair of traces) and the stacked ABR waveforms (bottom pair of traces) for the right ear (left) and the left ear (right) from an individual with a small intracanalicular tumor on the left side. While the amplitudes of wave V for both ears are not appreciably different for the standard ABR, the stacked ABR for the left ear shows a much smaller wave V amplitude compared to the wave V amplitude for the right ear. The plotting of the stacked ABR amplitude values on the cumulative amplitude function (bottom of Figure 6–15) clearly shows that the stacked ABR wave V amplitude for the left ear falls in the lower 20 percentile box (consistent with the presence of a small tumor), while the right ear wave V stacked amplitude value falls in the normal range.

The rationale for this method is that acoustic tumors, regardless of size or location, reduce the number of active neural elements and/or desynchronize the neural activity resulting in a reduction in response amplitude. However, the averaged standard ABR reflects the sum of primary activity along the cochlea that is not temporally aligned due to cochlear contributions with different delays. Thus, it represents a suboptimal neural output of all active auditory nerve fibers that may not accurately reflect the reduction in amplitude due to the presence of a tumor. To get an amplitude measure that is a true reflection of the auditory nerve output, the temporal canceling effects must be eliminated by aligning the responses from different cochlear regions as done with stacked ABR recordings. Thus, if any high-frequency fiber response is compromised due to the acoustic tumor pressure on the nerve, it will be reflected in reduced amplitude of the response below the 20% criterion. Don, Kwong, Tanaka, et al., (2005) observed a mean amplitude reduction of 50% in individuals with

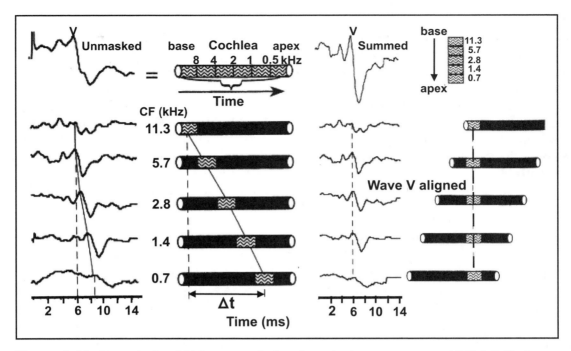

Figure 6–14. Unmasked and high-pass masked auditory brainstem responses (ABRs) (*left*) show a systematic increase in wave V latency as high-pass masking cutoff frequency decreases as the cochlear contribution to the response is increasingly restricted to the apical portion. *Second panel:* The derived narrowband regions (*gray stippled rectangles*) contributing to the ABR moving systematically from base to apex. *Third and fourth panels:* Temporal alignment of the different derived narrowbands before the waveforms are summed to produce the stacked ABR with larger amplitude shown at the top of the aligned derived-band waveforms (*third panel*). Data from "Successful Detection of Small Acoustic Tumors Using the Stacked Derived-Band Auditory Brain Stem Response Amplitude," by M. Don, A. Masuda, R. Nelson, and D Brackmann, 1997, *American Journal of Otology, 18*(5), pp. 608–621.

small acoustic tumors (less than 1 cm; $n = 54$) compared to nontumor and normal ears ($n = 78$) even before these patients sought medical attention. This stacked ABR method significantly improved the sensitivity of the ABR to detect small tumors that were missed by standard ABR (Don & Kwong, 2002; Don, Kwong, Tanaka, Brackmann, & Nelson, 2005; Don et al., 1997). In their initial study, Don, Masuda, Nelson, and Brackmann (1977) showed that stacked wave V amplitude in all five cases of small intracanalicular tumors was significantly smaller compared to a group of normal-hearing individuals without tumors (Figure 6–15, top and bottom panels). Subsequently, Don et al. (2005) compared the sensitivity of the SABR and standard ABR method to detect MRI-confirmed small acoustic neuromas (equal to or less than 1 cm) in 54 patients (in whom the tumor went undetected using standard ABR) and 78 patients in the nontumor normal-hearing control group. They found that SABR showed 95% sensitivity and 88% specificity, whereas the standard ABR measures were poorer in detecting these tumors, consistent with previous findings. Based on these results, they concluded that the SABR can be a sensitive, cost-effective, and easily recordable measure for screening for small acoustic tumors. In terms of when SABR is indicated, Don and Kwong (2002) suggest that SABR should be performed only when the ILDv appears normal and the clinician feels that retrocochlear involvement cannot be ruled out.

Given the typical large variability associated with the standard wave V amplitude recorded at intensities higher (Picton, 2011; Schwartz & Berry, 1985) than those used in the stacked ABR protocol (60 dB nHL), it is not surprising that the relatively smaller amplitudes for stacked ABR also show large intersubject variability, which might limit the clini-

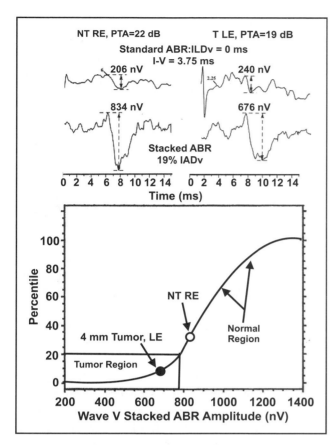

Figure 6–15. Comparison of standard and tacked auditory brainstem response (ABR) amplitude in an individual with a small intracanalicular tumor on the left side. Puretone averages indicated normal hearing sensitivity. ABR waveforms for the standard click ABR (top pair, RE on the left and LE on the right in each pair) and the stacked ABR (bottom pair of waveforms in the *top panel*). Wave V amplitude is provided for both ABRs. It is clear from the waveform data that the stacked ABR wave V amplitude is much larger for both ears compared to wave V amplitude obtained for the standard click ABR. However, wave V amplitude for the left ear (676 nV) falls within the lower 20% (shown by the white diamond symbol) of the cumulative percentile curve (*bottom panel*) suggesting an acoustic tumor. Data from "Successful Detection of Small Acoustic Tumors Using the Stacked Derived-Band Auditory Brain Stem Response Amplitude," by M. Don, A. Masuda, R. Nelson, and D Brackmann, 1997, *American Journal of Otology*, *18*(5), pp. 608–621.

cal utility of this procedure. Additionally, not all commercially available evoked potential systems are equipped to perform SABR, and the lengthy test protocol may discourage its use in the clinic.

Many clinicians report both high false-positive rates (low specificity) and lengthy test time. These issues, at least in part, reflect an inadequate understanding of the fundamental principles of SABR and general inattention to certain technical details, including (1) *criterion for subjects* (e.g., older subjects and subjects with hearing loss will have smaller amplitude responses prone to variability, and higher false-positive rates). In fact, Don et al. (2005) suggest that SABR not be performed in individuals with hearing loss greater than 50 dB HL; (2) *higher electrode impedances* that produce poorer SNR and may lengthen test time, so care should be taken to obtain electrode impedances well below 3000 ohms; (3) choice of *transducer*: the stacked ABR was developed using Etymōtic ER-2 earphones to optimize activation of higher-frequency fibers compromised by tumors and therefore use of any other transducer (e.g., Etymōtic, ER-3, often used clinically) will change the frequency response and stimulus level such that HF fibers are not activated adequately, thus reducing both sensitivity and specificity; (4) *test environment*: recordings made outside a sound booth could be smaller in amplitude due to masking by background environmental noise; (5) *high residual noise* during recording that can contaminate the ABR and lengthen test time—care should be taken to have the subject relaxed; and (6) use of *published criterion values and/or reliance on norms provided by the manufacturer* may lead to misinterpretation and higher false-positive rates. Generally, it is recommended that clinicians develop their own in-house norms on normal-hearing individuals. Thus, while recording the stacked ABR may appear simple, these are important steps that have to be attended to and optimized to improve both the sensitivity and specificity of the measure.

Don, Kwong, and Tanaka (2010) attempted to address the large intersubject variability in the SABR amplitude, and the poor specificity of SABR. Although SABR has been effective in improving the detection of small tumors overall, the poor specificity is primarily due to smaller than expected amplitudes in nontumor ears (Don et al., 1997, 2005). Based on their observation of lower variability in wave V amplitude between the right and left ears within individuals, they proposed the use of the less variable measure of interaural amplitude difference in wave V (ISABR). Like the ILDv for latency, the smaller wave V amplitude from the tumor side is subtracted from the usually larger wave V amplitude from the nontumor side and then divided by the amplitude of the nontumor side to obtain a normalized interaural amplitude difference. They reasoned that since this is a relative measure, it will be less influenced by factors that affect the absolute amplitude. It has the additional advantage of evaluating tumor and nontumor patients with large and small absolute wave V amplitudes, respectively; and the interaural measure uses the patient as their own control. Applying this method to nontumor/normal-hearing individuals and 17 individuals with small acoustic tumors (less than 1 cm), they found that the ISABR wave V amplitude differences were greater for patients with tumors (mean = 43%, SD = 21.3% at the 50% point) compared to the mean for the nontumor/normal groups (mean less than 1%, SD = 9% at the 50% point). This suggests that a small tumor will reduce the amplitude by ~43% compared to the nontumor side. They showed that an interaural wave V amplitude difference of only about 8% will result in a sensitivity of 95% and a specificity of nearly 83% (Figure 6–16)—comparable to their SABR data (Don et al., 2005). Since the interaural difference is much greater for confirmed tumor patients than nontumor patients, it is possible that nontumor/normal-hearing individuals with SABR amplitudes falling in the lower 20%, and interaural differences close to zero will be incorrectly identified as having a tumor. In contrast, the ISABR will show little or no interaural difference and accurately identify the absence of a tumor. Thus, ISABR provides an additional measure that will increase specificity by reducing the false-positive rate based on using just SABR. The bar plot in Figure 6–17 clearly shows that a small normalized SABR and a large interaural difference (IASBR difference) are indeed due to a tumor. That is, the almost linear function in Figure 6–17 (black bars) shows that for individuals with a small tumor, the smaller the normalized SABR amplitude, the larger will be the interaural amplitude difference. Note that ISABR differences for normal individuals hover around zero since the wave V amplitude from each ear will not be very different.

Kochanek et al. (2015) compared the sensitivity and relative effectiveness of tone burst elicited ABRs, standard ABR to click, and the stacked ABR in detecting small acoustic neuromas to determine if tone burst ABR could be a faster alternative to stacked ABR. They reasoned that the less robust

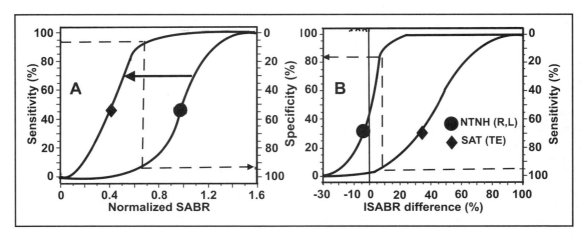

Figure 6–16. Comparison of the cumulative distribution of the normalized SABR amplitude (A) and the cumulative distribution of the percent interaural difference in the ISABR amplitudes (B) for the nontumor normal hearing (NTNH) and small acoustic tumor (SAT) populations. For SABR, a criterion that achieves 95% sensitivity results in 93% specificity (*dashed lines*). For ISABR, for a criterion that achieves 95% sensitivity (the interaural difference is about 8%), the specificity is about 83%. ISABR provides an additional measure that increases the specificity by reducing the false-positive rate associated with using SABR alone. Data used with permission from Don, Kwong, and Tanaka (2012).

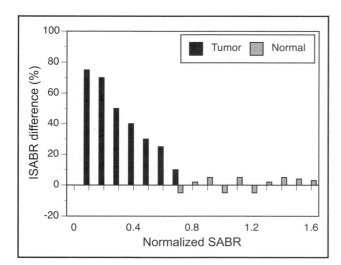

Figure 6–17. ISABR amplitude difference (in percentage) is plotted as a function of normalized SABR amplitude for the tumor patients (*black bar on the left*) as well as the nontumor (*gray bars on the right*). Only the tumor patients show an inverse linear relationship where the ISABR difference decreases as normalized SABR amplitude increases because of the tumor. In contrast, there is no such relationship for the normal group, and the values as expected hover around the zero point. Data used with permission from Don, Kwong, and Tanaka (2012).

wave V response amplitude to frequency specific tone bursts with gradual rise-fall times would be more susceptible to desynchronization results from compression of the auditory nerve by the tumor. They compared ABRs using the three methods in individuals with small (*n* = 16 ears, less than 1 cm in size) and medium/large (*n* = 13 ears, between 1.5 and 2 cm in size) tumors, with essentially normal hearing sensitivity, and individuals (*n* = 265 ears) without retrocochlear lesions. As expected, the results using stacked ABR showed high sensitivity (96.6%) to detect small tumors, but the large variability in the wave V amplitude resulted in very low specificity (26%), indicating a high false-positive rate. Figure 6–18 illustrates the comparisons between the three procedures. The standard ABR results showed good specificity (98%) but poor sensitivity (44.8%). That is, it detected only large tumors and missed detecting all the small tumors. Tone burst ABR results showed the best sensitivity (89.7%—detected 26 and missed 3 small tumors) and specificity (89.4%). Based on these results, the authors suggest the use of a two-stage acoustic neuroma screening procedure consisting of a standard ABR initially followed by tone burst ABR. In our view, this approach would be more effective if higher-frequency (3000, 4000, and 6000 Hz) tone bursts were utilized with an ER-2 transducer (which activates higher frequencies more effectively compared to the ER-3) to activate higher-frequency fibers that may be compromised earlier in small auditory nerve tumors.

The stacked ABR technique also sheds some important light on the source of the ILDv. By comparing click alone and derived-band responses from tumor cases, Don, Kwong, and Tanaka (2010) demonstrated the dependence of the ILDv measure on activity in the high-frequency regions of the cochlea. Specifically, when there is no high-frequency contribution to the ABR (above 8000 Hz) from the tumor side, ILDv will be large because of the differences in the primary place of activity —more apical for the tumor side (longer latency) and basal dominant activity (shorter latency) for the nontumor side resulting in a significant ILDv. If the tumor does not sufficiently eliminate the high-frequency activity, then the ILDv should be approaching zero, since there should not be any difference in the cochlear places contributing to the response. Therefore, in the case of the former, the ILDv is due to a difference in the cochlear places providing the primary contribution to the ABR and does not reflect a neural conduction delay due to compression of the nerve. Don et al. (2010) reason persuasively that ILDv will be normal and miss detecting tumors if there is no sufficient compromise of a subset of high-frequency fibers that normally dominate the latency of wave V in the click alone response. In light of this, the assumption that the ILDv provides a clean measure of neural conduction delay is questionable. However, this account of the ILDv source is not entirely consistent with the observation of essentially normal wave V latency in sloping high-frequency cochlear losses, the significant ILDs sometimes observed with little or no hearing loss (e.g., Bauch et al., 1996; Musiek et al., 1996), and the ability of the ILDv to clearly distinguish cochlear and auditory nerve and brainstem lesions (Musiek, Johnson, Gollegly, et al., 1989).

Another appropriate stimulus to consider here is the emergent broadband chirp. ABRs elicited by

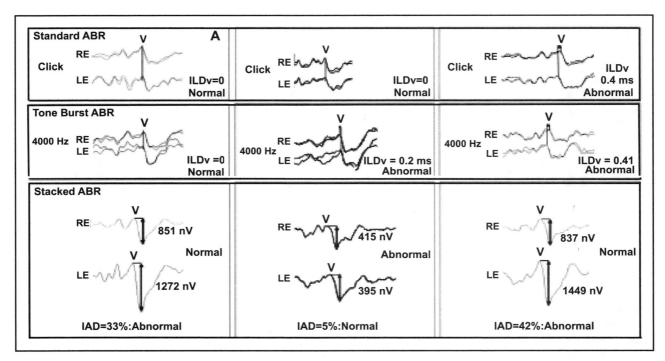

Figure 6–18. Comparison between standard click auditory brainstem response (ABR) (*top row*), tone burst ABR (*middle row*), and stacked ABR (*bottom row*) for three subjects with confirmed small acoustic tumors. In the first case on the left, standard tone burst and stacked ABR results were all normal except for abnormal ISABR amplitude. For the second case in the middle, only standard ABR was normal with both tone burst and stacked ABR abnormal. For the third case on the right, standard, tone burst, and ISABR amplitudes were abnormal. These examples suggest that the combined use of these procedures may improve small acoustic tumor detection. Data used with permission from "Comparison of 3 ABR Methods for Diagnosis of Retrocochlear Hearing Impairment," by K. M. Kochanek, L. Sliwa, M. Gotebiowski, A. Pitka, and H. Skarzynski, 2015, *Medical Science Monitor, 21*, pp. 3814–3824.

broadband chirps reflect the sum of cochlear contributions that are temporally aligned by virtue of the stimulus components compensating for the cochlear delay to produce a more synchronous neural activity. Thus, the phase cancellation effects seen with standard click ABRs due to cochlear contributions with different cochlear delays are eliminated. It has been well established that ABRs elicited by these chirps are more robust and exhibit larger amplitudes compared to standard click-elicited ABRs. Given this, it is reasonable to propose that, like the stacked ABR (which also removes the smearing effects of cochlear delay by the process of time aligning the derived responses), the chirp ABR might better reflect the effects of desynchronization due to tumor-induced compression of the auditory nerve, thus improving detection of smaller tumors.

Importantly, this stimulus will allow recording of the responses at higher levels, which will enable sufficient activation of higher-frequency regions that are compromised by the tumor (and therefore would better reflect the auditory nerve output) and enable more stable responses with less amplitude variability. Because there is no need for high-pass masking, this stimulus will also significantly reduce test time, without the need for the subsequent derivation steps, and summing the temporally aligned derived-band responses. The availability of narrowband chirps has the potential of evaluating the sensitivity of high-frequency chirps in detecting small acoustic tumors. However, to date, we are not aware of any published reports evaluating the clinical utility of chirp-elicited ABRs in the detection of small acoustic tumors.

Relationship Between ABR and Auditory Nerve Tumor Size

There is strong evidence that the ABR wave V latency and its derivatives, the I–V IPL and ILDv, increase as a function of tumor size (Bauch et al., 1996 Musiek, Josey, & Glasscock, 1986a, 1986b). However, the evaluation of the correlation between different ABR metrics and tumor size has produced equivocal findings. Several studies (Grabel, Zapulla, Ryder, Wang, & Malis, 1991; Shih, Tseng, Yeh, Hsu, & Chen, 2009; Zapulla, Greenblatt, & Karmel, 1982) show at least a moderate correlation (e.g., relationship between IPL I–V and tumor size in Figure 6–19), while others show either a weak or no correlation between ABR changes and tumor size (Bauch et al., 1996; Musiek et al., 1986a, 1986b). However, examining the ILDv data from Bauch et al. (1996), there appears to be a clear trend that the ILDv increases with tumor size, albeit the data are only for 10 subjects. Evaluating the relationship between the I–III IPL and tumor size in 56 individuals with confirmed acoustic tumors (10 intracanalicular, and 46 extracanalicular), Zappulla et al. (1982) found a significant positive correlation between ipsilateral I–III IPL and tumor size as well as between contralateral III–V IPL and tumor size. The III–V prolongations on the contralateral side were for larger tumors that displaced the brainstem. Similarly, Shih et al. (2009) also observed a positive correlation between ipsilateral/contralateral ABR indices and tumor size.

Bilateral Effects of Auditory Nerve and Lower Brainstem Lesions

Most auditory nerve and lower brainstem tumors characteristically produce abnormalities in the ear ipsilateral to the tumor side with normal ABR elicited by stimulation of the contralateral ear. However, large tumors (greater than 2 cm in size) can displace, compress, and stretch the brainstem in a caudorostral direction affecting the contralateral rostral brainstem. The result is abnormal ABRs with stimulation of either ear. Specifically, in addition to the typical I–III and I–V IPL prolongation on ipsilateral stimulation, the contralateral ear will likely show a I–V IPL prolongation mostly resulting from an increase in the III–V IPL (wave IV and/or wave V abnormality), or an absent wave V with only waves I–IV present (Figure 6–20) with normal I–III IPL (Musiek & Kibbe, 1986; Nodar & Kinney, 1980; Selters & Brackmann, 1977; Shih et al., 2009; Zapulla et al., 1982). Moffat, Baguley, Hardy, and Tsui (1989) reported contralateral ABR abnormalities in only 16.4% of their 79 patients with unilateral acoustic neuroma. Contralateral ABR abnormalities in these patients included abnormal III–V prolongation in six patients and abnormal I–III IPL in seven patients. Also, they found contralateral abnormalities in 25.6% of patients with large tumors (greater than 2.5 cm), 14% of patients with medium tumors (1.0–2.5 cm), and no contralateral abnormalities in patients with small intracanalicular tumors. In some large tumors (greater than 4 cm), it is also possible that only wave IV may be present with the absence of wave V. These changes in the contralateral ABR suggest that the enlarged

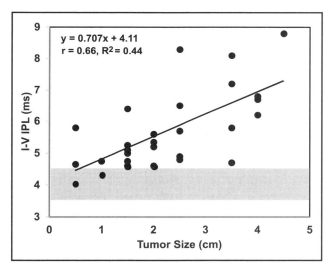

Figure 6–19. Scatterplot and regression line depicting the relationship between I–V interpeak latency (IPL) and tumor size from 28 individuals with confirmed acoustic neuroma. There is a trend indicating that the I–V IPL increases with tumor size. The shaded light gray area represents the normal range for the I–V IPL. I–V IPL tolerance is 4.55 ms. ABR was absent in 13 other individuals with a tumor. Created using data from "Electrocochleography and Auditory Brainstem Electric Responses in Patients With Pontine Angle Tumors," by J. J. Eggermont, M. Don, and D. E. Brackmann, 1980, *Annals of Otology, Rhinology, and Laryngology*, 89(6, Pt. 2), pp. 1–19.

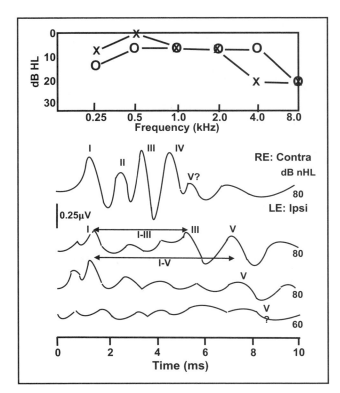

Figure 6–20. Representative auditory brainstem responses (ABRs) from a young adult patient with a large left side (4 cm) cerebellopontine angle tumor displacing the brainstem and producing bilateral ABR abnormality. Audiograms were normal with excellent word recognition bilaterally. The left ear shows abnormally delayed wave V (7.3 ms), thus producing an abnormal I–III and I–V interpeak latency (IPL). The poorly defined response at 60 dB nHL is inconsistent with the essentially normal hearing sensitivity. The right ear (contralateral to the lesion) shows robust waves I–IV and only an abnormally small wave V. The brainstem displacement produced by the large tumor compromises the wave V generator on the contralateral side. Waveform rendering based on data from "ABR in the Eighth Nerve and Low Brainstem Lesions," by F. E. Musiek and K. M. Gollegly. In *The Auditory Brainstem Response*, by J. T. Jacobson (Ed.), 1985, Chapter 10, p. 193. Copyright 1985 by College Hill Press, San Diego, CA.

tumor is affecting the rostral brainstem neural generator sites for waves IV and V. In addition to the changes in absolute latencies and IPLs on the contralateral side, Zapulla et al. (1982), observed that contralateral response latency changes were correlated with tumor size and reflected the extent of brainstem compression by the tumor. Nodar and Kinney (1980) also demonstrated prolonged latencies, reduced amplitudes, and poor morphology and repeatability of contralateral responses in 12 patients with large tumors (greater than 2 cm) in the vicinity of the VIIIth nerve. Similarly, Shih et al. (2009) showed longer contralateral wave V absolute latency, and III–V IPL in individuals with vestibular schwannoma equal to or greater than 2 cm compared to individuals with tumors less than 2 cm in size. They concluded that the presence of an abnormal contralateral wave V absolute latency and III–V IPL indicated a tumor size potentially larger than 2 cm. Given these consistent results of contralateral ABR abnormalities in individuals with VIIIth nerve tumors equal to or larger than 2 cm, it is important to evaluate ABRs from both ears.

Use of V/I Amplitude Ratio in the Detection of Auditory Nerve and Lower Brainstem Lesions

Since the peak-to-trough amplitude of the ABR components exhibits large intersubject variability, it does not appear to be a valid metric in clinical differential diagnosis. To overcome this problem of amplitude variability, a relative measure expressing the ratio between wave V and wave I amplitude, the V/I amplitude ratio, is more commonly used in differential diagnosis (Chiappa, Harrison, Brooks, & Young, 1980; Hall, 1992; Musiek et al., 1996; Rosenhall, Hedner, & Björkman, 1981; Stockard & Rossiter, 1977). As mentioned earlier in this chapter, wave V amplitude is typically 1.5 to 1.7 times larger than wave I. However, in retrocochlear lesions, particularly upper brainstem lesions involving demyelination, wave V shows poor repeatability and appreciably smaller amplitude than wave I, resulting in a V/I amplitude ratio that is much lower than 1 (that is, wave I is bigger than wave V). A V/I amplitude ratio of less than 0.75 is suggestive of a retrocochlear pathology. While this measure is considered in the detection of acoustic neuromas, it has shown poor test sensitivity but high specificity (Musiek et al., 1996). These authors point out a strong association between the presence of a vestibular schwannoma and a V/I amplitude ratio of less than 0.75. However, in their evaluation of the relative effectiveness of six different ABR indices, the V/I amplitude ratio and the III–V IPL had the lowest sensitivity (43% and 30%, respectively). It is likely that this metric is more sensitive in the detection of upper brainstem lesions that typically show amplitude reduction for the IV/V complex due to functional compromise of their neural generators. The reader is cautioned here that the choice of electrodes is an important variable. Electrodes such as tiptrodes or intrameatal electrodes enhance wave I amplitude and therefore could change the V/I amplitude relationship compared to the use of the standard electroencephalograph-type scalp electrodes.

IV. ABR IN AUDITORY NEUROPATHY (AN) AND COCHLEAR SYNAPTOPATHY

Introduction

Other non-mass auditory nerve anomalies include the rare condition of total absence of the auditory nerve: cochlear nerve aplasia (Casselman, Offeciers, & Govaerts, 1997); reduced number of spiral ganglion neurons (Nadol & Young, 1989; Otte, Schunknecht, & Kerr, 1978); neural transmission/dyssynchrony (auditory neuropathy—more commonly labeled as auditory neuropathy spectrum disorders [ANSD]); and a reduction in the synaptic ribbons associated with IHC-auditory nerve synapses (cochlear synaptopathy). Here we focus on AN and cochlear synaptopathy. While both these disorders typically show normal function of the OHC subsystem, as reflected by normal otoacoustic emissions (OAE), their manifestation in the ABR is distinct, consistent with the compromise of presumably different neural mechanisms.

ABRs in Auditory Neuropathy

As described in an earlier chapter, AN operationally is an auditory nerve dysfunction characterized by abnormal neural transmission along the auditory nerve resulting from dyssynchronous neural activity (reflected in abnormal or absent ABR components) in individuals with hearing loss and normal OHC subsystem (reflected by normal OAE and the presence of a cochlear microphonic). Seen in about 1% to 8% of individuals with hearing loss, the locus of the lesion may include the IHC/auditory nerve presynaptic region of transmitter release, the postsynaptic region that initiates the development of excitatory postsynaptic potentials (EPSPs), and/or the spiral ganglion cells that disrupt neural transmission along the auditory nerve to the cochlear nucleus in the brainstem. The dyssynchrony in neural activity disrupts fine-grained temporal processing of sounds, which is believed to cause the difficulty experienced in speech perception and sound localization (which is exacerbated in the presence of noise) by these individuals. In terms of etiology, both environmental (e.g., hyperbilirubinemia, thiamine deficiency, and hypoxia in the newborn) and genetic factors have been associated with AN. AN due involving gene mutation often manifests as a hereditary syndrome including hearing loss and other neuropathies (e.g., Charcot-Marie-Tooth disease [CMT]) that affect not only the spiral ganglion cells but other peripheral neurons as well). While over 80 genes have been identified to cause CMT, altered expressions of two genes, MPZ (Myelin Protein Zero) and PMP22 (Peripheral Myelin Protein 22) have been specifically associated with AN. These two proteins expressed in Schwann cells are involved in the proper formation and maintenance of compact myelin. Mutations that disrupt the function of these proteins can lead to deficient expression of myelin and degeneration of the myelin sheath in the peripheral nervous system (Kirschner, Inouye, & Saavedra, 1996; Watila & Balarabe, 2015).

Common audiometric findings in patients with AN include mild to severe hearing loss (Wang, Gu, Han, & Yang, 2015); word recognition reduced disproportionately to the degree and configuration of hearing loss; difficulty in understanding speech, particularly in adverse listening conditions; absent acoustic reflexes (in 90% of the cases) or elevated when present; absent OAEs in about 25% of the cases; and absent OAE suppression (the normal reduction in OAE amplitude when a sound is introduced in the contralateral ear) in the ipsilateral ear only suggesting the involvement of the afferent pathway (Hood, Berlin, Bordelon, & Rose, 2003) and not the efferent system. Clinical diagnosis is primarily made using ABR and OAE, demonstrating a combination of abnormal ABR suggesting auditory nerve dysfunction, and normal OAEs using either the broadband click-evoked transient otoacoustic emissions (TROAEs) or the frequency-specific distortion product otoacoustic emissions (DPOAEs), suggesting normal functional integrity of the OHC subsystem. In addition, derivation of the receptor cochlear microphonic (CM) response from the ABR also provides a measure of the functional integrity of the OHC subsystem. Thus, the typical results consistent with an AN diagnosis will show abnormal or absent ABR and the presence of OAE and CM (Figure 6–21). The absence of both ABR and OAE obscures such a definitive diagnosis of AN. However, a combination of absent ABR, present CM, and absent OAE could still point to AN.

The use of alternating stimulus polarity, which essentially averages the response to each polarity, will eliminate the CM, and in the absence of the ABR is not very useful diagnostically. The test strategy then is to record ABRs to each onset polarity (condensation and rarefaction) to derive the cochlear microphonic. Specifically, subtraction of the independent responses to each polarity will yield a real biologic CM if stimulus artifact can be ruled out. Even with a single polarity recording, a sustained CM can be visualized in some individuals with AN (Sininger & Oba, 2001; Starr et al., 2001). There are several ways to determine if the result of the subtraction process is indeed a true CM and not a stimulus artifact. Since the stimulus artifact should show no measurable latency, and the CM has a latency of about 0.6 ms plus the almost 1-ms acoustic delay due to the tubing of the insert earphone, the resulting temporal separation between the two responses could be used to separate them. This is not an ideal method since the two responses could overlap if there is any ringing in the stimulus. A better method to rule out stimulus artifact and confirm a true biologic response is to block the stimulus to the ear by pinching the insert ear tubing while the transducer is in place and energized. Thus, if a response is still present in this condition, it must be a stimulus artifact since no audible stimulus is presented to generate a true CM. Ideally, the use of a magnetically shielded earphone is the best solution because it will eliminate stimulus artifact. Given that AN may fluctuate over time, particularly in the newborn, care should be taken to repeat measures over time to confirm the diagnosis before intervention is planned.

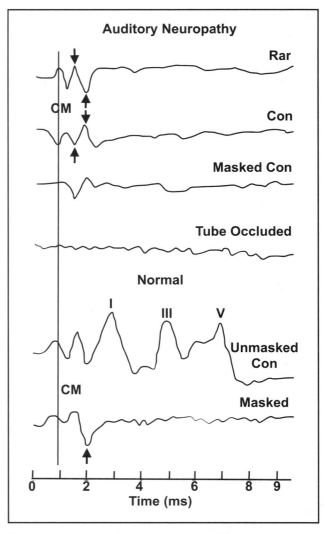

Figure 6–21. Cochlear microphonic (CM) and auditory brainstem responses (ABRs) in an individual with auditory neuropathy (top four traces) and a normal individual. ABRs are absent with only the CM (indicated by up and down arrows) present. The CM polarity reverses when onset polarity is reversed. The addition of masking still shows the CM present. The absence of CM with insert earphone tube occlusion confirms that the observed response is a true biologic CM. For the normal ear, clear ABR components (I through V) are present, which are then completely masked in the presence of noise, again leaving the receptor potential unchanged. Created using data from "Auditory Neuropathy," by A. Starr, T. W. Picton, Y. Sinninger, L. Hood, and C. Berlin, 1996, *Brain, 119*(3), pp. 741–753.

Outcomes with traditional amplification or cochlear implants (CIs) depend on the nature of the auditory nerve/synapse dysfunction. Since dyssynchrony and neural transmission is the problem in AN, amplifying sounds via hearing aids may be of little or no benefit. Shearer and Hanson (2019), based on data from their timely review of the effects of both qualitative and quantitative auditory nerve deficits (using a precise description of the site of the lesion) on cochlear implant outcomes, showed that patients with lesions primarily limited to the cochlear sensory system and the synapse (cochlea, IHCs, ribbon synapse's presynaptic and postsynaptic sites) showed optimal CI outcomes because these elements are bypassed by the CI. In contrast, individuals with lesions that directly involve the auditory nerve showed poor outcomes with CIs because of disrupted neural transmission. It is unlikely that any ABR component would be present unless the distal portion of the auditory nerve is not affected, in which case only wave I would be present. However, absent ABRs with the presence of cochlear microphonics are more common in individuals with AN.

ABRs in Cochlear Synaptopathy

There is compelling evidence from recent animal studies that even moderate levels of noise exposure can substantially reduce the number of synaptic ribbons (Figure 6–22A and B) between the IHCs and auditory nerve fibers (cochlear synaptopathy) without affecting audiometric thresholds (Furman, Kujawa, & Liberman, 2013; Hickox, Larsen, Heinz, Shinobu, & Whitton, 2017; Kujawa & Liberman, 2009; Lin, Furman, Kujawa, & Liberman, 2011; Maison, Usubuchi, & Liberman, 2011; Valero et al., 2017). Since there is no measurable hearing loss in the presence of reported hearing deficits, this phenomenon has also been labeled as a hidden hearing loss (HHL). The IHC ribbon synapse consists of a long tether anchored to the presynaptic cell membrane that holds the synaptic vesicles proximal to the presynaptic release point at the synaptic cleft. The synaptic component includes both pre- and postsynaptic sites. Cochlear synaptopathy-induced reduction in the synaptic ribbons compromises this structural arrangement believed to facilitate optimal transmission with high temporal precision and likely disrupts neural transmission.

In animals, wave I amplitude appears to be a sensitive noninvasive measure to evaluate and detect cochlear synaptopathy since its reduction and shallower growth have been shown to strongly correlate with the number of surviving spiral ganglion

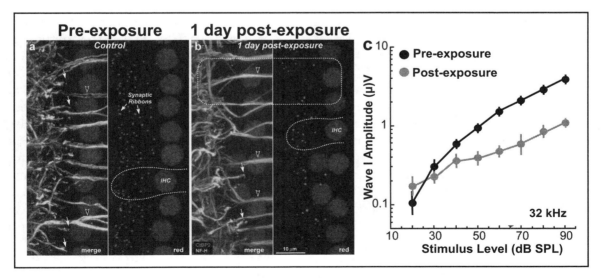

Figure 6–22. A. Intact synaptic ribbons. **B.** Loss of synaptic ribbons after noise exposure. **C.** Consistent with this, the VIII nerve compound action potential postexposure (*gray symbols*) shows reduced amplitude compared to preexposure (*black symbols*) amplitude. Data from "Adding Insult to Injury: Cochlear Nerve Degeneration After 'Temporary' Noise-Induced Hearing Loss," by S. G. Kujawa and M. C. Liberman, 2009, *Journal of Neuroscience*, *29*(45), pp. 14077–14085 and "Primary Neural Degeneration in the Guinea Pig Cochlea After Reversible Noise-Induced Threshold Shift," by H. W. Lin, A. C. Furman, S. G. Kujawa, and M. C. Liberman, 2011, *Journal of the Association for Research in Otolaryngology*, *12*, pp. 605–616.

neurons (Liberman & Kujawa, 2017). Also, the relatively unaltered ABR wave V amplitude in the presence of reduced wave I amplitude suggests central compensation for the reduced peripheral output (Shaheen, Valero, & Liberman, 2015). However, not all human studies have uniformly shown wave I amplitude reduction in individuals with a history of noise exposure and normal hearing sensitivity (Fulbright, Le Prell, Griffiths, & Lobarinas, 2017; Grinn, Wiseman, Baker, & Le Prell, 2017; Grose, Buss, & Hall III, 2017; Liberman, Epstein, Cleveland, Wang, & Maison, 2016; Prendergast et al., 2017; Stamper & Johnson, 2015). For example, Valderrama et al. (2018), Bramhall, Konrad-Martin, McMillan, and Griest (2017), and Stamper and Johnson (2015) showed a correlation between wave I amplitude reduction and noise exposure. Several other studies, while not specifically showing wave I amplitude reduction, have observed alterations in other ABR indices that support noise exposure–induced cochlear synaptopathy. For example, Liberman et al. (2016) observed enhanced SP/AP (summating potential/action potential) ratio in their high-risk group (college-age musicians) that was correlated with speech deficits in noise, reverberation, and time compression; Grose, Buss, and Hall III (2017) showed reduced wave V/I amplitude ratio in the high-risk group; Valderrama et al. (2018), observed a correlation between wave I–V IPL and word recognition scores; Ridley, Kopun, Neely, Gorga, and Rasetshwane (2018) suggest that the SP/AP ratio, wave I, wave V and the threshold-in-noise residual may be useful measures for predicting HHL in humans; and more recently, Mepani et al. (2020) found evidence suggesting neural deficits (elevated SP or SP/AP ratio). Several factors could account for the lack of uniform findings in human studies, including the inherent difficulty in accurately defining the experimental and control groups to be sufficiently distinct based on less than optimal noise exposure history; differences in susceptibility to noise damage among humans—tough versus tender ears (Attanasio et al., 1999; Henderson, Subramaniam, Spongr, & Attanasio, 1996; Subramaniam, Campo, & Henderson, 1991); variability of ABR wave I amplitude in human ABRs due to factors such as age, sex, audiometric thresholds, and head size (Burkard & Don, 2007; Gorga, Worthington, et al., 1985; Mitchell, Phillips, & Trune, 1989); and the possibility that transducer type and stimulus paradigms utilized to date may not have been optimally sensitive to reveal consequences of noise-induced cochlear synaptopathy.

In an effort aimed at identifying more sensitive stimulus manipulations that produce reliable changes in human ABR that reliably reflect consequences of cochlear synaptopathy, Suresh and Krishnan (2021) evaluated the effects of stimulus level and background noise on the amplitude and latency of ABRs obtained from individuals at low and high risk for music–induced cochlear synaptopathy using a transducer (Etymōtic, ER-2) with extended high-frequency response. For the stimulus-level experiment, they evaluated click-elicited ABRs in the two groups across a range of intensities (30–90 dB nHL in 10-dB steps). The rationale here is that amplitude reduction for ABR wave I in the high-risk group may be limited to moderate and higher-level sounds (60 dB nHL and greater) since cochlear synaptopathy is believed to functionally compromise low spontaneous rate (LSR) and medium spontaneous rate (MSR) fibers at these levels (Furman et al., 2013). Thus, no wave I amplitude difference between the groups is expected at lower levels since responses largely reflect activation of the functionally intact high spontaneous rate (HSR) fibers in both groups. However, it should be noted here that the loss of LSR fibers alone is insufficient to appreciably reduce the amplitude of the auditory nerve compound action potential (Bourien et al., 2014). They also predicted that this reduced auditory nerve output in the high-risk group may increase the I–III and I–V IPLs due to an increase in synaptic integration time, and the triggering of central compensatory gain mechanisms (Bramhall et al., 2017; Shaheen et al., 2015) will increase the V/I amplitude ratio (decrease in wave I amplitude with no appreciable decrease in wave V amplitude).

As predicted, Suresh and Krishnan (2021) observed that only wave I amplitude was significantly smaller in the high-risk group for levels above about 60 dB nHL with no group differences below this level (Figure 6–23A and B). These findings are consistent with both noise-induced and

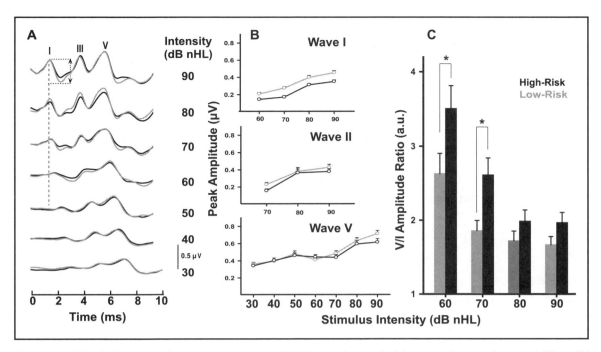

Figure 6–23. A. Auditory brainstem response (ABR) waveforms. **B.** Mean amplitude of waves I, III, and V. **C.** The mean V/I amplitude ratio plotted as a function of stimulus level for the low-risk (*light gray*) and the high-risk (*black*) groups. It is clear from (A) and (B) that only wave I shows smaller amplitude for the high-risk group compared to the low-risk group at stimulus levels above about 50 dB nHL. This results in a V/I amplitude ratio (C) that is consistently larger for the high-risk group compared to the low-risk group at 60 and 70 dB nHL. Used with permission from "Search for Electrophysiological indices of Hidden Hearing Loss in Humans: Click Auditory Brainstem Response Across Sound Levels and in Background Noise," by C. Suresh and A. Krishnan, 2021, *Ear and Hearing, 42*(1), pp. 53–67.

age-related cochlear synaptopathy in animals (Furman et al., 2013; Kujawa & Liberman, 2009; Liberman et al., 2016; Lin et al., 2011; Sergeyenko, Lall, Liberman, & Kujawa, 2013) despite complete recovery of cochlear thresholds (Kujawa & Liberman, 2009), and in humans with a history of noise exposure (Bramhall et al., 2017; Stamper & Johnson, 2015). The reduced wave I amplitude at moderate to high stimulus levels in all of these human studies has been interpreted to suggest a loss of synapses at the IHCs and/or reduced auditory nerve fibers, consistent with the data from the animal models of noise-induced cochlear synaptopathy. Specific mechanisms for ABR wave I amplitude reduction include a reduction in the number of active neural elements and the degree of synchrony in these active neural elements. However, Suresh and Krishnan (2021) do not rule out the possibility that wave I amplitude reduction may be associated with sub-clinical changes in OHC function not revealed in DPOAE tests, damage to IHCs, or the auditory nerve unrelated to the IHC-auditory nerve synapse.

The increased V/I amplitude ratio (due to the lack of wave V amplitude change in the presence of wave I amplitude reduction) for the high-risk group in this study may suggest the operation of compensatory gain mechanisms (Figure 6–23C). This finding is similar to observations in animal studies of synaptopathy. For example, in mice with noise or age-related cochlear synaptopathy, reduced auditory nerve drive, as indicated by a wave I amplitude reduction, did not result in wave V amplitude reduction (Hickox & Liberman, 2013; Möhrle et al., 2016; Sergeyenko et al., 2013), suggesting that some form of homeostatic gain control mechanism, proximal to the generator sites of wave III and V, is engaged to compensate for the reduced input from the auditory nerve.

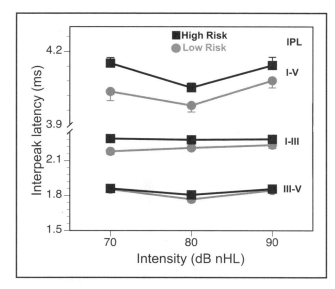

Figure 6–24. Mean I–V, I–III, and III–V interpeak latencies (IPLs) plotted as a function of stimulus level for the low-risk (gray) and high-risk (black) groups. Both IPLs I–III and I–V are longer for the high-risk group. Used with permission from "Search for Electrophysiological indices of Hidden Hearing Loss in Humans: Click Auditory Brainstem Response Across Sound Levels and in Background Noise," by C. Suresh and A. Krishnan, 2021, *Ear and Hearing*, *42*(1), pp. 53–67.

In addition, Suresh and Krishnan (2021) observed that the high-risk group showed prolonged I–III and I–V IPLs (Figure 6–24), suggesting longer synaptic integration time and/or neural conduction time between the generators of wave I (distal part of the auditory nerve) and wave III (cochlear nucleus). This longer conduction time may reflect reduced auditory nerve output which, in turn, may have introduced synaptic delays due to disruption in neural timing for more rostral responses (waves III and V). Since neural conduction time, reflected in the IPLs, is dependent on both fiber diameter and extent of myelination, the increased IPLs may represent consequences of cochlear synaptopathy that produce anterograde changes (including reduced fiber diameter and/or demyelination) in the auditory nerve (Tagoe, Barker, Jones, Allcock, & Hamann, 2014) and brainstem pathways. It is also possible that these changes could be the consequence of changes occurring earlier than the distal portion of the auditory nerve (the presumed generator site of wave I) in the neural components of the SP (Pappa et al., 2019).

There is evidence of neurotransmitter-mediated inhibition beginning at the level of ventral and dorsal cochlear nucleus regulating input to higher levels of the auditory system (Caspary, Havey, & Faingold, 1983; Caspary et al., 2008; Caspary, Rybak, & Faingold, 1985; Caspary et al., 2005). The central compensatory gain likely reflects a selective loss of inhibition (disinhibition) due to changes in the balance of excitatory and inhibitory inputs at the level of the brainstem consequent to reduced central inputs resulting from cochlear synaptopathy (Chambers et al., 2016; Möhrle et al., 2016; Salvi et al., 2017; Salvi, Wang, & Ding, 2000). A similar mechanism is thought to account for reduced wave I amplitude and unaltered wave III and wave V amplitude in individuals with normal pure-tone thresholds who report tinnitus (Gu, Herrmann, Levine, & Melcher, 2012; Schaette & McAlpine, 2011). This similarity in findings in individuals with tinnitus and individuals with ABR changes consistent with cochlear synaptopathy suggests that tinnitus may be a potential perceptual consequence of synaptopathy. Thus, the lack of group differences for ABR amplitudes III and V in the presence of group differences in wave I amplitude may suggest the operation of central compensatory gain mechanisms (Chambers et al., 2016; Eggermont, 2017; Salvi et al., 2017; Sheppard et al., 2017; Suresh & Krishnan, 2020).

Cochlear synaptopathy may also degrade neural representation of certain acoustic features important for speech perception, particularly in noise (e.g., Lopez-Poveda, 2014). There is some indirect evidence suggesting a correlation between changes in different brainstem electrophysiologic indices and deficits in speech perception in noise (Bharadwaj et al., 2014; Bramhall et al., 2019; Liberman & Kujawa, 2017; Liberman et al., 2016; Lobarinas, Spankovich, & Le Prell, 2017; Mepani et al., 2020; Plack, Barker, & Prendergast, 2014; Valderrama et al., 2018). Evaluating the effectiveness of ABR in noise measures (in both humans and a mice model), Mehraei et al. (2016) showed that the human ABR wave V latency prolongation with an increase in ipsilateral broadband masking noise mimicked the growth in the amplitude of wave I between 60 and 100 dB pe dB SPL. These results suggest that changes in the latency shift of wave V in noise may, at least in part, reflect changes in the more peripheral auditory nerve response. Based on their results in animals showing smaller wave IV (equivalent to wave V in humans) latency shift in noise, they reasoned that reduced wave V latency shift with increasing levels of ipsilateral masking noise could reflect the activity of LSR and MSR fibers given their delayed onset response (Bourien et al., 2014; Rhode & Smith, 1985) and greater resistance to masking (Costalupes, 1985; Young & Barta, 1986). More recently, Suresh and Krishnan (2021) examined if ABR components are more susceptible to noise degradation (that is greater changes in response latency and amplitude) for the high-risk group compared to the low-risk group. They reasoned that the selective loss of LSR and MSR fibers (which normally show greater suppressive effects at high intensities) in cochlear synaptopathy will reduce the suppressive masking effects provided by both LSR and MSR fibers (Cai & Geisler, 1996a, 1996b; Delgutte, 1990; Fahey & Allen, 1985) and should therefore produce smaller wave I amplitude reduction in background noise. The reduction of the suppressive masking effect may also degrade neural representation of formant peaks in noise (Sachs & Young, 1979), thereby producing speech perception deficits in noise. Consistent with their predictions, increasing noise level produced greater latency shift for wave V compared to wave I resulting in an increased I–V IPL that was similar for both groups (Figure 6–25A). However, wave I amplitude decrement with increase in background noise level was relatively smaller for the high-risk group (Figure 6–25B and C) with no group difference in amplitude change for wave V, suggesting that masking effects are reduced for individuals in the high-risk group. Unlike previous studies, there was no group difference in wave V latency shift in noise. These authors attribute the wave V latency shift in noise in both groups to be a consequence of increased synaptic integration time that is cumulative along the several synapses leading to the generator(s) of wave V.

The smaller wave I amplitude change in noise for the high-risk group, although counterintuitive at first glance, is consistent with the smaller wave I amplitude change with increasing background noise observed in older adults, and no difference in wave V amplitude change between young and older individuals (Burkard & Sims, 2002). These results suggest that, like cochlear synaptopathy, aging also results in greater loss of LSR and MSR fibers (Schmiedt, Mills, & Boettcher, 1996). The observation of a relatively smaller change in wave I amplitude for the high-risk group may be interpreted to suggest reduced susceptibility to masking. That is, the reduction in LSR and MSR fibers in the high-risk group may reduce the suppressive masking effects, particularly at moderate levels of masking noise (Delgutte, 1990; Rhode, 1978). The shallower slope of amplitude reduction for the high-risk group observed by Suresh and Krishnan (2021) may suggest that the upward spread of masking, largely due to suppression, is more gradual (Delgutte, 1990). Thus, the reduced/shallower wave I reduction in noise for the high-risk group may be related to a reduction in MSR and LSR fibers and/or the absence of the central component of suppression (Cai & Geisler, 1996; Delgutte, 1990). Additionally, there is also the possibility of HSR fiber damage/loss following noise overexposure that produces cochlear synaptopathy. Recordings from auditory nerve fibers following moderate noise exposure in chinchillas show reduced driven rates in HSR fibers (Muthaiah, Walls, & Heinz, 2017), suggesting that the pathophysiology of hidden hearing loss could be more complex.

Given the observation that suppression at moderate to high levels helps in retaining clear formant peaks at higher levels (Sachs & Young, 1979), it is tempting to speculate that the reduced suppressive masking effects observed here for the high-risk individuals may indeed degrade representation of formant peaks in the presence of noise, thereby producing deficits in speech perception in noise. While other electrophysiologic metrics have also advanced an association between noise exposure and speech-in-noise perception (Liberman et al., 2016; Mepani et al., 2020; Valderrama et al., 2018) suggesting functional deficits, the fundamental difficulty is that they do not provide a coherent explanation of how a limited population neural activity synchronized to the onset of a brief stimulus could be used to predict speech perception in noise,

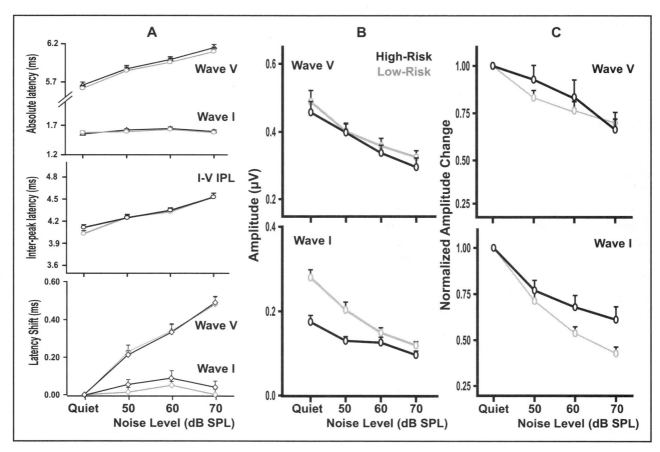

Figure 6–25. **A.** (*Top*) Mean absolute latency for waves V and I; (*middle*) mean I–V interpeak latency (IPL); and (*bottom*) mean latency shift for waves V and I plotted for the quiet and noise conditions for the low-risk (*gray*) and high-risk (*black*) groups. Absolute latencies of waves I and V, and the I–V show essentially similar changes with increase in noise level, with only wave I latency showing a slightly greater latency shift with increase in noise level. **B.** The mean amplitude of (*top*) wave V and (*bottom*) wave I are plotted for the quiet and noise conditions for the two groups. While wave V amplitude changes with increasing noise level are essentially the same for both groups, wave I amplitude shows a shallower slope of amplitude change for the high-risk group compared to the low-risk group. **C.** The normalized amplitude changes for (*top*) wave V and (*bottom*) wave I show that wave I amplitude changes less with noise level compared to the change observed for the low-risk group. Used with permission from "Search for Electrophysiological indices of Hidden Hearing Loss in Humans: Click Auditory Brainstem Response Across Sound Levels and in Background Noise," by C. Suresh and A. Krishnan, 2021, *Ear and Hearing*, *42*(1), pp. 53–67.

which presumably recruits a vast network involving cortical and subcortical structures. Plainly put, the neural activity underlying the brainstem electrophysiologic measures used and the neural networks involved in speech perception in quiet and noise cannot be directly compared. While the reduction in wave I amplitude observed in human studies cannot be confirmed with certainty to be associated with cochlear synaptopathy, an examination of harvested human temporal bones does show an age-related reduction in both synaptic ribbons and spiral ganglion neurons that show a strong correlation with an age-related reduction in ABR wave I amplitude (Konrad-Martin et al., 2012; Makary, Shin, Kujawa, Liberman, & Merchant, 2011; Wu et al., 2018). Given the equivocal nature of ABR results in humans presumed to have cochlear synaptopathy, the recent experimental approach by Suresh and Krishnan (2021) may be a step in the right direction, utilizing optimal methods including a clearer separation of the control and the experimental group; use of extended high-frequency transducers to better capture neural contributions from higher-frequency neurons that may be more functionally compromised by cochlear synaptopathy; and stimulus manipulations that may better tap at specific physiological changes consequent to cochlear synaptopathy.

V. ABR IN UPPER (ROSTRAL) BRAINSTEM LESIONS

ABR Characteristics

In our classification dichotomy, rostral brainstem lesions involve structures and neural tracts in the brainstem from the midpontine level to the midbrain (IC) that primarily contribute to the generation of the later ABR components (the IV/V complex) while sparing the auditory nerve and lower brainstem structures. Hall (2006) provides an excellent review of the characteristics and clinical manifestation of a wide range of brainstem disorders with different etiologies. Since pure-tone thresholds in individuals with upper brainstem lesions are likely to be normal, the recommendation for ABR testing may result from a reported history of persistent neurologic symptoms (e.g., dizziness or balance problems, facial numbness, or spasms, blurred vision, and other sensory-motor deficits). Unfortunately, lesions are typically diffuse, involving multiple structures and extending into the caudal brainstem. Consequently, they do not conform to our convenient dichotomy of caudal and rostral brainstem lesions. Lesions could be tumors (which may produce pressure effects that result in neural conduction block), demyelinating disorders like multiple sclerosis (which slow neural conduction and disrupt neural timing), or cardiovascular disorders (that could alter physiology due to less than optimal blood flow to the ABR neural generators). While it is clear that ABR does not identify the specific site or laterality of the lesion, it is a sensitive measure of brainstem pathology involving the auditory pathways and can reliably differentiate between levels of lesions (Hall, 2007; Hosford-Dunn, 1985; Stockard, Rossiter, Wiederholt, & Kobayashi, 1976). For example, the different patterns of IPL and amplitude changes in the ABR can differentiate auditory nerve/caudal brainstem lesions from midpontine/midbrain lesions.

If lesions are diffuse and involve both the caudal and rostral brainstem, then it is likely that both the I–III and III–V IPLs would be abnormal (Stockard et al., 1976). However, if lesions are confined to the rostral brainstem, then waves I, II, and III would appear robust with normal absolute and IPLs and amplitude, while the IV/V complex would exhibit longer latency (and therefore longer III–V and I–V IPL), amplitude reduction (resulting in an abnormal V/I amplitude ratio), poor waveform morphology (Figure 6–26, upper brainstem tumor; and Figure 6–27, multiple sclerosis), and poor repeatability (Benna, Gilli, Ferrero, & Bergamasco, 1982; Gilroy, Lynn, & Pellerin, 1977; Parving, Elberling, & Smith, 1981). There is also some evidence of increased susceptibility to stimulus rate in indi-

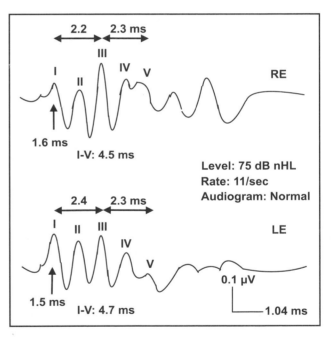

Figure 6–26. Representative auditory brainstem responses (ABRs) from a young adult with a confirmed tumor in the midbrain. The patient reported a history of vertigo and diplopia. Hearing sensitivity was normal for both ears. Waves I, II, III, and IV are robust bilaterally. III–V and I–V interpeak latencies (IPLs) are abnormal for both ears and slightly longer with left ear stimulation. I–III IPL in the left ear is borderline normal. V/I amplitude ratio is abnormal for both ears. Waveform rendering based on replotted data from "ABR in the Eighth Nerve and Low Brainstem Lesions," by N. P. Lynn and G. E. Verma. In *The Auditory Brainstem Response*, by J. T. Jacobson (Ed.), 1985, Chapter 11, p. 213. Copyright 1985 by College Hill Press, San Diego, CA.

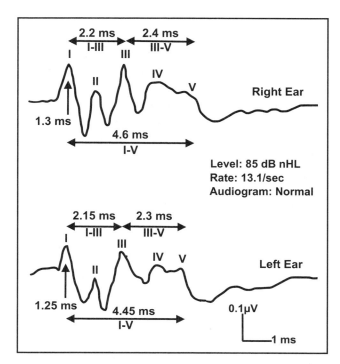

Figure 6–27. Representative auditory brainstem responses (ABRs) from a patient diagnosed with multiple sclerosis. History presented included left extremity weakness, left eyelid twitch, and blurred vision. Robust wave I–III with essentially normal absolute latency for waves I, III, and normal I–III interpeak latency (IPL). Abnormal III–V and I–V IPL binaurally. Poor morphology with reduced amplitude for wave V (resulting in an abnormal V/I amplitude ratio). Note the increased separation of the IV–V interval. Waveform rendering based on data from "ABR in the Eighth Nerve and Low Brainstem Lesions," by N. P. Lynn and G. E. Verma. In *The Auditory Brainstem Response*, by J. T. Jacobson (Ed.), 1985, Chapter 11, p. 213. Copyright 1985 by College Hill Press, San Diego, CA.

viduals with upper brainstem lesions, particularly in individuals with a demyelinating disorder like multiple sclerosis (Jacobson, Murray, & Deppe, 1987; Musiek et al., 1989; Stockard, Sharbrough, & Stockard, 1977). Un-like auditory nerve and caudal brainstem lesions, rostral brainstem lesions show characteristically bilateral effects (Benna et al., 1982; Musiek & Geurkink, 1982)—that is, the presence of abnormal ABR indices with stimulation of either ear. Overall, the pattern of ABR results changes depending on the location and extent of involvement of auditory structures and tracts along the brainstem (Baran, Catherwood, & Musiek, 1995).

VI. ABR TEST STRATEGY FOR NEURODIAGNOSTIC EVALUATION OF SITE(S) OF LESION

Since we described the test strategy for hearing screening and threshold determination in the previous chapter, we focus here on the optimal ABR test strategy to identify lesion(s) beyond the cochlea —that is, retrocochlear pathology involving the auditory nerve and/or the brainstem. The specific aim is to choose the optimal stimulus and recording parameters to obtain a robust repeatable ABR ideally with all components easily identifiable, from both ears. This allows the evaluation of all the ABR indices that are sensitive indicators of retrocochlear pathology, including absolute latency of all components, IPLs I–III, III–V, and I–V, ILDv, and the V/I amplitude ratio. A soft qualitative index is the response morphology that simply provides an overall impression of whether the response looks "normal."

Choice of Stimulus Parameters

Stimulus

It is well established that the broadband click stimulus with its brief duration and abrupt rise-fall times is the most ideal stimulus to excite the entire cochlear partition and produce synchronous activity in a population of neural elements in the auditory nerve and brainstem to produce a robust ABR with all components clearly discernible. While the conventional choice in most clinical practice is the click, the broadband chirp stimulus with its ability to improve neural synchrony by stimulating all cochlear regions simultaneously (and thereby eliminating the disruptive effects of cochlear delays on ABR generation) should be considered as a potential first choice. Furthermore, the chirp stimuli in effect produce "stacked ABRs" that have been shown to increase the sensitivity to de-tect small tumors missed by the conventional click-evoked ABR that is subject to smearing due to the different delays of cochlear regional contributions.

Stimulus intensity should be set to as high a level as permissible (without causing discomfort to the individual) to obtain a robust response. This is typically around 80 to 85 dB nHL. In the presence of a significant unilateral loss and the danger of contralateralization, a 50 dB SPL broadband noise should be used to mask the nontest ear. Contralateralization usually produces a very delayed wave V with no wave I when the test ear is being stimulated at high intensities (greater than 70 dB nHL).

Onset Polarity

Either an alternating or separate rarefaction and condensation *onset polarities* may be utilized, whichever produces the best response. In the presence of a high-frequency hearing loss, the use of alternating polarity may smear the response (due to the addition of responses with different latencies for each polarity), making it difficult to identify the response peaks, particularly wave V. This, in turn, will adversely influence response interpretation.

Stimulus Repetition Rate

Comparison of recordings at a slower (about 29.9 clicks/s) and a faster (89.9/s) rate will allow evaluation of neural adaptation effects. Certain auditory nerve and brainstem lesions may be more susceptible to rate effects (e.g., individuals with a demyelinating disorder, like multiple sclerosis, involving the auditory brainstem structures) and may show increased susceptibility to rate, which may produce abnormal response morphology and abnormal absolute and interpeak latencies. If the response morphology is very poor at the above rates, a much slower rate (5–10 clicks/s) should be used to see if the response morphology improves and the components become more identifiable. Remember, we need a response with all components clearly identifiable for accurate interpretation.

Transducer

Almost all early studies using the ABRs to evaluate auditory nerve and brainstem lesions have utilized transducers with frequency response characteristics similar to the now commonly used transducer, the Etymōtic ER-3A. The frequency response of this transducer is essentially flat out to 4000 Hz and then rolls off at about 35 to 40 dB/octave, thus potentially not permitting evaluation of the higher-frequency regions that may be compromised by the pathology. The use of the Etymōtic ER-2 transducer, with its extended frequency response out to at least 10 kHz, will allow evaluation of higher-frequency contributions to the ABR and thus may increase sensitivity to detect a neural abnormality.

Choice of Recording Parameters

Electrode Configuration

Most commonly, a single *vertical-ipsilateral channel* with an electrode on the high forehead at the hairline serving as the noninverting input (positive); an electrode on the ipsilateral mastoid serving as the inverting input (negative); and an electrode on the midforehead (about an inch below the location of the noninverting electrode) serving as the common ground electrode. This is the best electrode configuration for clearly identifying all ABR components of interest. However, a three-channel simultaneous recording would increase the accuracy of wave identification that, in turn, enables a more accurate measurement of the response indices important for the interpretation of the ABR. In addition to the vertical-ipsilateral channel described earlier, the second channel is set up to record between the same high forehead electrode and an inverting electrode on the contralateral mastoid. This *vertical-contralateral* channel with wave I absent and clear separation of the IV–V complex can enable a more accurate measure of wave V latency. The third channel is set to record between the electrode on the contralateral mastoid and the ipsilateral mastoid (horizontal configuration). This configuration yields enhanced waves I and III that will facilitate accurate identification of these components. Overall, use of these additional channels will increase the accuracy of peak identification. The few minutes of additional time required to place these electrodes is, in our minds, worthwhile. Finally, if postauricular muscle potential affects wave V measurement, the individual can be instructed to shift position and relax and/or the electrodes from the mastoid can be moved to either the earlobe or the preauricular region anterior to the tragus. Alternatively, the use of ear canal tiptrodes may not only solve this problem but also enhance the amplitude of wave I.

Other Recording Parameters

To record the click-evoked ABR with the best morphology and definition of all response components, the most commonly used analog filter band-pass setting is 100 to 3000 Hz.

Typically, an amplification factor between 100,000 and 200,000 is sufficient and commonly used. Digitization is done using an analysis epoch of 15 to 20 ms and a sampling frequency between 20 and 40 kHz. Two replicates of 1,500 sweeps of averaging are commonly used. With a greater degree of hearing loss, additional sweeps may be required.

Response Interpretation

For both ears, the ABR indices required to determine the site(s) of lesion include absolute latencies of waves I, III, and V; IPLs I–III, I–V, and III–V; ILDv; and the V/I amplitude ratio. ABRs in auditory nerve and lower brainstem lesions are characterized by abnormal waveform morphology, delayed absolute latencies of waves III and V resulting in abnormal I–III (greater than 2.4 ms) and I–V IPLs (greater than 4.5 ms) with normal III–V IPL (1.8–2.0 ms). These abnormalities are typical when the affected ear is stimulated. However, contralateral and/or bilateral ABR abnormalities are common for larger auditory nerve tumors that displace the brainstem, usually seen as absent wave V or abnormal III–V IPL. In addition to IPLs, ILDv is also a reliable response index to differentiate cochlear and retrocochlear lesions. ILDv (greater than 0.4 ms) is also a reliable metric to flag auditory nerve and brainstem abnormalities. The ABR abnormalities in upper brainstem lesions are often bilateral and characterized by robust waves I, III, and IV but poorly defined wave V that may be difficult to identify. IPL III–V is abnormal (greater than 2.3 ms), and IPL I–III is typically normal. Also, wave V amplitude is significantly smaller than wave I amplitude, resulting in an abnormal V/I amplitude ratio (V/I ratio less than 0.75). Comparisons of the differences in ABR changes in conductive, cochlear, and auditory nerve and brainstem lesions are provided in the following summary.

VII. SUMMARY

- ABRs can be reliably used to differentiate middle ear, cochlear, auditory nerve, lower brainstem, and upper brainstem lesions by carefully evaluating the pattern of changes in the response indices. Thus, they play an important role in differential diagnosis.

- CHL essentially attenuates the sound reaching the cochlea and results in prolonged absolute latencies of all components with normal IPLs. The slope of the wave V LI function is similar to that recorded from normal-hearing individuals but shifted to the right by the amount of the conductive component. This property may allow estimation of the magnitude of the conductive component when used with wave V latency for bone-conducted stimuli as the reference, although the reliability of this approach has been questioned. Even in CHL, the slope of the wave V latency-intensity function depends on the configuration of the hearing loss.

- In cochlear hearing loss, robust ABRs, better than predicted by the degree of hearing loss, may be observed at high intensities only 10 to 15 dB above threshold, suggesting recruitment associated with cochlear loss. Generally, cochlear losses produce normal wave V latency at high intensities and abnormally prolonged latencies at low intensities, particularly for sloping high-frequency losses. Consequently, the slope of the wave V LI function is much steeper than observed in individuals with normal hearing or CHL. While IPLs are generally normal in cochlear hearing losses, IPLs may not be a pure measure of the neural conduction time since data exist to show that the latencies of waves V and I are differentially altered by degree and configuration of hearing loss and therefore could produce I–V IPL changes.

- ABRs in auditory nerve and lower brainstem lesions are characterized by abnormal waveform morphology, delayed absolute latencies of waves III and V resulting in abnormal I–III and I–V IPLs with normal III–V. Most ABR changes are ipsilateral to the site of the lesion. However, larger auditory nerve tumors can displace the brainstem and produce abnormal contralateral responses, usually absent wave V or abnormal III–V IPL. In addition to IPLs, ILDv is a reliable response index to differentiate cochlear and retrocochlear lesions. Both IPLs and ILDv tend to increase as tumor size increases.

- While ABR shows high sensitivity in the detection of acoustic tumors, it tends to miss small acoustic tumors. The use of stacked ABRs (SABRs) and ISABR have appreciably increased the sensitivity of the ABR to detect small tumors. Further research is required with chirp stimuli as a possible simpler alternative to stacked ABR in the detection of small tumors.

- ABRs may also be a potentially useful tool to identify the new clinical phenomenon of hidden hearing loss associated with cochlear synaptopathy. Wave I amplitude appears to be a sensitive noninvasive measure to evaluate and detect cochlear synaptopathy since its reduction and/or shallower growth has been shown to strongly correlate with the number of surviving spiral ganglion neurons. However, to date, results from human studies do not uniformly show wave I amplitude reduction. Further research using stimulus manipulations that produce changes in human ABR that reliably reflect consequences of cochlear synaptopathy is needed to develop a reliable and valid clinical tool to identify hidden hearing loss.

- ABR in upper brainstem lesions is characterized by response waveforms that show robust waves I, III, and IV but poorly defined wave V that may be difficult to identify. IPL I–III is typically normal, while IPL III–V is abnormal (which could also result in an abnormal I–V IPL). These changes are often bilateral, unlike the unilateral abnormalities seen with auditory nerve and lower brainstem lesions. More commonly, wave V is appreciably smaller than wave I, resulting in an abnormal V/I amplitude ratio. Some demyelinating disorders localized to the brainstem may be more susceptible to abnormal stimulus rate effects.

REFERENCES

Anteby, I., Hafner, H., Pratt, H., & Uri, N. (1986). Auditory brainstem evoked potentials in evaluating the central effects of middle ear effusion. *International Journal of Pediatric Otorhinolaryngology, 12*(1), 1–11.

Antonelli, A. R., Bellotto, R., & Grandori, F. (1987). Audiologic diagnosis of central versus eighth nerve and cochlear auditory impairment. *Audiology, 26,* 209–226.

Attanasio, G., Barbara, M., Buongiorno, G., Cordier, A., Mafera, B., Piccoli, F., . . . Filipo, R. (1999). Protective effect of the cochlear efferent system during noise exposure. *Annals of the New York Academy of Sciences, 884*(1), 361–367.

Baran, J. A., Catherwood, K. P., & Musiek, F. E. (1995). Negative ABR findings in an individual with a large brainstem tumor: Hit or miss? *Journal of the American Academy of Audiology, 6,* 211–216.

Barrs, D. M., Brackmann, D. E., Olson, J. E., & House, W. F. (1985). Changing concepts of acoustic tumor diagnosis. *Archives of Otolaryngology-Head and Neck Surgery, 111,* 17–21.

Bauch, C. D., & Olsen, W. O. (1986). The effect of 2000–4000 Hz hearing sensitivity on ABR results. *Ear and Hearing, 7,* 314–317.

Bauch, C. D., & Olsen, W. O. (1989). Wave V interaural latency differences as a function of asymmetry in 2000–4000 Hz hearing sensitivity. *American Journal of Otology, 10*(5), 389–392.

Bauch, C. D., Olsen, W. O., & Harner, S. G. (1983). Auditory brain-stem response and acoustic reflex test. Results for patients with and without tumor matched for hearing loss. *Archives of Otolaryngology-Head and Neck Surgery, 109,* 522–525.

Bauch, C. D., Olsen, W. O., & Pool, A. F. (1996). ABR indices: Sensitivity, specificity, and tumor size. *American Journal of Audiology, 5,* 97–104.

Bauch, C. D., Rose, D. E., & Harner, S. G. (1982). Auditory brainstem response results from 255 patients with suspected retrocochlear involvement. *Ear and Hearing, 3,* 83–86.

Benna, P., Gilli, M., Ferrero, P., & Bergamasco, B. (1982). Brainstem auditory evoked potentials in supratentorial tumors. *Electroencephalography and Clinical Neurophysiology, 54*, 8–9.

Bharadwaj, H. M., Verhulst, S., Shaheen, L., Liberman, M. C., & Shinn-Cunningham, B. G. (2014). Cochlear neuropathy and the coding of supra-threshold sound. *Frontiers in Systems Neuroscience, 8*, 26.

Borg, E., & Löfqvist, L. (1982). Auditory brainstem response (ABR) to rarefaction and condensation clicks in normal and abnormal ears. *Scandinavian Audiology, 11*, 227–235.

Bourien, J., Tang, Y., Batrel, C., Huet, A., Lenoir, M., Ladrech, S., . . . Wang, J. (2014). Contribution of auditory nerve fibers to compound action potential of the auditory nerve. *Journal of Neurophysiology, 112*(5), 1025–1039.

Bramhall, N. F., Konrad-Martin, D., McMillan, G. P., & Griest, S. E. (2017). Auditory brainstem response altered in humans with noise exposure despite normal outer hair cell function. *Ear and Hearing, 38*(1), e1.

Bramhall, N., Beach, E. F., Epp, B., Le Prell, C. G., Lopez-Poveda, E. A., Plack, C. J., . . . Canlon, B. (2019). The search for noise-induced cochlear synaptopathy in humans: Mission impossible? *Hearing Research, 377*, 88–103.

Brooks, G. B., & Woo, J. (1994). Hearing preservation in acoustic neuroma surgery. *Clinical Otolaryngology, 19*, 204–214.

Burkard, R. F., & Don, M. (2007). The auditory brainstem response. In R. F. Burkard, M. Don, & J. J. Eggermont (Eds.), *Auditory evoked potentials* (pp. 254–274). Baltimore, MD: Lippincott Williams & Williams.

Burkard, R. F., & Sims, D. (2002). A comparison of the effects of broadband masking noise on the auditory brainstem response in young and older adults. *American Journal of Audiology, 11*(1), 13–22.

Bush, M. L., Shinn, J. B., Young, A. B., & Jones, R. O. (2008). Long-term hearing results in gamma knife radiosurgery for acoustic neuromas. *Laryngoscope, 118*(6), 1019–1022.

Cai, Y., & Geisler, C. D. (1996a). Suppression in auditory-nerve fibers of cats using low-side suppressors. I. Temporal aspects. *Hearing Research, 96*(1–2), 94–112.

Cai, Y., & Geisler, C. D. (1996b). Suppression in auditory-nerve fibers of cats using low-side suppressors. II. Effect of spontaneous rates. *Hearing Research, 96*(1–2), 113–125.

Cashman, M., & Rossman, R. (1983). Diagnostic features of the auditory brainstem response in identifying cerebellopontine angle tumors. *Scandinavian Audiology, 12*, 35–41.

Caspary, D. M., Havey, D. C., & Faingold, C. L. (1983). Effects of acetylcholine on cochlear nucleus neurons. *Experimental Neurology, 82*(2), 491–498.

Caspary, D. M., Ling, L., Turner, J. G., & Hughes, L. F. (2008). Inhibitory neurotransmission, plasticity and aging in the mammalian central auditory system. *Journal of Experimental Biology, 211*(11), 1781–1791.

Caspary, D. M., Rybak, L. P., & Faingold, C. L. (1985). The effects of inhibitory and excitatory amino acid neurotransmitters on the response properties of brainstem auditory neurons. *Auditory Biochemistry*, 198–226.

Caspary, D. M., Schatteman, T. A., & Hughes, L. F. (2005). Age-related changes in the inhibitory response properties of dorsal cochlear nucleus output neurons: Role of inhibitory inputs. *Journal of Neuroscience, 25*(47), 10952–10959.

Casselman, J. W., Offeciers, F. E., & Govaerts, P. J. (1997). Aplasia and hypoplasia of the vestibulocochlear nerve: Diagnosis with MR imaging. *Radiology, 202*, 773–781.

Chambers, A. R., Resnik, J., Yuan, Y., Whitton, J. P., Edge, A. S., Liberman, M. C., & Polley, D. B. (2016). Central gain restores auditory processing following near-complete cochlear denervation. *Neuron, 89*(4), 867–879.

Chambers, R. (1989). Auditory brain-stem responses in children with previous otitis media. *Archives of Otolaryngology-Head and Neck Surgery, 115*, 452–457.

Chandrasekhar, S. S., Brackmann, D. E., & Devgan, K. K. (1995). Utility of auditory brainstem response audiometry in diagnosis of acoustic neuromas. *American Journal of Otology, 16*(1), 63–67.

Chiappa, K. H., Harrison, J. L., Brooks, E. B., & Young, R. R. (1980). Brainstem auditory evoked responses in 200 patients with multiple sclerosis. *Annals of Neurology, 7*, 135–143.

Clarkson, C., Antunes, F. M., & Rubio, M. E. (2016). Conductive hearing loss has long-lasting structural and molecular effects on presynaptic and postsynaptic structures of auditory nerve synapses in the cochlear nucleus. *Journal of Neuroscience, 36*(39), 10214–10227.

Clopton, B. M., & Silverman, M. S. (1977). Plasticity of binaural interaction, II: Critical period and changes in midline response. *Journal of Neurophysiology, 40*, 1275–1280.

Clopton, B. M., & Silverman, M. S. (1978). Changes in latency and duration of neural responding following developmental auditory deprivation. *Experimental Brain Research, 32*(1), 39–47.

Coats, A. C. (1978). Human auditory nerve action potentials and brain stem evoked responses latency—Intensity functions in detection of cochlear and retrocochlear abnormality. *Archives of Otolaryngology, 104*(12), 709–717.

Coats, A. C., & Martin, J. L. (1977). Human auditory nerve action potentials and brainstem evoked responses: Effects of audiogram shape and lesion location. *Archives of Otolaryngology, 103*, 605–622.

Costalupes, J. A. (1985). Representation of tones in noise in the responses of auditory nerve fibers in cats. I. Comparison with detection thresholds. *Journal of Neuroscience, 5*(12), 3261–3269.

Delgutte, B. (1990). Two-tone rate suppression in auditory-nerve fibers: Dependence on suppressor frequency and level. *Hearing Research, 49*(1–3), 225–246.

Don, M., & Eggermont, J. J. (1978). Analysis of the click-evoked brainstem potentials in man using high-pass noise masking. *Journal of the Acoustical Society of America, 63*, 1084–1092.

Don, M., & Kwong, B. (2002). Differential diagnosis. In W. Katz (Ed.), *Handbook of clinical audiology* (5th ed., pp. 274–279). Baltimore, MD: Lippincott Williams & Wilkins.

Don, M., Kwong, B., & Tanaka, C. (2012). Interaural stacked auditory brainstem response measures for detecting small unilateral acoustic tumors. *Audiology and Neuro-otology, 17*, 54–68.

Don, M., Kwong, B., Tanaka, C., Brackmann, D., & Nelson, R. (2005). The stacked ABR: A sensitive and specific screening tool for detecting small acoustic tumors. *Audiology and Neuro-otology, 10*(5), 274–290.

Don, M., Masuda, A., Nelson, R., & Brackmann, D. (1997). Successful detection of small acoustic tumors using the stacked derived-band auditory brain stem response amplitude. *American Journal of Otology, 18*(5), 608–621.

Don, M., Ponton, C. W., Eggermont, J. J., & Kwong, B. (1998). The effects of sensory hearing loss on cochlear filter times estimated from auditory brainstem response latencies. *Journal of the Acoustical Society of America, 104*, 2280–2289.

Dornhoffer, J. L., Helms, J., & Hoehmann, D. H. (1994). Presentation and diagnosis of small acoustic tumors. *Otolaryngology-Head and Neck Surgery, 111*(3P1), 232–235.

Dornhoffer, J. L., Helms, J., & Hoehmann, D. H. (1995). Hearing preservation in acoustic tumor surgery: Results and prognostic factors. *Laryngoscope, 105*, 184–187.

Dornhoffer, J. L., Helms, J., & Hoehmann, D. H. (1999). Presentation and diagnosis of small acoustic tumors. *Otolaryngology-Head and Neck Surgery, 111*(3, Pt. 1), 232–235.

Eggermont, J. J. (1979). Narrow-band AP latencies in normal and recruiting human ears. *Journal of the Acoustical Society of America, 65*, 463–470.

Eggermont, J. J. (1982). The inadequacy of click-evoked auditory brainstem responses in audiological applications. *Annals of the New York Academy of Sciences, 388*, 707–709.

Eggermont, J. J. (2017). Effects of long-term non-traumatic noise exposure on the adult central auditory system. Hearing problems without hearing loss. *Hearing Research, 352*, 12–22.

Eggermont, J. J., Don, M., & Brackmann, D. E. (1980). Electrocochleography and auditory brainstem electric responses in patients with pontine angle tumors. *Annals of Otology, Rhinology, and Laryngology Supplement, 89*(6, Pt. 2), 1–19.

Fahey, P. F., & Allen, J. B. (1985). Nonlinear phenomena as observed in the ear canal and at the auditory nerve. *Journal of the Acoustical Society of America, 77*, 599–612.

Ferguson, M. O., Cook, R. O., Hall, J. W. III, Grose, J. J., & Pillsbury, H. C. (1998). Chronic conductive hearing loss in adults: Effects on the auditory brainstem response and masking-level difference. *Archives of Otolaryngology-Head and Neck Surgery, 124*(6), 678–685.

Folsom, R. C., Weber, B. A., & Thompson, G. (1983). Auditory brainstem responses in children with early recurrent middle ear disease. *Annals of Otology, Rhinology, and Laryngology, 92*, 249–253.

Fortnum, H., O'Neill, C., Taylor, R., Lenthall, R., Nikolopoulos, T., Lightfoot, G., . . . Mulvaney, C. (2009). The role of magnetic resonance imaging in the identification of suspected acoustic neuroma: A systematic review of clinical and cost effectiveness and natural history. *Health Technology Assessment, 13*(18), 1–154.

Fowler, C. G., & Durrant, J. D. (1994). The effects of peripheral hearing loss on the auditory brainstem response. In J. Jacobson (Ed.), *Principles and applications in auditory evoked potentials* (pp. 237–250). Boston, MA: Allyn & Bacon.

Fowler, C. G., & Mikami, C. M. (1993). Effects of cochlear hearing loss on the ABR latencies to clicks and 1000 Hz tone pips. *Journal of the American Academy of Audiology, 3*, 324–330.

Fria, T. J., & Sabo, D. L. (1979). Auditory brainstem responses in children with otitis media with effusion. *Annals of Otology, Rhinology, and Laryngology Supplement, 89*, 200–206.

Fulbright, A. N., Le Prell, C. G., Griffiths, S. K., & Lobarinas, E. (2017). Effects of recreational noise on threshold and suprathreshold measures of auditory function. *Seminars in Hearing, 38*(4), 298–318.

Furman, A. C., Kujawa, S. G., & Liberman, M. C. (2013). Noise-induced cochlear neuropathy is selective for fibers with low spontaneous rates. *Journal of Neurophysiology, 110,* 577–586.

Gilroy, J., Lynn, G. E., & Pellerin, R. J. (1977). Auditory evoked brainstem potentials in a case of "locked-in" syndrome. *Archives of Neurology, 34,* 492–495.

Glasscock 3rd, M. E., Jackson, C. G., Josey, A. F., Dickins, J. R., & Wiet, R. J. (1979). Brain stem evoked response audiometry in a clinical practice. *Laryngoscope, 89*(7 Pt 1), 1021–1035.

Godey, B., Morandi, X., Beust, L., Brassier, G., & Bourdiniere, J. (1998). Sensitivity of auditory brainstem response in acoustic neuroma screening. *Acta Otolaryngology, 118*(4), 501–504.

Gordon, M. L., & Cohen, N. L. (1995). Efficacy of auditory brainstem response as a screening test for small acoustic neuromas. *American Journal of Otology, 16*(2), 36–39.

Gorga, M. P., Reiland, J. K., & Beauchaine, K. A. (1985). Auditory brainstem responses in a case of high-frequency conductive hearing loss. *Journal of Speech and Hearing Disorders, 50,* 346–350.

Gorga, M. P., Worthington, D. W., Reiland, J. K., Beauchaine, K. A., & Goldgar, D. E. (1985). Some comparisons between auditory brain stem response thresholds, latencies, and the pure-tone audiogram. *Ear and Hearing, 6,* 105–112.

Grabel, J. C., Zappulla, R. A., Ryder, J., Wang, W., & Malis, L. I. (1991). Brain-stem auditory evoked responses in 56 patients with acoustic neurinoma. *Journal of Neurosurgery, 74*(5), 749–753.

Grinn, S. K., Wiseman, K. B., Baker, J. A., & Le Prell, C. G. (2017). Hidden hearing loss? No effect of common recreational noise exposure on cochlear nerve response amplitude in humans. *Frontiers in Neuroscience, 11,* 465.

Grose, J. H., Buss, E., & Hall, J. W. III. (2017). Loud music exposure and cochlear synaptopathy in young adults: Isolated auditory brainstem response effects but no perceptual consequences. *Trends in Hearing, 21,* 2331216517737417.

Gu, J. W., Herrmann, B. S., Levine, R. A., & Melcher, J. R. (2012). Brainstem auditory evoked potentials suggest a role for the ventral cochlear nucleus in tinnitus. *Journal of the Association for Research in Otolaryngology, 13*(6), 819–833.

Gunnarson, A. D., & Finitzo, T. (1991). Conductive hearing loss during infancy: Effects on later brain stem electrophysiology. *Journal of Speech and Hearing Research, 34,* 1207–1215.

Hall, J. W. (1992). In J. W. Hall (Ed.), *Handbook of auditory evoked response.* Boston, MA: Allyn & Bacon.

Hall, J. W. (2006). Adult diseases and disorders and clinical applications. In J. W. Hall (Ed.), *New handbook of auditory evoked response* (pp. 366–431). Boston, MA: Pearson.

Hall, J. W. III. (2007). Adult diseases and disorders and clinical applications. In J. W. Hall (Ed.), *New handbook of auditory evoked responses* (pp. 396–424). Boston, MA: Allyn & Bacon.

Hall, J. W., & Derlacki, E. D. (1986). Binaural hearing after middle ear surgery. *Journal of Otology, Rhinology, and Laryngology, 95,* 118–124.

Hall, J. W., & Grose, J. H. (1993). The effect of otitis media with effusion on the masking level difference and the auditory brainstem response. *Journal of Speech and Hearing Research, 36,* 210–217.

Hall, J. W., Grose, J. H., & Pillsbury, H. C. (1990). Predicting binaural hearing after stapedectomy from pre-surgery results. *Archives of Otolaryngology-Head and Neck Surgery, 116,* 946–950.

Hall, J. W., Grose, J. H., & Pillsbury, H. C. (1995). Long-term effects of chronic otitis media on binaural hearing in children. *Archives of Otolaryngology, 121,* 847–852.

Hashimoto, S., Kawese, T., Furukawa, K., & Takasaka, T. (1991). Strategy for the diagnosis of small acoustic neuromas. *Acta Oto-Laryngologica, 481,* 567–569.

Henderson, D., Subramaniam, M., Spongr, V., & Attanasio, G. (1996). Biological mechanisms of the "toughening" phenomenon. In *Auditory plasticity and regeneration* (pp. 143–154). New York, NY: Thieme Medical.

Henry, K. S., Kale, S., Scheidt, R. E., & Heinz, M. G. (2011). Auditory brainstem responses predict auditory nerve fiber thresholds and frequency selectivity in hearing impaired chinchillas. *Hearing Research, 280,* 236–244.

Hickox, A. E., Larsen, E., Heinz, M. G., Shinobu, L., & Whitton, J. P. (2017). Translational issues in cochlear synaptopathy. *Hearing Research, 349,* 164–171.

Hickox, A. E., & Liberman, M. C. (2013). Is noise-induced cochlear neuropathy key to the generation of hyperacusis or tinnitus? *Journal of Neurophysiology, 111*(3), 552–564.

Hood, L. J., Berlin, C. I., Bordelon, J., & Rose, K. (2003). Patients with auditory neuropathy/dys-synchrony lack efferent suppression of transient evoked otoacoustic emissions. *Journal of the American Academy of Audiology, 14,* 302–313.

Hosford-Dunn, H. (1985). Auditory brainstem response audiometry. Applications in central disorders. *Otolaryngologic Clinics of North America, 18*(2), 257–284.

Jacobson, J. T., Murray, T. J., & Deppe, U. (1987). The effects of ABR stimulus repetition rate in multiple sclerosis. *Ear and Hearing, 8*(2), 115–120.

Jerger, J., & Johnson, F. (1988). Interactions of age, gender, and sensorineural hearing loss on ABR latency. *Ear and Hearing, 9*, 168–176.

Jerger, J., & Mauldin, L. (1978). Prediction of sensorineural hearing level from the brainstem evoked response. *Archives of Otolaryngology-Head and Neck Surgery, 104*, 456–461.

Josey, A. F., Glasscock, M. E., & Jackson, C. G. (1988). Preservation of hearing in acoustic tumor surgery: Audiologic indicators. *Annals of Otology, Rhinology, and Laryngology, 97*, 626–630.

Josey, A. F., Glasscock, M. E., & Musiek, F. E. (1988). Correlation of ABR and medical imaging in patients with cerebellopontine angle tumors. *American Journal of Otology, 9*(Suppl.), 12–16.

Kanzaki, J., Ogawa, K., Ogawa, S., Yamamoto, M., & Ikeda, S. (1991). Audiological findings in acoustic neuroma. *Acta Oto-Laryngologica Supplementum, 487*, 125–132.

Keith, W. J., & Greville, K. A. (1987). Effects of audiometric configuration on the auditory brain stem response. *Ear and Hearing, 8*(1), 49–55.

Kemink, J. L., LaRouere, M. J., Kileny, P. R., Telian, S. A., & Hoff, J. T. (1990). Hearing preservation following suboccipital removal of acoustic neuromas. *Laryngoscope, 100*, 597–602.

Kirschner, D. A., Inouye, H., & Saavedra, R. A. (1996). Membrane adhesion in peripheral myelin: Good and bad wraps with protein P0. *Structure, 4*(11), 1239–1244.

Klein, A. J. (1986). Masking effects on ABR waves I and V in infants and adults. *Journal of the Acoustical Society of America, 79*(3), 755–759.

Kochanek, K. M., Sliwa, L., Gotebiowski, M., Pitka, A., & Skarzynski, H. (2015). Comparison of 3 ABR methods for diagnosis of retrocochlear hearing impairment. *Medical Science Monitor, 21*, 3814–3824.

Konrad-Martin, D., Dille, M. F., McMillan, G., Griest, S., McDermott, D., Fausti, S. A., & Austin, D. F. (2012). Age-related changes in the auditory brainstem response. *Journal of the American Academy of Audiology, 23*, 18–35.

Kujawa, S. G., & Liberman, M. C. (2009). Adding insult to injury: Cochlear nerve degeneration after "temporary" noise-induced hearing loss. *Journal of Neuroscience, 29*(45), 14077–14085.

Lapsiwala, S. B., Pyle, G. M., Kaemmerle, A. W., Sasse, F. J., & Badie, B. (2002). Correlation between auditory function and internal auditory canal pressure in patients with vestibular schwannomas. *Journal of Neurosurgery, 96*(5), 872–876.

Lasek, J. M., Klish, D., Kryzer, T. C., Hearn, C., Gorecki, J. P., & Rine, G. P. (2008). Gamma knife radiosurgery for vestibular schwannoma: Early hearing outcomes and evaluation of the cochlear dose. *Otology and Neurotology, 29*(8), 1179–1186.

Lenhardt, M. L., Shaia, F. T., & Abedi, E. (1985). Brainstem evoked response waveform variation associated with recurrent otitis media. *Archives of Otolaryngology, 111*, 315–316.

Lewis, J. D., Kopun, J., Neely, S. T., Schmid, K. K., & Gorga, M. P. (2015). Tone-burst auditory brainstem response wave V latencies in normal-hearing and hearing-impaired ears. *Journal of the Acoustical Society of America, 138*(5), 3210–3219.

Liberman, M. C., Epstein, M. J., Cleveland, S. S., Wang, H., & Maison, S. F. (2016). Toward a differential diagnosis of hidden hearing loss in humans. *PLOS One, 11*(9), e0162726.

Liberman, M. C., & Kujawa, S. G. (2017). Cochlear synaptopathy in acquired sensorineural hearing loss: Manifestations and mechanisms. *Hearing Research, 349*, 138–147.

Liberman, M. C., Liberman, L. D., & Maison, S. F. (2015). Chronic conductive hearing loss leads to cochlear degeneration. *PLOS One, 10*, e0142341.

Lin, H. W., Furman, A. C., Kujawa, S. G., & Liberman, M. C. (2011). Primary neural degeneration in the Guinea pig cochlea after reversible noise-induced threshold shift. *Journal of the Association for Research in Otolaryngology, 12*, 605–616.

Lobarinas, E., Spankovich, C., & Le Prell, C. G. (2017). Evidence of "hidden hearing loss" following noise exposures that produce robust TTS and ABR wave-I amplitude reductions. *Hearing Research, 349*, 155–163.

Lopez-Poveda, E. A. (2014). Why do I hear but not understand? Stochastic undersampling as a model of degraded neural encoding of speech. *Frontiers in Neuroscience, 8*, 348.

Mackersie, C. L., & Stapells, D. R. (1994). Auditory brainstem response wave I prediction of conductive component in infants and young children. *American Journal of Audiology, 3*(2), 52–58.

Magliulo, G., Gagliardi, M., Muscatello, M., & Natale, A. (1990). Masking level difference before and after surgery in unilateral otosclerosis. *British Journal of Audiology, 24*(2), 117–121.

Maison, S. F., Usubuchi, H., & Liberman, i M. C. (2011). Efferent feedback minimizes cochlear neuropathy from moderate noise exposure. *Journal of Neuroscience, 33*, 5542–5552.

Makary, C. A., Shin, J., Kujawa, S. G., Liberman, M. C., & Merchant, S. N. (2011). Age-related primary cochlear neuronal degeneration in human temporal bones. *Journal of the Association for Research in Otolaryngology, 12*, 711–717.

McGee, T. J., & Clemis, J. D. (1982). Effects of conductive hearing loss on auditory brainstem response. *Annals of Otology, Rhinology, and Laryngology, 91*, 304–309.

Mehraei, G., Hickox, A. E., Bharadwaj, H. M., Goldberg, H., Verhulst, S., Liberman, M. C., & Shinn-Cunningham, B. G. (2016). Auditory brainstem response latency in noise as a marker of cochlear synaptopathy. *Journal of Neuroscience, 36*(13), 3755–3764.

Mepani, A., Kirk, S., Hancock, K., Bennett, K., de Gruttola, V., Liberman, M. C., & Maison, S. F. (2020). Middle ear muscle reflex and word recognition in "normal-hearing" adults. Evidence for cochlear synaptopathy? *Ear and Hearing, 41*(1), 25–38.

Mitchell, C., Phillips, D. S., & Trune, D. R. (1989). Variables affecting the auditory brainstem response: Audiogram, age, gender and head size. *Hearing Research, 40*(1–2), 75–85.

Moffat, D. A., Baguley, D. M., Hardy, D. G., & Tsui, Y. N. (1989). Contralateral auditory brainstem response abnormalities in acoustic neuroma. *Journal of Laryngology and Otology, 103*(9), 835–838.

Möhrle, D., Ni, K., Varakina, K., Bing, D., Lee, S. C., Zimmermann, U., Knipper, M., & Rüttiger, L. (2016). Loss of auditory sensitivity from inner hair cell synaptopathy can be centrally compensated in the young but not old brain. *Neurobiology of Aging, 44*, 173–184.

Møller, K., & Blegvad, B. (1976). Brainstem responses in patients with sensorineural hearing loss. *Scandinavian Audiology, 5*, 15–27.

Moller, M., & Moller, A. (1983). Brainstem auditory evoked potentials in patients with cerebellopontine angle tumors. *Annals of Otology, Rhinology, and Laryngology, 92*, 645–650.

Moore, D. R., Hutchings, M. E., King, A. J., & Kowalchuk, N. E. (1989). Auditory brainstem of the ferret: Some effects of hearing with unilateral ear plug on the cochlea, cochlear nucleus, and projections to the inferior colliculus. *Journal of Neuroscience, 9*, 1213–1222.

Moore, D. R., Hutchings, M. E., & Meyer, S. E. (1991). Binaural masking level differences in children with a history of otitis media. *Audiology, 30*(2), 91–101.

Moore, D. R., & Irvine, D. R. F. (1981). Plasticity of binaural interaction in the cat inferior colliculus. *Brain Research, 208*, 198–202.

Murphy, M. R., & Selesnick, S. H. (2002). Cost-effective diagnosis of acoustic neuromas: A philosophical, macroeconomic, and technological decision. *Otolaryngology-Head and Neck Surgery, 127*(4), 253–259.

Musiek, F. E., & Geurkink, N. A. (1982). Auditory brainstem and central auditory test findings for patients with brainstem lesions: A preliminary report. *Laryngoscope, 92*, 891–900.

Musiek, F. E., Gollegly, K. M., Kibbe, K. S., & Reeves, A. G. (1989). Electrophysiologic and behavioral auditory findings in multiple sclerosis. *American Journal of Otology, 10*(5), 343–350.

Musiek, F. E., Johnson, G. D., Gollegly, K. M., Josey, A. F., & Glasscock, M. E. (1989). The auditory brain stem response interaural latency difference (ILD) in patients with brainstem lesions. *Ear and Hearing, 10*, 131–134.

Musiek, F. E., Josey, A. F., & Glasscock, M. E. (1986a). Auditory brain stem response: Interwave measurements in acoustic neuromas. *Ear and Hearing, 7*, 100–105.

Musiek, F. E., Josey, A. F., & Glasscock, M. E. (1986b). Auditory brain-stem response in patients with acoustic neuromas: Wave presence and absence. *Archives of Otolaryngology, 112*, 186–189.

Musiek, F. E., & Kibbe, K. (1986). Auditory brain stem response wave IV–V abnormalities from the ear opposite large cerebellopontine lesions. *American Journal of Otology, 7*(4), 253–257.

Musiek, F. E., McCormick, C. A., & Hurley, R. M. (1996). Hit and false-alarm rates of selected ABR indices in differentiating cochlear disorders from acoustic tumors. *American Journal of Audiology, 5*(1), 90–96.

Muthaiah, V. P. K., Walls, M., & Heinz, M. (2017). Effects of cochlear-synaptopathy inducing moderate noise exposure on auditory-nerve-fiber responses in chinchillas. *Journal of the Acoustical Society of America, 141*, 3814.

Nadol, J. B. Jr., & Young, Y. S. (1989). Survival of spiral ganglion cells in profound sensorineural hearing loss: Implications for cochlear implantation. *Annals of Otology, Rhinology, and Laryngology, 98*(6), 411–416.

Nodar, R. H., & Kinney, S. E. (1980). The contralateral effects of large tumors on brain stem auditory evoked potentials. *Laryngoscope, 90*(11), 1762–1768.

Okada, M., Welling, D. B., Liberman, C. M., & Maison, S. F. (2020). Chronic conductive hearing loss is associated with speech intelligibility deficits in patients with normal bone conduction thresholds. *Ear and Hearing, 41*, 500–507.

Otte, J., Schunknecht, H. F., & Kerr, A. G. (1978). Ganglion cell populations in normal and pathological human cochleae. Implications for cochlear implantation. *Laryngoscope, 88*(8), 1231–1246.

Pappa, A. K., Hutson, K. A., Scott, W. C., Wilson, J. D., Fox, K. E., Masood, M. M., . . . Fitzpatrick, D. C. (2019). Hair cell and neural contributions to the cochlear summating potential. *Journal of Neurophysiology, 121,* 2163–2180.

Parving, A., Elberling, C., & Smith, T. (1981). Auditory electrophysiology: Findings in multiple sclerosis. *Audiology, 20,* 123–142.

Picton, T. W. (2011). Auditory brainstem responses. Peaks along the way. In T. Picton (Ed.), *Human auditory evoked potentials* (pp. 214–284). San Diego, CA: Plural Publishing.

Pillsbury, H. C., Grose, J. H., & Hall, J. W. (1991). Otitis media with effusion in children. Binaural hearing before and after corrective surgery. *Archives of Otolaryngology, 117,* 718–723.

Plack, C. J., Barker, D., & Prendergast, G. (2014). Perceptual consequences of "hidden" hearing loss. *Trends in Hearing, 18,* 2331216514550621.

Polley, D. B., Thompson, J. H., & Guo, W. (2013). Brief hearing loss disrupts binaural integration during two early critical periods of auditory cortex development. *Nature Communications, 4,* 25–47.

Popescu, M. V., & Polley, D. B. (2010). Monaural deprivation disrupts development of binaural selectivity in auditory midbrain and cortex. *Neuron, 65,* 718–731.

Prendergast, G., Guest, H., Munro, K. J., Kluk, K., Léger, A., Hall, D. A., Heinz, M. G., & Plack, C. J. (2017). Effects of noise exposure on young adults with normal audiograms I: Electrophysiology. *Hearing Research, 344,* 68–81.

Prosser, S., & Arslan, E. (1987). Prediction of auditory brainstem response wave V latency as a diagnostic tool of sensorineural hearing loss. *Audiology, 26,* 179–187.

Prosser, S., Arslan, E., & Pastore, A. (1984). Auditory brainstem responses and hearing threshold in cerebellopontine angle tumors. *Archives of Otolaryngology-Head and Neck Surgery, 239,* 183–189.

Rad, M. F. (2011). Acoustic neurinomas. *Iranian Journal of Otorhinolaryngology, 23,* 1–10.

Rhode, W. S., & Smith, P. H. (1985). Characteristics of tone-pip response patterns in relationship to spontaneous rate in cat auditory nerve fibers. *Hearing Research, 18*(2), 159–168.

Ridley, C. L., Kopun, J. G., Neely, S. T., Gorga, M. P., & Rasetshwane, D. M. (2018). Using thresholds in noise to identify hidden hearing loss in humans. *Ear and Hearing, 39*(5), 829–844.

Robinette, M. S., Bauch, C. D., Olsen, W. O., & Cevette, M. J. (2000). Auditory brainstem responses and magnetic resonance imaging for acoustic neuromas: Costs by prevalence. *Archives of Otolaryngology-Head and Neck Surgery, 126*(8), 963–966.

Rosenhall, U., Hedner, M. L., & Björkman, G. (1981). ABR in brain stem lesions. *Scandinavian Audiology, Supplementum, 13,* 117–123.

Rosenhamer, H. J. (1981). The auditory evoked brainstem electric response (ABR) in cochlear hearing loss. *Scandinavian Audiology, Supplementum, 13,* 83–93.

Rosenhamer, H. J., Lindstrom, B., & Lundborg, T. (1981). On the use of click-evoked electric brainstem responses in audiological diagnosis: Latencies in cochlear hearing loss. *Scandinavian Audiology, 10,* 3–11.

Rowe, M. J. III. (1978). Normal variability of the brainstem auditory evoked response in young and old adult subjects. *Electroencephalography and Clinical Neurophysiology, 44,* 459–470.

Sachs, M. B., & Young, E. D. (1979). Encoding of steady-state vowels in the auditory nerve: Representation in terms of discharge rate. *Journal of the Acoustical Society of America, 66,* 470–479.

Salvi, R., Sun, W., Ding, D., Chen, G.-D., Lobarinas, E., Wang, J., . . . Auerbach, B. D. (2017). Inner hair cell loss disrupts hearing and cochlear function leading to sensory deprivation and enhanced central auditory gain. *Frontiers in Neuroscience, 10,* 621.

Salvi, R. J., Wang, J., & Ding, D. (2000). Auditory plasticity and hyperactivity following cochlear damage. *Hearing Research, 147*(1–2), 261–274.

Schaette, R., & McAlpine, D. (2011). Tinnitus with a normal audiogram: Physiological evidence for hidden hearing loss and computational model. *Journal of Neuroscience, 31*(38), 13452–13457.

Schmidt, R. J., Sataloff, R. T., Newman, J., Spiegel, J. R., & Myers, D. L. (2001). The sensitivity of auditory brainstem response testing for the diagnosis of acoustic neuromas. *JAMA Otolaryngology-Head and Neck Surgery, 127*(1), 19–22.

Schmiedt, R. A., Mills, J. H., & Boettcher, F. A. (1996). Age-related loss of activity of auditory nerve fibers. *Journal of Neurophysiology, 76*(4), 2799–2803.

Schwartz, D. M., & Berry, G. A. (1985). Normative aspects of the ABR. In J. T. Jacobson (Ed.), *The auditory brainstem response* (pp. 65–70). London, UK: Taylor and Francis.

Selters, W. A., & Brackmann, D. E. (1977). Acoustic tumor detection with brain stem electric response audiometry. *Archives of Otolaryngology, 103*(4), 181–187.

Selters, W., & Brackmann, D. (1979). Brainstem electric response audiometry in acoustic tumor detection.

In W. House & C. Luetje (Eds.), *Acoustic tumors* (pp. 225–235). Baltimore, MD: University Park Press.

Sergeyenko, Y., Lall, K., Liberman, M. C., & Kujawa, S. G. (2013). Age-related cochlear synaptopathy: An early-onset contributor to auditory functional decline. *Journal of Neuroscience, 33*(34), 13686–13694.

Serpanos, Y. C., O'Malley, H., & Gravel, J. S. (1997). The relationship between loudness intensity functions and the click-ABR wave V latency. *Ear and Hearing, 18*(5), 409–419.

Shaheen, L. A., Valero, M. D., & Liberman, M. C. (2015). Towards a diagnosis of cochlear neuropathy with envelope following responses. *Journal of the Association for Research in Otolaryngology, 16*(6), 727–745.

Shearer, A. E., & Hansen, M. R. (2019). Auditory synaptopathy, auditory neuropathy, and cochlear implantation. *Laryngoscope, Investigative Otolaryngology, 4*, 429–440.

Shelton, C., Brackmann, D. E., House, W. F., & Hitselberger, W. E. (1989). Acoustic tumor surgery: Prognostic factors in hearing conservation. *Archives of Otolaryngology-Head and Neck Surgery, 115*, 1213–1216.

Sheppard, A. M., Chen, G.-D., Manohar, S., Ding, D., Hu, B.-H., Sun, W., . . . Salvi, R. (2017). Prolonged low-level noise-induced plasticity in the peripheral and central auditory system of rats. *Neuroscience, 359*, 159–171.

Shih, C., Tseng, F.-Y., Yeh, T.-H., Hsu, C.-J., & Chen, Y.-S. (2009). Ipsilateral and contralateral acoustic brainstem response abnormalities in patients with vestibular schwannoma. *Otolaryngology-Head and Neck Surgery, 141*(6), 695–700.

Shohet, J. A. (2012). Skull base tumor and other CPA tumors. *Medscape.* Retrieved from http://emedicine.medscape.com/article/883090-overview

Sininger, Y., & Oba, S. (2001). Patients with auditory neuropathy: Who are they and what can they hear? In Y. Sininger & A. Starr (Eds.), *Auditory neuropathy: A new perspective on hearing disorders* (pp. 15–35). San Diego, CA: Singular Publishing.

Sohmer, H., Kinarti, R., & Gafni, M. (1981). The latency of auditory nerve-brainstem responses in sensorineural hearing loss. *Archives of Otorhinolaryngology, 230*, 189–199.

Stamper, G. C., & Johnson, T. A. (2015). Auditory function in normal-hearing, noise-exposed human ears. *Ear and Hearing, 36*(2), 172–184.

Stapells, D. R. (1989). Auditory brainstem response assessment of infants and children. *Seminar in Hearing, 10*, 229–251.

Starr, A., Picton, T. W., Sininger, Y., Hood, L., & Berlin, C. (1996). Auditory neuropathy. *Brain, 119*, 741–753.

Starr, A., Sininger, Y., Nguyen, T., Michalewski, T., Oba, S., & Abdala, C. (2001). Cochlear receptor (microphonic and summating potentials, otoacoustic emissions) and auditory pathway (auditory brainstem potentials) activity in auditory neuropathy. *Ear and Hearing, 22*, 91–99.

Stockard, J. J., & Rossiter, V. S. (1977). Clinical and pathologic correlates of brainstem auditory response abnormalities. *Neurology, 27*, 316–325.

Stockard, J. J., Rossiter, V. S., Wiederholt, W. C., & Kobayashi, R. M. (1976). Brainstem auditory evoked responses in suspected central pontine myelinolysis. *Archives of Neurology, 33*, 726–728.

Stockard, J. J., Sharbrough, F. W., & Stockard, F. E. (1977). Detection and localization of occult lesions with brainstem auditory responses. *Mayo Clinic Proceedings, 52*, 761–769.

Strelcyk, O., Christoforidis, D., & Dau, T. (2009). Relation between derived-band auditory brainstem response latencies and behavioral frequency selectivity. *Journal of the Acoustical Society of America, 126*, 1878–1888.

Sturzebecher, E., Kevanishvili, Z., Werbs, M., Meyer, E., & Schmidt, D. (1985). Interpeak intervals of auditory brainstem response, interaural differences in normal hearing subjects and patients with sensorineural hearing loss. *Scandinavian Audiology, 14*, 83–87.

Subramaniam, M., Campo, P., & Henderson, D. (1991). The effect of exposure level on the development of progressive resistance to noise. *Hearing Research, 52*(1), 181–187.

Suresh, C. H., & Krishnan, A. (2021). Search for electrophysiological indices of hidden hearing loss in humans: Click auditory brainstem response across sound levels and in background noise. *Ear and Hearing, 42*(1), 53–67.

Tagoe, T., Barker, M., Jones, A., Allcock, N., & Hamann, M. (2014). Auditory nerve perinodal dysmyelination in noise-induced hearing loss. *Journal of Neuroscience, 34*(7), 2684–2688.

Telian, S. A., Kileny, P. R., Niparko, J. K., Kemink, J. L., & Graham, M. D. (1989). Normal auditory brainstem response in patients with acoustic neuroma. *Laryngoscope, 99*, 10–14.

Terkildsen, K., Osterhammel, P., & Thomsen, J. (1981). The ABR and the MLR in patients with acoustic neuromas. *Scandinavian Journal of Audiology (Supplement), 13*, 103–107.

Timmer, F. C. A., Hanssens, P. E. J., van Haren, A. E. P., Mulder, J. J. S., Cremers, C. W. R. J., Beynon, A. J., . . . Graamans, K. (2009). Gamma knife radiosurgery for vestibular schwannomas: Results of hearing preservation in relation to the cochlear radiation dose. *Laryngoscope, 119*(6), 1076–1081.

Valderrama, J. T., Beach, E. F., Yeend, I., Sharma, M., Van Dun, B., & Dillon, H. (2018). Effects of lifetime noise exposure on the middle-age human auditory brainstem response, tinnitus and speech-in-noise intelligibility. *Hearing Research, 365*, 36–48.

Valero, M. D., Burton, J. A., Hauser, S. N., Hackett, T. A., Ramachandran, R., & Liberman, M. C. (2017). Noise-induced cochlear synaptopathy in rhesus monkeys (*Macaca mulatta*). *Hearing Research, 353*, 213–223.

Van der Drift, J. F., Brocaar, M. P., & von Zanten, G. A. (1988). Brainstem response audiometry. I. Its use in distinguishing between conductive and cochlear hearing loss. *Audiology, 27*, 260–270.

Van der Drift, J. F., von Zanten, G. A., & Brocaar, M. P. (1989). Brainstem electric response audiometry: Estimation of the amount of conductive hearing loss with and without use of the response threshold. *Audiology, 28*, 181–193.

Verhulst, S., Bharadwaj, H. M., Mehraei, G., Shera, C. A., & Shinn-Cunningham, B. G. (2015). Functional modeling of the human auditory brainstem response to broadband stimulation. *Journal of the Acoustical Society of America, 138*(3), 1637–1659.

Verhulst, S., Jagadeesh, A., Mauermann, M., & Ernst, F. (2016). Individual differences in auditory brainstem response wave characteristics: Relations to different aspects of peripheral hearing loss. *Trends in Hearing, 20*, 1–20.

Wang, Q., Gu, R., Han, D., & Yang, W. (2015). Familial auditory neuropathy. *Laryngoscope, 113*, 1623–1629.

Watila, M. M., & Balarabe, S. A. (2015). Molecular and clinical features of inherited neuropathies due to PMP22 duplication. *Journal of the Neurological Sciences, 355*(1–2), 8–24.

Wilson, D. F., Hodgson, R. S., Gustafson, M. F., Hogue, S., & Mills, L. (1992). The sensitivity of auditory brainstem response testing in small acoustic neuromas. *Laryngoscope, 102*, 961–964.

Wu, P. Z., Liberman, L. D., Bennett, K., de Gruttola, V., O'Malley, J. T., & Liberman, M. C. (2018). Primary neural degeneration in the human cochlea: Evidence for hidden hearing loss in the aging ear. *Neuroscience, 407*, 8–20.

Yamada, O., Kodera, K., & Yagi, T. (1979). Cochlear processes affecting wave V latency of the auditory evoked brain stem response. *Scandinavian Audiology, 8*, 67–70.

Yamada, O., Yagi, T., Yamane, H., & Suzuki, J.-I. (1975). Clinical evaluation of the auditory evoked brain stem response. *Aurix-Nasus-Larynx, 2*, 97–105.

Yamakami, I., Yoshinori, H., Saeki, N., Wada, M., & Oka, N. (2009). Hearing preservation and intraoperative auditory brainstem response and cochlear nerve compound action potential monitoring in the removal of small acoustic neurinoma via the retrosigmoid approach. *Journal of Neurosurgery and Psychiatry, 80*(2), 218–227.

Young, E. D., & Barta, P. E. (1986). Rate responses of auditory nerve fibers to tones in noise near masked threshold. *Journal of the Acoustical Society of America, 79*(2), 426–442.

Zappia, J. J., O'Connor, C. A., Wiet, R. J., & Dinces, E. A. (1997). Rethinking the use of auditory brainstem response in acoustic neuroma screening. *Laryngoscope, 107*(10), 1388–1392.

Zapulla, R. A., Greenblat, E., & Karmel, B. Z. (1982). The effects of acoustic neuromas on ipsilateral and contralateral brainstem auditory evoked potentials during stimulation of the unaffected ear. *American Journal of Otology, 4*, 118–122.

Zhuang, X., Sun, W., & Xu-Friedman, M. A. (2017). Changes in properties of auditory nerve synapses following conductive hearing loss. *Journal of Neuroscience, 37*(2), 323–332.

Neurotologic Applications: Electrocochleography (ECochG) and Intraoperative Monitoring (IOM)

SCOPE

In the preceding chapters, we focused on describing the scalp-recorded auditory brainstem response (ABR) and its clinical applications in hearing screening, threshold estimation, and differential diagnosis of sites of lesion. Here we focus on the use of cochlear receptor potentials (cochlear microphonic [CM] and summating potential [SP]) and the auditory nerve compound action potential (AN-CAP) that occur in the first few milliseconds poststimulus onset to evaluate the functional integrity of the inner ear/outer hair cell subsystem and the auditory nerve for differential diagnosis and for neural function monitoring during surgeries that involve the auditory nerve and brainstem. Because the sources of these potentials include outer hair cells, the inner hair-nerve synapse, and the auditory nerve, they may be useful in differentiating different types of sensorineural hearing losses, for example, differentiating Ménière's disease from auditory neuropathies. Collectively, the evaluation of these responses falls under the umbrella of electrocochleography (ECochG) using electrodes that are typically closer to the generator site(s) of these responses. The eCAP, electrical counterpart of the AN-CAP, recorded within the cochlea using electrodes of the user's cochlear implant (CI) and elicited by electrical stimulation has the potential to evaluate the neural survival and neural representation of spectral and temporal cues important for speech perception in CI users—both are important for prediction of CI outcomes. Finally, we describe the use of the AN-CAP directly from the auditory nerve and/or the cochlear nucleus, as well as the scalp-recorded ABR in intraoperative monitoring to minimize injuries from surgical manipulation and attempt preservation of hearing.

I. ELECTROCOCHLEOGRAPHY (ECochG)

The scalp-recorded ABR components, occurring in the first 10 ms post onset of brief auditory stimuli provide a noninvasive electrophysiological assay of the functional integrity of the auditory nerve and brainstem structures. In contrast, the combined recording of cochlear receptor potentials (CM, SP) and the AN-CAP occurring during the first 3 to 5 ms poststimulus onset is called ECochG. The recording is done using far-field electrodes placed at the opening of the ear canal (tiptrode) or, more commonly, an intrameatal electrode ("tymptrode") contacting the tympanic membrane; or using a more near-field transtympanic electrode placed on the promontory. These three potentials (Figure 7–1) can be used to assess the functional integrity of the outer hair cell (OHC) subsystem (CM), inner hair cell (IHC), IHC/auditory nerve synapse, postsynaptic events (SP), auditory nerve drive, and neural conduction (AN-CAP). The potentials are all associated with sequential transduction of the stimulus-elicited mechanical events along the cochlear partition to chemical and electrical responses of the OHCs, IHCs, and auditory nerve. While the structural differences between the two types of cochlear receptor cells (OHC and IHC) are clear, their specific functional differences and respective roles in hearing are still not clear. One school of thought is that acoustic stimulation shunts the ionic current from the OHCs to the IHCs to excite the IHCs and their drive of the auditory nerve. This transduction process could also be the contributing source for the backpropagated reflections of cochlear nonlinearity identified as otoacoustic emissions (OAEs) in the ear canal. There is renewed interest in ECochG fueled by its usefulness in identifying auditory neuropathy; its revival in identifying Ménière's disease following better diagnostic use of all information in the recorded waveforms; as an intraoperative test for cochlear implantation; and in using the cochlear implant electrodes to perform multichannel ECochG. We first describe each of the ECochG components and their clinical utility in diagnosis and intraoperative monitoring. A major long-term goal of ECochG is to help differentiate OHC from IHC or presynaptic losses, and from auditory nerve fiber (ANF) or postsynaptic losses, which are all presently combined together as sensorineural hearing loss. Differential diagnosis of different forms of sensorineural hearing loss could prove useful in improving hearing aid fitting, in predicting cochlear implantation outcomes, and in individualized regenerative medicine (McLean, McLean, Eatock, & Edge, 2016).

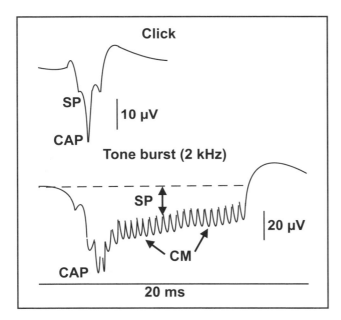

Figure 7–1. Evoked response waveforms elicited by clicks (*top*) and a longer 2-kHz tone burst (*bottom*) illustrating the VIIIth nerve compound action potential (CAP), cochlear microphonic (CM), and summating potential (SP). Unlike the CAP, which is an onset response, the receptor potentials are sustained over the duration of the stimulus. Note the CM is an alternating current potential, while the SP is a DC potential, which is simply seen as a positive or negative shift from the baseline. The large amplitude of these potentials is consistent with transtympanic electrocochleography with a recording electrode on the cochlear promontory.

Cochlear Microphonic (CM)

The CM is a sustained alternating current (AC) potential that is thought to reflect the receptor currents of OHCs that follow the basilar membrane displacement pattern (Dallos & Cheatham, 1976) during transduction (Figure 7–1, bottom trace). Although the CM is measured as a steady-state response elicited by frequency-specific pure tones, it is not a place-specific response as measured by electrodes placed in the round window niche, promontory, or at the tympanic membrane. This is because the CM reflects a complex sum of contributions from all hair cells excited along the cochlear partition by the stimulus-elicited basilar membrane (BM) displacement pattern. However, the cochlear place of generation of the CM remains unclear. At high frequencies, due to the fast changes in phase in the BM displacement, OHC currents from this active region tend to cancel and thereby contribute minimally to the measured CM. Thus, Dallos (1973) inferred that the measured CM largely reflects contributions from the passive apical region where the relatively smaller phase change allows a more effective sum of the components. However, Patuzzi, Yates, and Johnstone (1989b) demonstrated that ablation of the apical turn of the cochlea did not alter the round-window recorded CM using a low-frequency tone that engages the apical end. Therefore, the CM recorded at the promontory or in the ear canal arises primarily from OHCs in the more basal portions of the cochlea, while the apical regions make a negligible contribution to its generation (Johnstone, & Johnstone, 1966; Patuzzi, Yates, & Johnstone, 1989b; Withnell, 2001). However, there is also evidence suggesting that the promontory recorded CM for low frequencies may not only reflect basal activity but also include neural contributions (Chertoff, Earl, Diaz, & Sorensen, 2012; Chertoff et al., 2014; Kamerer, Diaz, Peppi, & Chertoff, 2016).

Pierson and Møller (1980) describe the CM as having two components—a more sensitive, low-intensity response with a limited linear operating range that is susceptible to fatigue or hypoxia, and a high-intensity component that is out of phase with the more sensitive response. Their conclusions are similar to those of Karlan, Tonndorf, and Khanna (1972) and generally concur with Dallos and Wang's (1974) view that the more sensitive component is generated by the OHCs and the second component by the IHCs. Experiments in kanamycin-treated guinea pigs with the OHCs destroyed showed that the CM produced by the IHCs was about 30 to 40 dB less sensitive than that generated by the OHCs (Dallos & Wang, 1974). Selective kanamycin-induced loss of OHCs in the basal region, and loss of IHCs with some retention of the OHCs in the apical region showed minimal changes in CM and SP from the apical regions (Dallos & Cheatham, 1976). Since the OHCs are largely implicated in the generation of cochlear receptor potentials and have very little contribution to the auditory nerve drive, these authors suggest that the OHCs may act to control current flow in the organ of Corti. It should be noted here that the observation of CM even in cases of severe to profound sensorineural hearing loss (therefore damage to the OHCs) poses a challenge to the widely accepted view that the CM is strictly related to OHC electrical activity with only a minor contribution from IHCs (Arslan, Turrini, Lupi, Genovese, & Orzan, 1997; Eggermont, 1979c; Santarelli, Scimemi, Dal Monte, & Arslan, 2006; Schoonhoven, Lamoré, de Laat, & Grote, 1999; Patuzzi et al., 1989a).

The characteristics of the CM also depend on the location of the recording electrode relative to its generator(s)—the greater the distance between the electrode and the generation site, the smaller will be the amplitude of the recorded cochlear potentials (Chertoff et al., 2012) because CM sources more distant from the recording electrode contribute less to the measured response than proximal ones. Thus, for an electrode placed at the round window (RW), contributions from more apical sources are de-emphasized compared to those near the base, an effect that may compromise the place-specificity of the CM (Patuzzi et al., 1989b). At high intensities, CM recorded with RW or ear canal electrodes may also be more basally biased. These uncertainties have limited the clinical utility of the CM. The CM is currently used primarily as a gross indicator of the integrity of OHC function across the cochlea (e.g., Gibson & Sanli, 2007; Radeloff, Shehata-Dieler, & Scherzed, 2012) in confirming auditory neuropathy, particularly when OAEs, the typically relied upon measure, are absent. (The specific use of CM in confirming auditory neuropathy is described in Chapter 6.) However, since place-specific CM could potentially shed more light on OHC functional integrity, several experimental approaches have been proposed (Charaziak, Shera, & Siegel, 2017; Chertoff et al., 2012; Ponton, Don, & Eggermont, 1992). Chertoff et al. (2012) monitored the level of CM evoked with a high-intensity, low-frequency tone burst in the presence of high-pass masking noise to detect regions of missing OHCs. They reasoned that the CM amplitude would increase as the high-pass noise cutoff is increased until the noise cutoff frequency overlaps the region of the missing OHCs (Figure 7–2). The growth of amplitude with increasing distance from the apex (that is, responses from increasingly more basal regions along the cochlear partition) is clearly shown in the right panel of Figure 7–2. While this is a clever approach, it may not be sensitive to detect lesions in the apical portions of the cochlea. Ponton et al. (1992) also found similar results using high-pass

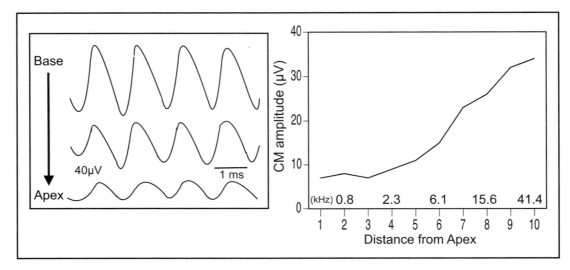

Figure 7–2. Cochlear microphonic (CM) response waveforms plotted from base to apex (*left*) show amplitude decrement. Mean CM amplitude plotted from apex to base (low to high frequency). The frequencies along the x-axis are also shown. Response amplitude grows from low frequency to high frequency with a steep increase above about 16 kHz. Data from "Analysis of the Cochlear Microphonic to a Low-Frequency Tone Embedded in Filtered Noise," by M. E. Chertoff, B. R. Earl, F. J. Diaz, and J. L. Sorensen, 2012, *Journal of the Acoustical Society of America*, *132*, pp. 3351–3362.

masking noise to mask out basal contributions to evaluate the residual CM from more apical regions. However, experimental validation of this method is lacking, and it is not clear if this method provides a sensitive index of apical OHC damage.

Using an innovative experimental approach, Charaziak, Shera, and Seigel (2017) demonstrated that round-window measures of CM in chinchilla may serve as sensitive indicators of the place-specific reduction in OHC-dependent cochlear gain resulting from acoustic trauma. They measured CMs before and after inducing notched hearing loss (4-kHz notched acoustic trauma) using low-intensity pure tones (probe tone) presented alone or with a saturating tone (ST) ranging in frequency from 1 to 2.6 times the probe tone frequency. To evaluate the place-specific CM generated at the ST place, they derived the residual CM (rCM), which represents the complex difference between the CM measured with and without the ST. While acoustic trauma produced little change in the probe-alone CM (black trace in Figure 7–3A), rCM levels were reduced in a frequency-specific manner (shades of gray traces in Figure 7–3A and B). The level shifts in the rCM correlated well with the frequency range of shifts in neural thresholds reflected in the CAP, suggesting that rCMs are place-specific (originating near the cochlear place tuned to the ST frequency) and thus can be used to assess OHC function in a specific cochlear place instead of the basally biased conventional CM. The authors speculate that the combined use of CM and rCM may provide insights on OHC-dependent phenomena like temporary threshold shift (TTS) and the medial olivocochlear reflex, and the potential to use rCM to monitor the functional integrity of the OHCs in a place-specific manner. They also indicate that the combined measures may broaden the diagnostic utility of ECochG. Specifically, the rCM provides a sensitive index of changes in the active cochlear gain, and the conventional CM may be an independent index of the transduction status.

Clinical Applications of the CM

There has been very little successful clinical use of CM in assessing OHC functional status in sensorineural hearing loss. This is in part due to the observation that robust CM can be present even

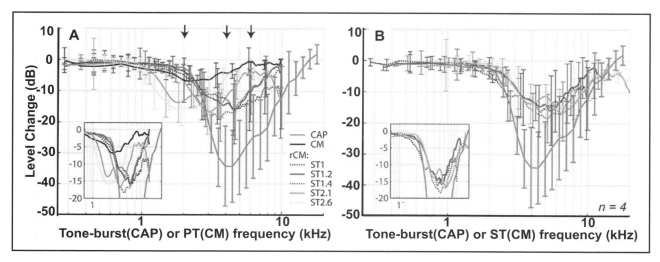

Figure 7–3. Mean changes in cochlear microphonic (CM; *solid black*) and residual CM (rCM) levels (*shades of gray, dotted and dashed lines*); see legend in (A) compared to mean shifts in compound action potential (CAP) thresholds (*light trace*) resulting from acoustic trauma in four chinchillas. **A.** rCM changes are plotted against the probe tone (PT) frequency. **B.** rCM changes are plotted against the saturating tone (ST) frequency. The error bars represent the standard deviation of a mean (for the CM data, error bars are shown every ~0.4 octave). The black arrows in (A) indicate frequencies at which data were compared to the model. The insets in each panel show the same data plotted with the error bars omitted to emphasize the alignment with the CAP data. Adapted from "Using Cochlear Microphonic Potentials to Localize Peripheral Hearing Loss," by K. K. Charaziak, C. A. Shera, and J. H. Siegel, 2017, *Frontiers in Neuroscience, 11*(169), pp. 1–13.

in the presence of significant hearing loss that would involve the OHCs ((Santarelli, Scimemi, Dal Monte, & Arslan, 2006; Liberman et al., (2002); Schoonhoven et al., 1999; Arslan et al., 1997; Eggermont, 1979a); and the reduced signal-to-noise ratio (SNR) observed with conventional noninvasive far-field electrode recordings. The main current application of CM is in the evaluation of a presynaptic, IHC-auditory nerve synapse, or auditory nerve dysfunction with functional integrity of the OHC subsystem as in auditory neuropathy (see Chapter 6 for more details).

Santarelli et al. (2006) described three patterns of CM and CAP responses in individuals with normal hearing, cochlear hearing loss, and auditory neuropathy (Figure 7–4). As expected, for individuals with normal hearing (and some individuals with mild cochlear hearing loss), they observed a normal click CAP threshold with CM present down to 50 dB nHL; for the cochlear loss group, they found elevated CAP and CM thresholds; and for the auditory neuropathy group, they found absent CAP and present CM suggesting functioning OHCs. Another interesting finding in individuals with normal hearing and a central auditory system pathology is the enhancement of CM amplitude and the prolonged ringing of the response (Gibbin, Mason, & Kent, 1983; Liu, Chen, & Xu, 1992; Santarelli et al., 2006), presumably due to enhanced cochlear gain resulting from reduced inhibitory influence of the medial efferents on the OHCs.

While individuals with auditory neuropathy may show varying degrees of hearing loss and a disproportionate decrease in speech perception abilities than predicted from the audiogram, the underlying etiology includes both genetic mutations and altered peripheral hearing mechanisms that are consistent with cochlear synaptopathy, which primarily involves a reduction in synaptic ribbons at the IHC-nerve junction (more about synaptopathy in Chapter 6). In acquired synaptopathy resulting from noise/music exposure, OAEs are normal, CM is present, and ABR waveforms are robust with normal thresholds and only a reduction in the amplitude of wave I at higher intensities (although this latter change is not observed across all human studies). In contrast, in auditory neuropathy, ABR is absent, and only OAEs and CM are present.

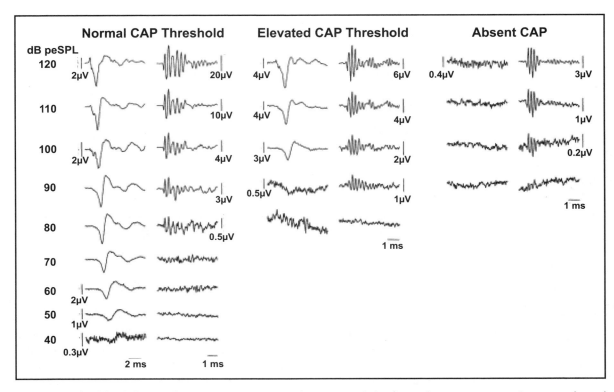

Figure 7–4. ECochG waveforms in response to alternating clicks from three representative ears plotted as a function of decreasing intensity for normal compound action potential (CAP) threshold, elevated CAP threshold, and the absence of neural response at maximum stimulation intensity (120 dB peSPL). Note the presence of cochlear microphonics (CM) and absence of CAP in the right-most row consistent with auditory neuropathy. Data from "Cochlear Microphonic Potential Recorded by Transtympanic Electrocochleography in Normally-Hearing and Hearing-Impaired Ears," by R. Santarelli, P. Scimemi, E. Dal Monte, and E. Arslan, 2006, *Acta Otorhinolaryngology Italy, 26*, pp. 78–95.

Summating Potential (SP)

The SP is a direct current potential with a positive (SP⁺) or a negative (SP⁻) polarity presumably resulting from asymmetric depolarization-hyperpolarization of the cochlear response associated with the OHCs (Russell, 2008). Dallos, Schoeny, and Cheaham (1972) characterize the SP as a product of CM distortions. However, there is considerable uncertainty about the source(s) of this rather enigmatic response. There is some recent evidence that OHCs, IHCs, and the auditory nerve contribute to the SP. Using combinations of ototoxins and neurotoxins to disentangle the relative contributions of the hair cells and the auditory nerve, Pappa et al. (2019) have shown that both the cochlear receptors (IHC and OHC) and the auditory nerve contribute to the SP, differ in polarity, and vary in amplitude across stimulus levels and frequency.

Human ECochG recordings using a promontory electrode and click stimulus typically show a negative DC shift with an inflection point separating the SP and the onset of the initial negative peak of the CAP. For longer-duration tone bursts, this DC potential is sustained for the duration of the stimulus and therefore is easier to identify (Figure 7–5). A change in response polarity (see Figure 7–5, response waveforms on the right) has been observed when the frequency of a constant intensity tone burst is increased (Dauman, Aran, Charlet de Sauvage, & Portmann, 1988; Eggermont, 1976c; Hornibrook, 2017; Hornibrook, Gourley, & Vraich, 2020). Unlike the amplitude of the neural CAP that decreases with increased repetition rate

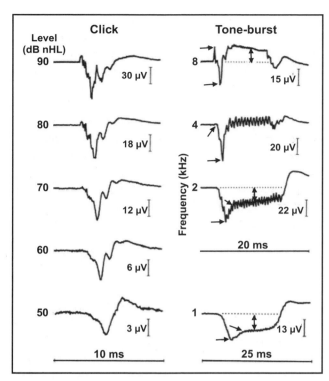

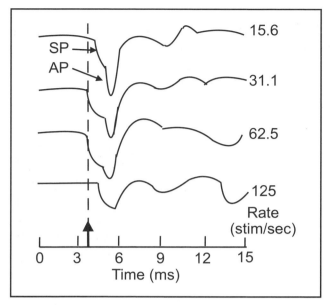

Figure 7–5. Transtympanic summating potential (SP) and compound action potential (CAP) to clicks plotted as a function of level (*left column*) and to tone burst at 1, 2, 4, and 8 kHz using a stimulus level of 90 dB SPL. The magnitude of the longer duration cochlear microphonics (CM)/SP for the tone burst is measured from the midpoint of the SP to the baseline. The SP and action potential (AP) can be clearly seen using the longer tone burst stimuli with the CM prominent at 2000 and 4000 Hz. The click response is dominated by the compound action potential that decreases in amplitude and shows latency prolongation as intensity is decreased. Adapted from "Tone Burst Electrocochleography for the Diagnosis of Clinically Certain Ménière's Disease," by J. Hornibrook, 2017, *Frontiers of Neuroscience*, *16*(11), p. 301 (originally from Dauman & Aran, 1991).

Figure 7–6. Auditory nerve compound action potentials showing clear summating potentials (SPs) plotted as a function of stimulus repetition rate (15.6, 31.1, 62.5, and 125 stimuli/sec). As the rate is increased, the action potential (AP) adapts (amplitude reduction and latency prolongation), leaving only the SP that is not affected by rate-induced adaptation. Data from "Electrocochleography," by J. J. Eggermont. In *Handbook of Sensory Physiology*, by W. D. Keidel and W. D. Neff (Eds.), 1976b, Vol. 5, Part 3, pp. 626–705. Copyright 1976 by Springer-Verlag, New York, NY.

of the stimulus, SPs are not susceptible to adaptation with an increase in the rate of stimulation (Figure 7–6). Therefore, this manipulation can be used to better isolate the fast and slow components of the SP from the CAP. In endolymphatic hydrops, the increased pressure in the scala media stretches the basilar membrane restricting its downward displacement, thereby enhancing the normal upgoing asymmetry resulting in an increased SP amplitude (Gibson, 1978). Thus, this enhancement of the SP and the decrease in CAP amplitude as the disease progresses, indicating distortion of the basilar membrane, is used as an index of inner ear endolymphatic hydrops (Dauman et al., 1988; Eggermont, 1976b; Gibson, Moffat, & Ramsden, 1977; Hornibrook, 2017; Hornibrook et al., 2020). Consistent with this, several studies have shown a decrease in SP amplitude with or without a change in CAP amplitude postadministration of glycerol as a treatment (Coats & Alford, 1981; Dauman, Aran, & Portmann, 1986 Gibson & Morrison, 1983; Moffatt, Gibson, Ramsden, & Booth, 1978), suggesting a pressure decrease in the scala media. However, Takeda and Kakigi (2010) failed to see any changes in the enhanced SP in patients with Ménière's disease post glycerol treatment, suggesting the SP enhancement in Ménière's disease may be related to hair cell dysfunction rather than a restricted displacement of the basilar membrane.

Since the SP increases relative to the CAP, Eggermont (1976c) suggested the use of a measure expressing the amplitude ratio between the two, the SP/AP ratio where the magnitude of each peak is measured initially (from a prestimulus baseline to their respective peaks) followed by the derivation of the SP/AP ratio. In normal ears, the mean SP/AP ratio (using transtympanic or extratympanic electrodes) in response to clicks is about 0.27 (SD = 0.027), with an upper limit of about 0.48 (SD = 0.082). This relative measure appears to be more stable for clicks compared to tone bursts. With tone bursts, the sustained SP response makes it is easier to measure either the amplitude (baseline to the peak shift) or an integrated area for the sustained SP rather than the conventional SP/AP ratio. For clicks, responses are typically obtained for both onset polarities (condensation and rarefaction) separately so that response components can be isolated. Addition of the responses to the two onset polarities will isolate the CAP (cancel the SP and CM that invert with polarity), and subtraction of the two will isolate the CM and SP.

Clinical Applications of SP

The SP's clinical application is primarily in the confirmation of a diagnosis of Ménière's disease. Ménière's disease is an inner ear disorder with symptoms including *vertigo attacks* (with or without hearing deficits) that are associated with combinations of fluctuating hearing (typically showing a unilateral rising hearing loss configuration with significantly reduced word recognition ability), *tinnitus*, and *aural fullness*. The exact mechanism of this hydrops, which produces an increase in pressure in the scala media, is unknown and presumably involves either overproduction, decreased absorption, or mechanical obstruction of endolymph.

Much of the earlier published work on the clinical application of the SP/AP ratio used click-evoked responses. Several of these studies showed an enhanced SP and the expected larger SP/AP ratio in the affected ear compared to the SP/AP ratio from the normal contralateral ear (e.g., Coats 1981; Gibson, 1978; Schmidt, Eggermont, & Odenthal, 1974). The SP/AP ratio criterion consistent with a diagnosis of Ménière disease ranged from 0.33 to 0.5, with sensitivity and specificity ranging from 40% to 85%, and 94% to 97%, respectively (see table from Hornibrook, 2017). For example, Gibson, Prasher, and Kilkenny (1983), using an SP/AP ratio criterion of 0.30, were successful in differentiating individuals with normal hearing, sensorineural hearing loss, and Ménière's disease when the hearing loss exceeded 40 dB HL. As can be seen in Table 7–1, the sensitivity values are generally low and quite variable across published reports. Ziylan, Smeeing, Stegeman, and Thomeer (2016), using a click SP/AP criterion of greater than 0.33, also found low sensitivity and predictive value of click SP in confirming the diagnosis of Ménière's disease. To increase both sensitivity and specificity, the SP/AP areal ratio measure was advanced by Ferraro and Tibbils (1999) using extratympanic recordings. Although this measure showed high sensitivity and specificity (Murad, Al-momani, Ferraro, Gajewski, & Ator, 2009), it could not be replicated when using transtympanic recordings (Ikino & de Almeida, 2006; Marcio et al., 2006). The reliability of the click SP/AP ratio used in the diagnosis of Ménière's disease remains an area of contention (because of variability in electrode type and location) that has largely contributed to the lack of widespread consistent use of ECochG. Hornibrook, Bird, Flook, and O'Bierne (2016) suggest that the use of click-elicited ECochG should be abandoned as it has failed to be a reliable index to confirm Ménière's disease.

All is not lost though. There is compelling evidence that the tone burst elicited SP recorded using a transtympanic electrode, with its easier recording and amplitude measurement, is superior to click-elicited SPs and a more reliable metric in confirmation of the diagnosis of Ménière's disease (Claes, De Valck, Van de Heyning, & Wuyts, 2011; Conlon & Gibson, 2000; Dauman & Aran, 1991; Hornibrook, 2017; Hornibrook et al., 2020). The previously cited studies showed that SPs recorded with transtympanic electrode in patients with Ménière's disease were significantly larger compared to control subjects (Figure 7–7), with the largest SPs observed at 1 and 2 kHz (Figure 7–8). To further demonstrate the better sensitivity of the tone burst SP compared to click SP, Gibson (2009) compared these two responses in individuals with Ménière's disease and individuals with equivalent degree of sensorineural hearing loss. He found that only the tone burst

Table 7–1. SP/AP Ratio Tolerance Values Used to Confirm Endolymphatic Hydrops and the Associated Sensitivity and Specificity Scores Across Studies

Authors	Electrode	SP/AP Criterion	Sensitivity (%)	Specificity (%)
Mori et al. (1987)	ET	0.44	68	
Aso et al. (1991)	TT	0.37	58	
Pou et al. (1996)	ET	0.35	57	94
Filipo et al. (1997)	TT	0.43	64	
Sass (1998)	TT	0.41	62	95
Ferraro & Tibbils (1999)	ET	0.41	60	
Camilleri et al. (2001)	TT	0.33	85	
Chung et al. (2004)	ET	0.34	71	96
Gibson (2005)	TT	0.47	40	97
Marcio et al. (2006)	TT	0.37	52	
Takeda & Kakigi (2010)	ET	0.40	56	
Claes et al. (2011)	TT	0.36	56	

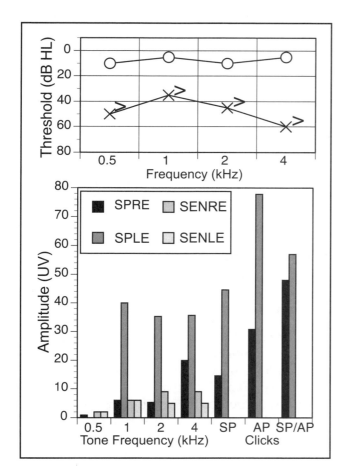

Figure 7–7. Summary of tone burst electrocochleographic results from an individual with confirmed Ménière's disease in the left ear. *Top:* Audiograms showing normal hearing sensitivity for the right ear and a mild-to-moderate sensorineural hearing loss in the left ear. *Bottom:* The amplitude of summating potential (SP) for the right ear (SPRE) and the left ear (SPLE) plotted as a function of frequency (500, 1000, 2000, and 4000 Hz). The SP/action potential (AP) ratio is also plotted at the extreme right of the figure. Both ears, particularly the left ear, showed enhanced SP and SP/AP ratio. Provisional diagnosis suggested hydrops in both ears. Data from "Tone Burst Electrocochleography Disproves a Diagnosis of Ménière's Disease Treated Aggressively," by J. Hornibrook, G. Gourley, and G. Vraich, 2020, *HNO, 68,* pp. 352–358.

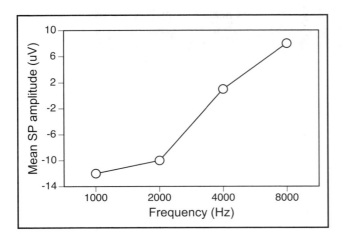

Figure 7–8. Mean summating potential (SP) amplitude plotted for four different tone burst frequencies in 75 patients confirmed with Ménière's disease. Note the large negative amplitudes at 1 and 2 kHz and the robust positive amplitudes at 4 and 8 kHz. Data from "Tone Burst Electrocochleography Disproves a Diagnosis of Ménière's Disease Treated Aggressively," by J. Hornibrook, G. Gourley, and G. Vraich, 2020, *HNO, 68*, pp. 352–358.

SP differentiated the two groups. Further analysis of their data revealed a sensitivity of 35% and specificity of 91% for the click SP/AP ratio, and a 95% sensitivity and 79% sensitivity for the tone burst SP/AP ratio (Iseli & Gibson, 2010). Hornibrook, George, Spellerberg, and Gourley (2011) compared the relative sensitivity of intratympanic magnetic resonance imaging (MRI) and tone burst ECochG in the diagnosis of Ménière's disease. In 30 patients with confirmed Ménière's disease, the ECochG was positive in 83% using tone bursts; positive in 30% using clicks; and positive in 47% using the intracranial MRI. The authors concluded that tone burst ECochG was the most sensitive index for confirming endolymphatic hydrops. Finally, a series of three studies by Hornibrook and colleagues (Hornibrook et al., 2010, 2011; Johnson, O'Beirne, Lin, Gourley, & Hornibrook, 2016) showed that in individuals with a clinical certainty of Ménière's diagnosis, transtympanic ECochG using tone bursts provided objective proof of hydrops (see Figure 7–8). There appears to be a consensus that a SP amplitude not less than 3 mV is diagnostic for endolymphatic hydrops (Claes et al., 2011; Gibson, 2005, 2009).

Although the move to use tone burst SP has improved the sensitivity of electrophysiological testing to identify Ménière's disease, the official diagnosis continues to be based on symptoms with very little use of ECochG among practitioners. A survey done by Nguyen, Harris, and Nguyen (2010) on the usefulness of ECochG for diagnosing Ménière's disease revealed a high reluctance among practitioners to use positive ECochG results to make a decision contrary to their clinical impression or a preference to use the videonystagmography (VNG) caloric test or vestibular evoked myogenic potentials (VEMPs). Only about 45% of practitioners used ECochG, with a majority of them using the less sensitive extratympanic approach (only 30% used the transtympanic approach). This lack of interest is in part due to the unrealized expectations from the unreliable click ECochG and a general lack of agreement on the choice of recording technique and choice of stimulus. However, given the growing compelling evidence that the transtympanic ECochG using tone bursts is still the simplest, most cost-effective, and most sensitive electrophysiological measure to confirm Ménière's disease diagnosis (Hornibrook, 2017), efforts should be made to promote the use of this technique. One other issue that needs to be addressed here is that most clinical practitioners for hearing care are audiologists; therefore, efforts should be made to improve the more practical noninvasive ECochG techniques, for example, the use of intrameatal tympanic membrane electrodes. There is some evidence that both transtympanic and tympanic membrane electrodes produce similar response patterns and are equally effective in the confirmation of Ménière's disease (Ferraro, Thedinger, Mediavilla, & Blackwell, 1994).

Whole-Nerve Compound Action Potential (CAP)

Response Characteristics

While both the CM and SP are presynaptic cochlear receptor potentials, the CAP recorded using transtympanic or extratympanic electrodes reflects neural activity from a population of neural fibers, in the distal portion of the auditory nerve, synchronized to the stimulus onset (Ozdamar & Dallos, 1978; Versnel, Prijs, & Schoonhoven, 1990). Like the ABR components, the CAP amplitude and latency depend on the cochlear regions contributing to the CAP, which in turn are dependent on stimulus bandwidth and intensity. The CAP is thought to represent the sum of single unit responses (Elberling & Hoke, 1978; Versnel, Prijs, & Schoonhoven, 1990). Since only the initial well-synchronized neural activity contributes to the development of the CAP, a click stimulus with its abrupt onset and broad spectrum would be an optimal stimulus (albeit, the recent arrival of chirps which could be more effective), and the basal cochlear region with the best synchronized neural activity will dominate the response. For both clicks and tone bursts, the CAP consists of a prominent short-latency negative component (N1) followed by a later smaller negative component (N2). While both components show amplitude increment and shortening of latency with an increase in stimulus intensity, the N1 component is increasingly prominent for stimulus levels above about 55 to 65 dB HL, while only a delayed broader N2 is clearly preserved at lower stimulus levels (Eggermont, 1976a; Elberling, 1973; Schoonhoven, 2007; Yoshie, 1976). It can be clearly seen in Figure 7–9 that the N1 response shows amplitude decrement and latency prolongation as stimulus intensity is reduced for both click-elicited (left) and 2000-Hz tone burst elicited (right) response; with the response still discernible close to threshold (Schoonhoven, 2007). Also, note the transition to a single broader and later peak at levels below 65 dB HL—presumably the N2 component. One interpretation for this double component is that the two components reflect contributions from two populations of ANFs—one a long latency low (better) threshold response, and the other a short latency higher threshold (poorer) response (Bourien

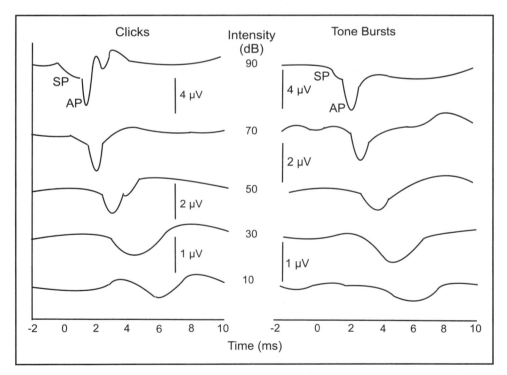

Figure 7–9. Compound action potentials (CAPs) to clicks and tone bursts are plotted as a function of stimulus intensity. The CAP for both stimuli decreases in amplitude and increases in latency as the stimulus level is decreased. Responses are clearly discernible down to 10 dB. Note the relatively smaller amplitude of the tone burst response. Data from "Responses From the Cochlea. Cochlear Microphonic, Summating Potential and Compound Action Potential," by R. Schoonhoven. In *Auditory Evoked Potentials: Basic Principles and Clinical Applications*, by R. F. Burkard, M. Don, and J. J. Eggermont (Eds.), 2007, pp. 180–198. Copyright 2007 Lippincott Williams & Wilkins, Baltimore, MD.

et al., 2014). It is also tempting to speculate that they represent predominantly high spontaneous and low spontaneous rate fibers, respectively.

Similar to the ABR to clicks, CAPs elicited by clicks are not place-specific in that they represent the sum of contributions along a broad region of the cochlear partition. High-pass masking techniques originally developed (Teas et al., 1962) to analyze click-evoked CAPs (later applied to the scalp recorded ABRs) can extract narrowband place-specific contributions to the transtympanic CAP (Eggermont, 1976a, 1979a, 1979b). Frequency-specific tone burst stimuli have also been used to obtain place-specific CAPs (Eggermont, 1976a; Eggermont, Spoor, & Odenthal, 1976; Schoonhoven, Fabius, & Grote, 1995; Sohmer & Feinmesser, 1973). However, with increasing stimulus levels, cochlear mechanics dictate a more basal spread of contributions even for frequency-specific tone bursts, particularly high-intensity, low-frequency tone bursts. Just like for clicks, an increase in stimulus intensity shortens the response latency and increases response amplitude. Also, increasing the frequency of the tone burst produces the expected shortening of latency, as the activity shifts from apical to basal regions, and a frequency-dependent increase in amplitude suggesting increasing synchrony of the neural activity. One other stimulus parameter that is of interest is the stimulus rate. The use of rapid stimulus rates will adapt the neural CAP, without altering the receptor potentials (see Figure 7–6), thereby providing an effective method to isolate these receptor potentials (Eggermont 1976b; Eggermont & Odenthal, 1974; Wilson & Bowker, 2002).

Recording Methods

Electrode Types and Placement. There are essentially three different extratympanic (ET) electrodes used to record the ECochG components: ear canal (tiptrode), intrameatal tympanic membrane, and transtympanic (TT) electrodes. The tiptrode, the least invasive of the three, and the most used by audiologists, is simply a gold foil wrapped around the insert earphone foam ear tip that makes contact with the skin of the ear canal. The tympanic membrane electrode (TM-wick electrode or tymptrode) is made up of a very small-diameter (about 0.1–0.2 mm) Teflon-coated silver wire encased in a flexible plastic tubing ending with a silver ball covered by a cotton wick saturated in a conductive gel. This electrode is slowly advanced along the posterior wall of the ear canal (after irrigating the canal with alcohol) until the cotton wick makes contact with the lateral portion of the tympanic membrane in the posterior inferior quadrant (Figure 7–10, thin black line along the floor of the ear canal). The electrode is held in place by the foam ear tip compressing on the cable as it is led out to the amplifier. The TT method uses a thin, insulated needle electrode that is advanced through the posterior inferior quadrant of the TM and the middle ear cavity until the exposed tip of the needle electrode rests on the cochlear promontory between the oval and round windows (see Figure 7–10). The ET electrodes (tiptrode and tympanic membrane electrodes) have a lower impedance (less than 20 kΩ) due to their relatively larger contact areas compared to the smaller contact area of the TT electrode (50–100 kΩ). The TT electrode, being the most proximal recording electrode to the response generators, produces the largest CAP (about 15 µV) followed by the tymptrode (3–5 µV), with the tiptrode producing the smallest response magnitude (1–2 µV)—this magnitude is still bigger than recording with a mastoid electrode (300–500 nV). Several studies have consistently shown that the CAP amplitude is appreciably greater (Figure 7–11) for the TT electrode compared to the tymptrode (Ferraro et al., 1994; Mori, Sacki, Matsunaga, & Asai, 1982; Noguchi, Komatsuzaki, & Nishida, 1999; Roland, Yellin, Meyerhoff, & Frank, 1995; Shoonhoven et al., 1995). Schoonhoven et al. (1995) demonstrated that tymptrode CAP amplitude was smaller by a factor of 0.43 compared to TT CAP amplitude. However, response detection and the slope of the amplitude change with intensity were similar for both types of recordings (Noguchi et al., 1999; Schoonhoven et al., 1995).

Response Recording

ECochG responses are recorded differentially between the recording electrode (tiptrode, TM, or TT electrode) and the mastoid. The recording electrode serves as the noninverting electrode with an electrode on the ipsilateral or contralateral mastoid serving as the inverting input, and an electrode on the forehead serving as the common ground.

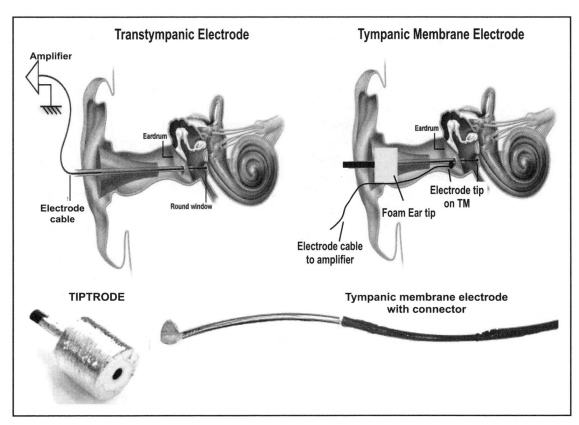

Figure 7–10. Electrode types used in electrocochleography. *Top left:* Transtympanic electrode that rests on the promontory. *Top right:* Intrameatal tympanic membrane electrode guided along the posterior wall of the ear canal and just contacts the tympanic membrane. *Bottom left:* TIPtrode gold foil wrapped around the foam tip serves as the electrode. *Bottom right:* TM electrode with its red connector cable.

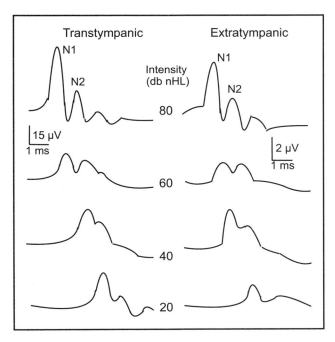

Figure 7–11. Compound action potential (CAP) waveforms plotted as a function of click level using transtympanic (*left*) and extratympanic-tympanic membrane electrodes (*right*). Note the big difference in amplitude with transtympanic recordings showing response amplitudes several orders of magnitude greater than responses recorded with the extratympanic electrode. For both recordings, the amplitude of the responses decreases, and the latency increases as stimulus intensity is decreased. Responses are clearly discernible down to 20 dB nHL for both recordings. Figure rendered using data from "Comparison Between AP and SP Parameters in Transtympanic and Extratympanic Electrocochleography," by N. Mori, K. Sacki, T. Matsunaga, and H. Asai, 1982, *Audiology, 21,* pp. 228–241.

Analog filtering is set to bandpass between 1 to 5 and 3 kHz, the amplifier gain is lower for the TT recording (10,000×) compared to the tympanic membrane electrode (25,000–50,000×) and tiptrodes (100,000–150,000×); and responses are averaged over a 15 to 20-ms analysis window. The number of sweeps required to obtain a reliable recording with good SNR is greater for the ET electrodes (500–1,000 sweeps) compared to the TT electrodes (250–400 sweeps). Thus, greater acquisition time will be needed for ET recordings. However, ET electrodes, unlike TT electrodes, can be placed by the audiologist and do not require a physician or an anesthetic to manage the pain resulting from piercing the tympanic membrane. See Chapter 10 for suggested protocol considerations for ECochG.

Clinical Applications of the CAP

Threshold Estimation. The CAP threshold is within about −8 to +2 dB of the behavioral threshold for tone bursts with octave frequencies from 500 to 8000 Hz for both extratympanic and transtympanic recordings for normal ears and a slightly smaller difference for individuals with cochlear hearing loss (Schoonhoven, Prijs, & Grote, 1996). The CAP-behavioral threshold difference is due to differences in the stimulus duration used, and differences in thresholds between normal and cochlear impaired ears due to differences in temporal integration. An earlier study by Spoor and Eggermont (1976) showed no difference between the two measures for tone bursts at 1, 2, and 4 kHz, and a −10-dB difference at 500 and 8000 Hz. ECochG can be used to estimate behavioral thresholds and has the added advantage of evaluating the functional integrity of OHC subsystem. However, the real or perceived invasive nature of recording ECochG either via tympanic membrane electrodes, or particularly, with transtympanic electrodes compared to the relative ease of recording ABR and ASSR have unfortunately dampened interest in considering these measures for clinical use. Lichtenhan et al. (2013) used a novel frequency–specific neural response called the auditory nerve overlapped waveform (ANOW) elicited by alternating polarity tones to estimate low-frequency cochlear thresholds. Essentially, when the overlapping receptor CM elicited by tone bursts with alternating onset phase are averaged (Figure 7–12A, top two traces), the CM cancels out, and the neural responses that occur mostly at a half-cycle of the tone bursts are "overlapped" in time (Figure 7–12A, bottom trace). The ANOW thus oscillates at twice the probe fre-

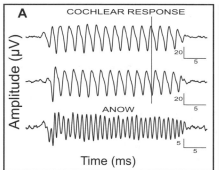 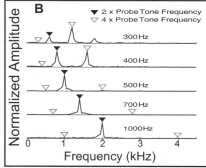 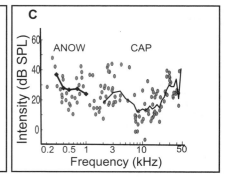

Figure 7–12. A. Cochlear responses (*top two traces*) and the auditory nerve overlapped response (ANOW) were recorded from a round-window electrode in cats in response to a 500-Hz tone presented at 50 dB SPL (*bottom trace*). The ANOW is derived by averaging the cochlear responses to opposite polarities and is twice the frequency of that of the cochlear response. The solid vertical line illustrates the polarity inversion of the cochlear response. **B.** Spectra of ANOW responses to tones of different frequencies. Consistent with the response, waveform spectra show peaks at two times the stimulus frequency and at integer multiples of the ANOW response. Response decreases in amplitude as frequency increases. **C.** Thresholds estimated for the low frequencies using ANOW, and thresholds at the high frequencies using the compound action potential (CAP) closely approximate the thresholds of single auditory nerve fibers (gray data points). Data shared by "Auditory Threshold Estimation Technique for Low Frequencies: Proof of Concept," by J. T. Lichtenhan, N. P. Cooper, and J. J. Guinan, Jr., 2013, *Ear and Hearing, 34*, pp. 42–51.

quency (Figure 7–12, bottom trace, and the spectral data shown in the middle panel (Figure 7–12B). ANOWs evoked from 300- to 1000-Hz tones are place-specific (Lichtenhan, Hartsock, Gill, & Guinan, 2014) and have thresholds (Figure 7–12C) that are 10 to 20 dB more sensitive, or better, than onset-CAP thresholds evoked from the same probe tones, suggesting a potential for use to determine low-frequency thresholds objectively. The ANOW is distinct from auditory neurophonic responses, which are evoked using higher-level tones and have cellular or spatial origins along the cochlear length that have yet to be fully understood (Henry, 1995; Lichtenhan et al. 2014; Snyder & Schreiner, 1984).

Differential Diagnosis

Most hearing losses consequent to a cochlear lesion exhibit elevated thresholds, reduced frequency selectivity, and a disrupted temporal pattern of neural activity (Harrison & Prijs, 1984; Liberman & Dodds, 1984; Versnel, Prijs, & Schoonhoven, 1997). Changes in ECochG components can reliably distinguish between presynaptic, postsynaptic, and neural dysfunction in these cochlear lesions. In normal-hearing individuals, the CAP amplitude growth function is characterized by a linear growth to about 40 to 50 dB HL, followed by a region of plateau or slow growth (50–60 dB) and then a resumption of the linear growth at higher levels (Figure 7–13, gray trace). In contrast, in cochlear losses, CAPs are robust (almost comparable to normal responses) with normal latency at high intensities but are difficult to reliably identify at lower intensities still above threshold. Consistent with this, the rate of amplitude change shows an abnormally steep slope (slope values greater than 0.037 log[pV]/dB for either tone burst or click responses is considered abnormal [Schoonhoven et al., 1995]). The steeper amplitude growth function in cochlear hearing loss (Figure 7–13, black trace) may be associated with loudness recruitment (Wang & Dallos, 1972). In Ménière's disease, the specific enhancement of the SP/AP ratio may distinguish it from sensorineural hearing loss with other etiologies.

Acoustic neuromas can also produce cochlear dysfunction by compromising blood supply to the cochlea resulting in ECochG changes similar to those observed in typical sensorineural hearing

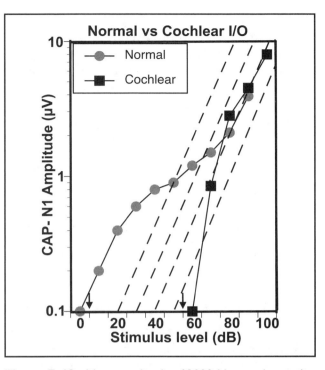

Figure 7–13. Mean amplitude of 2000-Hz tone burst elicited compound action potentials (CAPs) plotted as a function of intensity in an ear with normal hearing (*gray*) and an ear with cochlear hearing loss (*black*). For the normal hearing, individual responses are present down to 10 dB (*downward arrow*), whereas for the individual with cochlear impairment, robust responses are present down to 60 dB with responses above 60 dB tending to show much greater amplitude. Consistent with this, the amplitude growth function for cochlear loss shows an elevated threshold and a steeper slope compared to the normal-hearing group. Data from "Responses From the Cochlea. Cochlear Microphonic, Summating Potential and Compound Action Potential," by R. Schoonhoven. In *Auditory Evoked Potentials: Basic Principles and Clinical Applications*, by R. F. Burkard, M. Don, and J. J. Eggermont (Eds.), 2007, pp. 180–198. Copyright 2007 by Lippincott Williams & Wilkins, Baltimore, MD.

loss—that is, reduction or loss of cochlear receptor potentials. If the consequences of the lesion are restricted to the auditory nerve producing a neural conductive block and neural desynchronization, then CAPs will show prolonged latency, reduced amplitude, and broader response waveforms (Dauman, Aran, & Portman, 1988; Morrison, Gibson, & Beagley, 1976). That the nature of response change is dependent on which pre- or postsynaptic mechanisms are involved is also reflected in the selective presence of receptor potentials (CM and SP) and the reduction of CAP amplitude in auditory neuropathy (Starr et al., 2001); and the presence of receptor potentials with a reduction in CAP amplitude, and normal thresholds in cochlear synaptopathy (Kujawa & Liberman, 2009, 2015). In summary, a robust normal latency CAP response at high intensity, absent CM, and an abnormally steep CAP amplitude growth function is consistent with a cochlear site of lesion and loudness recruitment (Figure 7–12). Delayed CAP latency, broad waveforms, reduced amplitude, and the presence of receptor potentials are consistent with either an IHC-auditory nerve synapse dysfunction or an auditory nerve lesion (see Figure 7–4, middle row).

II. ABR DIAGNOSTIC MEASURE FOR COCHLEAR HYDROPS: COCHLEAR HYDROPS ANALYSIS MASKING PROCEDURE (CHAMP)

Changes in the response properties of the cochlear partition resulting from endolymphatic hydrops associated with Ménière's disease can produce alterations in the effects of high-pass masking of click-evoked ABR, resulting in a differential noise-induced latency change in normal and Ménière's ears. The increased stiffness of the basilar membrane due to increased endolymphatic volume presumably increases the cochlear traveling wave velocity (Donaldson & Ruth, 1996; Thornton, Farrell, & Haacke, 1991). Based on this rationale, Don, Kwong, and Tanaka (2005) developed a high-pass masking technique (called the cochlear hydrops analysis masking procedure [CHAMP]), wherein click-evoked ABR wave V latency in quiet and in the presence of high-pass noise masking were compared. Specifically, they recorded ABR to clicks in quiet and in the presence of masking noise high-pass filtered at 8, 4, 2, 1, and 0.5 kHz in non-Ménière's, normal-hearing individuals and individuals with Ménière's disease. Their results showed that the level of masking noise sufficient to mask the response to clicks in the normal-hearing individuals was insufficient to mask the responses in the individuals with Ménière's disease, thus producing an undermasked component. Comparison of the wave V latency shift between the quiet and the 500-Hz high-pass masking condition showed a mean latency shift of 4.8 ms for the normal-hearing individuals and only between a 0- and 0.2-ms shift in the individuals with Ménière's disease. Figure 7–14 shows an appreciably greater wave V latency shift as the high-pass filter cutoff is lowered for the normal group (left panel) compared to the little or no change in wave V latency for the Ménière's group (right panel). Importantly, no overlap in the results was observed at the individual level (100% sensitivity and specificity), thus making it a valuable clinical tool.

Don et al. (2005), instead of using the traveling wave velocity explanation, interpret their results to suggest that the early latency in the Ménière's group in the 500-Hz high-pass masking condition reflects primary activity originating from the basal high-frequency regions that are undermasked because of the mechanical effects of endolymphatic hydrops. The undermasking may also be due to the relatively lesser power of the pink noise in the high-frequency region. Another limitation is the difficulty in reliably measuring the appreciably smaller wave V response in the 500-Hz high-pass masking condition. Subsequent attempts at the validation of the CHAMP protocol in confirming endolymphatic hydrops have shown much lower sensitivity of the measure (DeValck, Claes, Wuyts, & Van de Heyning, 2007; Kingma & Wit, 2010; Lee et al., 2011; Ordóñez-Ordóñez et al., 2009). Lee et al. (2011) reported a sensitivity of 64% for the latency measure, which improved to 91% for the amplitude ratio measure, with specificity of 98% for latency and 83% for the amplitude ratio. They also found that CHAMP fared much better than ECochG in identifying Ménière's disease. The prospective validation study by Ordóñez-Ordóñez et al. (2009) in three groups of patients (vestibulopathy, neuropathy, and normal) showed 100% specificity but only 31% sensitivity. Kingma and Wit (2010) evaluated results from patients with unilateral Ménière's disease (with hearing loss greater than 60 dB accompanied by tinnitus and periodic vertigo attacks) and reported a sensitivity of only 32%. DeValck et al. (2007), in a retrospective study of 45 patients with otovestibular problems, found that 49% of the performed tests were uninterpretable, and in those with an interpretable result, the sensitivity was 31% and specificity was 28%. Thus, the CHAMP

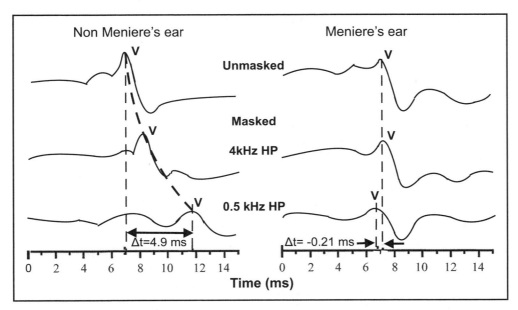

Figure 7–14. Representative auditory brainstem response (ABRs) from one individual to clicks plotted for the unmasked condition and high-pass masked conditions (4- and 0.5-kHz high-pass noise) are shown for the non-Ménière's ear (*left*) and Ménière's ear (*right*). The vertical dashed line aligned with wave V provides a reference to illustrate the amount of wave V latency shift as high-pass cutoff is decreased. While ABRs from the non-Ménière's ear show a large wave V latency shift (4.87 ms), there is virtually no wave V latency shifts (−0.2 ms) in the Ménière's ear. The absence of latency shift is consistent with the presence of Ménière's disease. Created using data from "A Diagnostic Test for Ménière's Disease and Cochlear Hydrops: Impaired High-Pass Noise Masking of Auditory Brainstem Responses," by M. Don, B. Kwong, and C. Tanaka, 2005, *Otology and Neurotology, 26*(4), pp. 711–722.

protocol appears to show consistent abnormalities in confirmed Ménière's patients, but its sensitivity and specificity are low in patients with no clear diagnosis. Therefore, its clinical utility is rather limited. In an attempt to address these limitations (presumably related to the difficulty in reliably identifying the small masked response), Don et al. (2007) proposed using the peak-to-trough amplitude. Specifically, wave V amplitude was measured on the difference waveform (quiet—500-Hz high-pass masked response). This amplitude was then normalized to the unmasked wave amplitude, thus providing a complex amplitude ratio measure. An amplitude ratio close to 1 reflects no undermasking and is consistent with a normal finding. An amplitude ratio of less than 1 is consistent with undermasking and points to Ménière's disease. This amplitude ratio measure provides a much higher sensitivity (100%) and specificity measure (75%) compared to the initial latency-based measure.

III. THE ELECTRICAL COMPOUND ACTION POTENTIAL (eCAP) AND ITS APPLICATION IN COCHLEAR IMPLANTS: INTRACOCHLEAR ECochG

Response Characteristics

Like its acoustical counterpart, the electrically evoked compound action potential (eCAP) represents synchronous firing in a population of ANFs in response to intracochlear electrical stimulation (see review by He, Teagle, & Buchman, 2017). Since the auditory nerve is used to encode and transmit information to higher centers along the auditory neuraxis, a direct measure of the eCAP using electrical stimulation should be relevant to CI outcomes. That is, a neural metric of the number of active neural elements and their responsiveness will provide useful information relevant to CI outcomes (Pfingst et al., 2015). In the last decade, there has been growing interest in utilizing eCAP to assess different aspects of auditory nerve responsiveness and the relevance to CI outcomes in adults and children (He, Abbas, Doyle, McFayden, & Mulherin, 2016; Hughes, Castioni, Goehring, & Baudhuin, 2012; Lee, Friedland, & Runge, 2012). The eCAP can be recorded directly from the exposed nerve trunk during surgery or from an intracochlear electrode in the cochlear implant using the reverse telemetry capability implemented in most current cochlear implants. It is a reliable stable response that can be easily recorded using the telemetry function implemented in the CI and the software provided by the manufacturer. The intracochlear recorded eCAP in human CI users is characterized by a robust biphasic response consisting of a negative peak N1 with a latency of 0.2 to 0.4 ms, followed by a positive peak P2 with a latency of 0.6 to 0.8 ms (Abbas et al., 1999), with an amplitude between 1 and 2 mV (Figure 7–15). A less common eCAP (type II) with two later positive peaks, P1 (axonal action potential) and P2 (dendritic action potential), has also been described (Stypulkowski & van den Honert, 1984). It should be noted here that the amplitude and latency of the eCAP are influenced by factors such as stimulation level (amplitude increases with stimulus level) (see Figure 7–15), intracochlear test electrode location (apical electrodes show large eCAP compared to recordings from basal electrodes presumably due to better neural survival and the shorter separation between the stimulating and recording electrodes in the apex [Tejani, Abbas, & Brown, 2017]), and stimulus polarity (shorter latency and greater amplitude latency for an anodic-leading biphasic pulse compared to a cathodic-leading biphasic pulse) (Baudhuin, Hughes, & Goehring, 2016). Also, the amplitude growth function shows a lower threshold and steeper slope for P1 compared to P2 (Figure 7–16). The steeper growth slopes in animal models have been interpreted to suggest higher spiral ganglion density (e.g., Pfingst et al., 2015), while the shallower eCAP amplitude growth slope in humans has been associated with a longer duration of hearing loss (Schvartz-Leyzac & Pfingst, 2016). However, the association between these factors and speech per-

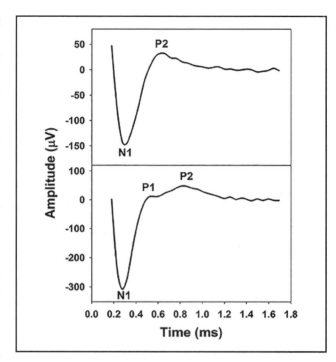

Figure 7–15. Intracochlear electrical compound action potential (eCAP) recordings from pediatric cochlear nucleus cochlear implant (CI) users with prelingual deafness. Typical eCAP waveform with only the N1-P2 biphasic morphology (*top*) and the less common eCAP with two positive peaks (*bottom*). Reprinted from "The Electrically Evoked Compound Action Potential: From Laboratory to Clinic," by S. He, H. F. Teagle, and C. A. Buchman, 2017, *Frontiers in Neuroscience, 11*, p. 339.

ception is not clear and has not been systematically evaluated to date. As with all evoked potentials, and particularly with the very short latency eCAP, the response can be potentially distorted by stimulus artifact given the proximity of the stimulating and recording electrodes. The use of alternating polarity and/or template subtraction using forward masking (Brown, Abbas, & Gantz, 1990) has been considered to eliminate the dominant stimulus artifact. However, since the response latency and amplitude are different for each polarity, the use of alternating polarity to eliminate stimulus artifact still leaves the response distorted. Since these responses arise from the peripheral portion of the auditory nerve, they are not influenced by the neural maturation effects typically observed for ABR components. Consequently, there are no major

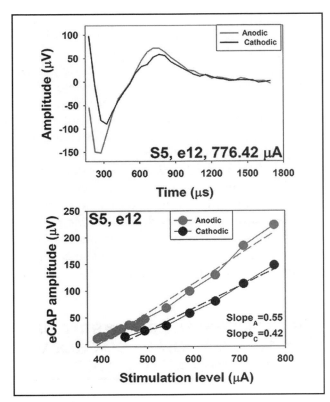

Figure 7–16. Electrical compound action potential (eCAP) waveforms for the anodic (*gray*) and cathodic (*black*) leading biphasic pulse (*top*) and the amplitude growth function for the two polarities (*bottom*). Response amplitude is consistently larger for the anodic phase and exhibits a steeper slope compared to the cathodic lead. Data from "The Electrically Evoked Compound Action Potential: From Laboratory to Clinic," by S. He, H. F. Teagle, and C. A. Buchman, 2017, *Frontiers in Neuroscience, 11*, p. 339.

morphological differences in eCAPs recorded from adult and pediatric CI users (Brown et al., 1990; Gordon, Papsin, & Harrison, 2004).

Clinical Applications

Earlier studies primarily focused on using the eCAP to determine program levels for individual CI electrodes (e.g., Brown et al., 1998; McKay, Chandan, Akhoun, Siciliano, & Kluk, 2013), but more recently the focus has shifted to using eCAP to evaluate neural survival (e.g., Kim et al., 2010; Pfingst, 2015), and spectral and temporal coding strategies and their relationship with auditory perception in CI users (e.g., DeVries, Scheperle, & Bierer, 2016; He et al., 2016; Tejani et al., 2017). Most studies have confirmed that the stimulus is audible at levels approximating the eCAP threshold. While the eCAP can provide an objective initial estimate of program levels, particularly in the absence of reliable behavioral response, its limited predictive power for detection (T level) and comfort (C or M level) estimation severely limit its application in setting program levels for individual patients. With respect to *spectral resolution*, it is known that CI implant users have poor spectral resolution that limits their speech perception ability (e.g., Winn & Litovsky, 2015; Winn, Won, & Moon, 2016). Unfortunately, the electrical fields created by each CI electrode of a multichannel device overlap and effectively reduce the number of independent spectral channels, resulting in unresolved spectral components that are detrimental to speech perception (e.g., Friesen, Shannon, Baskent, & Wang, 2001; Noble, Labadie, Gifford, & Dawant, 2013). Recent studies using improved quantification of the spread of excitation (SOE) pattern at the electrode-neural interface using the eCAP have shown an improved correlation between the eCAP SOE function and behavioral measures. However, it is important to note that the eCAP measure does not provide information about more central processes involved in speech perception. Scheperle and Abbas (2015) observed that eCAP SOE functions accounted for only part of the variance in the neural encoding of spectral information in the central auditory system. Thus, the utility of the eCAP measure to predict speech perception is questionable, although it can still provide useful information about channel interactions.

In addition to spectral resolution, *temporal cues* like response onset and rapid changes in response spectra and amplitude, well represented in the temporal pattern of neural activity in the ANFs, are also important for speech perception (e.g., Delgutte & Kiang, 1984). There is evidence to suggest that the temporal response properties of the auditory nerve fibers like refractory recovery (absolute and relative refractory periods), neural adaptation (decrease in firing rate after the initial vigorous onset response) and recovery from adaptation, and amplitude modulation (phase locking to envelope periodicity) detection of ANFs reflected in eCAP can represent speech envelope cues (e.g., Tejani et al., 2017). All of these temporal properties play an important role in speech encoding. For example, abnormal adaptation and recovery from adaptation could result in poor representation of the temporal envelope essential for optimal speech perception in CI users (Nelson & Donaldson, 2002). However, it is still not clear if or how temporal properties reflected in the eCAP are relevant to speech and language outcomes in CI users. It remains unclear the extent to which neural adaptation and recovery from this adaptation of the auditory nerve influence auditory temporal processing and speech perception capabilities in CI users. Similarly, although there is clear evidence of eCAP encoding amplitude modulation using sinusoidally amplitude-modulated pulse trains, the relationship between how the auditory nerve responds to AM stimuli and auditory perception in human CI users is not well understood.

Another area of eCAP application is the evaluation of the pattern and degree of **neural survival** of ANFs to determine the number of functional channels available. While it is not possible to directly determine the spiral ganglion (SG) density in humans using eCAP, evaluation of eCAP changes to certain stimulus manipulations that are sensitive to SG density is thought to provide this information, albeit indirectly. These measures include examining the slope of eCAP amplitude growth with increase in stimulus level (the rationale here is that steeper slopes will indicate higher SG density, whereas shallower slopes would be associated with lower SG density), examining changes in the interphase gap (IPG) producing changes in eCAP (poor SG survival indicated by elevated threshold and reduced eCAP amplitude when IPG is increased), and evaluating eCAP's polarity. Results from studies examining eCAP amplitude slope in CI users have not been consistently uniform; while some studies show better speech perception associated with steeper amplitude growth slopes (Brown, Abbas, & Gantz, 1990; Kim et al., 2010), other studies fail to show an association between amplitude growth slope and speech perception (e.g., Turner, Mehr, Hughes, Brown, & Abbas, 2002). Pfingst et al. (2017) showed that SG density only accounted for 50% of the variance in the slope of eCAP I/O function in an animal model. Schvartz-Leyzac and Pfingst (2016) observed an increase in eCAP amplitude and steeper slopes of the amplitude growth function with an increase in IPG. However, these effects show considerable intersubject and electrode location variability. Also, it is not known whether these changes in eCAP with changes in IPG influence speech perception or CI outcomes. Considerable research efforts are under way to understand how these measures influence speech perception, but are not at a point where most of these measures can be used in the clinic reliably. Nevertheless, these experimental advances are necessary stepping-stones to realize the clinical applications outlined earlier.

IV. ELECTRICAL ABR (eABR) AND ITS APPLICATION IN COCHLEAR IMPLANT EVALUATION

Scalp recordable ABRs can also be elicited by electrical stimulation of the auditory nerve using either extracochlear or intracochlear electrodes and are referred to as electrical ABRs (eABRs). The eABR, commonly recorded before cochlear implant (CI) or auditory brainstem implant (ABI) surgery (Sennaroğlu et al. (2016), serves as a preimplant prognostic test to verify the functional integrity of the auditory nerve and the brainstem. eABR threshold measures obtained from postoperative recordings using the array of CI electrodes could assist in CI programming (Brown et al., 1994; Lo, Chen, Horng, & Hsu, 2004; Shallop, VanDyke, Goin, & Mischke, 1991). While comparisons between ABR wave V and eABR eV are difficult given the differences in the expression of the levels of the stimuli and nature of their generation (the former involving broad or place-specific cochlear activation; the latter bypassing cochlear activation), place-specific ABR wave V amplitude is smaller than eV amplitude, presumably due to greater synchronization of the neural activity producing the eABR. The eABR components eIII and eV are thought to be generated in the mid-brainstem and upper brainstem, respectively (van den Honert & Stypulkowski, 1986).

Response Characteristics of the Normal eABR

Response Morphology

The normal eABR waveform morphology, like the acoustically elicited ABR, is characterized by a similar sequence of three or four positive peaks, each followed by a negative trough, labeled as eII, eIII, and eV (Figure 7–17) that occur about 1.5 ms earlier than responses to a high-intensity acoustically elicited ABR. Like the acoustic ABR, eABR may also show a wave IV shoulder occasionally. A large stimulus artifact is typically caused by the injection of electrical current into the cochlea and lasts through the first 2 ms of the analysis epoch, thereby obscuring the early components I and II. To avoid this large stimulus artifact that occurs when using a vertex-ipsilateral montage, it is common practice to record eABRs using a contralateral recording electrode montage (vertex/high forehead—contralateral mastoid).

Response Latency

Unlike the large (3–5 ms) intensity-induced latency changes in the scalp-recorded wave V, eABR eV shows little or no latency shift with changes in current levels except for a small shift (about 0.5 ms) near threshold (Abbas & Brown, 1988; Shallop, Beiter, Goin, & Mischke, 1990, van den Honert, & Stypulkowski, 1986). The eV latency prolongation near threshold (see Figure 7–17) is thought to reflect the time taken to build adequate charge to spread from the round-window membrane to the spiral ganglion. Response latency also varies with the location of the stimulating electrode. Using an extracochlear electrode (e.g., the transtympanic electrode located on the promontory) showed relatively longer eV latency (around 4.6–5.6 ms;

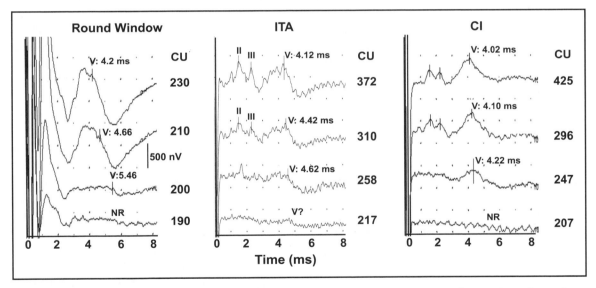

Figure 7–17. Representative electrical auditory brainstem response (eABR) waveforms plotted as a function of stimulus levels, expressed as current units (CU), from an individual obtained using an extracochlear (round-window electrode [*left*]) and two intracochlear stimulation types (ITA [*middle*], CI [*right*]). Response components and the current levels (CU) are identified in each panel. While the large stimulus artifact (and the use of contralateral montage in the round-window recording obscures wave I and II, a robust wave V is present. For the intracochlear recordings, waves eII, eIII, and eV are easily identifiable down to threshold levels. In all three recordings, wave V amplitude appears to show amplitude reduction and latency prolongation as stimulus intensity is decreased. Figure created from supplemental data in "Extracochlear Stimulation of Electrically Evoked Auditory Brainstem Responses (eABRs) Remains the Preferred Pre-implant Auditory Nerve Function Test in an Assessor-Blinded Comparison," by A. Causon, M. O'Driscoll, E. Stapleton, S. Lloyd, S. Freeman, and K. J. Munro, 2018, *Otology and Neurotology, 40*, pp. 47–55.

Causon et al., 2018; Mason, O'Donoghue, Gibbin, Garnham, & Jowett, 1997) compared to intracochlear electrodes like the intracochlear test array (ITA) and the CI electrode array. It is not clear why normal eABR latencies are longer using the extracochlear electrode. It is possible that the significantly larger charge (almost six times more) required to reach a threshold level eABR using the extracochlear electrode may account for the latency discrepancy between extracochlear and intracochlear electrodes. Since eABR is produced by direct electrical activation of the ANFs in the spiral ganglion, the response latency does not include the transducer acoustic delay, cochlear traveling wave delay, the hair cell-auditory nerve synaptic delay, and the delay associated with the initiation of stimulus driven synchronous neural activity in the auditory nerve. Using intracochlear electrodes, the absolute latency of wave eII is between 1.3 and 15.5 ms, wave eIII 2 and 2.4 ms, and wave eV 3.9 and 5.1 ms with no latency differences between ITA and CI electrodes. eABRs elicited using intracochlear apical electrodes show more robust and shorter latency for eV compared to basal electrodes with little or no latency difference for eII and eIII (Abdelsalam & Afifi, 2015; Causon et al., 2018; Firszt, Chambers, Kraus, & Reeder, 2002; Gordon, Papsin, & Harrison, 2007; Shallop et al., 1991). While the mechanism underlying this discrepancy is not known, some etiologies of hearing loss may render the basal region with fewer spiral ganglion neurons compared to the apical region resulting in the smaller amplitude and delayed basal response.

Similar to the decrease in the ABR interpeak latencies from birth to 2 years, suggesting ongoing neural maturation in the brainstem, eABR interpeak intervals also decrease over the first year of implant use for both apical and basal electrodes (Gordon, Papsin, & Harrison, 2007; Thai-Van, Cozma, & Boutitie, 2007). These developmental eABR changes, like the ABR developmental changes in the first two years, likely reflect neural maturation involving myelinization and improvement of synaptic efficiency in the brainstem.

Response Amplitude

Unlike the relatively small latency changes with intensity, eV amplitude exhibits a rapid growth (Figure 7–18) with increase in stimulus level (Abbas & Brown, 1988; Causon et al., 2018; Hughes, 2013; Starr & Brackmann, 1979) with a maximum amplitude of between 0.5 and 3 µV for stimulus intensities near the C-level. Although the response amplitude tends to asymptote here, it is not a reliable index for setting the C-level because of patent discomfort. Also, the amplitude growth function is steeper for the apical electrodes compared to the basal electrodes, reflecting the relative differences in the density of surviving neural elements in the cochlea. Smith and Simmons (1983) found shallow amplitude growth curves in cats with only 5% to 10% of spiral ganglion cells surviving after surgical ablation of the spiral ganglion. Their results suggest that the slope of the ABR eV amplitude growth function is dependent on spiral ganglion cell density and could act as a predictor index of postoperative CI performance. Abbas and Brown (1991) reported different eV amplitude growth functions for Nucleus and Symbion devices and attributed these to the differences in the artifacts generated by these devices. More recently, Causon et al. (2018) reported essentially similar eV amplitude growth functions for extracochlear (round-window) and intracochlear (ITA, and Medel CI) electrode arrays with the extracochlear growth functions showing more variability (Abbas & Brown, 1991).

Threshold

The electrical stimulation current needed to produce a repeatable threshold level eV response varies with implants but is about 0.1 to 0.2 mA. Like the ABR threshold, eABR thresholds are also higher than the perceptual threshold for the specific stimulus used. Causon et al. (2018) found that the charge required to produce a threshold-level response using extracochlear stimulation was significantly (about six times) greater than that needed for intracochlear electrodes. They explained that the extracochlear electrodes require a much larger charge to breach the round window and reach the spiral ganglion cells within the modiolus. Causon et al. (2018), comparing eABR recordings using a round-window electrode and two other intracochlear stimulation electrodes (ITA and CI stimulation), reported that the amplitude of eV at the threshold for the round-window electrode was 0.22 µV, 0.33 µV for the ITA electrode, and 0.26 µV for the CI electrode.

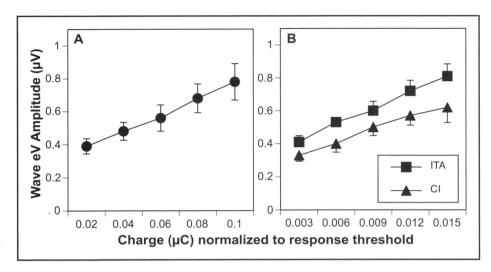

Figure 7–18. Electrical auditory brainstem response (eABR) eV amplitude plotted as a function of stimulus level (expressed as Charge, μC) for the round-window stimulation (A), and the two (ITA, *solid squares*; CI, *solid triangle*) steadily growing amplitude-intensity functions are essentially parallel for all three types of electrical stimulation (B). The CI amplitudes are the smallest among the three recordings. Note the larger variability (particularly at the higher levels) and the greater intensity required to elicit the round-window eABR. C = Coulomb, a common unit of electrical charge/sec; C = maximum amplitude of the current (amperes) in a pulse; X is the pulse width in seconds. Created using data from "Extracochlear Stimulation of Electrically Evoked Auditory Brainstem Responses (eABRs) Remains the Preferred Pre-implant Auditory Nerve Function Test in an Assessor-Blinded Comparison," by A. Causon, M. O'Driscoll, E. Stapleton, S. Lloyd, S. Freeman, and K. J. Munro, 2018, *Otology and Neurotology*, *40*, pp. 47–55.

Methods to Record and Analyze the eABR

Electrical Stimulation Methods

Unlike the relatively easy noninvasive procedure for recording the ABR, acquisition of the eABR is rather complex and requires specialized equipment, expertise, and sedated or very still patients, and the procedure can be more time consuming. eABRs can also be recorded during cochlear implant surgery while participants are under general anesthesia. Both extracochlear and increasingly intracochlear methods of stimulation are used to record the eABR. The conventional extracochlear method (commonly used preoperatively since the early days of cochlear implants) uses a transtympanic approach postmyringotomy with a stimulating electrode placed either on the promontory or the round window (Causon et al., 2018; Kileny, & Zwolan, 2004; Mason et al., 1997; Pau, Gibson, & Sanli, 2006; Sauvaget, Péréon, Nguyen The Tich, & Bordure, 2002). The round-window electrode stimulation appears to be better compared to promontory placement (Pau et al., 2006). This perioperative eABR approach via extracochlear stimulation uses either a needle electrode or a needle electrode with a ball tip (golf-club electrode) placed at the round window near the cochlea or on the promontory (Chouard, Koca, Meyer, & Jacquier, 1994; Meyer, Drira, Gegu, & Chouard, 1984). For intracochlear recordings, typically, two locations (both for ITA and CI) are used as the stimulation electrodes: one located near the basal end of the implant electrode array (electrode 5) and the other at the apical end (electrode 20). As mentioned earlier, the apical electrode elicits shorter latency and lower-threshold eABRs compared to the basal electrode. Causon et al. (2018) reported that the morphological characteristics of the ITA and CI elicited responses are similar but not very different from the extratympanic elicited responses. Based on a comparison between the eABRs elicited using intracochlear (ITA and CI) and extracochlear electrode stimulation, Causon et al. (2018) concluded that both approaches can be used to record an eABR that is representative of the one elicited by the CI. However, the extracochlear stimulation appears to be the preferred approach for preimplant evaluation given the invasive nature of the intracochlear methods.

Data Acquisition Methods

The electrical stimuli used to evoke the eABR are generated by a computer-controlled speech processor interface. The software generates and controls the sequence of radiofrequency bursts required to activate the implant device and to provide the appropriate trigger pulse for digitization. The software also allows the tester to choose the level (in current units), onset polarity, duration, and repetition rate of the stimulus. Typically, a biphasic current pulse with a negative to positive polarity and pulse duration between 50 and 200 μs is chosen and presented at a relatively slow rate of about 21 Hz in a monopolar stimulation mode. For threshold determination responses are recorded first using a level close to a comfortable level and reduced in steps of 20 units until a level is reached for which there is no discernible eV response component. The stimulus attenuation step can be reduced as threshold is approached to obtain a better estimate of eABR threshold.

As with the conventional ABR, two to three replicates of 1,000 sweeps are obtained. Artifact rejection is also used to eliminate sweeps with excessive noise. To reduce the large electrical stimulation-induced stimulus artifact, the first few milliseconds at the onset of the analysis time epoch are digitally blocked and further offline filtering is used to appreciably reduce this artifact. A filter setting of 20 to 3000 Hz is recommended to enable the detection of smaller delayed responses and to reduce temporal splatter of the artifact (please see Mason et al., 1997 for details on eABR procedures). To proceed with the recording (with minimal contamination of responses in the presence of the large stimulus artifact), several steps have to be taken, including the setting of the artifact rejection window past the first 2 ms to avoid continuous rejection of sweeps (which prevents saturation of the amplifier-blanking wherein the amplifier inputs are disabled for the first 2 ms); the use of alternating polarity to cancel the artifacts, which may not remove the artifact completely but is surely worth considering; and the use of a low high-pass filter setting to reduce the temporal scatter of the artifact.

Recording Montage and Response Analysis

The recording montage used for eABR is essentially the same as the one used for conventional ABR recording with one difference. The responses are commonly recorded differentially between a noninverting electrode placed at high forehead and an inverting electrode placed on the contralateral mastoid (instead of ipsilateral) with a ground electrode placed on the nape. For recording during CI surgery under general anesthesia, disposable subdermal needle electrodes are placed on the vertex (noninverting), contralateral mastoid (inverting), and forehead (common ground). Response components are visually identified using superimposed replicates. Absolute latencies of eII, eIII, and eV and the eIII–eV interpeak latencies are measured to assess the integrity of neural conduction in the brainstem. Normalized peak-to-peak amplitude, while quite variable, may provide useful information about neural synchrony in the responding neural elements. As described earlier, characterization of the slope of the eV amplitude growth function may be useful in assessing neural density. The eABR threshold is defined as the lowest stimulus level that elicits a replicable and identifiable eV with amplitude greater than 400 nV and with residual noise not exceeding one-third the size of the response waveform (Stevens, Booth, Brennan, Feirn, & Meredith, 2013). A growth in response amplitude and shortening of latency at levels higher than threshold will also confirm that the response is neural.

V. APPLICATION OF AUDITORY NERVE AND BRAINSTEM RESPONSES IN INTRAOPERATIVE MONITORING

Introduction and Rationale

Intraoperative monitoring (IOM), as the name implies, is the continuous monitoring of the integrity of neural function during intracranial surgery to reduce the potential risk of permanent damage that may compromise function. IOM of brain and nerve function, aided by technological surgical advances (e.g., two- and three-dimensional image-guided surgery, gamma-knife radiosurgery and stereotaxic radiosurgery), has now become routine with almost all surgical procedures to remove tumors along the auditory nerve, cerebellopontine angle, and brainstem. The increased use of IOM in VIIIth nerve tumor surgery has reduced the incidence of hearing loss and facial nerve dysfunction. The rationale for use of IOM is to alert the surgeon to make corrections in the surgical approach while the changes noted in the responses are still reversible. The assumptions are that surgical manipulations cause measurable changes in neural conduction and/or synaptic transmission before permanent injury sets in. Hearing and facial nerve function are at risk during a surgical procedure that involves resection of VIIIth nerve tumor, vestibular division resection, and microvascular decompression, which are prone to drilling- or retraction-induced mechanical damage caused by compression, stretching, cutting, or tearing; ischemia due to vasospasms or ligation; and noise-induced temporary hearing loss due to the drilling noise proximal to the cochlea. However, potential nonsurgical factors such as effects of body temperature, anesthesia, effects of drill noise, and other electrical interferences that could potentially alter the response properties should be ruled out first. By providing timely feedback on the functional status of the nerve to the surgeon, permanent damage to the structures and consequent postsurgical hearing loss and/or facial nerve dysfunction can be averted.

Surgical Approaches

Several different surgical approaches are considered for auditory nerve tumor resection. The decision to utilize a particular approach is dependent on the location and size of the tumor, as well as consideration of preservation of hearing and facial nerve function. The *translabyrinthine* approach is the most direct, relatively fast, and commonly used approach through the ear canal–mastoid–semicircular canals and the internal auditory meatus. This approach provides an excellent view of the tumor and facial nerve, thereby reducing the risk of injury to the facial nerve. However, this approach results in a complete loss of hearing and vestibular apparatus in almost all patients. The *middle fossa* approach bypasses the inner ear and approaches the tumor from the top of the internal auditory canal and carries a greater risk of damage to the facial nerve (Figure 7–19). Since it provides a very good view

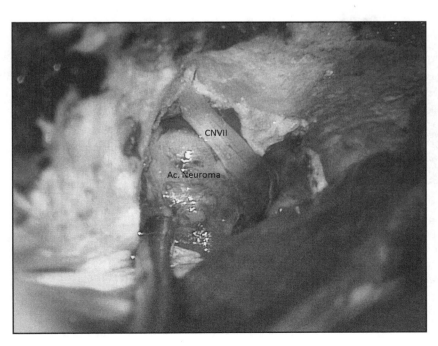

Figure 7–19. A midposterior fossa surgical approach view of an acoustic neuroma. The internal auditory canal has been partly drilled to expose the intracanalicular portion of the acoustic tumor (identified with label) with the facial nerve clearly visible to the right of the tumor. From *The Audiologist's Handbook of Intraoperative Neurophysiological Monitoring* (p. 67) by Paul R. Kileny. Copyright 2018 Plural Publishing, Inc. All rights reserved.

of the internal auditory canal, it is mainly used for small intracanalicular acoustic neuromas (tumors less than 2 cm in size) in patients with intact hearing. Two risk factors associated with this approach are the increased risk for facial nerve damage, and risks posed by retraction of the temporal lobe. The craniotomy created for *retrosigmoidal or occipital* approach offers a panoramic view of the posterior fossa (Figure 7–20). This approach involves retraction of the cerebellum to access extra-axial tumors; cranial nerve neurectomy and vascular decompression; and vertebrobasilar vascular disorders. Advantages of the retrosigmoidal approach are the potential for hearing preservation and a clear exposure of the inferior portion of the cerebellopontine angle (CPA). The main disadvantages are an appreciably higher incidence of persistent postoperative headache, a higher incidence of cerebrospinal fluid (CSF) leaks, and potential for cerebellar damage.

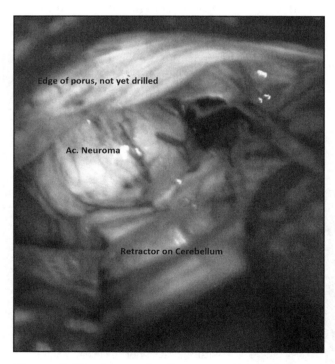

Figure 7–20. A posterior fossa retrosigmoidal surgical approach view of an acoustic neuroma. The internal auditory canal opening (porus acousticus) overhanging the acoustic tumor (identified by a label) has not yet been drilled. The cranial nerves are anterior to the tumor and not visible in this view. Adapted from *The Audiologist's Handbook of Intraoperative Neurophysiological Monitoring* (p. 68) by Paul R. Kileny. Copyright 2018 Plural Publishing, Inc. All rights reserved.

Commonly Used Measures for IOM

Our focus here is on the description of IOM of auditory structures with the desired goal of preservation of hearing. Auditory electrophysiological measures that provide a continuous monitoring of the functional status of the auditory nerve and brainstem during surgical removal of an VIIIth nerve tumor include the most commonly used scalp-recorded ABR to monitor the functional integrity of the brainstem structures and tracts; transtympanic electrocochleography (ECochG) to record both the cochlear receptor potentials and the auditory nerve CAP; and direct recording from the exposed auditory nerve (AN-CAP; Møller & Jannetta, 1981, 1983a) and/or from the surface of the cochlear nucleus (CN-CAP; Møller & Jannetta, 1983b) to monitor neural conduction in the auditory nerve. As an example, Figure 7–21 shows the comparison of pre- and postsurgical manipulation on the scalp-recorded ABR, and the directly recorded AN-CAP. Surgical manipulation broadens the AN-CAP and reduces ABR amplitude. ECochG captures the receptor components (CM and SP—not typically evaluated in IOM) and CAP from the distal portion of the auditory nerve, thus providing information about the functional status of the cochlea and distal portion of the auditory nerve, respectively. However, ECochG is most useful in monitoring cochlear functional integrity, and less useful during IOM because most of the changes resulting from surgical manipulations will be reflected in the measures from more proximal portions of the auditory nerve and brainstem. For optimal results, ECochG is performed using a transtympanic approach with an electrode placed on the promontory, closest to the CAP generator site. Given the appreciably higher response SNR with a promontory and intrameatal electrodes, response acquisition time can be significantly reduced.

The AN-CAP is recorded directly from the exposed intracranial portion of the nerve near the tumor site and provides real-time information about the functional status of the whole auditory nerve (see Figure 7–21). With its large amplitude (about 50 µV) and short acquisition time (only 10–20 stimulus sweeps), it continues to be used successfully in IOM during neurosurgery for vestibular schwannoma (Colletti, Bricola, Fiorino, &

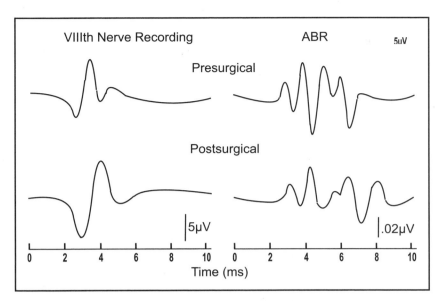

Figure 7–21. The effects of pre- (*top*) and postsurgical (*bottom*) manipulation on the auditory nerve compound action potential (AN-CAP) (*left*) and auditory brainstem response (ABR) (*right*) waveforms. The postmanipulation of the auditory nerve results in a broadening of the CAP response waveform, latency prolongation, and the loss of the P2, N2 components, suggesting a neural conduction block. ABRs show reduced amplitude and longer latency. Data from Møller, A. R., and Jannetta, P. J. (1983a). Monitoring auditory functions during cranial nerve microvascular decompression operations by direct recording from the eighth nerve. *Journal of Neurosurgery, 59*, 493–499.

Bruni, 1994; Colletti & Fiorino, 1998) and microvascular decompression (MVD) (Møller & Jannetta, 1983a; Møller, & Møller, 1989). The waveform of the AN-CAP is characterized by an initial small positive peak followed by a prominent negative peak, and then a smaller positive peak that is followed by a second negative peak reflecting neural activity from the cochlear nucleus (Figure 7–22). In terms of the effects of surgical manipulation on this response, auditory nerve stretching (Figure 7–22A) will delay the latency of the negative peak (reflecting reduction in conduction velocity), a neural conduction block affecting some fibers will tend to decrease the amplitude of the large negative peak, and a total neural conduction block (as in a severed nerve) will eliminate the negative peak with the CAP showing "only a positive component (Figure 7–22A and B). The use of a coagulation probe that results in heating the auditory nerve may also produce similar results (Figure 7–22B). Since the intracranial portion of the auditory cranial nerve is easily prone to damage due to pressure, a Teflon insulated wire surrounded by a cotton wick is used as a recording electrode. Since electrodes placed on the exposed nerve can be dislodged due to surgical manipulations or may limit access to the operating field, CAP recordings are made with the same Teflon wick electrode placed on the cochlear nucleus (CN) surface. Both the AN-CAP and the CN-CAP reflect the neural conduction in the nerve and provide the same information. Unlike the recording from the exposed nerve, the amplitude of the CN recording is smaller, and the complex waveform is characterized by an initial rapid biphasic component followed by a broad slow wave (Møller, Jho, & Janetta, 1994). Case examples with a description of the use of

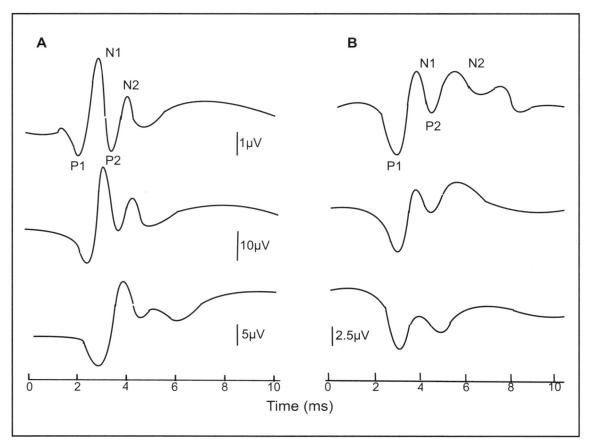

Figure 7–22. Effects of auditory nerve stretching on the auditory nerve compound action potential (AN-CAP) during surgery (waveforms in [**A**]) that may produce a neural conduction block. Stretching of the auditory nerve will progressively delay the response latency, reduce response amplitude of the later peaks (P2 and N2), and result in the eventual loss of the later negative component over time. **B.** Sequential recordings of AN-CAP during microvascular decompression surgery show that heating due to coagulation changes the triphasic response to a response with only the initial positive peak. The absence of the later components is taken to reflect a total conduction block. Created using data from Møller, A. R. (2010). Intraoperative neurophysiological monitoring. Springer Science & Business Media. (3rd ed., pp. 142A–143B).

AN-CAP monitoring with an aim of hearing preservation are shown in Figures 7–23, 7–24, 7–25, and 7-26.

The ABR provides information about the functional integrity of the entire auditory pathway from the auditory nerve to the midbrain. Since several auditory nuclei and tracts are manipulated during surgery, the ABR components may be more susceptible to change and show earlier changes than other metrics like changes in heart rate and blood pressure (Angelo & Møller, 1996). The combination of the two auditory nerve recordings (AN-CAP and CN-CAP) monitors real-time changes in auditory nerve function, and the scalp-recorded ABR monitors real-time changes in both auditory nerve and brainstem functional integrity. This real-time feedback alerts the surgeon to take corrective actions to prevent permanent damage.

7. Neurotologic Applications: Electrocochleography (ECochG) and Intraoperative Monitoring (IOM)   203

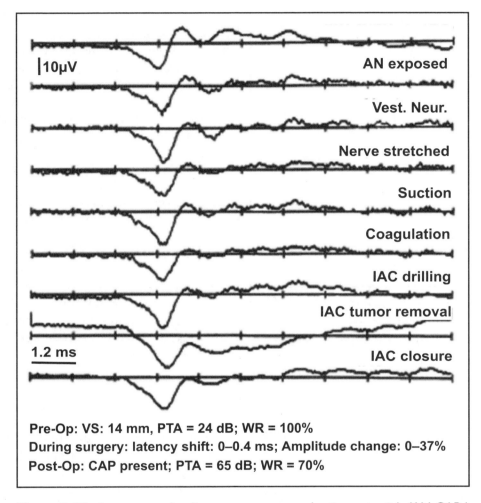

Figure 7–23. A sequence of auditory nerve compound action potentials (AN-CAPs) was recorded during surgery to remove a 14-mm vestibular schwannoma using a retrosigmoidal approach to preserve hearing. The pre-op audiometric results, changes in response latency and amplitude during surgery, and the post-op CAP and audiometric results are summarized at the bottom of the traces. Responses were generally stable during the different phases of surgery (labeled to the right of each trace). Postoperatively, AN-CAP was present with hearing preserved but showing an elevation in threshold and reduction in word recognition ability. Reprinted with permission from "Changes in Directly Recorded Cochlear Nerve Compound Action Potentials During Acoustic Tumor Surgery," by V. Colletti, A. Bricolo, F. G. Fiorino, and L. Bruni, 1994, *Skull Base Surgery, 4,* pp. 1–9.

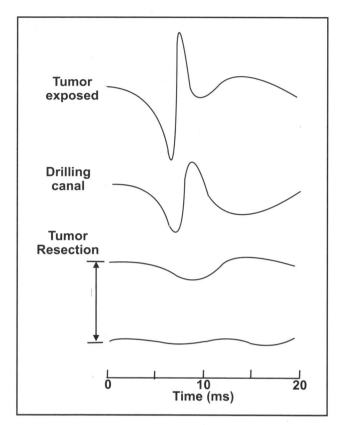

Figure 7–24. A sequence of auditory nerve compound action potentials (AN-CAPs) was recorded closer to the brainstem during surgery to remove a 2.5-cm vestibular schwannoma at the cerebellopontine angle using a retrosigmoidal approach with a goal to preserve hearing. Pre-op audiometric tests revealed high-frequency hearing loss, reduced word recognition ability, and abnormal auditory brainstem responses with prolonged I–III and I–V interpeak latencies. When the tumor was exposed during surgery, a clear AN-CAP was observed. However, as seen, the response suddenly disappeared during resection of the nerve presumably as a result of tearing of the nerve. Post-op testing revealed a profound hearing loss. Created using data from Dr. W. Martin.

IOM Procedures and Interpretation of Changes in Response During Surgery

Preliminary Considerations

There are a few important preliminary considerations prior to performing IOM. Both an audiologic workup, including pure-tone thresholds, word recognition testing, and ABR testing must be completed just before surgery to serve as a baseline. If responses are absent preoperatively, then it is very unlikely these responses will appear during IOM. Also, an otoscopic evaluation should be done to rule out excessive cerumen or other debris in the ear canal that may attenuate the signal reaching the cochlea. Care should be taken to perform a trial run before the event to ensure that all pieces of equipment are functioning properly. There are several stimulus and recording factors to consider in setting up for IOM in a challenging recording environment. The goal is to record clear, robust, interpretable responses as rapidly as possible to provide almost real-time feedback to the surgeon. Thus, stimulus and recording parameters have to be optimized to achieve this goal and sustain it throughout the monitoring session. Overall, the choice of stimuli and acquisition parameters is not very different from the procedure typically used to obtain ABRs in threshold assessment and/or differential diagnosis for site of the lesion. The main difference is that in IOM, the focus is on change in the response amplitude or latency relative to a baseline recording before the start of the surgery or during surgery.

Stimulus

It is not surprising that the stimulus of choice is the click, since it is the ideal stimulus to elicit a robust ABR. One drawback with click ABR acquisition, in particular, is that it takes a relatively long time to average the sweeps required to see a robust and stable response. However, more recently, chirp elicited ABRs have been successfully used in IOM during surgery for vestibular schwannomas, CPA tumors, and meningiomas (Di Scipio & Mastronardi, 2015, 2018; Mastronardi, Di Scipio, Cacciotti, & Roperto, 2018). These authors report that chirp-elicited ABR wave V amplitude is two times larger than that elicited by conventional clicks, reducing the number of sweeps required for a robust average response from 1,024 to 256 sweeps—one-fourth the time needed for the click ABR acquisition allowing for faster feedback (10–15 seconds). Responses are recorded using insert earphones using high-intensity stimuli (80–90 dB nHL) with fixed or alternating onset polarity and a rapid rate repetition rate (29–38/sec) to obtain a robust response in a short time. The specific stimulus level used may depend on pre-operative hearing thresholds. Although not commonly used, a binaural interleaved stimulation strategy will allow a comparison of responses from both ears in individuals with large tumors displacing the brainstem. The transtympanic or intrameatal electrodes should be placed before the insert eartip is positioned to keep the electrode cable from the ear canal and transtympanic electrode in place. Insert earphones are usually placed after the individual has been anesthetized. Care should be taken to place the transducers farther away from the electrodes to minimize stimulus artifact.

Response Recording

Acquisition parameters have to be optimized to improve SNR at each step so that response morphology is good, response detection is easy, and responses are obtained quickly. The first step is to ensure that electrode impedances are low and balanced across electrodes to optimize the common-mode rejection to obtain a favorable SNR. A two-channel recording is used with stainless steel EEG-type needle electrodes placed on the vertex (Cz)/high forehead (noninverting), on each earlobe/mastoid (inverting), and on the mid-forehead (common ground). More commonly, the inverting electrode on the affected (tumor) side is placed anterior to the tragus since the mastoid cannot be accessed. For ECochG recording, the inverting electrode is placed on the promontory (by the surgeon) or at the tympanic membrane by a trained audiologist with the noninverting electrode on the contralateral mastoid. The wire leading to the amplifier and the electrode can be held in place by the eartip. Only the surgeon can place the AN-CAP (usually on the most proximal portion of the nerve) and CN-AP electrodes (recording electrode placed either in the lateral recess of the fourth ventricle or near the vagus nerve as it enters the brainstem [Møller, 2020]) after the exposure of the auditory nerve and CN. Analog filter bandwidth is typically set between 150/200 Hz for the high-pass setting and 1500 Hz for the low-pass setting to minimize extraneous noise—a much narrower bandwidth than typically used in normal clinical settings. The biological amplifier used for response recording in IOM should be optically isolated to prevent electrocution, should have a high common-mode rejection ratio (greater than 100 dB), and have a quick recovery from saturation. Less amplifier gain is needed for the larger-amplitude ECochG and the intracranial recording (between 25,000 and 50,000—much lower gain may be required for the direct recording from the nerve) compared to the relatively higher gain needed for the much smaller scalp-recorded ABR (typically gain factor is 100,000–150,000). Artifact reject should be judiciously used to ensure interpretable responses and short acquisition time. Instead of the typical amplitude-based artifact rejection, software is available to provide near real-time recording using artifact rejection based on spectral analysis (Schmerber, Lavieille, Dumas, & Herve, 2004). Response-averaging parameters are essentially the same as in typical clinical ABR recordings. The intracranial recordings (AN-AP and CN-AP) requires the least number of sweeps (10–20 sweeps), followed by ECochG (100–150 sweeps), and ABR, which requires the greatest number of sweeps (250–1,000 sweeps) and therefore takes the longest time. As mentioned earlier, the use of chirps may substantially speed up ABR data acquisition.

Recently, a new system called the cerebellopontine angle (CPA) Master for IOM of auditory nerve function has been designed for surgery of cerebellopontine angle tumors while attempting to preserve hearing. This system allows continuous, almost real-time monitoring of cochlear nerve function using evoked dorsal cochlear nucleus potentials (DNAPs) by a specially designed DNAP electrode placed directly on the brainstem (Miyazaki & Caye-Thomasen, 2018). Another advantage of this system is the ability to precisely locate and track the entire trajectory of the auditory nerve from the brainstem back to the internal auditory canal. Additionally, the system's ability to evaluate the electrical functional integrity of an intact auditory nerve in translabyrinthine surgery enables the prediction of the benefits of cochlear implantation, should that be considered in the future.

Response Interpretation and Reporting

Unlike clinical testing, the strategy during IOM is to identify and report latency and amplitude changes that exceed baseline values and are deemed greater than the normal variability of the measure as quickly as possible to minimize the risk of permanent damage and postoperative hearing loss. While there are no specific standard values of tolerance for changes in latency and amplitude that should be reported, a 0.5-ms change in latency and a 50% reduction in amplitude are commonly used. Møller (2020) recommends reporting a wave V latency change as small as 0.25 ms, which reflects a change larger than the small random variations observed when the structure is not being surgically manipulated, to reduce the risk of postoperative permanent hearing loss. This emphasizes the importance of reporting even small changes in responses to the surgeon during IOM. Møller's (2020) view is that there is no established minimum latency change to predict risk of permanent postoperative hearing loss. When present, changes in the absolute latencies of waves I, III, and V; IPLs I–III, I–V, and III–V; and the V/I amplitude ratio should be reported. When ABR wave I is not identifiable, then the amplitude enhancement provided by ECochG and AN-CAP could be used to monitor changes. As covered in the section on the effects of upper brainstem lesions on the ABR, surgical manipulations that affect the rostral brainstem will likely produce III–V IPL prolongation and a reduced V/I amplitude ratio. Prolongation of the I–III IPL is also consistent with a surgical manipulation–induced neural conduction delay. Deterioration and/or absence of wave III is also a strong indicator of imminent damage to caudal brainstem structures. Wave V is the only component that is more commonly preserved, and deterioration in the amplitude of wave V has been associated with postoperative hearing loss. AN-CAP, with its generators more likely to bear the brunt of surgical manipulations, is a more sensitive index of surgical manipulation–related changes. For example, stretching of the auditory nerve will cause a conduction delay reflected as latency prolongation; partial blocking of the nerve will reduce the negative components of AN-CAP; and complete blocking of the nerve, resulting from tearing, will change the triphasic morphology of the AN-CAP, showing only a positive component (Møller, 2020). It should be noted here that a decrease in core body temperature (below about 35°C) during surgery could also significantly alter the response morphology, increase IPLs, and reduce amplitude. Once these changes are observed, they should be communicated to the surgeon clearly and promptly. A presurgery meeting of the entire team should rehearse the IOM plan and be very clear about the objectives. There should be a real-time stamp record of all events during the monitoring process.

Hearing Preservation (HP) in IOM

Only about 10% to 15% of individuals with auditory nerve tumors meet the pre-operative criteria for hearing preservation, with higher priority given to facial nerve function preservation and complete tumor removal. Most of the successes in hearing preservation are limited to individuals with relatively small acoustic tumors (less than 1.5 cm). In individuals with small tumors, all three measures (ECochG, AN-CAP, and ABR) are possible. The selection criteria of individuals for hearing preservation are mainly based on preoperative hearing (HP most commonly attempted in class A [pure-tone average ≤30 dB and word recognition ≥70%] and class B [pure-tone average >30 and ≤ 50 dB and word recognition ≥50%] of the AAO-HNS [1995] classification of hearing). A second criterion is tumor size of ≤1.5 cm but not to exceed 2.0 cm. Other factors relevant to attempting hearing preservation include the presence of OAEs, short duration of hearing loss, and the presence of ABR wave III (Ferber-Viart, Laoust, Boulud, Duclaux, & Dubreuil, 2000). Socially useful hearing preservation (class A and B) rates for small auditory nerve tumors range from 61% to 78% (de Freitas, Russo, Sequino, Piccirillo, & Sanna, 2012; Mastronardi et al., 2018; Rueβ et al., 2017; Tamara et al., 2009; Wanibuchi et al., 2014; Watanabe et al., 2016; Yamakami, Ito, & Higuchi, 2014). Most of these studies showed that HP success rate is inversely related to tumor size with large tumors (greater than 2 cm) showing poorer outcomes compared to tumors less than 2 cm (in general, about 50% of individuals with small tumors have better preoperative hearing, and they tend to maintain hearing postsurgery). For example, Mastronardi et al. (2018) found a success rate of 61.5% for tumors smaller than 2 cm and 41.7% for tumors greater than 2 cm in size. Yamakami et al. (2014) observed that better preoperative hearing resulted in a higher rate of postoperative HP. Also, they found that the consistent use of IOM was associated with better HP rates. Finally, long-term (median: 7 years) follow-up of their patients showed only a minimal decline in hearing and no recurrence of the tumor. Compared to ABR, the CN-CAP has been shown to provide more reliable auditory monitoring by reflecting auditory function almost in real time, with better prediction of postoperative hearing, and overall is a more useful metric during the removal of small auditory nerve tumors with good hearing preservation (Yamakami, Yoshinori, Saeki, Wada, & Oka, 2009). Case examples with the description of the use of AN-CAP monitoring with an aim of hearing preservation are shown in Figures 7–22, 7–23, and 7–24. The next set of cases illustrates the use of simultaneous recordings of ECochG, AN-CAP, and ABR to enable assessment of the integrity of cochlear, auditory nerve, and auditory brainstem function (Figures 7–25, 7–26, and 7–27). It is clear from these case illustrations that continuous monitoring of auditory function using these evoked potentials provides an effective tool to minimize damage to auditory structures and improves the ability to preserve postoperative hearing (Youssef & Downes, 2009).

VI. SUMMARY

- Unlike the scalp-recorded ABR, ECochG measures the cochlear receptor potentials (CM and SP) and the AN-CAP that occur in the first few milliseconds post–stimulus onset to evaluate the functional integrity of the OHC subsystem and the auditory nerve.

- Renewed interest in ECochG is fueled by its potential to differentiate OHC from IHC or presynaptic losses, and from ANF or postsynaptic losses, which are all presently grouped together as sensorineural hearing loss. Differential diagnosis of different forms of sensorineural hearing loss could prove useful

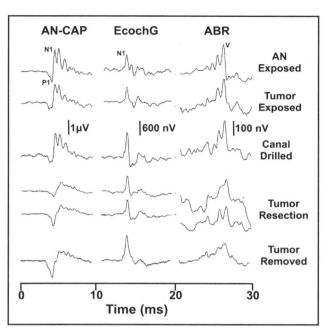

Figure 7–25. A sequence of auditory nerve compound action potential (AN-CAP) (*left*), ECochG action potential (AP) (*middle*), and auditory brainstem responses (ABR) (*right*) recorded simultaneously during surgery from an individual with a 2.0-cm vestibular schwannoma using a retrosigmoidal approach with a goal to preserve hearing. Pre-op pure-tone thresholds, word recognition scores, and ABR were all normal. Responses showed no change when the auditory nerve and tumor were exposed. The start of drilling produced small changes that resulted in a pause in surgical manipulations until the responses recovered. Marked changes were observed when the vestibular nerve was sectioned to remove the tumor. ABR showed marked deterioration later in surgery with partial recovery at the end of surgery. Post-op hearing thresholds and word recognition score remained unchanged. Created using data from Dr. W. Martin.

in improving hearing aid fitting, in predicting cochlear implantation outcomes, and in individualized regenerative medicine.

- CM are sustained OHC receptor AC potentials that reflect the complex sum of contributions from all hair cells excited along the cochlear partition by the stimulus-elicited basilar membrane (BM) displacement pattern. Thus, they can be used to differentiate cochlear from neural pathology. However, there is also the possibility that CM could have at least two components—a more sensitive component

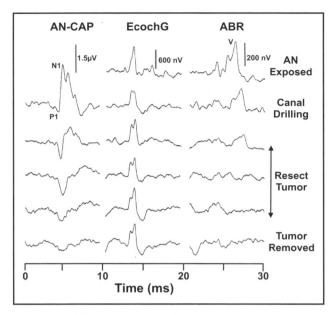

Figure 7–26. A sequence of auditory nerve compound action potential (AN-CAP) (*left*), ECochG action potentials (AP) (*middle*), and auditory brainstem response (ABR) (*right*) recorded simultaneously during surgery from an individual with a 1.5-cm intracanalicular vestibular schwannoma using a retrosigmoidal approach with a goal to preserve hearing. Pre-op pure-tone thresholds showed a mild high-frequency hearing loss, excellent word recognition, and normal ABR. The tumor was found to involve both the auditory and the vestibular portions. Even though a careful approach was followed, the AN-CAP and the ABR deteriorated during resection of the tumor and were unidentifiable. In contrast, the AP from the distal portion (ECochG) remained stable and unchanged. Post-op audiometry revealed a profound hearing loss. Created using data from Dr. W. Martin.

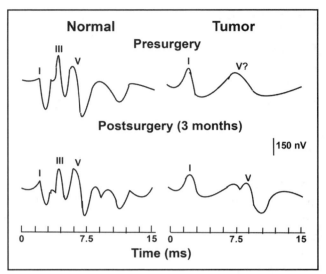

Figure 7–27. Pre-op (*top pair*) and 3 months post-op auditory brainstem responses (ABRs) (*bottom pair*) from the normal ear (*left*) and the affected ear (*right*) in an individual with a 2.5-cm cerebellopontine angle meningioma. Pre-op audiometry revealed a mild-to-profound sensorineural hearing loss with poor word recognition in the affected ear. ABR was abnormal in the ear ipsilateral to the tumor. Transient evoked otoacoustic emission was present and indicated normal cochlear function. ABRs were continuously monitored during surgery. Three-month postoperative rerecording of the ABR showed discernible waves I and V with delayed latencies. Audiogram obtained at this time showed that hearing thresholds had recovered to within normal limits. Created using data from Figure 3b (p. 252) and Figure 6b (p. 254) in Kileny, P. R., Edwards, B. M., Disher, M. J., & Telian, S. A. (1998). Hearing improvement after resection of cerebellopontine angle meningioma: case study of the preoperative role of transient evoked otoacoustic emissions. *Journal of the American Academy of Audiology, 9,* 251–256.

reflecting the activity of the OHCs and a less sensitive component from the IHCs.

- The basal bias of the CM at high-intensities using promontory or round-window electrodes limits its clinical utility. However, since place-specific CM could potentially shed more light on OHC functional integrity, several recent experimental approaches have shown promise in recording place-specific CM. The main clinical application of the CM currently is in the confirmation of auditory neuropathy.

- The SP is a negative DC shift receptor potential that is associated temporally with the neural CAP and presumably reflects asymmetric depolarization-hyperpolarization of the cochlear response associated with the OHCs. However, unlike the neural action potential, the SP is not adapted by rapid rate of stimulation.

- The SP has been shown to be enhanced relative to the auditory nerve compound potential in endolymphatic hydrops resulting in an increased SP/AP ratio. The sustained SP to tone bursts is more reliable for the diagnosis of Ménière's disease.

- In order to encourage more clinical audiologists to use ECochG, efforts should be made to improve the more practical noninvasive techniques, for example, intrameatal tympanic membrane electrodes. There is some evidence that both transtympanic and tympanic membrane electrodes produce similar response patterns and the same rates of diagnosis confirmation of Ménière's disease.

- The CAP recorded using transtympanic or extratympanic electrodes reflects neural activity from a population of neural fibers, in the distal portion of the auditory nerve, synchronized to the stimulus onset. Like the ABRs, place-specific CAPs can be recorded using frequency-specific tone bursts. Transtympanic electrodes show the largest CAP amplitude followed by tympanic membrane electrode, with the tiptrode CAP being the smallest.

- CAP thresholds are within 5 dB of behavioral thresholds. The use of the novel ANOW response holds the potential for low-frequency place-specific responses. A robust normal latency CAP response at high intensity, absent CM, and an abnormally steep CAP amplitude growth function are consistent with a cochlear lesion and loudness recruitment. Delayed CAP latency, broad waveforms, reduced amplitude, and presence of the receptor potentials are consistent with either an IHC-auditory nerve synapse dysfunction or an auditory nerve lesion.

- The electrically evoked compound action potential (eCAP) represents synchronous firing in a population of auditory nerve fibers in response to intracochlear electrically stimulated auditory nerve fibers in CI users. Since it provides a neural metric of the number of active neural elements and their responsiveness, and representation of spectral and temporal cues important for speech perception, there is growing interest in utilizing eCAP to assess different aspects of auditory nerve responsiveness and their relevance to CI outcomes in adults and children. Considerable research efforts are being made to understand how these measures influence speech perception, but additional research is required before these measures can be used in the clinic reliably. Nevertheless, these experimental advances are necessary stepping-stones to realize the clinical applications outlined earlier.

- The electrically evoked ABR (eABR) provides a robust measure of the functional integrity of the auditory nerve and brainstem neural elements and can be used as both a pre-implant verification of the neural density and post-implant monitoring of changes in auditory function to monitor for cochlear implant outcomes.

- IOM is the continuous monitoring of the integrity of neural function during intracranial surgery in order to reduce the potential risk of permanent damage that may compromise function. One of the primary goals of intraoperative monitoring is to preserve hearing.

- Auditory electrophysiological measures that provide continuous monitoring of the functional status of the auditory nerve and brainstem during surgical removal of VIIIth nerve tumors include the ABR to monitor the functional integrity of the brainstem structures and tracts, transtympanic electrocochleography (ECochG) to record both the cochlear receptor potentials and the auditory nerve CAP, and direct recording from the exposed auditory nerve and/or from the surface of the cochlear nucleus to monitor neural conduction in the auditory nerve (AN-CAP and CN-CAP).

- Auditory nerve stretching will delay the latency of the negative peak (reflecting reduction in conduction velocity); neural conduction block affecting some fibers will tend to decrease the amplitude of the large negative peak, and a total neural conduction block (as in a severed nerve) will eliminate the negative peak with the CAP showing only a positive component.

- The combined use of CAP (AN-CAP, CN-CAP) and ABR provides monitoring of real-time changes in auditory nerve function, and the relatively time-delayed assessment of brainstem functional integrity, respectively. Unlike clinical testing, the strategy here is to identify and report latency and amplitude changes that exceed baseline values and are deemed greater than the normal variability of the measure as quickly as possible to the surgeon to minimize the risk of permanent damage and postoperative hearing loss. While there are no specific standard values of tolerance for change in latency and amplitude that should be reported, a 0.25-ms change in latency and a 50% reduction in amplitude are commonly used.

- The hearing preservation success rate is better in small tumors compared to larger tumors, in individuals with better preoperative hearing, and when a consistently reliable IOM method is used. Long-term follow-up of patients with post-operative hearing preservation showed little decline in hearing and no recurrence of the tumor. Thus, continuous monitoring of auditory function using these evoked potentials provides an effective tool to minimize damage to auditory structures and improves the ability to preserve postoperative hearing.

REFERENCES

Abbas, P., & Brown, C. (1988). Electrically evoked brainstem potentials in cochlear implant patients with multi-electrode stimulation. *Hearing Research, 36*, 153–162.

Abbas, P., & Brown, C. (1991). Electrically evoked auditory brainstem response: Growth of response with current level. *Hearing Research, 51*, 123–137.

Abbas, P. J., Brown, C. J., Shallop, J. K., Firszt, J. B., Hughes, M. L., Hong, S. H., & Staller, S. J. (1999). Summary of results using the nucleus CI24M implant to record the electrically evoked compound action potential. *Ear and Hearing, 20*, 45–59.

Abdelsalam, N. M. S., & Afifi, P. O. (2015). Electric auditory brainstem response (E-ABR) in cochlear implant children: Effect of age at implantation and duration of implant use. *Egyptian Journal of Ear, Nose, Throat and Allied Sciences, 16*, 145–150.

American Academy of Otolaryngology-Head and Neck Surgery Foundation I. (1995). Committee on hearing and equilibrium guidelines for the evaluation of hearing preservation in acoustic neuroma (vestibular schwannoma). *Otolaryngology-Head and Neck Surgery, 113*(3), 179–180.

Angelo, R., & Møller, A. R. (1996). Contralateral evoked brainstem auditory potentials as an indicator of intraoperative brainstem manipulation in cerebellopontine angle tumors. *Neurological Research, 18*, 528–540.

Arslan, E., Turrini, M., Lupi, G., Genovese, E., & Orzan, E. (1997). Hearing threshold assessment with auditory brainstem response (ABR) and electrocochleography (ECochG) in uncooperative children. *Scandinavian Audiology Supplement, 46*, 32–37.

Aso, S., Watanabe, Y., & Mizukoshi, K. (1991). A clinical study of electrocochleography in Meniere's disease. *Acta oto-laryngologica, 111*(1), 44-52.

Baudhuin, J. L., Hughes, M. L., & Goehring, J. L. (2016). A comparison of alternating polarity and forward masking artifact-reduction methods to resolve the electrically evoked compound action potentials. *Ear and Hearing, 4*, 247–255.

Bourien, J., Tang, Y., Batrel, C., Huet, A., Lenoir, M., Ladrech, S., . . . Wang, J. (2014). Contribution of auditory nerve fibers to compound action potential of the auditory nerve. *Journal of Neurophysiology, 112*, 1025–1039.

Brown, C., Abbas, P., Fryauf-Bertschy, H., Kelsay, D., & Gantz, B. (1994). Intraoperative and postoperative electrically evoked auditory brain stem responses in nucleus cochlear implant users: Implications for the fitting process. *Ear and Hearing, 15*, 168–176.

Brown, C. J., Abbas, P. J., & Gantz, B. (1990). Electrically evoked whole nerve action potentials: Data from human cochlear implant users. *Journal of the Acoustical Society of America, 88*, 1385–1391.

Camilleri, A. E., & Howarth, K. L. (2001). Prognostic value of electrocochleography in patients with unilateral Meniere's disease undergoing saccus surgery. *Clinical Otolaryngology & Allied Sciences, 26*(3), 257–260.

Causon, A., O'Driscoll, M., Stapleton, E., Lloyd, S., Freeman, S., & Munro, K. J. (2018). Extracochlear stimulation of electrically evoked auditory brainstem responses (eABRs) remains the preferred pre-implant auditory nerve function test in an assessor-blinded comparison. *Otology and Neurotology, 40*, 47–55.

Charaziak, K. K., Shera, C. A., & Siegel, J. H. (2017). Using cochlear microphonic potentials to localize peripheral hearing loss. *Frontiers in Neuroscience, 11*(169), 1–13.

Chertoff, M. E., Earl, B. R., Diaz, F. J., & Sorensen, J. L. (2012). Analysis of the cochlear microphonic to a low-frequency tone embedded in filtered noise. *Journal of the Acoustical Society of America, 132*, 3351–3362.

Chertoff, M. E., Earl, B. R., Diaz, F. J., Sorensen, J. L., Thomas, M. L. A., Kamerer, A. M., & Peppi, M. (2014). Predicting the location of missing outer hair cells using the electrical signal recorded at the round window. *Journal of the Acoustical Society of America, 136*(3), 1212–1224.

Chouard, C., Koca, E., Meyer, B., & Jacquier, I. (1994). Test of electrical stimulation of the round window. Diagnostic and prognostic value of the rehabilitation of total deafness by cochlear implant. *Annals d'oto-laryngologie Chir cervico faciale, 111*, 75–84.

Chung, W. H., Cho, D. Y., Choi, J. Y., & Hong, S. H. (2004). Clinical usefulness of extratympanic electrocochleography in the diagnosis of Meniere's disease. *Otology & Neurotology, 25*(2), 144–149.

Claes, G. M. E., De Valck, C. F., Van de Heyning, P., & Wuyts, F. L. (2011). The Ménière's disease index: An objective correlate of Ménière's disease, based on audiometric and electrocochleographic data. *Otology and Neurotology, 32*, 887–892.

Coats, A. C. (1981). The summating potential and Ménière's disease. I. Summating potential amplitude in Ménière's ears and non-Ménière's ears. *Archives of Otolaryngology, 107*, 199–208.

Coats, A. C., & Alford, B. R. (1981). Ménière's disease and the summating potential. III. Effect of glycerol administration. *Archives of Otolaryngology, 107*, 469–473.

Colletti, V., Bricolo, A., Fiorino, F. G., &Bruni, L. (1994). Changes in directly recorded cochlear nerve compound action potentials during acoustic tumor surgery. *Skull Base Surgery, 4*, 1–9.

Colletti, V., & Fiorino, F. G. (1998). Advances in monitoring of seventh and eighth cranial nerve function during posterior fossa surgery. *American Journal of Otology, 19*, 503–512.

Conlon, B. J., & Gibson, W. P. R. (2000). Electrocochleography in the diagnosis of Ménière's disease. *Acta Otolaryngology, 120*, 480–483.

Dallos, P. (1973). *The auditory periphery: Biophysics and physiology*. New York, NY: Academic Press.

Dallos, P., & Cheatham, M. A. (1976). Production of cochlear potentials by inner and outer hair cells. *Journal of the Acoustical Society of America, 60*, 510–512.

Dallos, P., Schoeny, Z. G., & Cheatham, M. A. (1972). Cochlear summating potentials: Descriptive aspects. *Acta Oto-laryngologica, Supplementum, 302*, 1–46.

Dallos, P., & Wang, C. Y. (1974). Bioelectric correlates of kanamycin intoxication. *Audiology, 13*, 277–289.

Dauman, R., & Aran, J. M. (1991). Electrocochleography and the diagnosis of endolymphatic hydrops: Clicks and tone bursts. In I. Kaufman Arenberg (Ed.), *Inner ear surgery* (pp. 123–133). Amsterdam/ New York, NY: Kugler.

Dauman, R., Aran, J. M., Charlet de Sauvage, R., & Portmann, M. (1988). Clinical significance of the summating potential in Ménière's disease. *American Journal of Otology, 9*, 31–38.

Dauman, R., Aran, J. M., & Portmann, M. (1986). Summating potential and water balance in Ménière's disease. *Annals of Otology, Rhinology, and Laryngology, 95*, 389–395.

de Freitas, M. R., Russo, A., Sequino, G., Piccirillo, E., & Sanna, M. (2012). Analysis of hearing preservation and facial nerve function for patients undergoing vestibular schwannoma surgery: The middle cranial fossa approach versus the retrosigmoid approach. Personal experience and literature review. *Audiology and Neuro-otology, 17*(2), 71–81.

Delgutte, B., & Kiang, N. Y. S. (1984). Speech coding in the auditory nerve: IV. Sounds with consonant-like dynamic characteristics. *Journal of the Acoustical Society of America, 75*, 897–907.

De Valck, C. F. J., Claes, G. M. E., Wuyts, F. L., & Van de Heyning, P. H. (2007). Lack of diagnostic value of high-pass noise masking of auditory brainstem responses in Ménière's disease. *Otology and Neurotology, 28*(5), 700–707.

DeVries, L., Scheperle, R., & Bierer, J. A. (2016). Assessing the electrode-neuron interface with the electrically evoked compound action potential, electrode position, and behavioral thresholds. *Journal of the Association for Research in Otolaryngology, 17*, 237–252.

Di Scipio, E., & Mastronardi, L. (2015). CE-Chirp ABR in cerebellopontine angle surgery neuromonitoring: Technical assessment in four cases. *Neurosurgery Reviews, 38*(2), 381–384.

Di Scipio, E., & Mastronardi, L. (2018). Level specific CE-Chirp BAEPs: A new faster technique in neuromonitoring cochlear nerve during cerebellopontine angle tumor surgery. *Interdisciplinary Neurosurgery, 11*, 4–7.

Don, M., Kwong, B., & Tanaka, C. (2005). A diagnostic test for Ménière's disease and cochlear hydrops: Impaired high-pass noise masking of auditory brainstem responses. *Otology and Neurotology, 26*(4), 711–722.

Don, M., Kwong, B., & Tanaka, C. (2007). An alternative diagnostic test for active Ménière's disease and cochlear hydrops using high-pass noise masked responses: The complex amplitude ratio. *Audiology and Neuro-otology, 12*(6), 359–370.

Donaldson, G. S., & Ruth, R. A. (1996). Derived-band auditory brain-stem response estimates of traveling wave velocity in humans: II. Subjects with noise-induced hearing loss and Ménière's disease. *Journal of Speech and Hearing Research, 39*(3), 534–545.

Eggermont, J. J. (1976a). Analysis of compound action potential responses to tone bursts in the human and guinea pig cochlea. *Journal of the Acoustical Society of America, 60,* 1132–1139.

Eggermont, J. J. (1976b). Electrocochleography. In W. D. Keidel & W. D. Neff (Eds.), *Handbook of sensory physiology* (Vol. 5, Part 3, pp. 626–705). New York, NY: Springer-Verlag.

Eggermont, J. J. (1976c). Summating potentials in electrocochleography. Relation to hearing pathology. In R. J. Ruben, C. Elberling, & G. Salomon (Eds.), *Electrocochleography* (pp. 67–87). Baltimore, MD: University Park Press.

Eggermont, J. J. (1977). Electrocochleography and recruitment. *Annals of Otology, Rhinology, and Laryngology, 86*(2), 138–149.

Eggermont, J. J. (1979a). Compound action potentials: Tuning curves and delay times. *Scandinavian Audiology, Supplementum,* (9), 129–139.

Eggermont, J. J. (1979b). Narrow-band AP latencies in normal and recruiting human ears. *Journal of the Acoustical Society of America, 65,* 463–470.

Eggermont, J. J. (1979c). Summating potentials in Ménière's disease. *Archives of Otorhinolaryngology, 222,* 63–74.

Eggermont, J. J., & Odenthal, D. W. (1974). Electrophysiological investigation of the human cochlea: Recruitment, masking and adaptation. *Audiology, 13,* 1–22.

Eggermont, J. J., Spoor, A., & Odenthal, D. W. (1976). Frequency specificity of tone burst electrocochleography. In R. J. Ruben, C. Elberling, & G. Salomon (Eds.), *Electrocochleography* (pp. 215–246). Baltimore, MD: University Park Press.

Elberling, C. (1973). Transitions in cochlear action potentials recorded from the ear canal in man. *Scandinavian Audiology, 2,* 151–159.

Elberling, C., & Hoke, M. (1978). Decoding of human compound action potentials. *Scandinavian Audiology, 7,* 171–175.

Ferber-Viart, C., Laoust, L., Boulud, B., Duclaux, R., & Dubreuil, C. (2000). Acuteness of preoperative factors to predict hearing preservation in acoustic neuroma surgery. *Laryngoscope, 110,* 145–150.

Ferraro, J. A., Thedinger, B. S., Mediavilla, S. J., & Blackwell, W. L. (1994). Human summating potential to tone bursts: Observations on tympanic membrane versus promontory recordings in the same patients. *Journal of the American Academy of Audiology, 5,* 24–29.

Ferraro, J. A., & Tibbils, P. (1999). SP/AP area ratio in the diagnosis of Ménière's disease. *American Journal of Audiology, 8,* 21–27.

Firszt, J. B., Chambers, R. D., Kraus, N., & Reeder, R. M. (2002). Neurophysiology of cochlear implant users I: Effects of stimulus current level and electrode site on the electrical ABR, MLR, and N1-P2 response. *Ear and Hearing, 23*(6), 502–515.

Filipo, R., Cordier, A., Barbara, M., & Bertoli, G. A. (1997). Electrocochleographic findings: Meniere's disease versus sudden sensorineural hearing loss. *Acta Oto-Laryngologica, 117*(sup526), 21-23.

Forgues, M., Koehn, H. A., Dunnon, A. K., Pulver, S. H., Buchman, C. A., Adunka, O. F., & Fitzpatrick, D. C. (2014). Distinguishing hair cell from neural potentials recorded at the round window. *Journal of Neurophysiology, 111,* 580–593.

Friesen, L. M., Shannon, R. V., Baskent, D., & Wang, X. (2001). Speech recognition in noise as a function of the number of spectral channels: Comparison of acoustic hearing and cochlear implants. *Journal of the Acoustical Society of America, 110,* 1150–1163.

Gibbin, K. P., Mason, S. M., & Kent, S. E. (1983). Prolongation of the cochlear microphonic in man. Cochlear microphonic ringing. *Acta Otolaryngology, 95,* 13–18.

Gibson, W. P. R. (1978). Electrocochleography (EcochG). In W. P. R. Gibson (Ed.), *Essentials of clinical electric response audiometry* (pp. 59–106). London, UK: Churchill Livingstone.

Gibson, W. P. R. (2005). The role of transtympanic electrocochleography in the diagnosis of Ménière's disease: A comparison of click and 1 kHz tone burst stimuli. In D. J. Lim (Ed.), *Ménière's disease and Inner Ear Homeostasis Disorders* (pp 140-142). Los Angeles, CA: House Ear Institute.

Gibson, W. P. R. (2009). A comparison of two methods of using transtympanic electrocochleography for the diagnosis of Ménière's disease: Click summating potential/action potential ratio measurements compared with tone burst summating potential measurements. *Acta Otolaryngology, 129,* 38–42.

Gibson, W. P., Moffat, D. A., & Ramsden, R. T. (1977). Clinical electrocochleography in the diagnosis and management of Ménière's disorder. *Audiology, 16,* 389–401.

Gibson, W. P., & Morrison, A. W. (1983). Electrocochleography and the glycerol dehydration test: A case study. *British Journal of Audiology, 17,* 95–99.

Gibson, W. P. R., Prasher, D. K., & Kilkenny, G. P. G. (1983). Diagnostic significance of transtympanic electrocochleography in Ménière's disease. *Annals of Otology, Rhinology, and Laryngology, 92,* 155–159.

Gibson, W. P. R., & Sanli, H. (2007). Auditory neuropathy: An update. *Ear and Hearing, 28,* 102S–106S.

Gordon, K. A., Papsin, B. C., & Harrison, R. V. (2004). Toward a battery of behavioral and objective measures to achieve optimal cochlear implant stimulation levels in children. *Ear and Hearing, 25*, 447–463.

Gordon, K. A., Papsin, B. C., & Harrison, R. V. (2007). Auditory brainstem activity and development evoked by apical versus basal cochlear implant electrode stimulation in children. *Clinical Neurophysiology, 118*, 1671–1684.

Harrison, R. V., & Prijs, V. F. (1984). Single cochlear fibre responses in guinea pigs with long-term endolymphatic hydrops. *Hearing Research, 14*, 79–84.

He, S., Abbas, P. J., Doyle, D. V., McFayden, T. C., & Mulherin, S. (2016). Temporal response properties of the auditory nerve in children with auditory neuropathy spectrum disorder and implanted children with sensorineural hearing loss. *Ear and Hearing, 37*, 397–411.

He, S., Teagle, H. F., & Buchman, C. A. (2017). The electrically evoked compound action potential: From laboratory to clinic. *Frontiers in Neuroscience, 11*, 339. https://doi.org/10.3389/fnins.2017.00339.

Henry, K. R. (1995). Auditory nerve neurophonic recorded from the round window of the Mongolian gerbil. *Hearing Research, 90*, 176–184.

Hornibrook, J. (2017). Tone burst electrocochleography for the diagnosis of clinically certain Ménière's disease. *Frontiers of Neuroscience, 16*(11), 301.

Hornibrook, J., Bird, P., Flook, E., & O'Beirne, G. A. (2016). Electrocochleography for the diagnosis of Ménière's disease: The wrong stimulus. *Otology and Neurotology, 37*, 1677–1678.

Hornibrook, J., George, P., & Gourley, J. (2010). Vasopressin in definite Ménière's disease with positive electrocochleographic findings. *Acta Otolaryngology, 13*, 613–617.

Hornibrook, J., George, P., Spellerberg, M., & Gourley, J. (2011). HSP70 antibodies in 80 patients with "clinically certain" Ménière's disease. *Annals of Otology, Rhinology, and Laryngology, 120*, 651–655.

Hornibrook, J., Gourley, G., & Vraich, G. (2020). Tone burst electrocochleography disproves a diagnosis of Ménière's disease treated aggressively. *HNO, 68*, 352–358. https://doi.org/10.1007/s00106-019-0722-7

Hughes, M. (2013). Part III physiological objective measures. In T. Zwolan, & J. Wolfe (Eds.), *Objective measures in cochlear implants* (pp. 93–149). San Diego, CA: Plural Publishing.

Hughes, M. L., Castioni, E. E., Goehring, J. L., & Baudhuin, J. L. (2012). Temporal response properties of the auditory nerve: Data from human cochlear-implant recipients. *Hearing Research, 285*, 46–57.

Ikino, C. M. Y., & de Almeida, E. R. (2006). Summating potential-action potential waveform amplitude and width in the diagnosis of Ménière's disease. *The Laryngoscope, 116*(10), 1766-1769.

Iseli, C., & Gibson, W. P. R. (2010). A comparison of three methods of using transtympanic electrocochleography for the diagnosis of Ménière's disease: Click summating potential measurements, tone burst summating potential measurements amplitude measures, and biasing of the summating potential with a low tone. *Acta Otolaryngology, 130*, 95–101.

Johnstone, J. R., & Johnstone, B. M. (1966). Origin of the summating potential. *Journal of the Acoustical Society of America, 40*, 1405–1413.

Kamerer, A. M., Diaz, F. J., Peppi, M., & Chertoff, M. E. (2016). The potential use of low-frequency tones to locate regions of outer hair cell loss. *Hearing Research, 342*, 39–47.

Karlan, M. S., Tonndorf, J., & Khanna, S. M. (1972). Dual origins of the cochlear microphonics—Inner and outer hair cells. *Annals of Otolaryngology, 81*, 696–704.

Kileny, P. R., Edwards, B. M., Disher, M. J., & Telian, S. A. (1998). Hearing improvement after resection of cerebellopontine angle meningioma: Case study of the preoperative role of transient evoked otoacoustic emissions. *Journal of the American Academy of Audiology, 9*, 251–256.

Kileny, P., & Zwolan, T. (2004). Perioperative, transtympanic electric ABR in pediatric cochlear implant candidates. *Cochlear Implants International, 5*(Suppl. 1), 23–25.

Kim, J. R., Abbas, P. J., Brown, C. J., Etler, C. P., O'Brien, S., & Kim, L. S. (2010). The relationship between electrically evoked compound action potential and speech perception: A study in cochlear implant users with short electrode array. *Otology and Neurotology, 31*, 1041–1048.

Kingma, C. M., & Wit, H. P. (2010). Cochlear hydrops analysis masking procedure results in patients with unilateral Ménière's disease. *Otology and Neurotology, 31*(6), 1004–1008.

Kujawa, S. G., & Liberman, M. C. (2009). Adding insult to injury: Cochlear nerve degeneration after "temporary" noise-induced hearing loss. *Journal of Neuroscience, 29*(45), 14077–14085.

Kujawa, S. G., & Liberman, M. C. (2015). Synaptopathy in the noise-exposed and aging cochlea: Primary neural degeneration in acquired sensorineural hearing loss. *Hearing Research, 330*(Part B), 191–199. https://doi.org/10.1016/j.heares.2015.02.009

Lee, J. B., Choi, S. J., Park, K., Park, H. Y., Hong, J. J., Hwang, E., . . . Choung, Y.-H. (2011). Diagnostic efficiency of the cochlear hydrops analysis masking procedure in Ménière's disease. *Otology and Neurotology, 32,* 1486–1491.

Lee, E. R., Friedland, D. R., & Runge, C. L. (2012). Recovery from forward masking in elderly cochlear implant users. *Otology and Neurotology, 33,* 355–363.

Liberman, M. C., & Dodds, C. W. (1984). Single neuron labeling and chronic pathology: III. Stereocilia damage and alteration of threshold tuning curves. *Hearing Research, 16,* 55–74.

Lichtenhan, J. T., Cooper, N. P., & Guinan, J. J., Jr. (2013). Auditory threshold estimation technique for low frequencies: Proof of concept. *Ear and Hearing, 34,* 42–51.

Lichtenhan, J. T., Hartsock., J. J., Gill, R. M., & Guinan, J. J., Jr. (2014). The auditory nerve overlapped waveform (ANOW) originates in the cochlear apex. *Association for Research in Otolaryngology, 15,* 395–411.

Liu, C., Chen, X., & Xu, L. (1992). Cochlear microphonics and recruitment. *Acta Otolaryngology, 112,* 215–220.

Lo, T., Chen, Y., Horng, M., & Hsu, C. (2004). Efficacy of EABR and ECAP in programming children with Nucleus-24 cochlear implants. *Cochlear Implants International, 5*(Suppl. 1), 47–49.

Marcio, C., Ikino, Y., & de Almeida, R. (2006). Summating potential-action potential waveform amplitude and width in the diagnosis of Ménière's disease. *Laryngoscope, 116,* 1766–1769.

Mason, S., O'Donoghue, G., Gibbin, K., Garnham, C., & Jowett, C. (1997). Perioperative electrical auditory brain stem response in candidates for pediatric cochlear implantation. *American Journal of Otology, 18,* 466–471.

Mastronardi, L., Di Scipio, E., Cacciotti, G., & Roperto, R. (2018). Vestibular schwannoma and hearing preservation: Usefulness of level specific CE-Chirp ABR monitoring. A retrospective study on 25 cases with preoperative socially useful hearing. *Clinical Neurology and Neurosurgery, 165,* 108–115.

McKay, C. M., Chandan, K., Akhoun, I., Siciliano, C., & Kluk, K. (2013). Can ECAP measures be used for totally objective programming of cochlear implants? *Journal of the Association for Research in Otolaryngology, 14,* 879–890.

McLean, W. J., McLean, D. T., Eatock, R. A., & Edge, A. S. (2016). Distinct capacity for differentiation to inner ear cell types by progenitor cells of the cochlea and vestibular organs. *Development, 143,* 4381–4393.

Meyer, B., Drira, M., Gegu, D., & Chouard, C. (1984). Results of the round window electrical stimulation in 460 cases of total deafness. *Acta Otolaryngology, Supplement, 411,* 168–176.

Miyazaki, H., & Caye-Thomasen, P. (2018). Intraoperative auditory system monitoring. *Advances in Oto-rhino-laryngology, 81,* 123–132.

Moffat, D. A., Gibson, W. P. R., Ramsden, A. W., & Booth, J. B. (1978). Transtympanic electrocochleography using glycerol dehydration. *Acta Otolaryngology, 85,* 158–166.

Møller, A. R. (2010). *Intraoperative neurophysiological monitoring* (3rd ed., pp 142–143). Springer Science & Business Media.

Møller, A. R. (2020). Neurophysiology of the auditory system: Basics and IOM techniques. In V. Deletis, J. Shils, F. Sala, & K. Seidel (Eds.), *Neurophysiology in neurosurgery: A modern approach* (2nd ed., pp. 65–85). Amsterdam, the Netherlands: Elsevier.

Møller, A. R., & Jannetta, P. J. (1981). Compound action potentials recorded intracranially from the auditory nerve in man. *Experimental Neurology, 74,* 862–874.

Møller, A. R., & Jannetta, P. J. (1983a). Monitoring auditory functions during cranial nerve microvascular decompression operations by direct recording from the eighth nerve. *Journal of Neurosurgery, 59,* 493–499.

Møller, A. R., & Jannetta, P. J. (1983b). Auditory evoked potentials recorded from the cochlear nucleus and its vicinity in man. *Journal of Neurosurgery, 59,* 1013–1018.

Møller, A. R., Jho, H. D., & Jannetta, P. J. (1994). Preservation of hearing in operations on acoustic tumors: An alternative to recording ABR. *Neurosurgery, 34,* 688–693.

Møller, A. R., & Møller, M. B. (1989). Does intraoperative monitoring of auditory evoked potentials reduce incidence of hearing loss as a complication of microvascular decompression of cranial nerves? *Neurosurgery, 24,* 257–263.

Mori, N., Asai, H., Doi, K., & Matsunaga, T. (1987). Diagnostic value of extratympanic electrocochleography in Ménière's disease: Intérêt diagnostique de l'électrocochléographie extratympanique dans la maladie de Menière. *Audiology, 26*(2), 103–110.

Mori, N., Sacki, K., Matsunaga, T., & Asai, H. (1982). Comparison between AP and SP parameters in transtympanic and extratympanic electrocochleography. *Audiology, 21,* 228–241.

Morrison, A. W., Gibson, W. P., & Beagley, H. A. (1976). Transtympanic electrocochleography in the diagnosis of retrocochlear tumors. *Clinical Otolaryngology and Allied Sciences, 1,* 153–167.

Murad, O., Al-momani, Ferraro, J. A., Gajewski, B. J., & Ator, G. (2009). Improved sensitivity of electrocochleography in the diagnosis of Ménière's disease. *International Journal of Audiology, 48*(11), 811–819.

Nelson, D. A., & Donaldson, G. S. (2002). Psychophysical recovery from pulse-train forward masking in electrical hearing. *Journal of the Acoustical Society of America, 112,* 2932–2947.

Nguyen, L. T., Harris, J. P., & Nguyen, Q. T. (2010). Clinical utility of electrocochleography in the diagnosis and management of Ménière's disease. AOS and ANS membership survey data. *Otology and Neurotology, 31*(3), 455–459.

Noble, J. H., Labadie, R. F., Gifford, R. H., & Dawant, B. M. (2013). Image-guidance enables new methods for customizing cochlear implant stimulation strategies. *IEEE Transactions in Neural Systems Rehabilitation Engineering, 21,* 820–829.

Noguchi, Y., Komatsuzaki, A., & Nishida, H. (1999). Cochlear microphonics for hearing preservation in vestibular schwannoma surgery. *Laryngoscope, 109,* 1982–1987.

Ordóñez-Ordóñez, L. E., Rojas-Roncancio, E., Hernández-Alarcón, V., Jaramillo-Safón, R., Prieto-Rivera, J., Guzmán-Durán, J., . . . Angulo-Martínez, E. S. (2009). Diagnostic test validation: Cochlear hydrops analysis masking procedure in Ménière's disease. *Otology and Neurotology, 30*(6), 820–825.

Ozdamar, O., & Dallos, P. (1978). Synchronous responses of the primary auditory fibers to the onset of tone bursts and their relation to the compound action potentials. *Brain Research, 155,* 169–175.

Pappa, A. K., Hutson, K. A., Scott, W. C., Wilson, J. D., Fox, K. E., Masood, M. M., . . . Fitzpatrick, D. C. (2019). Hair cell and neural contributions to the cochlear summating potential. *Journal of Neurophysiology, 121*(6), 2163–2180.

Patuzzi, R. B., Yates, G. K., & Johnstone, B. M. (1989a). Changes in cochlear microphonic and neural sensitivity produced by acoustic trauma. *Hearing Research, 39,* 189–202.

Patuzzi, R. B., Yates, G. K., & Johnstone, B. M. (1989b). The origin of the low frequency microphonic in the first cochlear turn of guinea-pig. *Hearing Research, 39,* 177–188.

Pau, H., Gibson, W., & Sanli, H. (2006). Trans-tympanic electric auditory brainstem response (TT-EABR): The importance of the positioning of the stimulating electrode. *Cochlear Implants International, 7,* 183–187.

Pfingst, B. E., Colesa, D. J., Swiderski, D. L., Hughes, A. P., Strahl, S. B., Sinan, M., & Raphael, Y. (2017). Neurotrophin gene therapy in deafened ears with cochlear implants: long-term effects on nerve survival and functional measures. *Journal of the Association for Research in Otolaryngology, 18*(6), 731-750.

Pfingst, B. E., Zhou, N., Colesa, D. J., Watts, M. M., Strahl, S. B., Garadat, S. N., . . . Zwolan, T. A. (2015). Importance of cochlear health for implant function. *Hearing Research, 322,* 77–88.

Pierson, M., & Møller, A. (1980). Some dualistic properties of the cochlear microphonic. *Hearing Research, 2,* 135–150.

Ponton, C. W., Don, M., & Eggermont, J. J. (1992). Place-specific derived cochlear microphonics from human ears. *Scandinavian Audiology, 21,* 131–141.

Pou, A. M., Hirsch, B. E., Durrant, J. D., Gold, S. R, & Kamerer, D. B. (1996) Efficacy of tympanic electrocochleography in the diagnosis of endolymphatic hydrops. *American Journal of Otology, 17,* 607–611.

Radeloff, A., Shehata-Dieler, W., & Scherzed, A. (2012). Intraoperative monitoring using cochlear microphonics in cochlear implant patients with residual hearing. *Otology and Neurotology, 33,* 348–354.

Roland, P. S., Yellin, M. W., Meyerhoff, W. L., & Frank, T. (1995). Simultaneous comparison between transtympanic and extratympanic electrocochleography. *American Journal of Otology, 16,* 444–450.

Rueß, D., Pöhlmann, L., Grau., S., Hamisch, C., Hellerbach, A., Treuer, H., . . . Ruge, M. I. (2017). Long-term follow-up after stereotactic radiosurgery of intracanalicular acoustic neurinoma. *Radiation Oncology, 12*(1), 68–76.

Russell, I. J. (2008). Cochlear receptor potentials. In P. Dallos (Ed.), *The senses: A comprehensive reference* (Chapter 3.20, pp. 320–358). Amsterdam, the Netherlands: Elsevier.

Santarelli, R., Scimemi, P., Dal Monte, E., & Arslan, E. (2006). Cochlear microphonic potential recorded by transtympanic electrocochleography in normally-hearing and hearing-impaired ears. *Acta Otorhinolaryngology Italy, 26,* 78–95.

Sass K. 1998. Sensitivity and specifi city of transtympanic electrocochleogra-phy in Meniere's disease. *Acta Otolaringologica, 118*(2), 150–156.

Sauvaget, E., Péréon, Y., Nguyen The Tich, S., & Bordure, P. (2002). Electrically evoked auditory potentials: Comparison between transtympanic promontory and round-window stimulations. *Neurophysiology Clinics, 32,* 269–274.

Scheperle, R. A., & Abbas, P. J. (2015). Relationships among peripheral and central electrophysiological measures of spatial and spectral selectivity and speech perception in cochlear implant users. *Ear and Hearing, 36,* 441–453.

Schmerber, S., Lavieille, J. P., Dumas, G., & Herve, T. (2004). Intraoperative auditory monitoring in vestibular schwannoma surgery: New trends. *Acta Otolaryngology, 124*(1), 53–61.

Schmidt, P. H., Eggermont, J. J., & Odenthal, D. W. (1974). Study of Ménière's disease by electrocochleography. *Acta Oto-laryngologica, Supplementum, 316,* 75–84.

Schoonhoven, R. (2007). Responses from the cochlea. Cochlear microphonic, summating potential and compound action potential. In R. F. Burkard, M. Don, & J. J. Eggermont (Eds.), *Auditory evoked potentials: Basic principles and clinical applications* (pp. 180–198). Baltimore, MD: Lippincott Williams & Wilkins.

Schoonhoven, R., Fabius, M. A., & Grote, J. J. (1995). Input/output curves to tone bursts and clicks in extratympanic and transtympanic electrocochleography, *Ear and Hearing, 16,* 619–630.

Schoonhoven, R., Lamoré, P. J., de Laat, J. A., & Grote, J. J. (1999). The prognostic value of electrocochleography in severely hearing-impaired infants. *Audiology, 38,* 141–154.

Schoonhoven, R., Prijs, V. F., & Grote, J. J. (1996). Response thresholds in electrocochleography and their relation to the pure tone audiogram. *Ear and Hearing, 17,* 266–275.

Schvartz-Leyzac, K. C., & Pfingst, B. E. (2016). Across-site patterns of electrically evoked compound action potential amplitude-growth functions in multichannel cochlear implant recipients and the effects of the interphase gap. *Hearing Research, 341,* 50–65.

Sennaroğlu, L., Colletti, V., Lenarz, T., Manrique, M., Laszig, R., Rask-Andersen, H., . . . Polak, M. (2016). Consensus statement: Long-term results of ABI in children with complex inner ear malformations and decision making between CI and ABI. *Cochlear Implants International, 17*(4), 163–171.

Shallop, J. K., Beiter, A. L., Goin, D. W., & Mischke, R. E. (1990). Electrically evoked auditory brain stem responses (EABR) and middle latency responses (EMLR) obtained from patients with the nucleus multichannel cochlear implant. *Ear and Hearing, 11*(1), 5–15.

Shallop, J., VanDyke, L., Goin, D., & Mischke, R. (1991). Prediction of behavioral threshold and comfort values for nucleus 22-channel implant patients from electrical auditory brain stem response test results. *Annals of Otology, Rhinology, and Laryngology, 100,* 896–898.

Smith, L., & Simmons, F. (1983). Estimating eighth nerve survival by electrical stimulation. *Annals of Otology, Rhinology, and Laryngology, 92,* 19–23.

Snyder, R. L., & Schreiner, C. E. (1984). The auditory neurophonic: Basic properties. *Hearing Research, 15,* 261–280.

Sohmer, H., & Feinmesser, M. (1973). Routine use of electrocochleography (cochlear audiometry) on human subjects. *Audiology, 12,* 167–173.

Spoor, A., & Eggermont, J. J. (1976). Electrocochleography as a method for objective audiogram determination. In S. K. Hirsh, D. H. Eldredge, I. J. Hirsh, & S. R. Silverman (Eds.), *Davis and hearing: Essays honoring Hallowell Davis* (pp. 411–418). St. Louis, MO: Washington University Press.

Starr, A., & Brackmann, D. E. (1979). Brain stem potentials evoked by electrical stimulation of the cochlea in human subjects. *Annals of Otology, Rhinology, and Laryngology, 88,* 550–556.

Starr, A., Sininger, Y., Nguyen, T., Michalewski, H. J., Oba, S., & Abdala, C. (2001). Cochlear receptor (cochlear microphonic and summating potentials, otoacoustic emissions) and auditory pathway (auditory brainstem potentials) activity in auditory neuropathy. *Ear and Hearing, 22,* 91–99.

Stevens, J., Booth, R., Brennan, S., Feirn, R., & Meredith, R. (2013). Guidance for auditory brainstem response testing in babies. Version 2.1. In G. Sutton & G. Lightfoot (Eds.), *Newborn hearing screening and assessment* (NHS Antenatal and Newborn Screening Programmes).

Stypulkowski, P. H., & van den Honert, C. (1984). Physiological properties of the electrically stimulated auditory nerve. I. Compound action potential recordings. *Hearing Research, 14,* 205–223.

Takeda, T., & Kakigi, A. (2010). The clinical value of extratympanic electrocochleography in the diagnosis of Ménière's disease. *ORL Journal of Otorhinolaryngology Related Specialties, 72,* 196–204.

Tamura, M., Carron, R., Yomo, S., Arkha, Y., Muraciolle, X., Porcheron, D., . . . Régis, J. (2009). Hearing preservation after gamma knife radiosurgery for vestibular schwannomas presenting with high-level hearing. *Neurosurgery, 64,* 289–296.

Tejani, V. D., Abbas, P. J., & Brown, C. J. (2017). Relationship between peripheral and psychophysical measures of amplitude modulation detection in cochlear implant users. *Ear and Hearing, 38*(5), e268–e284.

Thai-Van, H., Cozma, S., & Boutitie, F. (2007).The pattern of auditory brainstem response wave V maturation in cochlear-implanted children. *Clinical Neurophysiology, 118,* 676–689.

Thornton, A. R., Farrell, G., & Haacke, N. P. (1991). A non-invasive, objective test of endolymphatic hydrops. *Acta Otolaryngology Supplement, 479,* 35–43.

Turner, C., Mehr, M., Hughes, M., Brown, C., & Abbas, P. (2002). Within-subject predictors of speech recognition in cochlear implants: A null result. *Acoustics Research Letters, Online, 3,* 95–100.

van den Honert, C., & Stypulkowski, P. H. (1986). Characterization of the electrically evoked auditory brainstem response (ABR) in cats and humans. *Hearing Research, 21,* 109–135.

Versnel, H., Prijs, V. F., & Schoonhoven, R. (1990). Single-fibre responses to clicks in relationship to the compound action potential in the guinea pig. *Hearing Research, 46,* 147–160.

Versnel, H., Prijs, V. F., & Schoonhoven, R. (1997). Auditory-nerve fiber responses to clicks in guinea pigs with a damaged cochlea. *Journal of the Acoustical Society of America, 101,* 993–1009.

Wang, C.-Y., & Dallos, P. (1972). Latency of whole-nerve action potential: Influence of hair-cell normalcy. *Journal of the Acoustical Society of America, 52,* 1678–1686.

Wanibuchi, M., Fukushima, T., Friedman, A. H., Watanabe, K., Akiyama, Y., Mikami, T., . . . Mikuni, N. (2014). Hearing preservation surgery for vestibular schwannomas via the retrosigmoid transmeatal approach: Surgical tips. *Neurosurgical Review, 37*(3), 431–444.

Watanabe, S., Yamamoto, M., Kawabe, T., Koiso, T., Yamamoto, T., Matsumura, A., & Kasuya, H. (2016). Stereotactic radiosurgery for vestibular schwannomas: Average 10-year follow-up results focusing on long-term hearing preservation. *Journal of Neurosurgery, 125*(Suppl. 1), 64–72.

Wilson, W. J., & Bowker, C. A. (2002). The effects of high stimulus rate on the electrocochleogram in normal-hearing subjects. *International Journal of Audiology, 41,* 509–517.

Winn, M. B., & Litovsky, R. Y. (2015). Using speech sounds to test functional spectral resolution in listeners with cochlear implants. *Journal of the Acoustical Society of America, 137,* 1430–1442.

Winn, M. B., Won, J. H., & Moon, I. J. (2016). Assessment of spectral and temporal resolution in cochlear implant users using psychoacoustic discrimination and speech cue categorization. *Ear and Hearing, 37,* e377–e390.

Withnell, R. H. (2001). Brief report: The cochlear microphonic as an indication of outer hair cell function. *Ear and Hearing, 22,* 75–77.

Yamakami, I., Ito, S., & Higuchi, H. (2014). Retrosigmoid removal of small acoustic neuroma: Curative tumor removal with preservation of function. *Journal of Neurosurgery, 121*(3), 554–563.

Yamakami, I., Yoshinori, H., Saeki, N., Wada, M., & Oka, N. (2009). Hearing preservation and intraoperative auditory brainstem response and cochlear nerve compound action potential monitoring in the removal of small acoustic neurinoma via the retrosigmoidal approach. *Journal of Neurology, Neurosurgery, and Psychiatry, 80,* 218–227.

Yoshie, N. (1976). Electrocochleographic classification of sensorineural defects: Pathological pattern of the cochlear nerve compound action potential in man. In R. J. Ruben, C. Elberling, & G. Salomon (Eds.), *Electrocochleography* (pp. 353–386). Baltimore, MD: University Park Press.

Youssef, A. S., & Downes, A. E. (2009). Intraoperative neurophysiological monitoring in vestibular schwannoma surgery: Advances and clinical implications. *Neurosurgical Focus, 27*(4), E9.

Ziylan, F., Smeeing, D. P. J., Stegeman, I., & Thomeer, H. G. (2016). Click stimulus electrocochleography versus MRI with intratympanic contrast in Ménière's disease: A systematic review. *Otology and Neurotology, 37,* 421–427.

8

Brainstem Evoked Responses to Complex Sounds: Characteristics and Clinical Applications

SCOPE

In the preceding chapters, we focused on the characteristics and clinical applications of the more commonly used auditory brainstem response (ABR), which reflects population neural activity synchronized to the onset of brief stimuli. When multiple, harmonically related frequency components are combined to form a complex sound, it is characterized by a slowly varying periodic envelope and rapidly varying frequency components contained in the envelope referred to as the temporal fine structure (Figure 8–1, identified as ENV and TFS, respectively, in the bottom trace). Here we focus on the characteristics and potential clinical applications of two related, but distinct types of brainstem evoked response generated by complex sounds including speech. One is the envelope following response (EFR), and the other is the frequency following response (FFR). While EFR reflects sustained neural phase-locking to the *envelope periodicity* of the stimulus waveform (Figure 8–1, middle trace showing a waveform largely representing the low-frequency envelope periodicity), *FFR* reflects sustained neural phase-locking to the *temporal fine structure* of complex sounds (the relatively higher frequency response shown as the FFR waveform in Figure 8–1). It should be noted here that the phase-locked activity elicited by a single-onset polarity stimulus is a combination of neural phase-locking to the envelope periodicity as well as to the temporal fine structure, with the more robust phase-locking to the envelope periodicity dominating the response waveform. Different labels have been used to identify these responses (e.g., EFR has been referred to as the auditory steady-state response [ASSR] when amplitude-modulated stimuli have been used, speech ABR [sABR] when speech stimuli have been used, or FFR$_{ENV}$ when complex sounds like speech and/or complex tones have been used). FFR been referred to FFR$_{SPEC}$ or FFR$_{TFS}$. We have chosen to use the more accurate descriptor EFR for the envelope following response because the response reflects neural phase-locking to the envelope periodicity, regardless of the type of complex sound used to elicit them; and FFR for responses representing neural phase-locking to the spectral components of the stimulus. Because both of these responses provide information about the nature of the temporal neural encoding of certain acoustic features important for the perception of complex sounds, they can potentially be effective electrophysiologic measures to evaluate the nature of degradation of these features in individuals with cochlear or

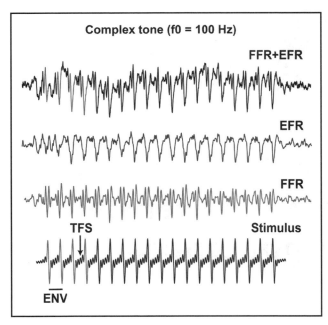

Figure 8–1. Waveforms representing combined frequency following response (FFR) and envelope following response (EFR) (FFR + EFR). EFR and FFR are elicited by a complex tone with a fundamental frequency (f0) of 100 Hz. The combined waveform (elicited using a single-onset polarity) shows phase-locking to both the envelope periodicity (100 Hz) and the spectral components (temporal fine structure) of the complex tone. In response to alternating polarity, only the EFR is seen. Subtraction of the response to each polarity will yield the FFR containing only phase-locking to the spectral components.

retrocochlear hearing impairment, monitor treatment outcomes with amplification, evaluate effects of auditory retraining, and test and evaluate optimal signal processing strategies for hearing prosthetic devices. This chapter focuses on potential clinical audiologic applications of these responses, and the next chapter considers the basic science and translational applications of these brainstem responses, particularly the FFR.

I. ENVELOPE FOLLOWING RESPONSE (EFR)

An EFR, as indicated earlier, is a class of evoked auditory evoked responses generated in the brainstem that reflect sustained phase-locked neural activity among a population of neural elements along the auditory neuraxis that follow the temporal envelope periodicity of a complex sound (Figure 8–1, second trace identified as EFR) (Aiken & Picton, 2006; Ananthakrishnan & Krishnan, 2018; Ananthakrishnan, Krishnan & Bartlett, 2016; Ananthakrishnan, Luo, & Krishnan, 2017; Campbell, Atkinson, Francis, & Green, 1977; Hall, 1979; Suresh, Krishnan, & Luo, 2020). In this section, we use the labels *EFR* and *ASSR* interchangeably. During cochlear transduction, each cochlear filter responds to a narrow band of frequencies that drive each auditory nerve fiber (ANF). The narrowband ANF frequency filters separate the input signals into ENV and TFS components. Since the broader high-frequency filters can contain more harmonics (which likely are unresolved), they interact to produce a modulation response corresponding to the fundamental periodicity that is sharper than a lower-frequency filter that contains fewer harmonics. The TFS response, as expected, fluctuates at a rate corresponding to the center frequency of each cochlear filter. The inability of the cochlea to follow very rapid TFS fluctuations restricts neural phase-locking to below 2000 Hz in humans with only a robust ENV locking observed at higher frequencies. Since both EFR and FFR overlap to produce a complex response waveform in response to a fixed-onset polarity stimulus, averaging the responses to alternating polarity will effectively isolate the EFR from the FFR as well as the cochlear microphonic (CM) and stimulus artifact, since the EFR does not change with polarity change (Aiken & Picton, 2008; Ananthakrishnan & Krishnan, 2018; Suresh & Krishnan, 2021; Greenberg, Marsh, Brown, & Smith, 1987; Krishnan, 2002). Thus, EFR alone is summed and preserved, while the other components are subtracted out (Figure 8–2). To extract the FFR (see Figure 8–2), the responses to opposite polarities are subtracted (Aiken & Picton, 2008; Ananthakrishnan & Krishnan, 2018; Suresh & Krishnan, 2021; Krishnan, 2002). This is similar to the compound histogram technique developed by Arthur, Pfeifer, and Suga (1971) and Goblick and Pfeifer (1969) for the temporal analysis of single-unit discharge patterns. The phenomenon of neural phase-locking has been well demonstrated at all levels along the auditory pathway, although the upper-frequency limit decreases from the auditory nerve (AN; close to

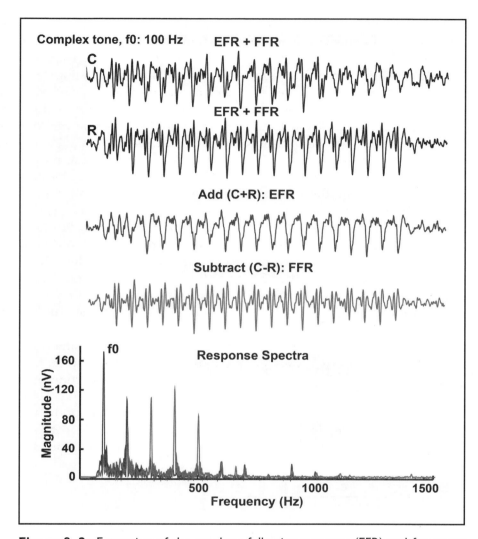

Figure 8–2. Extraction of the envelope following response (EFR) and frequency following response (FFR) using addition and subtraction of responses to condensation and rarefaction-onset polarities. The top waveforms represent responses to condensation (C) and rarefaction (R) stimulus-onset polarities. These responses contain both EFR and FFR. The addition of these two responses (*dark gray waveform*) results in the EFR, and subtraction (C − R) results in the FFR (*light gray waveform*). Note the lower-frequency periodicity of the EFR compared to the FFR. The spectra of the EFR (*black*) and FFR (*gray*) to a complex tone are shown at the bottom of the waveforms. The FFR components extend to several higher-frequency harmonics, while the EFR shows a prominent peak at f0. From "Language Experience Shapes Processing of Pitch Relevant Information in the Human Brainstem and Auditory Cortex: Electrophysiological Evidence," by A. Krishnan and J. T. Gandour, 2014, *Acoustics Australia, 42*(3), pp. 187–199. Reprinted with permission from Springer.

5000 Hz) to the auditory cortex (less than 200 Hz). Also, neural phase-locking ability (as indicated by the synchronization index) in the entire population of ANFs decreases with increasing frequency with the membrane time constant of the inner hair cell (IHC) being a limiting factor (Palmer & Russell, 1986). However, AN population response can follow the envelope of sinusoidally amplitude modulated (SAM) tones with high carrier frequencies provided the modulation frequency (envelope periodicity) is well below the phase-locking cutoff frequency (Rees & Moller, 1983; Yin & Kuwada, 1983). ASSR elicited by SAM sounds, essentially an EFR, is being used by some clinicians for threshold estimation (Dimitrijevic et al., 2002; Picton et al., 2003; Picton, van Roon, & John, 2009; also, please read clinical applications of ASSRs in Chapter 5). More recently, there is growing interest in the use of EFR elicited by speech stimuli to evaluate its clinical utility in indexing hearing aid benefits (Anderson & Kraus 2013; Easwar, Purcell, Aiken, Parsa, & Scollie, 2015b; Jenkins, Fodor, Presacco, & Anderson, 2018). We first describe the characteristics, recording, and analysis techniques for the EFR (ASSR) elicited by SAM stimuli followed by EFR to speech stimuli and complex sounds.

II. RESPONSE CHARACTERISTICS OF EFRS ELICITED BY SAM TONES

Because EFRs represent phase-locking to the envelope periodicity presented in the stimulus, it is useful to initially describe the temporal and spectral characteristics of the commonly used SAM tone to elicit these responses. The SAM tone is created by sinusoidally modulating the amplitude of a constant-amplitude higher-frequency carrier (f_c) tone using low-frequency modulation (f_m), whose modulation depth can be varied between 0% and 100%. A SAM tone with 100% modulation depth (Figure 8–3) provides the maximum amplitude modulation cue, and its spectrum is characterized by a maximum peak at f_c and harmonically related peaks below (at $f_c - f_m$) and above (at $f_c + f_m$) f_c at half the amplitude relative to f_c with no spectral energy in the SAM tone at f_m. During cochlear transduction, the AN response is rectified (Figure 8–3, bottom left) because the ANFs fire only during the unidirectional excitatory phase of the hair cell. The spectrum of this rectified neural response (Figure 8–3, bottom right) contains energy not only at f_c and its sidebands but also at the modulation frequency (f_m) and its harmonics (considered to be rectifier distortion products). Neurons along the auditory pathway in the brainstem can phase-lock to both the modulation frequency to produce the EFR (ASSR in this case) and to the spectral components (provided they are below the

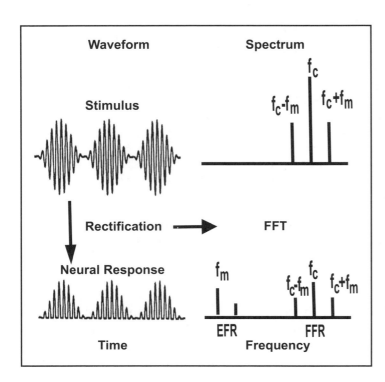

Figure 8–3. Waveform and spectra of a sinusoidally amplitude modulated (SAM) tone (A) and the resulting neural EFR and FFR components. The stimulus waveform shows the periodicity of the SAM tone, and its spectrum illustrates the frequency component at the carrier frequency (f_c) and the sidebands $f_c - f_m$, and $f_c + f_m$. The responses waveform (*bottom left*) shows the rectified neural response following the stimulus waveform periodicity. The response spectrum (*right*) shows the phase-locked components at f_c, and the sidebands. Also, the response spectrum shows a spectral component at the modulation frequency (corresponding to the periodicity).

upper-frequency limit for neural phase-locking of about 1700–2000 Hz) to produce the FFR. As mentioned earlier, this upper-frequency limit for neural phase-locking also decreases from about 5000 Hz at the AN level, to less than 2000 Hz at the midbrain (inferior colliculus [IC]) and less than 150 Hz in the auditory cortex. This poses a real challenge to the effectiveness of neural phase-locking based temporal encoding schemes of stimulus spectrum described for the ANF population. It is believed that a transformation from a temporal to a place-based discharge rate code occurs at the level of the midbrain that selectively increases the discharge rate for a specific modulation rate.

Effects of Intensity

The amplitude of the EFR to single and multiple SAM tones exhibits an almost linear growth with increasing intensity (Figure 8–4, left panel) independent of the modulation frequency (Ménard, Gallégo, Berger-Vachon, Collet, & Thai-Van, 2008; Picton, Skinner, Champagne, Kellett, & Maiste, 1987; Picton, van Roon, & Sasha John, 2007, 2009).

However, it should be noted here that for responses elicited by multifrequency stimuli, the amplitude growth function tends to saturate at higher intensities for the 1000 and 2000 Hz carrier frequency (Picton et al., 2007). The slope of the amplitude growth function has been shown to vary with a carrier frequency (1.30 nV at 500 Hz, 0.87 nV at 1000 Hz, 0.75 nV at 2000 Hz, and 1.40 nV at 4000 Hz). The average increase in amplitude across carrier frequencies is between 1.08 and 1.9 nV for multiple stimuli and single-carrier frequencies (Lins & Picton, 1995; Picton et al., 2007; Vander Werff & Brown, 2005). Since the EFR components can be reliably detected at levels close to behavioral threshold (between 4 and 17 dB above behavioral threshold in the 500- to 4000-Hz range) using both single-frequency and multifrequency SAM stimuli, they can be used to estimate behavioral thresholds reliably (Cone-Wesson, Dowell, Tomlin, Rance, & Ming, 2002; Dimitrijevic et al., 2002; Herdman & Stapells, 2003; Lins et al., 1996), with excellent test-retest reliability (D'Haenens et al., 2008). This difference is even smaller in individuals with cochlear hearing loss. Herdman and Stapells (2003) have also shown a 1 to 3 dB difference between the EFR threshold

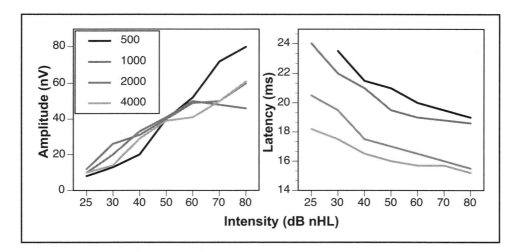

Figure 8–4. The effects of stimulus intensity on the mean amplitude (*left*) and mean latency (*right*) of the responses elicited by 500-, 1000-, 2000-, and 4000-Hz stimuli presented binaurally. The amplitude increases with increasing intensity, but at 1000 and 2000 Hz, the amplitude tends to saturate at the higher intensities. Response latencies, derived from the phase delay information, decrease with increasing intensity and with increasing carrier frequency. Figure created using data from "Human Auditory Steady-State Responses During Sweeps of Intensity," by T. W. Picton, P. van Roon, and M. Sasha John, 2007, *Ear and Hearing, 28*(4), pp. 542–557.

and behavioral threshold across carrier frequencies for both monaural and binaural multifrequency EFR acquisition. Given this favorable empirical evidence, its ease of recording, automatic response detection, and potential to significantly reduce test time, it is somewhat surprising to see its limited use in clinical threshold estimation. Like the behavior of ABR, ASSR response latency decreases and amplitude increases with stimulus intensity (Figure 8–4, right panel).

Effects of Carrier Frequency

EFRs to modulated SAM tones for clinical threshold estimation use single-frequency carriers or, more commonly, simultaneous presentation of multiple frequencies monaurally or binaurally. In order to isolate frequency-specific and ear-specific information, a unique modulation frequency between 80 and 110 Hz is assigned to each carrier frequency. Thus, the combined stimulus containing energy at each one of the carrier frequencies (typically 500, 1000, 2000, and 4000 Hz) activates four different cochlear regions in a frequency-specific manner (Figure 8–5). The unique modulation frequencies assigned to these tones elicit the EFRs resulting from the primary activity at distinct cochlear regions corresponding to the carrier frequency (Figure 8–5, spectrum on the right showing peaks at the four modulation frequencies). This multiple stimulus approach has been shown to enable the completion of testing both ears in about the time taken to complete testing of one stimulus frequency in one ear using the single-frequency stimulation technique (Lins et al., 1996).

For EFRs elicited by single frequency and multiple frequencies, carriers presented monotically or dichotically, the response amplitude does not vary appreciably across carrier frequencies (Figure 8–6, top panel) for stimulus levels 60 dB sound pressure level (SPL) or less (Herdman & Stapells, 2001; John, Lins, Boucher, & Picton, 1998; Korczak, Smart, Delgado, Strobel, & Bradford, 2012; Lins & Picton, 1995; Mo & Stapells, 2008; Picton, 2013). However, it is possible that interfrequency interaction effects

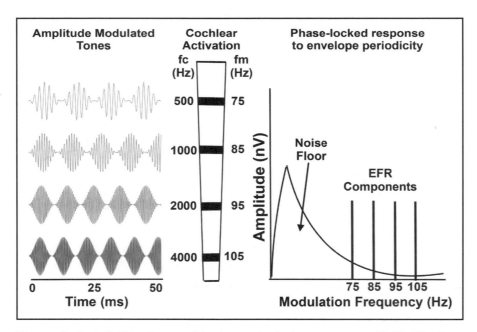

Figure 8–5. *Left:* Waveforms of the four individual carrier tones. *Middle:* The basilar membrane region activated by each frequency and the modulation rate used for each frequency. All tones are presented simultaneously and thus stimulate the frequency regions of the basilar membrane best tuned to these frequencies. *Right.* The energy present at the modulation frequency of each tone is shown in the response spectrum. Created using data from Dr. Peggy Karzak et al. (2012).

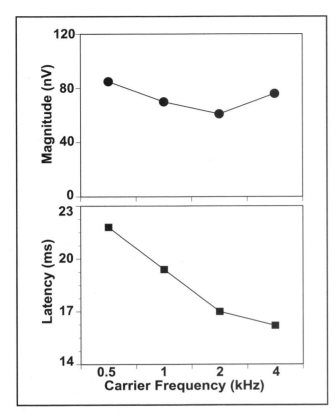

Figure 8–6. The mean amplitude (*top*) and latency (*bottom*) for the brainstem auditory stead-state responses plotted as a function of the carrier frequency of the multiple frequency stimuli presented dichotically. The amplitude of the responses at 1000 and 2000 Hz is smaller compared to responses obtained with single-frequency stimuli, suggesting interaction effects using multiple frequency stimuli. As expected, response latency decreases as the frequency is increased. Created using data from "Multiple Auditory Steady State Responses (80–101 Hz): Effects of Ear, Gender, Handedness, Intensity and Modulation Rate," by T. W. Picton, P. van Roon, and M. Sasha John, 2009, *Ear and Hearing, 30*, pp. 100–109.

like the upward spread of masking, suppression, and facilitation (Lins & Picton, 1995; Picton, van Roon, & John, 2007, 2009; Picton et al., 2003) may reduce the EFR amplitude, particularly for stimulus levels above 60 dB SPL. For example, John et al. (1998) showed that the responses became smaller with multiple stimulation when the intensity of the stimuli was increased from 60 to 75 dB SPL. Also, Dimitrijevic et al. (2002) reported that in some of their hearing-impaired subjects, ASSR threshold estimates for 2000 and 4000 Hz were more accurate using the single-frequency approach compared to the multifrequency approach, suggesting the presence of possible interfrequency masking. Finally, Picton, van Roon, and John (2009) showed that for a dichotically presented multifrequency stimuli at 73 dB SPL, the amplitude of the responses at 1000 and 2000 Hz was smaller compared to responses obtained with single-frequency stimuli. These authors also implicated the upward spread of masking effects for this amplitude reduction. However, this explanation does not account for the lack of amplitude reduction for the 4000-Hz response. Masking effects could likely decrease the response at higher frequencies, and two-tone suppression could account for the amplitude decrease at lower frequencies (John et al., 1998). These interaction effects could be minimized if fewer stimuli were used and/or with the use of greater frequency separation between the carriers. The small differences between the modulation frequencies could potentially generate a response following the beats. However, the typically higher high-pass setting of the amplifier and the much longer analysis epoch would preclude its recording. Consistent with the different cochlear traveling wave delays associated with stimulus frequency, EFR latency (Figure 8–6, bottom panel) decreases as the carrier frequency is increased (John & Picton, 2000b; Picton et al., 2009).

Effects of Modulation Rate

Systematic manipulation of the modulation frequency (rate) and/or modulation depth of SAM tones/noise may be used to evaluate the sensitivity of the auditory system to temporal changes. In humans, as the modulation rate of the amplitude-modulated swept tone is increased from 10 to 100 Hz, the EFR amplitude initially increases to a maximum around 40 to 50 Hz followed by a sharp drop in amplitude (Figure 8–7, top panel) at about 60 Hz (for these modulation rates, the response is dominated by cortical generators; thus, the amplitude of the response is several orders of magnitude greater than the responses from deep within the brainstem). For sinusoidally amplitude modulated tones, the EFR amplitude decreases steadily with an increase in modulation rate from 100 to 600 Hz with a plateau between 300 and 400 Hz (Figure 8–7,

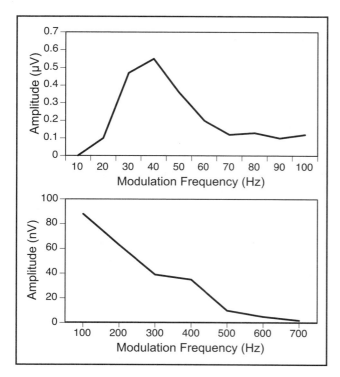

Figure 8–7. Effects of modulation rate on EFR amplitude. *Top:* A dominant envelope following response (EFR) amplitude peak at 40 Hz for responses elicited by swept modulation tones from 20 to 100 Hz with a constant modulation rate of 25%. The appreciably smaller amplitudes in the 100- to 600-Hz region are not plotted here. *Bottom:* Mean amplitude of the EFRs elicited by amplitude-modulated tones of increasing modulation frequency. Response amplitude steadily decreases with increasing modulation rate, with a plateau in the 300- to 400-Hz region. The responses are quite small above 500 Hz and barely above the noise floor. Thus, increasing the modulation rate decreases the EFR with no discernible response components present above about 500 Hz. The top panel figure was created using data from "Near-Threshold Recordings of Amplitude Modulation Following Responses (AMFR) in Children of Different Ages," by J. Pethe, R. Mühler, K. Siewert, and H. von Specht, 2004, *International Journal of Audiology, 43*, pp. 339–345.

perceptual measures, is similar to the modulation rate functions described for auditory neurons (Joris, Schreiner, & Rees, 2004). Part of the difficulty characterizing the sensitivity of the EFRs to changes in modulation rate is due to the multiple generator sources (rostral brainstem presumably IC; thalamus, and the auditory cortex) contributing to the scalp recorded EFR. The individual contributions of these sources to the EFR appear to change with modulation rate such that below about 50 Hz, the EFR is largely dominated by contributions from the auditory cortex (e.g., the 40-Hz EFR has a latency between 20 and 40 ms); as the modulation rate is increased beyond about 90 Hz, the response reflects neural activity primarily from the rostral brainstem latency between 8 and 10 ms (Herdman et al., 2002; Picton, John, Dimitrijevic, & Purcell, 2003).

Effects of Age

The EFRs generated at the cortical level (40 Hz) and the brainstem (above about 80 Hz) show changes with age during early development (birth to adulthood) and in later years (aging effects). Unlike the distinct large peak at 40 Hz in adults, infant EFRs are smaller in amplitude and about the same across modulation rates. Using amplitude-modulated noise in children ranging in age from 2 months to 14 years, Pethe, Mühler, Siewert, and von Specht (2004) observed an increase in the amplitude of EFRs with increasing age with the slope of amplitude growth steeper for the 40-Hz component compared to the 80-Hz component (Figure 8–8). That is, the 40-Hz component was equal in amplitude to the 80-Hz component below 1 year of age, but by age 14 years, the 40-Hz component was appreciably larger than the 80-Hz component (150 nV versus 80 nV). However, response detection was easier for the 80-Hz component compared to the 40-Hz component because of the higher noise floor for the 40-Hz response. The peak location of the 40-Hz response has been shown to increase with age (Poulsen, Picton, & Paus, 2009; Purcell et al., 2004). Poulsen et al. (2009) observed that the peak of the 40 Hz in the 10-year-old subjects was around 30 Hz and around 42 Hz in individuals ranging in age from 19 to 45 years. Similarly, Purcell et al. (2004)

bottom panel). For modulation frequencies above about 450 Hz, the responses are quite small and barely above the noise floor (Purcell, John, Schneider, & Picton, 2004; Shinn-Cunningham, Varghese, Wang, & Bharadwaj, 2017). The activity above about 90 Hz is thought to be of brainstem origin (Figure 8–7, bottom panel). This essentially low-pass sensitivity, while not entirely conforming to

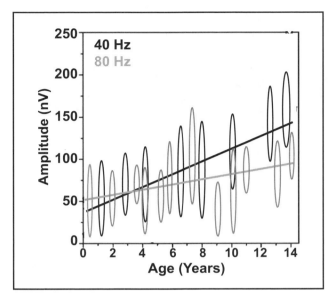

Figure 8–8. Amplitude growth functions for the 40-Hz envelope following response (EFR; *black*) and 80-Hz EFR (*gray*) at 50 dB are plotted as a function of age (birth to 14 years). While the amplitude of the 40-Hz EFR tends to increase with age (note the considerable variability indicated by the ellipses), the 80-Hz EFR amplitude changes very little with age. These results suggest the neural maturation time course for the 40-Hz cortical generators and the 80-Hz brainstem generators are different. Created using data from "Near-Threshold Recordings of Amplitude Modulation Following Responses (AMFR) in Children of Different Ages," by J. Pethe, R. Mühler, K. Siewert, and H. von Specht, 2004, *International Journal of Audiology*, *43*, pp. 339–345.

observed that the frequency of the 40-Hz response changed from 37 Hz in young adults (20–29 years) to 41 Hz in older adults (70–79 years). When summarizing the pattern of the shift in peak location of the 40-Hz response and its latency changes as a function of age, Picton (2011) showed that peak frequency increased gradually from age 10 to about 45 years and then decreased gradually above the age of 45 years. In contrast, the latency of the response showed a gradual linear increase as a function of age (at the rate of 0.08 ms/year). Purcell et al. (2004) found that in younger listeners, the detectable ASSR modulation frequency was higher (494 Hz) than that observed in older listeners (294 Hz), with the EFR amplitude versus modulation rate function diverging for the two groups at 100 Hz. Similarly,

Grose, Mamo, and Hall (2009) observed a smaller EFR amplitude for older listeners at a modulation rate of 128 Hz but not at 32 Hz, regardless of the carrier frequency. These results suggest that age-related deficits in temporal processing as reflected in the EFRs are restricted to high modulation frequencies. These changes in older adults may in part reflect aging-related cochlear hearing loss and/or central changes involving a decrease in neural conduction velocity and reduced synaptic efficiency.

III. USE OF EFR IN AUDITORY THRESHOLD ESTIMATION

Air-Conduction Threshold Estimation in Adults and Infants With Normal Hearing (AC-EFR)

While several studies have used the EFRs elicited by SAM tones to examine the effects of aging on temporal processing ability in young and older individuals, its primary clinical application is in threshold estimation. The narrowband-derived responses using high-pass masking at moderate stimulus levels show maximum amplitude within a half octave of the SAM tone across frequency for both single and multiple stimuli recordings suggesting good place specificity that is equal to or better than that observed for ABR (Herdman et al., 2002). Like tone burst ABR, EFRs also provide reliable, accurate, and place-specific estimates of air-conduction thresholds that are within 5 to 15 dB (for the multifrequency EFR) and 15 to 25 dB (for the single-frequency EFR) of behavioral thresholds in normal-hearing adults. Mean difference scores (MDSs), reflecting the difference between the poorer EFR threshold and the better behavioral pure-tone thresholds, are about 15 dB at 500 Hz, 10 dB at 1000 Hz, and 9.5 dB at 2000 and 4000 Hz (Cone-Wesson et al., 2002; D'Haenens et al., 2008; Dimitrijevic et al., 2002; Herdman & Stapells, 2003; Lins et al., 1996). Herdman and Stapells (2003) found MDS to be about 1–3 dB across test frequencies for both monaural and binaural conditions (Table 8–1, top). There is general agreement that simultaneous binaural multifrequency EFRs could

Table 8–1. Multifrequency 80-Hz Auditory Steady-State Response Behavioral Mean Difference Scores (MDSs) in Decibels and Standard Deviations (Within Parentheses) Across Studies for Normal-Hearing Adults, Hearing-Impaired Sdults, and Older Children Wsing Monaural Testing

Group	Study	Frequency (Hz) 500	1000	2000	4000
Normal adults	D'Haenens et al. (2008)	19 (12)	13.5 (10)	11 (9)	13.5 (9.3)
	Tlumak et al. (2007)	17 (12)	13 (12)	11 (10)	15 (10)
	Elberling et al. (2007)	11 (7)	10 (7)	6 (5)	13 (4)
	Picton et al. (2005)	21 (8)	7 (8)	10 (6)	13 (7)
	Luts & Wouters (2005)	12 (7)	7 (7)	12 (7)	13 (7)
	Herdman & Stapells (2003)	11 (11)	10 (11)	11 (10)	14 (10)
	Dimitrijevic et al. (2002)	17 (10)	4 (11)	4 (8)	11 (17)
	Herdman & Stapells (2001)	14 (10)	8 (7)	8 (9)	15 (9)
	Lins et al. (1996)	14 (11)	12 (11)	11 (8)	13 (11)
	Mean:	15.11	9.38	9.33	11.94
Hearing-impaired adults	Aimoni et al. (2018)				
	0–13 years	0.9 (13.6)	−1.8 (12.4)	−0.8 (14.6)	−1.5 (11.7)
	14–25 years	−2.2 (10.7)	−5.4 (11.4)	−8.6 (10.6)	−11.2 (11.2
	D'Haenens et al. (2009)				
	(Mild)	14 (11)	13 (8)	14 (7)	13 (6)
	(Moderate)	14 (7)	10 (10)	9 (6)	11 (9)
	Lin, Ho, & Wu (2009)	17 (14)	15 (9)	14 (8)	11 (8)
	Tlumak et al. (2007)	14 (13)	10 (13)	9 (12)	8 (13)
	Vander Werff & Brown (2005)	15 (8)	9 (6)	8 (6)	6 (5)
	Van Mannen & Stapells (2005)	17 (11)	15 (7)	19 (9)	4 (10)
	Picton et al. (2005)	11 (18)	−4 (9)	3 (11)	5 (12)
	Herdman & Stapells (2003)	14 (13)	8 (9)	5 (9)	3 (10)
	Dimitrijevic et al. (2002)	13 (11)	5 (8)	5 (9)	8 (11)
	Lins et al. (1996)	9 (9)	13 (12)	11 (10)	12 (13)
	Mean:	12.54	8.86	8.84	6.98

provide a faster and reliable objective estimate of thresholds.

Objective estimates of hearing thresholds are particularly important for early detection and remediation to minimize the deleterious effects of hearing loss on speech and language development. While the most recent Joint Committee on Infant Hearing (JCIH, 2019) continues to recommend the use of ABR as the gold standard for both hearing screening and threshold estimation, serious consideration should be given to the use of EFRs given their demonstrated accuracy and reliability. The reluctance to use ASSR is in part due to the lack of availability of the ASSR module in all commercially available auditory evoked potential systems, and the greater challenge posed by the recording environment and ambient noise levels that may elevate estimated thresholds by 5 to 20 dB (Lins et al., 1996; Savio, Cárdenas, Pérez Abalo, González, & Valdés, 2001) compared to recordings made in quieter sound-treated booths (Stroebel, Swanepoel, & Groenewald, 2007; Swanepoel & Steyn, 2005; Van Maanen & Stapells, 2009). Also, the considerably smaller EFR amplitudes in infants and young children (e.g., 17 nV in infants versus 35 nV in normal-hearing adults at 50 dB; John, Brown, Muir, & Picton, 2004) compared to adults makes response detection more difficult near threshold (John et al., 2004; Luts, Desloovere, & Wouters, 2006). Van Maanen and Stapells, (2009) demonstrated that the detectability of the ASSR in infants can be substantially increased across stimuli using a lower noise criterion (5 nV instead of 10 nV) that essentially enhances the response signal-to-noise ratio (SNR). Nevertheless, EFR thresholds in infants and young children are about 10 to 15 dB higher across frequencies compared to adults (Lins et al., 1996; Rance & Rickards, 2002; Van Maanen & Stapells, 2009). Comparison of EFR thresholds in younger and older babies shows an improvement in threshold suggesting neural maturational effects (John et al., 2004; Luts et al., 2006; Rance & Tomlin, 2006; Ribeiro, Carvallo, & Marcoux, 2010; Savio et al., 2001). For example, Savio et al. (2001) showed that thresholds were 10 to 15 dB better for older babies (7–10 months) compared to younger babies (0–1 month). Maturational differences also produce larger-amplitude EFRs in term babies compared to premature babies (John et al., 2004; Luts et al., 2006: Ribeiro et al., 2010). For example, John et al. (2004) observed larger response amplitudes at 1000, 2000, and 4000 Hz in full-term babies compared to premature infants. However, Ribeiro et al. (2010) found only that the 500- and 4000-Hz EFRs showed significant difference between the two groups. Luts et al. (2006), based on their observation of a systematic increase in EFR amplitude with age, suggested an optimal age (between 1 week and 4 months) for EFR testing. Clearly, more studies are needed to more completely characterize these maturational changes in EFR.

Threshold Estimation in Adults and Infants With Sensorineural Hearing Loss

In adults with sensorineural loss (Table 8–1, bottom) the mean MDS across frequency is 13 dB at 500 Hz, 9.15 dB at 1000 Hz, 9.3 dB at 2000 Hz, and 8.6 dB at 4000 Hz (Dimitrijevic et al., 2002; Herdman & Stapells, 2003; Lins et al., 1996; Rance, Rickards, Cohen, DeVidi, & Clarke, 1995). Variability in the threshold measures is similar across test frequency, with prediction accuracy slightly poorer at 500 Hz. With respect to the influence of degree and configuration of hearing loss on threshold prediction accuracy, Rance et al. (1995) observed that EFR was more accurate for hearing losses greater than 60 dB HL. In contrast, Herdman and Stapells (2003) reported that multifrequency EFR provides good estimates of the threshold for hearing losses ranging from mild to profound. Threshold estimates were within 20 dB of behavioral threshold in 83% to 100% of individuals with sensorineural hearing loss. Thus, it appears that the degree and configuration of hearing loss do not influence the accuracy of threshold prediction. Also, Luts and Wouters (2005) did not find any difference in the accuracy of threshold estimates (both within 8–13 dB of behavioral thresholds) provided by single-frequency and multifrequency testing techniques. The recommended normal hearing levels for screening using the multifrequency EFRs are 50 dB HL at 500 Hz, 45 dB HL at 1000 Hz, and 40 dB HL at 2000 and 4000 Hz (Van Maanen & Stapells, 2009, 2010). Dimitrijevic et al. (2002) found a strong correlation between EFR threshold and behavioral thresholds at 500, 1000, 2000, and 4000 Hz. The spectral responses plotted as a function of increasing level (left panel), estimated electrophysiologic and behavior thresholds (top right panel), and the EFR-behavioral threshold relationship for all carriers (bottom right panel) are shown in Figure 8–9. They noted a good correspondence between the electrophysiologic and behavioral thresholds. These authors observed a high correlation (0.92) between the electrophysiologic and the behavioral thresholds.

Relatively few studies have been published examining the relationship between EFR and behavioral thresholds in infants and young children using single-frequency stimuli (Cone-Wesson

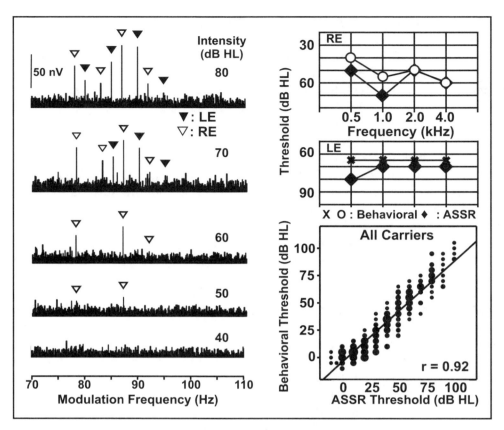

Figure 8–9. Envelope following responses (EFRs) elicited by the dichotic presentation of multifrequency stimuli. The spectral data are plotted as a function of increasing stimulus level (*left*) showing the response peaks for the right ear (*open inverted triangle*) and the left ear (*solid inverted triangle*). The audiograms (*top right*) show the comparison between behavioral (*open circles*) and EFR threshold estimates (*solid circles*). Spectral data for the right ear show peaks down to 50 dB HL with no response peak for the left ear below 70 dB HL. *Bottom right:* Good agreement was found between the behavioral and EFR threshold estimates with a strong correlation between the two measures. Created using data from "Estimating the Audiogram Using Multiple Auditory Steady-State Responses," by A. Dimitrijevic, M. S. John, P. Van Roon, D. W. Purcell, J. Adamonis, J. Ostroff, . . . T. W. Picton, 2002, *Journal of American Academy Audiology, 13*, pp. 205–224.

et al., 2002; Rance & Briggs, 2002; Rance et al., 1995) or multifrequency stimuli (Han, Mo, Liu, Chen, & Huang, 2006; Luts, Desloovere, Kumar, Vandermeersch, & Wouters, 2004; Rodrigues & Lewis, 2010; Van Maanen & Stapells, 2010). Results from studies using single-frequency stimuli and sensorineural hearing loss (ranging from normal to profound) have generally shown a strong correlation (between $r = 0.77$ and 0.96) between EFR threshold and behavioral thresholds from 250 to 4000 Hz. For example, Rance et al. (1995) reported a strong positive correlation ($r = 0.97$) between EFR threshold estimate and behavioral thresholds in young children (mean age 5 to 29 months) with moderate to severe sensorineural hearing loss. Based on the results of these studies, the authors concluded that the single-frequency EFRs provide reliable threshold estimates in young children and may assist in hearing aid fittings.

With respect to the use of multifrequency technique in studying the relationship between EFR threshold and behavioral threshold in hearing-impaired infants and young children, there are only a few published reports (Han et al., 2006; Luts et al., 2004; Rodrigues & Lewis, 2010; Van Mannen & Stappells, 2010). Like the results from the single-frequency studies, these multifrequency EFR studies also reported a strong correlation between EFR threshold and behavioral thresholds. Also, these studies showed a strong correlation between click or tone burst evoked ABR threshold and EFR threshold. For example, Rodrigues and Lewis (2010) found a strong correlation between tone burst ABR threshold and EFR threshold ($r = 0.7$), and between EFR threshold and behavioral thresholds (mean $r = 0.95$). ABR and ASSR were recorded on different days in this study. Van Mannen and Stapells (2010), recording tone-evoked ABR and multifrequency ASSR in the same session, also showed a strong positive correlation between ABR threshold and EFR threshold ($r = 0.97$) with ASSR thresholds 6–12 dB nHL higher than tone burst ABR threshold. Finally, Luts et al. (2004) found a positive correlation between EFR and click-evoked ABR ($r = 0.77$), and between EFR and behavioral thresholds ($r > 0.9$). These strong correlations notwithstanding, caution should be exercised in the use of binaural multifrequency ASSR to estimate hearing thresholds in infants and young children with a sensorineural hearing loss given the paucity of empirical data.

Bone-Conduction Threshold Estimation in Normal and Hearing-Impaired Individuals (BC-EFR)

A relatively few series of papers have been published by Small and colleagues exploring the clinical utility of ASSRs elicited by bone-conducted SAM tones (Small & Stapells, 2006, 2008a, 2008b; Small, Hatton, & Stapells, 2007) in mostly normal-hearing adults and young children. Small and Stapells (2006) reported that mean BC-EFR thresholds in normal-hearing adults were between 15 and 25 dB nHL at carrier frequencies of 500 to 4000 Hz with slightly better thresholds at higher frequencies. These authors also observed appreciably better thresholds (compared to adults at 500 and 1000 Hz) in infants less than 27 weeks of age. Following up on the possibility of maturational effects on BC-EFR thresholds, Small and Stapells (2008a) observed that the BC-EFR threshold increased with age at only the low frequencies, with high-frequency thresholds unaltered. The mean EFR thresholds in young infants/children (birth to 2 years) at low frequencies (500 and 1000 Hz) were 15 to 20 dB better compared to adults (also see Casey & Small, 2014).

Two recently published reports examined the utility of combining AC-EFR and BC-EFR to estimate thresholds in children with normal, conductive hearing loss and cochlear hearing loss (Garcia, de Azevedo, Biaggio, Didone, & Gurgel Testa, 2014; Ismaila, El-Saiid, El-Sebaii, & Fadel, 2016). Ismaila et al. (2016) reported that in children (3–6 years of age) with conductive hearing loss, the mean BC-EFR thresholds closely matched the values for the normal group (minimal normal levels for BC-EFR 23.5 dB HL at 500 Hz; 22.5 dB HL at 1000 Hz, 20 dB HL at 2000 Hz, and 25 dB HL at 4000 Hz), suggesting that BC-EFR is a reliable measure in children with normal and conductive hearing loss. The reliability of the BC-EFR in children with conductive hearing loss is also suggested by the similar results of Garcia et al. (2014). They evaluated 60 children ranging in age from birth to 6 months (30 normal hearing and 30 with conductive pathology). They found that the BC-EFR thresholds across carrier frequencies were similar for the two groups, while the AC-EFR threshold was elevated for the conductive loss group (producing a 20-dB difference in the AC-EFR and BC-EFR threshold), consistent with the presence of a conductive component.

The BC-EFR threshold estimates in children with sensorineural hearing loss appear to be less reliable, particularly for severe-to-profound losses. For mild-to-moderate losses, the BC-EFR was able to provide a reasonably good estimate of the threshold, although the contamination from the presence of spurious responses resulting from electromagnetic artifacts cannot be ruled out completely (Garcia et al., 2014; Swanepoel, Ebrahim, Friedland, Swanepoel, & Pottas, 2008). These authors conclude that BC-EFR may not be a reliable measure in children with a moderate or greater degree of hearing loss because the presence of spurious responses resulting from aliasing, stimulus artifacts, and/or vestibular responses precludes accurate determination of threshold. Collectively, these studies suggest that BC-EFR may complement the AC-EFR threshold in children with normal hearing or with conductive hearing loss. More studies are needed which adequately address the concerns of electromagnetic artifacts and/or aliasing problems during digitization that contaminate the responses, particularly at low frequencies (Picton & John., 2004; Small & Stapells, 2004), thus questioning its validity in estimating thresholds in individuals with a moderate or greater degree of sensorineural hearing loss. These spurious BC-EFR components can be observed as low as 45 dB HL at 500 Hz, 30 dB HL at 1000 Hz, 50 dB HL at 2000 Hz, and 50 dB HL at 4000 Hz (Jeng, Brownt, Johnson, & Vander Werff, 2004; Small & Stapells, 2004). Picton & John (2004) have suggested the use of antialiasing techniques and/or alternate stimulus polarity to minimize spurious responses contaminating the BC-EFR.

Several methodological considerations that could affect the EFR threshold include the method used to couple the bone vibrator to the skull, location of the vibrator placement, and differences in ipsilateral and contralateral recordings. Small et al. (2007) observed similar EFR thresholds using an elastic headband or handheld coupling of the bone vibrator; higher EFR thresholds (12–19 dB) when using forehead placement versus temporal or mastoid placements; and only infants showed better EFR thresholds (10–13 dB) across carrier frequencies for ipsilateral recordings compared to contralateral recordings with no differences observed in adults. From this discussion, BC-EFR currently offers limited clinical application as an excellent validation of tone-elicited ABR thresholds. More widespread clinical application in the estimation of reliable thresholds in infants and young children with different types and degrees of hearing loss will have to await sufficient and compelling AC-EFR and BC-EFR data.

IV. EFRS ELICITED BY SPEECH SOUNDS

Here we focus on the description of EFRs to speech syllables that presumably has greater potential to identify temporal processing deficits in a range of clinical population with language-based learning problems, including children with dyslexia, specific language impairment, and autism spectrum disorders. A wide range of speech stimuli has been used in the extant speech EFR literature to study EFR and FFR (Aiken & Picton, 2006, 2008; Ananthakrishnan, Krishnan, & Bartlett, 2016; Ananthakrishnan et al., 2017; Banai et al., 2009; Chandrasekaran et al., 2009; Hornickel & Kraus, 2013; Krishnan, 2002; Strait, Hornickel, & Kraus, 2011; Suresh & Krishnan, 2020; Suresh, Krishnan, & Luo, 2020). However, the consonant-vowel (CV) syllable /da/ is a commonly used stimulus to examine the EFR and its utility in different clinical populations as a metric of the integrity of neural response timing and neural synchronization (e.g., Banai et al., 2009; Chandrasekaran et al., 2009; Hornickel & Kraus, 2013; Jones et al., 2020; Kraus & Nicol, 2018; Krizman, Skoe, Marian, & Kraus, 2014; Otto-Meyer, Krizman, White-Schwoch, & Kraus, 2018; Strait et al., 2011; White-Schwoch et al., 2015). Recording and analysis software using this stimulus has been implemented in several commercially available auditory evoked potential systems, although it is not clear what specific audiologic applications these responses are appropriate for at an individual level. Although there is no clear compelling rationale for the specific choice of the CV syllable /da/, the spectrotemporal characteristics of speech sounds in general are quite distinct from nonspeech periodic complex sounds, although both have an envelope and temporal fine-structure components. It may be that this behaviorally relevant speech sound has the advantage to examine onset, dynamic, and steady-state neural activity that may show increased susceptibility to degradation in individuals with auditory temporal processing deficits.

Characteristics of Speech Stimuli

Natural speech sounds are produced by the airstream from the lungs setting the vocal cords into a complex periodic vibration. This complex source waveform is then shaped by changes in the vocal tract configuration using articulators. Different articulator configurations change the resonance characteristics of the vocal tract, resulting in amplification of certain harmonics (formants) and attenuation of other non-formant-related harmonics. Thus, speech sounds produced in this manner by imparting different vocal tract (filter) shapes will have distinct and unique formant patterns associated with a given sound but with the same fundamental periodicity for a given talker. For example, English vowels /a/ and /u/ can be differentiated based on the differences in the first two (male productions of vowel /a/: F1 is about 700 Hz, and F2 is about 1100 Hz; and for vowel /u/: F1 is about 300 Hz, and F2 is about 900 Hz with f0 equal to 100 Hz) to three formant frequency locations (Liberman, Cooper, & Gerstman, 1954). Similarly, CV syllables /ba/, /da/, and /ga/ can be distinguished based on their different F2 formant transition trajectories (Liberman, Cooper, & Gerstman, 1954). While steady-state speech sounds can be synthesized to better control spectrotemporal parameters for experimental studies, natural speech productions are inherently dynamic and time variant. That is, they may contain frication noise bursts at the onset and formant transitions (change in formant frequencies over time) as in the case of the CV syllable /da/. Shown in Figure 8–10 are the time waveform, spectrogram, and average spectrum of the CV syllable /da/. The 170-ms time waveform is characterized by an initial relatively small amplitude frication noise burst about 10 ms in duration (peak energy of this noise is around

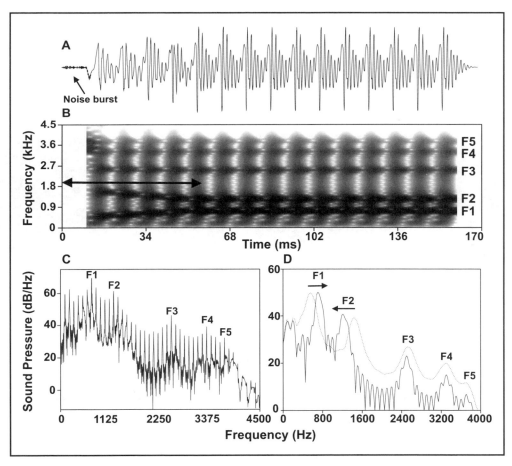

Figure 8–10. The waveform (**A**), spectrogram (**B**), average spectrum (**C**), and instant spectra at two different temporal points in the stimulus waveform (**D**) for the CV syllable /da/. The waveform shows the initial plosive noise burst followed by a voiced periodic segment. The spectrogram shows the time-variant first and second formant over the first 40 to 50 ms, followed by a steady-state period over the remaining segment. The formant frequencies are identified to the right. The instant spectra show the increase in F1 frequency and a decrease in F2 frequency (indicated by the right- and left-pointing arrows, respectively) over time.

4000 Hz) followed by the periodic voiced portion (envelope periodicity of 100 Hz, peaks 10 ms apart). As shown in the spectrogram in Figure 8–10, the F1 frequency increases from about 550 Hz at the onset of the sound to about 730 Hz; F2 decreases from about 1500 Hz at the onset to about 1220 Hz over the first 50 ms, and both remain unaltered thereafter, indicated by the essentially parallel bands for F1 and F2. F3 (2500 Hz) and F4 (3330 Hz) and the smaller F5 (3750 Hz) are time invariant throughout the duration of the stimulus. The f0 is constant at 100 Hz throughout the syllable. The average spectrum on the right in Figure 8–10 illustrates the spectral envelope wherein amplitude progressively decreases for successively higher formants.

Response Characteristics of the EFR to the CV Syllable /da/

General Description

Typically, EFRs are recorded either monaurally or binaurally at suprathreshold stimulus levels between 65 and 80 dB SPL. As shown in Figure 8–11, the complex waveform of the EFR to the CV syllable /da/ is characterized by an onset response to initial noise burst (the V-A component is essentially the onset wave V of the ABR to clicks but longer in latency due to smaller amplitude and more gradual rise-fall times) followed by sustained EFR to the envelope periodicity of the time-variant vowel

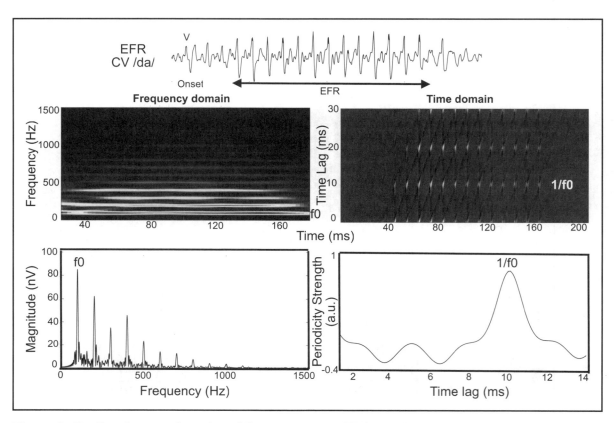

Figure 8–11. Grand averaged envelope following response (EFR) waveform in response to the CV syllable /da/ (*top*), and the frequency-domain (*left*) and time-domain (*right*) characterizations of the response. The spectrogram (*left, middle row*) shows robust bands of phase-locked activity at the f0 and lower harmonics over the duration of the stimulus. Consistent with this, the autocorrelogram (*right, middle row*), which measures the phase-locked periodicities over the duration of the stimulus, shows a clear band of activity at a delay of 10 ms, which is the period of the 100-Hz fundamental frequency of the stimulus. The average spectrum (*bottom row, left*) shows robust peaks at the f0 and several harmonics. The autocorrelation function (ACF), which measures the neural periodicity strength, shows a robust peak at 10 ms, which is the period of the 100-Hz f0.

/a/ (Akhoun et al., 2008; Hornickel, Skoe, Nicol, Zecker, & Krau, 2009; Johnson et al., 2008a). Based on the EFRs to a shorter (40 ms) version of the CV /da/, the onset response to the initial burst has been labeled as V and A, and a small offset response O (variable and not readily discernible in all individuals), with several cycles of the EFR, identified as D, E, and F. Frequency domain analysis reveals a robust peak at the fundamental frequency and several integer multiples of the f0 reflecting primarily rectifier distortion products and not phase-locking to the temporal fine structure of the sound. However, small contributions from the frequency doubling effect for neural components seen at low frequencies when responses to alternating polarities are added cannot be completely ruled out.

Effects of Stimulus Polarity on Speech-Evoked EFR

Since EFRs are derived by adding the responses to condensation and rarefaction polarity, one area of concern is the effects of asymmetry on the response to each polarity on the added EFR. Small polarity differences in EFR amplitude exist, and they show individual differences and tend to vary across stimuli (Aiken & Purcell, 2013; Easwar et al., 2015; Greenberg, 1980; Kumar, Bhat, D'Costa, Srivastava, & Kalaiah, 2013). Easwar et al. (2015) examined these differences in the EFRs to vowel /e/ in a natural hVd context, different vowels with or without the first harmonic, and carriers with resolved and unresolved harmonic components presented at 80 dB SPL. For vowel /e/, they found a difference of greater than 39 nV in 30% of their subjects. In addition, they found a significant EFR amplitude difference for vowels with lower F1 frequencies with the first harmonic present (like vowel /u/), and for carriers with resolved harmonics compared to a high-frequency carrier with unresolved harmonics. In contrast, using the shorter CV syllable /da/ (40 ms), Kumar et al. (2013) did not see any significant effect of polarity on the amplitude of the EFR. Asymmetry in the stimulus envelope relative to the baseline for the two polarities and overlap of FFR component at the first harmonic (h1) and the fundamental EFR periodicity likely contribute, at least in part, to these differences. Given that EFR amplitude may be influenced by polarity effects and consequently their detection in some individuals, it may be better to use the most robust response from a single polarity. However, it should be noted that a single polarity response reflects a combination of the EFR and FFR components, albeit dominated by the EFR.

Test-Retest Reliability of the EFRs

Stability and good repeatability of the response indices from session to session are crucial for the validity of EFRs in clinical and research applications. Song, Nicol, and Kraus (2011) examined the intrasubject test-retest reliability of the /da/ EFRs in two groups of young adults where measures were obtained in quiet and in the presence of two- and six-tasker babble in two different recording sessions separated by 41 to 58 days. Both the time domain (RMS amplitude, stimulus-to response correlation, and latency) and frequency domain (spectral analysis) response indices indicated that the EFR to the CV syllable was remarkably stable and replicated well from session to session both in quiet and in the presence of the multitasker babble. Bidelman, Pousson, Dugas, and Fehrenbach (2018) reported that the test-retest reliability of the speech-FFR is better than the ABR. More recently, Easwar, Scollie, Aiken, and Purcell (2020) examined the between-session test-retest reliability of the characteristics of the EFRs elicited in young adults using two different modulations contained in a speech token (/susaʃi/) presented at 65 dB SPL. Their results showed a good correlation between repeated measurements with no significant differences in EFR amplitude or phase coherence between sessions. The small variability that they did observe could not be explained by the differences in the noise variance between sessions, leading the authors to speculate that differences in efferent modulation of the brainstem response may be at play.

Stimulus Specificity of the EFR

A fundamental question is whether the spectrotemporal characteristics of the sustained EFR to different speech syllables with the same periodicity are distinct. To the extent that the EFR reflects primarily neural phase-locking to the temporal envelope periodicity, it is reasonable to assume that the brainstem neurons will simply follow the envelope periodicity without regard to the contents of the envelope for different complex sounds with the same envelope periodicity. To examine this, we recorded responses to a range of complex sounds including CV syllables /da/, /ba/, steady vowel /a/, a 15-harmonic complex tone, and iterated rippled noise (IRN) with a delay of 10 ms—all with a fundamental periodicity of 100 Hz. The IRN stimulus does not have a prominent envelope but imparts a temporal regularity. As expected, the spectrotemporal characteristics of the EFRs across stimuli were qualitatively similar (except for the EFRs to IRN) with robust response waveforms following the envelope periodicity (Figure 8–12, left). Time-domain autocorrelation functions (ACFs), reflecting the strength of phase-locking at the fundamental periodicity showed sharp peaks 10 ms (period of the 100-Hz periodicity) and progressively smaller peaks at delays corresponding to the periods of the 2f0 and 3f0 (Figure 8–12, middle). This pattern becomes even clearer in the frequency domain spectral data that show essentially similar spectral characteristics for all stimuli except IRN (Figure 8–12, right). The EFR to the IRN is relatively smaller in amplitude with no clear periodicity in the response, smaller ACF peaks (expected, since IRN does not have a prominent envelope), and distinct spectra compared to the other complex sounds.

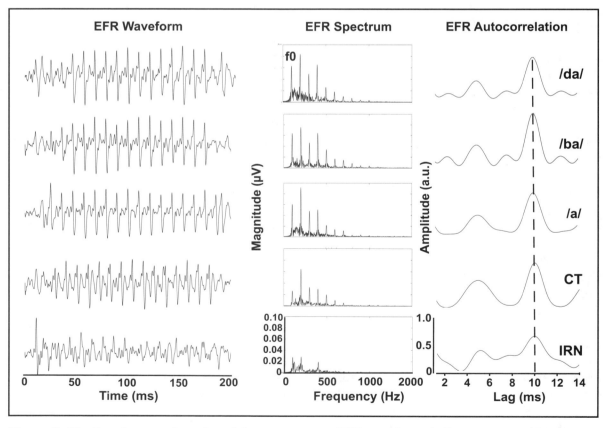

Figure 8–12. Grand averaged envelope following response (EFR) waveforms (*left*), spectra (*middle*), and autocorrelation functions (ACFs) for different complex sounds with the same f0. Except for the response to the IRN stimuli, the other complex stimuli elicit robust EFRs that are to a first approximation essentially similar in terms of the waveform, spectra, and ACFs. This is not surprising since the EFR represents largely neural phase-locking to envelope periodicity. Also, the weak response to the iterated rippled noise (IRN) stimulus is expected because they do not have a prominent envelope periodicity cue.

These findings suggest that the spectrotemporal characteristics of EFR are not stimulus specific but rather reflect primarily neural phase-locking to the temporal envelope periodicity.

Potential Clinical Applications of EFRs

While there are no specific EFR applications that are routinely used in clinics at the current time, we describe here potential clinical applications in characterizing the nature of the neural encoding degradation resulting from cochlear impairments and indexing hearing aid outcomes. EFRs have been used extensively to describe the disruption in neural timing and neural encoding at the brainstem level in populations with a variety of language-based learning problems, including specific language impairment, dyslexia, autism spectrum disorders, the influence of bilingualism, and in monitoring auditory training gains (Banai & Kraus, 2008; Banai et al. 2009; Banai, Nicol, Zecker, & Kraus, 2005; Chandrasekaran et al., 2009; Cunningham, Nicol, Zecker, Bradlow, & Kraus, 2001; Hornickel et al., 2009; Jones et al., 2020; Krizman et al., 2014; Krizman, Slater, Skoe, Marian, & Kraus, 2015; Otto-Meyer et al., 2018; Russo, Nicol, Trommer, Zecker, & Kraus, 2009; Song, Skoe, Wong, & Kraus, 2008).

Effects of Cochlear Impairment on Envelope Encoding

Both EFR and FFR represent sustained phase-locked neural activity in the brainstem that has been shown to preserve information about certain acoustic features important for auditory perception in general, and speech perception specifically. The reduced high-frequency audibility and/or broadened auditory filters consequent to cochlear hearing loss may account for the deterioration of neural representation of the envelope, which in turn may reduce the ability to discriminate differences in f0 (Bacon & Gleitmann, 1992; Bacon & Veimeister, 1985; Leek & Summers, 1996; Strickland & Viemeister, 1996). It is likely that in the presence of significant hearing impairment in the high frequencies, information about f0 is largely derived from the interactions between the multiple high-frequency unresolved multiple components falling in a widened auditory filter (Cariani & Delgutte, 1996a, 1996b; Meddis & O'Mard, 1997; Sayles & Winter, 2008). Speech perception deficits consequent to cochlear hearing loss, central auditory processing deficits, and age-related structural and functional changes in the auditory peripheral and central mechanisms may reflect, at least in part, a degradation or disruption in the neural representation of acoustic features important for speech perception. Ananthakrishnan et al. (2016) reported smaller EFR amplitude at f0 in individuals with a mild-to-moderate sensorineural hearing loss compared to normal-hearing individuals for a steady-state vowel stimulus presented at equal SPLs. Their observation of f0 amplitude increase with intensity (presented at equal SL) at the same rate in both groups suggests that the reduced f0 amplitude observed in the hearing-impaired group is likely due to reduced audibility in the impaired high frequencies (see Figure 8–25). Restoring audibility in the high frequencies will likely minimize the difference between the two groups. Hao et al. (2018) evaluated EFR and FFR elicited by the CV syllable /da/ in quiet and in noise in subjects with normal and cochlear hearing loss identified as presbycusis. Like Ananthakrishnan et al. (2016), they reported a significant decrease in the EFR amplitude and stimulus-response correlation in the hearing-impaired group, both in quiet and in the presence of noise. However, the reduction in the noise condition was greater for the normal group compared to the hearing-impaired group, suggesting possible differences in the effectiveness of suppressive masking in the two groups. These authors also observed a weak association between better performance on the SIN test and larger EFR amplitude, only for the quiet condition. Based on these findings, it is clear that EFR indices are sufficiently robust to capture alterations in the temporal encoding of the envelope resulting from cochlear hearing loss. Both reduced audibility and an alteration in the balance between the envelope and TFS encoding in adverse listening conditions in the hearing-impaired group may, at least in part, account for the difficulties in speech perception in noise.

In contrast to the results showing reduced envelope coding in hearing-impaired individuals, a couple of studies have reported enhanced envelope representation consequent to cochlear hearing loss (Anderson, Parbery-Clark, White-Schwoch, Drehobl, & Kraus, 2013; Kale & Heinz, 2010). Anderson et al. (2013) observed enhanced envelope representation in individuals with mild-to-moderate cochlear hearing loss presumably due to a reduction in inhibition, enhancement of the excitatory mechanisms, and the possibility of enhanced component interactions in the high-frequency regions due to widening of the auditory filter consequent to cochlear hearing loss (Vale & Sanes, 2002), These authors observed envelope enhancement only when the stimulus was adjusted for audibility and/or in the presence of background noise. Differences in the way equal audibility was defined in the Anderson et al. (2013) and Ananthakrishnan et al. (2016) studies could account for the absence of enhanced F0 in the latter study. Also, the enriched high-frequency content of the CV syllables used in the Anderson et al. (2013) study compared to the relatively restricted low-frequency spectrum of the vowel /u/ used in the Ananthakrishnan et al. (2016) study may elicit a more robust EFR component because of the greater contributions from the high-frequency regions. Kale and Heinz (2010) also reported enhanced envelope representation in chinchillas with noise-induced sensorineural hearing loss, which they attribute to the very steep rate-level functions resulting from a loss of a greater number of IHCs in moderate-severe hearing losses. Their suggestion that this envelope enhancement is minimized in mild-moderate hearing losses with lesser IHC involvement (and therefore more gradual rate-level functions) may account for the absence of envelope enhancement by Ananthakrishnan et al. (2016). It is also possible that the ensemble activity from a population of neurons with different thresholds and rate-level functions reflected in the scalp-recorded EFR could obscure the enhancement observed by Kale and Heinz (2010) at the single-unit level.

Utility of EFR in Hearing Aid Outcome Measure

The ability to record robust EFRs to long speech samples simulating running speech and its temporal envelope lends itself well to provide an objective metric to evaluate benefits from amplification. Such longer-duration stimuli with longer interstimulus intervals are optimal for use with hearing aids because they can more accurately capture the nonlinear properties of amplification implemented in hearing aids (Easwar, Purcell, & Scollie, 2012). Easwar and colleagues utilize an innovative approach that uses a series of consonant-vowel complexes that resemble the temporal envelope of running speech to elicit the EFRs. Frequency specificity and bandwidth are also important considerations in measuring hearing aid benefits, since hearing loss and hearing aid gain are frequency dependent, and speech intelligibility and quality are dependent on sufficiently wide bandwidth to represent a wide range of speech frequencies. Consistent with these considerations, Easwar, Purcell, Aiken, Parsa, and Scollie (2015a) created a speech stimulus (soosaashee) consisting of vowels and fricatives, where vowels carry the most energy at low and mid frequencies and fricatives carry the most energy at the high frequencies. To improve frequency specificity and to minimize cancellations resulting from latency differences resulting from differences in cochlear places contributing to the response, the f0 of each vowel in "soosaashee" was lowered in the low-frequency formant region without altering the f0 in the second and higher formant regions. The fricatives were amplitude modulated at the speaker's average f0 to be able to elicit an EFR. Thus, for each vowel, two robust EFRs with unaltered amplitude and detectability (Easwar, Scollie, & Purcell, 2019) are simultaneously elicited—one from the first formant and one from the higher formants with their amplitudes and detectability (an idea similar to the multifrequency EFRs described earlier). The final version of this stimulus could then elicit EFRs, representing low, mid, and high frequencies. EFRs elicited by this stimulus in unaided (using insert earphone) and aided (through individually fitted hearing aids) conditions at two levels (50- and 65-dB SPL, representing soft and conversational speech level) were used to measure hearing aid benefit in adults with mild-to-moderate sloping sensorineural hearing loss (Easwar et al., 2015b). Their results showed that aided conditions revealed a higher number of EFRs with greater amplitude compared to the unaided condition with more change observed for mid- to high-frequency stimuli compared to low-frequency stimuli (Figure 8–13). The larger change for mid- to high-frequency stimuli reflected the larger improvements in sensation level of stimuli, measured behaviorally. Also, as bandwidth increased, the number of detectable EFRs and their amplitude increased in a frequency-specific manner that correlated with improvements in speech understanding as well as sound quality rating (Figure 8–14). These findings suggest that EFRs are capable of measuring changes in both audibility and aided audible bandwidth.

Finally, the optimal utility of EFRs for aided applications depends on how accurately they differentiate audible from inaudible speech. Easwar et al. (2020) reported that the accuracy of EFRs appears to be *dependent on the specific statistical indicator* used to detect the EFRs. Relative to the F-ratio that compares the EFR amplitude with that of noise, Hotelling's T^2 and phase coherence that uses phase and amplitude, or only phase information, respectively, from every stimulus trial, improve the performance of EFRs in terms of sensitivity (true positive rate; detected when the stimulus is audible). While the sensitivity was ~68% for both Hotelling's T^2 and phase coherence, it was ~60% for the F-ratio. Stimulus levels in this study varied from 20 dB SPL (close to the threshold) to conversational-level speech (65 dB SPL). Likewise, the accuracy of EFRs is also *stimulus dependent*, with fricative stimuli providing the best sensitivity. The sensitivity was ~88% to 90% for the fricatives and ranged between 57% and 71% for the vowel stimuli. The stimulus dependency likely reflects the minimum sensation level needed to detect an EFR. EFRs elicited by fricative stimuli can be detected as close to 2 to 4 dB above threshold, whereas EFRs elicited by vowel F2+ stimuli need the level to be 8 to 12 dB above threshold. Likewise, EFRs elicited by vowel

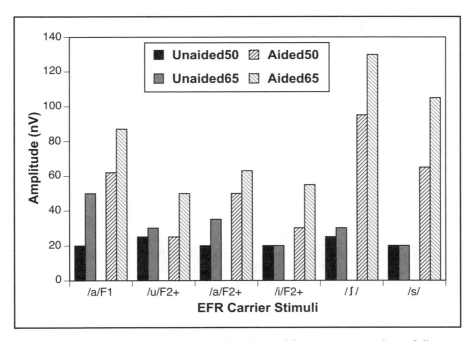

Figure 8–13. Effect of stimulus level and amplification on envelope following response (EFR) amplitude. At both levels (solid back and gray squares), significant improvement in EFR magnitude with amplification (stipples squares) is observed for almost all stimuli with the aided increase in EFR amplitude more pronounced for the fricatives. Data from "Evaluation of Speech-Evoked Envelope Following Responses as an Objective Aided Outcome Measure: Effect of Stimulus Level, Bandwidth, and Amplification in Adults With Hearing Loss," by V. Easwar, D. W. Purcell, S. J. Aiken, V. Parsa, and S. D. Scollie, 2015, *Ear and Hearing, 36*(6), pp. 635–652.

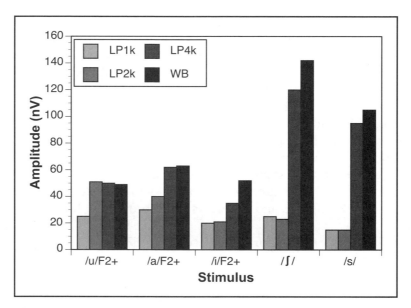

Figure 8–14. Effect of bandwidth on envelope following response (EFR) amplitude for individual F2+ carriers and fricatives. Individual F1 carriers for /u/, /a/, and /i/ did not show significant differences across bandwidth and therefore are not plotted here. Responses are generally larger for broader bandwidth stimuli and particularly for the fricatives. LP, low-pass filter; WB, full bandwidth. Created using data from "Evaluation of Speech-Evoked Envelope Following Responses as an Objective Aided Outcome Measure: Effect of Stimulus Level, Bandwidth, and Amplification in Adults With Hearing Loss," by V. Easwar, D. W. Purcell, S. J. Aiken, V. Parsa, and S. D. Scollie, 2015, *Ear and Hearing, 36*(6), pp. 635–652.

F1 stimuli needed the level to be 13 to 22 dB above the threshold. These estimates were obtained in normal-hearing individuals.

Jenkins, Fodor, Presacco, and Anderson (2018) evaluated the effects of amplification on neural encoding of a speech signal (CV syllable /ga/) in older hearing-impaired (mild-to-moderate sensorineural hearing loss [SNHL]) first-time users of hearing aids. They reasoned that amplification may result in improved neural representation of certain acoustic features (higher amplitudes, improved phase-locking, and earlier latencies), particularly features that are less audible. Free-field unaided and aided EFRs were recorded in sound-field quiet (65 dB SPL and 80 dB SPL) and in the presence of multitalker babble at +10 SNR. As predicted, amplification increased phase-locking and response amplitude (particularly for the less audible transition segments) while decreasing response latency. However, they observed substantial intersubject variability in the hearing-impaired individuals. While these approaches are well motivated and promising, additional studies in individuals with hearing loss (with and without hearing aids) across age are needed to validate these initial findings to move progressively toward effective clinical use. In addition, knowledge about how amplification characteristics selectively alter neural encoding would be useful to enable the application of these neural measures to optimize signal processing strategies that would be most appropriate at the individual level.

V. FREQUENCY FOLLOWING RESPONSE (FFR)

General Description

In the last decade, there has been a steady increase in utilizing the FFR/EFR to address clinical/

research questions as reflected by an appreciable increase in published studies on EFR and FFR using a variety of complex sounds. The focus clearly has shifted, rightfully so, in applying FFRs to evaluate the integrity of neural encoding of complex sounds as a metric of auditory temporal processing in normal and impaired ears, to explore age-related changes in neural encoding, and to understand the role of experience-dependent plasticity in shaping subcortical processing and its application to training and perceptual learning. The FFR, first described by Moushegian, Rupert, and Stillman (1973), is different from both ABR and EFR. Unlike the onset-sensitive ABR, the FFR reflects sustained neural activity among a population of neural elements that is phase-locked to the individual cycles of the stimulus waveform. Also, unlike EFR, which merely follows the envelope periodicity of a complex sound, the scalp-recorded FFR represents sustained phase-locking to the individual cycles of a pure tone (between 100 and 1700 Hz—the upper-frequency limit for FFR) and phase-locking to the TFS of complex sounds. Unlike the flat spectrum of a complex harmonic tone, the long-term average speech spectrum characteristically shows a 6-dB/octave decrease in spectral energy above about 500 Hz. Thus, the ability to generate a recordable FFR to a speech sound is constrained by both a frequency and a level limit.

Sustained neural phase-locking to low-frequency tones has been well demonstrated among a large proportion of brainstem neurons and in near-field recordings from almost all nuclei along the brainstem. Currently, the clinical uitility of the FFR is very limited. However, there is a substantial and growing interest in using the FFR to evaluate the functional integrity of temporal encoding of complex sounds and how they are altered by hearing impairment, and tonal language and music experience. Here we describe the characteristics of human FFR elicited by a variety of stimuli ranging from simple tone bursts to more complex sounds including tonal complexes, and steady-state and time-variant speech sounds with a focus on studies that have potential clinical applications. The use of the FFRs in addressing basic science questions relevant to the encoding of complex sounds, processing of pitch relevant information, and how it is shaped by experience and aging-related decline in neural encoding are discussed in the next chapter.

Response Characteristics

Frequency Following Response to Tone Bursts

Most tone burst–elicited evaluation of FFR has been largely limited to the 500-Hz stimulus with a handful of studies exploring the effects of stimulus frequency. The tone burst–evoked FFR, like the ABR, is rather small in amplitude (several hundred nanovolts) and can be recorded easily using the same data acquisition procedures used for ABR recording (Figure 8–15). However, care should be taken to ensure that overlapping contamination by CM and/or stimulus artifact is minimized. Worden and Marsh (1968) compared the FFRs recorded from multiple nuclei along the brainstem in cats, and the round window–recorded CM from the same animals. They observed several differences between the two measures: CM latency (1–2 ms) was much shorter than the FFR (3–6 ms), with FFR latency increasing with recordings from increasingly rostral structures along the brainstem; FFR spectra show robust peaks at harmonics of the fundamental frequency (presumably reflecting rectifier distortion products associated with cochlear transduction), while the more sinusoidal CM did not exhibit harmonic distortion; FFR appears to disappear earlier compared to CM in terminal anoxia, suggesting that the FFR is sensitive to changes in the normal metabolism of neural tissue; and FFR amplitude decreases gradually over the duration of the response, suggesting neural adaptation. The upper-frequency limit of FFR at the auditory nerve level is approximately 5 kHz, consistent with the upper limit of peripheral auditory phase-locking for single units (Rose, Brugge, Anderson, & Hind, 1967), while the CM was recordable out to 40 kHz in the cat; and FFR recorded from the ventral cochlear nucleus or medial superior olive is abolished after cochlear nerve section or cryogenic cooling of the ventral cochlear nucleus, whereas the CM remains unaltered by either manipulation (Marsh, Worden, & Smith, 1970).

Effects of Stimulus Level

Like the ABR, the FFR increases in amplitude with increasing signal level (Figure 8–16) up to about 65 to 75 dB SPL and then asymptotes or decreases

242 *Auditory Brainstem Evoked Potentials: Clinical and Research Applications*

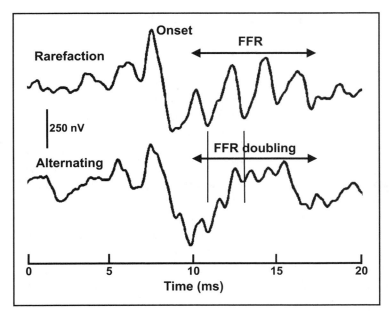

Figure 8–15. Frequency following response (FFR) waveforms elicited by 500-Hz tone burst with rarefaction onset polarity (*top*) and alternating onset polarity (*bottom*). The FFR to rarefaction polarity shows a robust onset response followed by a smaller amplitude but clear cycles of FFR. The response to the alternating phase shows an equally robust onset response, but the following FFR is even smaller in amplitude and doubles in frequency. The two vertical lines corresponding to one period (2 ms here) clearly show the doubling effect. Adapted with permission from "The Frequency Following Response and the Onset Response: Evaluation of Frequency Specificity Using a Forward-Masking Paradigm," by A. K. Ananthanarayan and J. D. Durrant, 1992, *Ear and Hearing*, *13*(4), pp. 228–233.

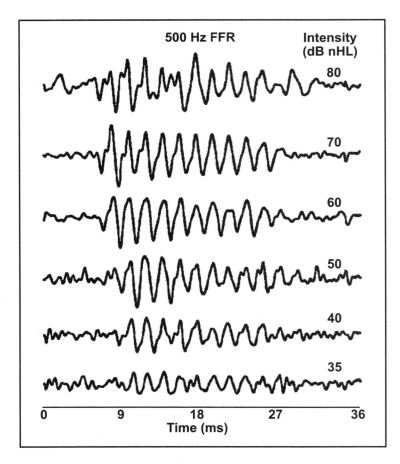

Figure 8–16. Frequency following responses (FFRs) elicited by a 500-Hz tone burst plotted as a function of stimulus level. Note the progressive decrease in amplitude and latency prolongation as stimulus intensity is decreased. Adapted with permission from *Auditory Evoked Potentials: Basic Principles and Clinical Application*, by R. Burkard, M. Don, and J. J. Eggermont, 2006, Wolters Kluwer Health, Inc, Philadelphia, PA.

with further increase in signal level (Krishnan, 2007; Marsh, Brown, & Smith, 1975). Similar amplitude behavior has been reported for the multiple components generated by complex stimuli (Krishnan, 1999, 2002; Pandya & Krishnan, 2004). Both an increase in synchronized discharge rate of auditory neurons and an increase in the number of neural elements phase-locked to the stimulus likely account for the amplitude growth with increasing stimulus level. Because of the increasing time delay in the traveling wave in more apical regions, high-frequency units will discharge sooner than will low-frequency units. Consequently, growth in FFR amplitude due to neural recruitment should be reflected in the onset latency of the FFR. Description of the behavior of FFR onset latency is complicated by the difficulty in accurately measuring the onset latency of the FFR. Two factors contribute to this difficulty. First, the longer rise times typically used for the stimulus to minimize the onset response makes it difficult to determine which stimulus cycle is effective in eliciting the response. Second, onset components can still overlap the initial portion of the FFR. Several studies report that the latency of the FFR is between 5.5 and 7 ms to a 500-Hz tone burst (Glaser, Suter, Dasheiff, & Goldberg, 1976; Greenberg et al., 1987). The few reports on FFR latency suggest that, unlike the ABR, the FFR onset latency to simple tone bursts does not change appreciably over a wide range of stimulus levels (Marsh, Worden, & Smith, 1975; Huis in't Veld, Osterhammel, & Terkildsen, 1977). Interestingly, the phase of single-unit synchronization remains constant as a function of stimulus level only for units tuned to the stimulus frequency (Anderson, Rose, Hind, & Brugge, 1971). However, Stillman, Crow, and Moushegian (1978) have shown that the fourth cycle of their FFR changed 2.2 ms over a 55-dB dynamic range. Later cycles of the FFR components have been shown to change in latency with changes in stimulus level. More recently, Bidelman and Powers (2018), characterized the input-output function and latency of FFRs elicited by both speech and tones. They reported that the FFR amplitude increased with stimulus level (25–80 dB SPL) with a steeper growth function for tones compared to speech. Response latency decreased 4 to 5 ms over the same range of intensity change with shorter latencies for speech compared to tones.

Effects of Stimulus Frequency

The scalp-recorded human FFR can be evoked by tones of frequencies below about 2000 Hz (Bidelman & Powers, 2018; Glaser et al., 1976; Moushegian et al., 1973). The upper-frequency limit for the FFR is consistent with decreases in the upper-frequency limit of phase-locking with ascending nuclei along the auditory brainstem pathway. The upper-frequency limit is approximately 5 kHz for the cochlear nucleus, 3 to 4 kHz for the trapezoid body and medial superior olive, and 1.5 to 2 kHz for lateral lemniscus and IC (Starr & Hellerstein, 1971). Preliminary unpublished findings from our laboratory indicate that shorter-latency FFR components, presumably from more caudal generators, may be recordable to frequencies as high as 3000 Hz using ear canal electrodes in a horizontal electrode montage (similar to King, Hopkins, & Plack, 2016). More robust higher-frequency FFRs have been reported for the horizontal montage than for the vertical montage (Galbraith, Bagasan, & Sulahian, 2001). The FFR threshold is approximately 45 to 50 dB SPL for a 500-Hz tone burst and increases appreciably with increasing frequency (Gardi, Salamy, & Mendelson, 1979; Glaser et al., 1976; Huis in't Veld, Osterhammel, & Terkildsen, 1977; Marsh et al., 1975; Stillman, Moushegian, & Rupert, 1976). However, FFR thresholds can be as low as 20 dB SPL for a 500-Hz tone burst for near-field recordings from within auditory brainstem nuclei. This is due in part to the properties of volume conduction. There can be a dramatic decrease in signal size from near-field to scalp responses in the simultaneous recording of FFR in the cat, making it often unnecessary to average the near-field FFR. Increased noise from cortical neural activity and muscle potentials also contributes to the decrease in the SNR for scalp recordings. FFR amplitude decreases with increasing frequency (Figure 8–17) for tone bursts, two-tone stimuli, increasing harmonic number of a multitone complex (Figure 8–18), and synthetic speech sounds (Gardi, Salamy, & Mendelson, 1979; Glaser et al., 1976; Greenberg et al., 1987; Krishnan & Parkinson, 2000; Marsh et al., 1975; Rickman, Chertoff, & Hecox, 1991). Since FFR amplitude provides an index of the degree of phase-locking in the neural elements that generate the FFR, this amplitude reduction may reflect a reduction in phase-locking ability with increasing frequency. Direct comparisons of phase-locking strength (Bidelman, 2018) revealed FFRs were modulated by stimulus frequency and anatomical level (see Figure 8–18). Amplitudes became progressively weaker in all sources with increasing frequency, consistent with

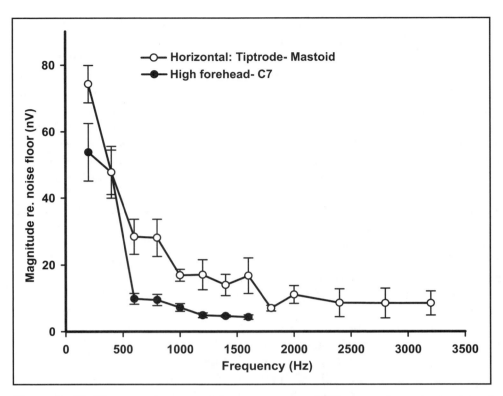

Figure 8–17. The mean frequency following response (FFR) spectral magnitude plotted as a function of stimulus frequency for the vertical electrode montage (*solid circles*) and the horizontal recording montage (*open circles*). For both, response amplitude decreases precipitously for frequencies above about 400 Hz. No repeatable response components were detectable above about 1600 Hz for the vertical montage. In contrast, a small but repeatable response was detectable up to about 3200 Hz. The higher upper-frequency limit observed in the horizontal montage may reflect a combination of the upper-frequency limit for more caudal FFR generators (reflected in the horizontal montage) and the possibility of cochlear microphonics contributing to these responses.

the roll-off of neural phase-locking at higher anatomical levels. Phase-locking strength progressively decreased from the AN to the IC, and from the IC to the primary auditory cortex (PAC).

VI. FREQUENCY FOLLOWING RESPONSES TO COMPLEX SOUNDS

Since phase-locked neural activity to complex sounds is dominated by EFR components to the envelope periodicity, the FFR to the temporal fine structure must be derived by subtracting the responses to condensation and a rarefaction onset polarity to minimize the EFR and enhance the TFS response component (Figure 8–19). The spectra of the subtracted TFS response to a two-tone stimulus not only contain phase-locked activity representing the two tonal frequencies but also the brainstem representation of the cochlear nonlinearity, the cubic difference tone at 2f1-f2 (Chertoff, Hecox, & Goldstein, 1992; Elsisy & Krishnan, 2008; Hall, 1979; Krishnan, 1999; Pandya & Krishnan, 2004; Rickman et al., 1991).

Frequency Following Responses Representing Cochlear Nonlinearity

Most of our understanding of the cochlear initiation sites and characteristics of the cubic distortion

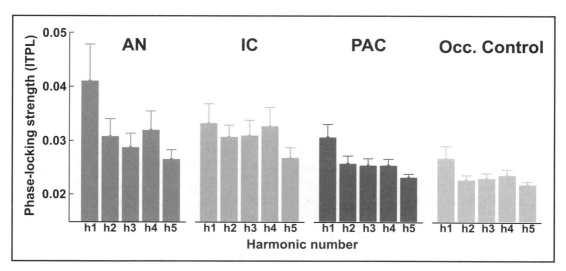

Figure 8–18. Mean frequency following response (FFR) phase-locking strength as a function of increasing harmonic number from different generator sources (auditory nerve [AN], brainstem [BS], primary auditory cortex [PAC], and occipital control response). The envelope following response (EFR) from the brainstem shows the strongest phase-locking at f0 (H1), with the cortical response indistinguishable from the control representing the noise floor. Note the decrease in phase-locking strength as the harmonic number increases consistent with the decrease in neural phase-locking ability as frequency increases. Unpublished figures courtesy of Dr. G. M. Bidelman.

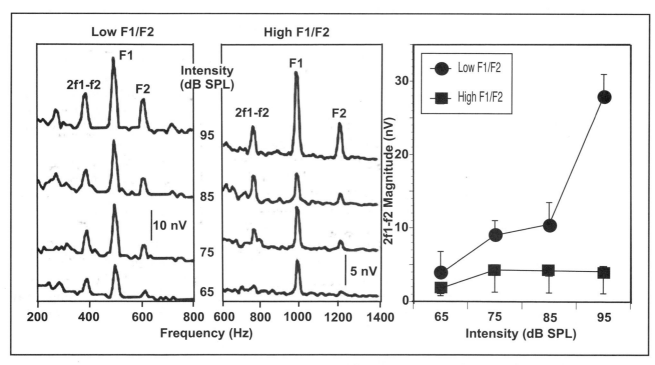

Figure 8–19. *Left, middle:* The frequency following response (FFR) spectra plotted as a function of intensity for a low F1/F2 and high F1/F2 primary pair, respectively. The rightmost panel depicts the mean distortion product plotted as a function of intensity for the two stimulus pairs. Spectral data clearly show the peak at 2f1-f2 across almost all levels. For both stimuli, the distortion product can be characterized as compressive, except for the sharp increase in amplitude at 95 dB SPL for the low F1/F2 stimulus. Reprinted with permission from "Human Frequency-Following Response Correlates of the Distortion Product at 2F1–F2," by P. K. Pandya and A. Krishnan, 2004, *Journal of the American Academy of Audiology, 15*(3), pp. 184–197. Copyright Georg Thieme Verlag KG.

product at 2f1-f2 is derived from animal and human studies using the distortion product otoacoustic emissions (DPOAEs). Several studies examined the characteristics of the neural response representing this cochlear nonlinearity (Chertoff & Hecox, 1990; Chertoff, Hecox, & Goldstein, 1992; Elsisy & Krishnan, 2008; Goldstein, 1967; Goldstein & Kiang, 1968; Kim, Molnar, & Matthews, 1980; Krishnan, 1999; Pandya & Krishnan, 2004; Rickman, Chertoff, & Hecox, 1991; Robertson & Johnstone, 1981). While the DPOAE represents the backpropagated response measured in the ear canal as an acoustic signal, the neural distortion product at 2f1-f2 (FFR_{DP}) reflects phase-locked neural activity to the distortion product frequency. Rickman et al. (1991) were the first to report the presence of neural FFR_{DP} at 2f1-f2 in the human FFR elicited by a two-tone stimulus (f1: 510 Hz; f2: 800 Hz) that increased in amplitude as the f2/f2 ratio was increased from 1.16 to 1.46. This FFR_{DP} behavior is somewhat consistent with DPOAE data except for the absence of a reduction in amplitude for f1/f2 ratios greater than 1.3 observed for the latter. Chertoff et al. (1992), recording from chinchillas, observed similar changes in amplitude for the FFR_{DP} in chinchillas elicited by a two-tone stimulus (500–800 Hz) as f2/f1 ratio was increased from 1.12 to 1.52. However, the FFR_{DP} amplitude for a two-tone stimulus with primaries at 800 and 1700 Hz was essentially unaltered with an increase in f2/f1 ratio. For a two-tone stimulus with primaries at 1100 and 1400 Hz, they observed maximum FFR_{DP} amplitude at f2/f2 ratios of 1.22, 1.32, and 1.42. Pandya and Krishnan (2004) examined the amplitude growth functions of the primaries and FFR_{DP} for responses elicited by three different two-tone stimuli (500, 610 Hz; 1000, 1220 Hz; and 1400, 1708 Hz) with a constant f2/f1 ratio of 1.22. The FFR spectral data (Figure 8–19, left) show clear peaks corresponding to f1, f2, and FFR_{DP} for both stimuli. The input-output behavior plotted in Figure 8–19 (right panel) shows that while FFRs at f1 and f2 tend to increase with intensity, the FFR_{DP} exhibits a nonmonotonic compressive growth function except for a sharp amplitude increase at 95 dB SPL for the lowest two-tone stimulus. Elsisy and Krishnan (2008) evaluated the amplitude growth functions of the simultaneously recorded acoustic distortion product otoacoustic emissions (DPOAE) and (FFR_{DP}) at 2f1-f2 to determine if the two measures showed similar intensity-dependent behavior that would suggest shared cochlear generators. Responses were recorded from normal-hearing adults for a tone burst stimulus pair at 40–70 dB nHL. DPOAE and FFR_{DP} in response to a two-tone stimulus (F1: 500 Hz; F2: 612 Hz) were recorded at 40 to 70 dB nHL. The amplitude growth function for FFR_{DP} revealed a compressive saturating nonlinearity, while the DPOAE amplitude growth function exhibited a compressive growth at moderate intensities changing to a linear growth at higher intensities. Results appear to suggest that cochlear generators may be contributing differentially to the acoustic and the neural distortion products. These findings of nonmonotonic behavior of FFR_{DP} in the studies by the Krishnan group are consistent with the extant DPOAE research literature (Harris, 1990; He & Schmiedt, 1993; Kimberley & Nelson, 1989; Lonsbury-Martin et al., 1990; Nelson & Kimberley, 1992; Popelka, Osterhammel, Nielsen, & Rasmussen, 1993; Stover, Neely, & Gorga, 1996) and likely reflects the result of destructive interactions between multiple components, frequency shifts in the DPOAE microstructure, and/or fundamental properties of the active and passive cochlear mechanisms (He & Schmiedt, 1997; Manley, Koppl, & Johnstone, 1990; Nelson & Kimberley, 1992; Norton & Rubel, 1990; Stover & Norton, 1993). Also, the observation of different amplitude behavior for the phase-locked activity at the two primaries and the FFR_{DP} may suggest differences in the cochlear processes generating these responses. Finally, FFR_{DP} responses appear more easily identifiable and less variable relative to DPOAE, particularly at lower stimulus levels and frequencies below about 1000 Hz. Taken together, FFR_{DP} might be a good complement to the less reliable DPOAE in determining the functional integrity of cochlear function at frequencies below 1000 Hz. Findings may point to a potential benefit of applying FFR testing to complement DPOAE in evaluating the cochlear function at low frequencies.

FFRs Elicited by Steady-State Speech-Like and Speech Sounds

It is well established that encoding of the first two formants of most vowels is sufficient for their identification (Brown, 1958; Carlson, Fant, & Granstrom, 1975; Peterson & Barney, 1952). A neural phase-locking based temporal-place scheme has been shown to play a dominant role in the neural encoding of the spectrum of steady-state sounds in the population response of single neurons in the AN and ventral cochlear nucleus (Caspary, Rupert, & Moushegian, 1977; Palmer, Winter, & Darwin, 1986; Recio & Rhode, 2000; Young & Sachs, 1979). The scalp-recorded FFR has also been shown to preserve spectral- and pitch-relevant information contained in speech and nonspeech complex stimuli (Aiken & Picton, 2008; Ananthakrishnan & Krishnan, 2018; Ananthakrishnan et al., 2016; Ananthakrishnan et al., 2017; Bidelman, Gandour, & Krishnan, 2011; Bidelman & Krishnan, 2009, 2011; Galbraith, Jhaveri, & Kuo, 1997; Greenburg, 1980; Krishnan, 1999, 2002; Krishnan & Agrawal, 2010; Krishnan, Bidelman, & Gandour, 2010; Krishnan & Gandour, 2014; Krishnan et al., 2016; Krishnan & Plack, 2011; Krishnan, Xu, Gandour, & Cariani, 2004, 2005; Smalt et al., 2012; Suresh, Krishnan, & Luo, 2020; Swaminathan, Krishnan, & Gandour, 2008).

There has been a steady increase in the number of studies that have used speech-elicited FFRs to examine neural encoding in normal and impaired ears to speech and speech-like stimuli (Ananthakrishnan & Krishnan, 2018; Ananthakrishnan et al., 2016; Ananthakrishnan et al., 2017; Anderson et al., , 2013; Bidelman et al., 2011; Bidelman & Krishnan, 2009, 2011; Galbraith et al., 1997; Greenburg, 1980; Krishnan & Agrawal, 2010; Krishnan et al., 2010; Krishnan & Gandour, 2014; Krishnan et al., 2016; Krishnan & Plack, 2011; Krishnan et al., 2004, 2005; Smalt et al., 2012; Suresh, Krishnan, & Luo, 2020; Swaminathan et al., 2008). However, to date, only a few studies have specifically addressed the neural encoding of spectra of speech sounds (Aiken & Picton 2008; Krishnan, 1999, 2002). Krishnan (1999) recorded FFRs elicited by three different two-tone approximations of English vowels (/u/, /ɔ/, and /a/) at 88, 75, 65, and 55 dB nHL to evaluate the neural encoding of spectra of these sounds. Spectral analyses of the FFRs revealed distinct peaks at frequencies corresponding to the first and second formants across all levels, suggesting that phase-locked activity among two distinct populations of neurons is indeed preserved in the FFR. In addition, the FFR spectrum for vowels /ɔ/ and /a/ revealed a robust FFR_{DP}. A comparison of FFRs to the vowel approximations and responses to the individual frequency components (F1, F2) revealed effects that may be suggestive of two-tone synchrony suppression and/or lateral inhibition. A follow-up study (Krishnan, 2002) using steady-state synthetic speech versions of these three vowels showed robust FFRs with clear spectral peaks at harmonics proximal to the first and second formant of each vowel at all levels (Figure 8–20, first four panels), with F1, F2 amplitude increasing with increasing intensity. However, the amplitude growth functions for the smaller F2 components were shallower compared to F1 (Figure 8–20, rightmost panel). These results were interpreted to suggest that the robust responses at the two formant-related harmonics represent phase-locked activity in two distinct populations of brainstem auditory neurons driven by their characteristic places along the cochlear partition. Support for this view is derived from the following observations: FFRs to moderate-intensity tone bursts are place-specific (Ananthanarayan & Durrant, 1992); distinct response peaks at f1, f2, and 2f-f2 peak for the two-tone vowel stimuli (Krishnan, 1999); and FFRs are able to accurately track the frequency change presented in either upward or downward swept tonal glide (Krishnan & Parkinson, 2000). In this framework, each harmonic in the complex stimuli would engage a specific place on the cochlea (therefore, a specific frequency) that would produce phase-locked activity in two distinct populations of brainstem neurons with characteristic frequencies proximal to F1 and F2. That is, the spectral peaks in the FFR harmonics close to F1 and F2 likely reflect phase-locked activity from distinct populations of neurons. Krishnan (2002) also observed that for each vowel, the F1 response was dominant at high stimulus levels, consistent with the phenomenon of formant capture. Young and Sachs (1979) demonstrated this in the responses of the ANFs to speech stimuli. Specifically, as the intensity increases, not only does the response at the F1 place increase, but also it progressively reflects increasing contributions from units with higher characteristic frequencies due to upward spread of excitation (synchrony spread). This process likely accounts for the observation of the dominant spectral peak at F1 in the FFR data. Finally, the observation of smaller FFR amplitudes for harmonics between the formants

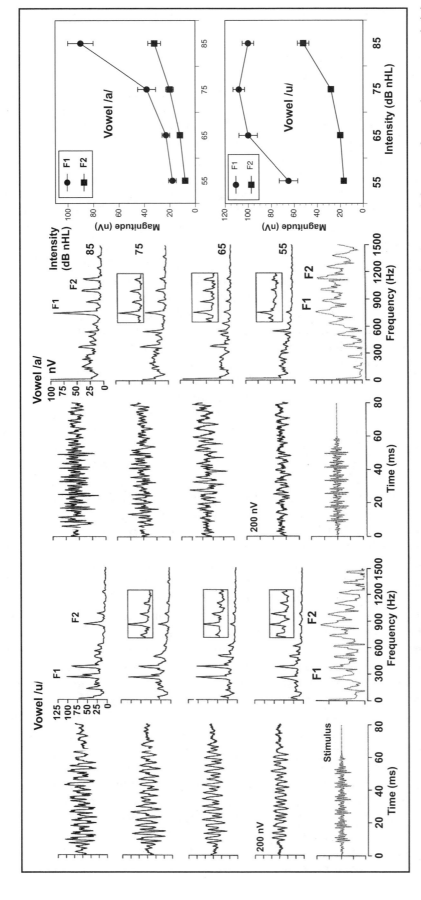

Figure 8–20. Frequency following response (FFR) waveforms, spectra (plotted as a function of intensity), and amplitude growth functions for steady-state vowels /u/ (*left pair*) and /a/ (*middle pair*). The mean amplitude growth of the F1 (*solid circle*) and F2 (*solid square*) response peaks with intensity for vowel /a/ (*top*) and vowel /u/ (*bottom*) are shown in the extreme right panels. The inset in the spectral data shows the magnified smaller F2-related spectral peaks. For both vowels, spectral components can be detected down to 55 dB nHL. For both vowels and both formants, amplitude grows with intensity with different characteristics. The stimulus waveforms and spectra (dotted traces) are shown at the bottom of the response waveforms and spectral for each vowel. From "Human Frequency Following Response: Representation of Steady-State Vowels," by A. Krishnan, 2002, *Hearing Research*, *166*, pp. 192–201. Copyright 2002, with permission from Elsevier.

seen in the FFR data suggests selective synchrony suppression to enhance spectral peaks at the formant frequencies (Krishnan, 2002). Taken together, these results clearly suggest that the phase-locked activity underlying the FFR can preserve certain acoustic features of speech sounds.

FFRs Elicited by Time-Variant Speech-Like and Speech Sounds

Most speech sounds in natural speech are inherently time-variant—that is, their spectrotemporal acoustic features change over time. There is compelling evidence that these time-varying acoustic features (e.g., formant transitions) of speech sounds play an important role in speech perception (Jacobson, Fant, & Halle, 1963). Thus, to be useful, phase-locked activity generating the FFR should be able to preserve some of these time-variant features. As an initial step to examine this, Krishnan and Parkinson (2000) evaluated the encoding of simple linearly rising (400–600 Hz) and falling (600–400 Hz) tonal glides, grossly approximating formant trajectories in real speech. The results of this study demonstrated that human FFR follows the trajectory of the rising and falling tones (Figure 8–21) in a robust fashion. The authors proposed that the changing frequency in the stimulus was encoded by a progressive shift in the population of neurons phase-locked to the changing stimulus frequency. Also, the decreasing amplitude with increasing frequency observed for the rising glide supports the view that neural phase-locking deteriorates with increasing frequency. Similar FFR findings have been reported by Billings, Bologna, Muralimanohar, Madsen, and Molis (2019): Clinard and Cotter (2015) in adults, and Madhavi, Krishnan, and Weber-Fox (2009) in children. The observation of smaller overall amplitude for the falling glide compared to the rising glide has been interpreted to suggest that the neural activity for rising frequency is more synchronous than for a falling frequency (Dau, 2003; Janssen, Steinhoff, & Bohnke, 1991). However, Billings et al. (2019) did not observe this differential sensitivity to the direction in their study. Plyler and Ananthanaraya (2001) also demonstrated that the phase-locked activity reflected in the FFR was able to track the formant transition in normal-hearing adults in response to CV syllables (Figure 8–22). However, smaller-duration formant transitions (50 ms or less) in shorter CV syllables do not appear to show a clear following in the FFR, probably obscured by the overlapping onset components. More recently, Suresh and Krishnan (2020) demonstrated that the FFR can follow the trajectory

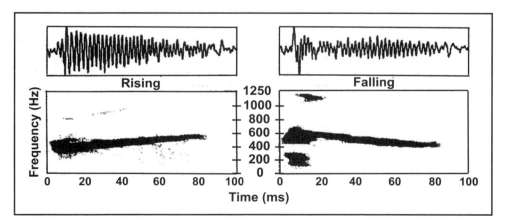

Figure 8–21. Frequency following response (FFR) waveforms and spectrograms to an upward (*left*) swept tone (400–600 Hz) and a downward (*right*) swept (600–400 Hz) tone. The rising and falling bands in the spectrogram clearly show the ability of the phase-locked activity to follow frequency change. Reprinted with permission from "Human Frequency-Following Response: Representation of Tonal Sweeps," by A. Krishnan and J. Parkinson, 2000, *Audiology and Neuro-otology, 5*, pp. 312–321. Copyright 2000 Karger Publishers, Basel, Switzerland.

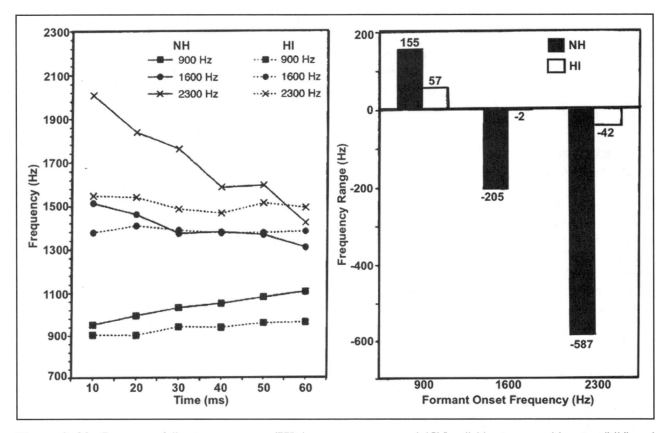

Figure 8–22. Frequency following responses (FFRs) to consonant-vowel (CV) syllables in normal-hearing (NH) and hearing-impaired (HI) individuals. For the NH group, the second formant tracking followed the stimulus formant transition. In contrast, phase-locked neural activity in the HI group failed to track the formant change faithfully as indicated by the flat lines (*left*). The frequency range of tracking is also significantly reduced in the hearing-impaired group (*right*). FFR tracking of formant transitions presented in three CV syllables in normally hearing (*solid line*) and hearing-impaired (*dotted line*) listeners. The bar graph on the right shows the range of frequency change reflected in the FFR for the two groups of subjects. Both graphs show that the formant transitions are well tracked by the phase-locked FFR in the normal-hearing listeners, but tracking remains essentially flat for the hearing-impaired subjects. Reprinted with permission from "Human Frequency Following Responses: Representation of Second Formant Transitions in Normal-Hearing and Hearing-Impaired Listeners," by P. N. Plyler and A. K. Ananthanarayan, 2001, *Journal of the American Academy of Audiology, 12*, pp. 423–533.

of decreasing frequencies of the first and second formant in a diphthong as the vowel moves from /a/ to /au/ to /u/ (Figure 8–23). Both the spectrogram (Figure 8–23, middle panel) and the instant spectra (Figure 8–23, bottom two panels) representing the earlier /a/ segment and the later /u/ clearly show that the phase-locked activity can follow the formants. Collectively, these results with time-varying signals suggest that the neural encoding of more complex time-varying speech stimuli, tapping at aspects of auditory temporal processing, may be more sensitive indicators of changes in temporal processing resulting from peripheral and central auditory disorders.

VII. COCHLEAR REGIONS CONTRIBUTING TO THE FFR

Since it takes relatively higher stimulus levels (40–45 dB above behavioral threshold) to elicit the FFR to low-frequency stimulus, higher-frequency regions may contribute appreciably to a high-intensity, low-frequency response due to the increased basal bias. For example, tones between 200 and 500 Hz presented at 65 to 75 dB excite the 6-kHz cochlear place (Rhode, 1978). Therefore, place-specific responses can be obtained only at a much lower level. In addition, the FFR is influenced by the various mechani-

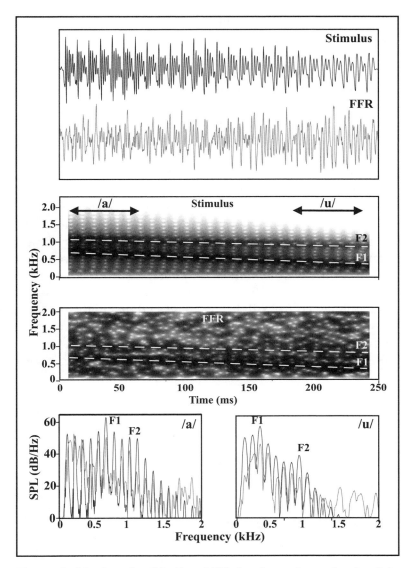

Figure 8–23. Stimulus (*black*) and FFR (*gray*) waveforms for the diphthong /au/ (*top pair*); spectrograms of the stimulus and FFR (middle pair); and instant spectra of the FFR and stimulus overlaid for time instants representing /a/ (*bottom left*), and a later time segment just before stimulus offset representing /u/. The FFR clearly shows the neural phase-locking tracking the time-varying F1 and F2 decreasing in frequency (indicated by the dotted white line). The instant spectra clearly show that formant-related harmonics shift down in frequency as the stimulus moves from /a/ to /u/.

cal and neural mechanisms in the cochlea and the auditory brainstem. For example, it is unlikely that the FFRs elicited by 200 to 500 Hz tones below 100 dB in the squirrel monkey reflect activity from higher frequencies, since high-frequency (near 6 kHz) ANFs in the squirrel monkey do not respond to these tones below 100 dB SPL (Geisler, Rhode, & Kennedy, 1974). It is more likely that ANFs with characteristic frequencies below 2 kHz that respond to 200 to 500 Hz tones at stimulus levels sufficient to elicit a robust FFR suggest that these low-frequency stimuli could be exciting cochlear regions about one to two octaves higher than the nominal value of the stimulus (Rose, Hind, Anderson, & Brugge, 1971).

Several investigators have sought to determine the place specificity of scalp-recorded FFR using cochlear and/or neural modeling, masking studies, or recordings from hearing-impaired listeners. Studies measuring the effect of noise masking on the FFR have established that at low and moderate intensities, the FFR is generated by low-frequency units with little or no contribution from the basal region. Narrowband noise centered on 4 kHz has no effect on the latency or amplitude of the 500-Hz FFR (Huis in't Veld et al., 1977). De Boer, Machiels, and Kruidenier (1977) observed that the FFR elicited by a 500-Hz tone burst at 50 and 60 dB SPL was masked only when the masker bandwidth overlapped the signal frequency (250–4000 Hz versus 800–4000 Hz). Comparable results were obtained by Yamada, Kodera, Hink, and Suzuki (1979), and Moushegian, Rupert, and Stillman (1978) with FFR masking occurring only when the high-pass masker cutoff was lowered to below 2 kHz. Similarly, a moderate-intensity 500-Hz FFR was only diminished when the tonal forward masker was between 500 and 1000 Hz (Figure 8–24, waveform left, and mean amplitude data right) and not above (Ananthanarayan & Durrant, 1992). The 500-Hz response amplitude was enhanced (Figure 8–24, right) in the presence of the higher-frequency maskers. Even for tone bursts presented at 60 dB above threshold, Huis in't Veld et al. (1977) observed that the 500-Hz FFR was reduced in amplitude only when narrowband noise was below 2000 Hz, suggesting that at this level, the 500-Hz FFR reflects the activity of neurons with characteristic frequencies below 2 kHz. However, for an FFR elicited by a 95 dB SPL low-frequency tone burst, comparison of high-pass masked response and model (incorporating filtering for BM transformations, IHC transduction, and a spike generation mechanism) responses suggested that highly synchronized neural activity in the high-frequency channels largely contributed to the high-intensity, low-frequency FFR with little contribution from the poorly synchronized low-

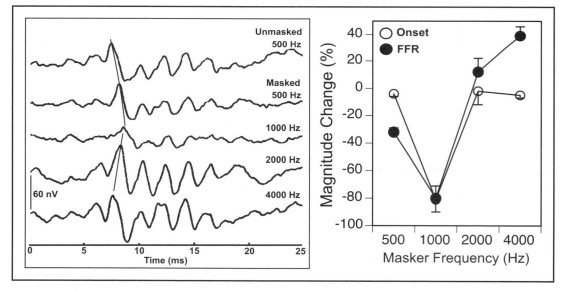

Figure 8–24. Frequency following response (FFR) waveforms elicited by a 500-Hz tone burst in unmasked and forward-masking conditions (*left*) and the mean amplitude change for the onset response (*open circle*) and the FFR (*solid circle*) plotted as a function of masker frequency. The tonal masker frequencies are identified to the right of each trace in the masked conditions. Both the waveform data and the mean amplitude data show that both the onset and the FFR components were maximally reduced in the presence of the 500- and 1000-Hz tonal maskers. The thin vertical lines follow the latency shift for the onset component. Error bars represent ±1 SEM. Adapted with permission from "The Frequency Following Response and the Onset Response: Evaluation of Frequency Specificity Using a Forward-Masking Paradigm," by A. K. Ananthanarayan and J. D. Durrant, 1992, *Ear and Hearing, 13*(4), pp. 228–233.

frequency channels (Janssen et al., 1991). Similar results have been described by another modeling study aimed at describing the cochlear and auditory nerve processes underlying the generation of both ABR and FFR (Dau, 2003).

Some masking experiments paradoxically have reported response enhancement for higher high pass masker cutoff frequencies which essentially minimized the basal contribution to the low frequency FFR (see Figure 8–24) (Ananthanarayan & Durrant, 1992; Davis & Hirsh, 1976; De Boer et al., 1977; Huis in't Veld et al., 1977). While the underlying basis for this enhancement is not clear, the FFR may have multiple sources with different phases, so enhancement could occur if masking eliminates some of the sources that are in opposition (Davis & Hirsh, 1976; De Boer et al., 1977). However, this explanation is unlikely given that FFR latency is not substantially altered by high-pass noise masking of varying cutoff frequencies. It is more likely that these results are consistent with a more discrete cochlear initiation site for the FFR.

Another way to determine the place specificity of the low-frequency FFR is to record from individuals with high-frequency hearing loss starting at different frequencies (akin to recording 500-Hz responses using high-pass masking). Results from several studies indicate that robust FFR to a low-frequency tone burst is present in individuals with a significant hearing loss above 2 kHz, suggesting that the basal cochlear region need not be intact to record an FFR (Gardi & Merzenich,1979; Huis in't Veld et al., 1977; Moushegian et al., 1978; Yamada, Kodera, Hink, & Yamane, 1978). Importantly, the 500-Hz FFR threshold has consistently been shown to be within normal limits when the behavioral threshold is normal at 500 Hz, even in the presence of a substantial hearing loss at 1 kHz (Yamada et al., 1978). Most of these studies have reported that the difference between the FFR threshold and behavioral thresholds is smaller in individuals with sensorineural hearing loss compared to normal-hearing individuals (Huis in't Veld et al., 1977).

In summary, the place specificity of low-frequency FFR is intensity dependent. For signal levels up to 55 dB above behavioral threshold, FFR is place-specific (i.e., primarily engaging low-frequency neurons), with cochlear contributions largely restricted to a place respresenting a narrow frequency region around the nominal frequency of the stimulus. As stimulus levels increase above about 60 dB above the behavioral threshold, the basal bias progressively increases, and increasingly neurons representing high-frequency channels will contribute to the response. For stimulus levels greater than about 75 dB, the activity could spread two or more octaves above the stimulus frequency.

VIII. HOW IS THE POPULATION RESPONSE REFLECTED IN THE FFR RELATED TO SINGLE-NEURON ACTIVITY?

It is generally accepted that the FFR is a true neural potential, representing the summation of synchronous phase-locked neural activity from a population of neural elements along the auditory brainstem. Indirect evidence supporting this view is suggested by the ability to record FFR from brainstem nuclei that have a substantial population of phase-locking neurons (Marsh, Brown, & Smith, 1975). These authors also showed that the upper-frequency limit for FFR at each nucleus corresponds to the upper limits of synchronized single-unit activity. Furthermore, FFR has not been recorded from the medial geniculate body and auditory cortex, where only a smaller number of units show phase locking (Marsh et al., 1975; Worden & Marsh, 1968). Using a more direct comparison of FFR and the underlying single-unit activity, Holstein, Buchwald, and Schwafel (1969) found that the time-integrated envelope of single-unit spike activity in the cochlear nucleus corresponds closely to FFR recorded from a small population of neurons in the same region. Further evidence relating FFR to single-unit activity is found in a study by Marsh, Smith, and Worden (1972). They simultaneously recorded the response of single units and FFR in the cochlear nucleus, as well as the CM, to tones presented with a variable amount of masking noise. At noise levels sufficient to attenuate or abolish the FFR, the synchrony of the single units was also disrupted, although the discharge rate was often unaffected. The CM, on the other hand, displayed little degradation with increasing noise levels.

IX. NEURAL GENERATORS OF THE EFR/FFR

While it is well established that phase-locked neural activity occurs throughout the auditory pathways, including the primary auditory cortex, most previous studies in humans and animals tend to favor the dominance of brainstem sites as sources of the scalp-recorded FFR. However, more recently there appears to be an emergence of a renewed debate about the possibility of the primary auditory cortex contributing to the scalp-recorded FFR (Bidelman, 2018; Bidelman & Momtaz, 2021; Coffey, Herholz, Chepesiuk, Baillet, & Zatorre, 2016).

Early Research Supporting Brainstem Origin of the FFR

Even earlier work on the FFR generators yielded conflicting results, mostly about a single dominant or multiple sources in the brainstem (Marsh et al., 1975; Starr & Hellerstein, 1971; Worden & Marsh, 1968). The discrepancies reflect the possibility of multiple brainstem sources with different strengths and orientations contributing to the FFR. Based on the results of these studies, the FFR could be generated by a single source, two distinct sources, or multiple sources (Bledsoe & Moushegian, 1980; Davis & Britt, 1984; Gerken, Moushegian, Stillman, & Rupert, 1975; Mair & Laukli, 1984; Scherg & Brinkmann, 1979; Smith, Marsh, & Brown, 1975; Sohmer & Pratt, 1977; Stillman, Crow, & Moushegian, 1978; Yamada, Marsh, & Potsic, 1980). The 6-ms latency of the scalp-recorded FFR corresponds closely to the latency of ABR wave V and suggests an upper brainstem source, presumably the IC. Smith, Marsh, and Brown (1975) tested this hypothesis by comparing scalp-recorded FFRs in cats with responses recorded from the brainstem nuclei in the same animals. They found that the response latency of both responses was almost identical (5.6 versus 5.3 ms, respectively), suggesting a common source in the IC. Also, cryogenic cooling of IC attenuated both IC and scalp-recorded FFR while leaving the medial superior olive (MSO)–recorded FFR unaltered, suggesting no significant contributions to the FFR from structures caudal to the IC. In contrast, Gardi and Merzenich (1979) reported little or no alteration in the scalp-recorded FFR in cats when the IC was ablated bilaterally. Instead, their results suggested that 50% of the FFR was due to cochlear nucleus activity, 20% to activity in the superior olivary complex (SOC), and 25% to the CM.

Several studies have reported FFRs with latencies much shorter than 6 ms suggesting a more caudal origin of the FFR (Davis & Britt, 1984; Mair & Laukli, 1984; Sohmer & Pratt, 1976; Sohmer, Pratt, & Kinarti, 1977; Stillman et al., 1978). For example, Sohmer and Pratt (1977) found two distinct scalp signals—one with a latency of 6 ms (upper brainstem origin as this potential is not recordable in patients with lesions confined to the upper medulla and midbrain), and the other with a short latency of 1 ms that was eliminated with alternating polarity (consistent with CM). Davis and Britt (1984) showed that their FFRs recorded in cats to 3000-Hz tone were unaltered by aspiration of IC, SOC, and cochlear nucleus, confirming a CM. Stillman et al. (1978) also differentiate two scalp potentials—one with a latency of 3.8 to 4.2 ms (FFP1) and the other with a latency of 6 ms (FFP2). The longer latency component presumably was from the IC (Moushegian & Rupert, 1970; Smith et al., 1975), and the shorter latency component (FFP1), which was prominent at higher stimulus levels, presumably was generated by the same source as wave III of the ABR (probably the cochlear nucleus) (Figure 8–25). Scherg and Brinkman (1979) have differentiated these two components based on their latency, amplitude behavior, and electrode montage. The latency of FFP1 ranges between 1.4 (70 dB HL) and 3.5 ms (40 dB HL), whereas FFP2 varies between 6.8 (70 dB HL) and 12.1 ms (30 dB HL). FFPl is present only using an ipsilateral vertex to earlobe electrode montage, suggesting an ipsilateral AN or cochlear nucleus generator site. Huis in't Veld et al. (1977) also reported two short-latency FFR components—one with a 2-ms latency and the other with a 3-ms (at 90 dB SPL) latency, again suggesting multiple sources including CM, AN, and cochlear nucleus. Galbraith, Bagasan, and Sulahian (2001) interpreted their more robust, shorter-latency (2.6 ms) FFR for the horizontal electrode montage compared to the less robust, longer-latency (4.38 ms) FFR for the vertical electrode montage to reflect phase-locked neural activity in

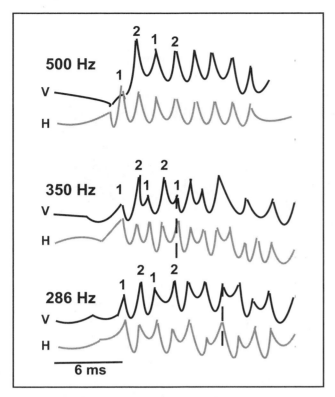

Figure 8–25. Comparison of FFRs recorded to several low-frequency tones using a vertical (*top black trace* in each pair) and a horizontal montage (the *bottom gray trace* in each pair). Two distinct components (FFP1 and FFP2) are clearly seen in all tracings. FFP2 appears to be prominent in the vertical montage and the FFP1 component in the horizontal montage. These results suggest that each component may have distinct neural generators. Data from "Components of the Frequency-Following Potential in Man," by R. D. Stillman, G. Crow, and G. Moushegian, 1978, *Electroencephalography and Clinical Neurophysiology, 44*, pp. 438–446.

the AN and brainstem, respectively. Krishnan and Chelluri (unpublished laboratory report) reasoned that if the horizontal derivation represented more caudal generators, higher-frequency FFRs should be detectable given the higher upper-frequency limit for phase-locking at more caudal levels in the auditory pathway. The observation of higher-frequency components (up to about 2500 Hz) for the horizontal recordings compared to about 1500 Hz for our vertical recordings appears to be consistent with this view. Collectively, these studies appear to support the notion that multiple sources between the AN and the IC contribute to the FFR that can be somewhat isolated using different recording electrode configurations. However, it is likely that the primary auditory cortex also contributes to the FFR for frequencies below about 120 Hz.

Current Views on the Neural Generators of the FFR

Notwithstanding the evidence presented earlier suggesting multiple sources in the brainstem contributing to the FFR, there has been an ongoing debate about the neural generators of the FFR with the recent emergence of a controversial point of view based on magnetoencephalography (MEG) data that the scalp-recorded FFR reflects phase-locked activity primarily originating in the primary auditory cortex with remarkably little contribution from the subcortical generators (Coffey et al., 2016). Clearly, this view is diametrically opposite and inconsistent with the long-held and the more recent view that the brainstem is the primary source of the FFR (Bidelman, 2018; Bidelman & Momtaz, 2021; Bidelman et al., 2015; Chandrasekaran & Kraus, 2010; Gardi et al., 1979; Krishnan, 2007; Smith et al., 1975; Sohmer et al., 1977). Recently, Bidelman (2018) applied sophisticated source imaging techniques (including discrete dipole modeling, distributed imaging, independent component analysis, and computational simulations) on the scalp-recorded FFRs elicited by speech sounds to determine the relative contributions of the periphery (AN), brainstem (IC), and primary auditory cortex (PAC) to the FFR. They reasoned that significant cortical contributions to the FFR would not be present above about 100 Hz given the known lower limits of neural phase-locking observed for cortical neurons (Brugge et al., 2009; Joris et al., 2004; Lu, Liang, & Wang, 2001; Wallace, Rutkowski, Shackleton, & Palmer, 2000). On the contrary, the FFR would be dominated by brainstem sources given that higher frequencies engage peripheral (AN) and brainstem generators, while low frequencies recruit mainly cortical neural ensembles (Herdman et al., 2002; Kuwada et al., 2002). Their results showed that neural activity from the AN, IC, dominantly contributed to the FFRs with very little contribution from the primary auditory cortex (Figure 8–26). The source phase-locked waveforms from the AN and IC are appreciably more robust compared to

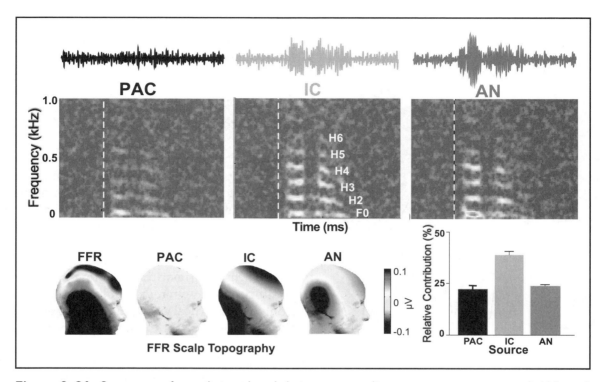

Figure 8–26. Source waveforms (*top row*) and their corresponding response spectrograms (*middle row*) from the auditory nerve (AN, *left*), brainstem (BS, *middle*), and primary auditory cortex (PAC, *right*) elicited by a speech syllable. The response is the strongest in the BS followed by the AN, with a weak response from PAC limited to the fundamental frequency (100 Hz). Darker colors reflect activity phase-locked from trial to trial (i.e., FFR) at each time and frequency. Consistent with this, the scalp distribution of voltage (*bottom left*) is strong for the BS and very weak for the PAC. Bar chart on the bottom right showing the mean relative contribution of these sources to the FFR again shows that the BS source is the primary contributor to the FFR. Error bars. ±1 SEM. Collectively, these results suggest that the primary source contributing to the generation of the scalp-recorded FFRs to speech syllables is the IC. Created using data from "Subcortical Sources Dominate the Neuroelectric Auditory Frequency-Following Response to Speech," by G. M. Bidelman, 2018, *NeuroImage*, *175*, pp. 56–69.

the noisy waveform from the PAC (Figure 8–26, waveforms at the top). This observation becomes clearer in the response spectrograms presented later—again very little activity at the f0 with no discernible components above f0 from the PAC. However, frequency-specific evaluation of source waveforms showed the relative contribution of these nuclei to the aggregate FFR varied across stimulus frequencies. While AN and BS sources produced robust FFRs up to ~700 Hz, PAC showed extremely weak phase-locking with little FFR energy above the speech fundamental (100 Hz). Distributed cortical source imaging further showed no measurable phase-locked activity for FFRs greater than 150 Hz, with only the subcortical sources remaining active (Figure 8–26, bottom). Further, their results showed that phase-locking in the primary auditory cortex was extremely weak and seen only in the grand average with phase-locking indistinguishable from the no response control or their own baseline indicating no reliable primary auditory cortex phase-locking to the fundamental periodicity. This is in sharp contrast to the EEG-derived FFR that revealed a rich spectrum with robust components detectable out to 1500 Hz. In addition, cross-correlation analysis of their source waveforms showed response latencies consistent with AN, IC, and auditory cortex activation sites. These findings are in sharp contrast with the findings of Coffey et al. (2016) for MEG derived FFRs. Based on these results, Bidelman (2018) suggests that the cortical dominance observed in the Coffey et al. (2016) MEG data is likely due to increased sensitivity of MEG to superficial brain tissue, decreased sensitivity to deep structures like the brainstem (Baillet, 2017; Baillet, Mosher, & Leahy, 2001; Cohen & Cuffin, 1983; Hillebrand & Barnes, 2002), and therefore underestimating subcortical structures that drive most of the FFRs elicited by speech stimuli. The brainstem dominance of the FFR generation is further reinforced by recent findings by Bidelman and Momtaz (2021), which showed that the f0 magnitudes of the FFRs elicited by speech in noise were largest in subcortical sources (BS > AN > PAC) with a weak FFR from the PAC (just above the noise floor) and limited to an f0 of about 100 Hz. Further, a brainstem-behavior regression analysis of their data revealed that the AN and BS FFRs were sufficient to describe listeners' QuickSIN scores with the FFRs from the auditory cortex (left or right PAC) unable to predict SIN performance. Thus, the subcortical FFR sources are not only dominant but also appear to be more strongly linked to the speech FFRs and SIN processing in normal-hearing adults as observed in previous EEG studies. Finally, the observation (White-Schwoch et al., 2019) of robust FFRs and absent cortical responses in individuals with bilateral primary auditory cortex lesions lends further support to the notion of primary brainstem sources for the FFR. Overall, these results are consistent with the views expressed in the previous section that the FFR is primarily a brainstem response for frequencies above 100 Hz. Cleanly separating subcortical from cortical FFRs can be achieved by ensuring stimulus frequencies are greater than 100 to 150 Hz, above the phase-locking limit of cortical neurons.

X. CLINICAL APPLICATIONS OF THE FFR

Peripheral SNHL produces changes in the processing of sounds in the brainstem and auditory cortex resulting from reduced fine-grained input to the central auditory system. For example, reduced cochlear output (and consequently the reduced neural drive to the central structures) can lead to tonotopic remapping in the IC (Willott, 1991) and other changes in central auditory processing (Aizawa & Eggermont, 2006) that reflect a change in the nature of central gain adjustments and alterations in the balance of excitatory and inhibitory neurotransmitters in the brainstem (Dong et al., 2010). Speech perception in individuals with SNHL is considerably reduced, particularly in adverse listening conditions, and cannot be completely restored with amplification. This occurs because cochlear damage, in addition to elevating audiometric thresholds, likely degrades the neural representation of envelope and temporal fine-structure information along the central auditory pathways including the brainstem. Here we describe some recent results that indicate that there are changes in the temporal representation of both envelope and temporal fine structure of speech sounds in individuals with SNHL.

Like the EFRs described earlier, FFRs have also been used to examine if cochlear impairment degrades the neural representation of certain temporal fine-structure features that may be important for speech perception (Ananthakrishnan et al., 2016; Anderson, Parbery-Clark et al. 2013; Plyler & Krishnan, 2001). Plyler and Ananthanarayan (2001) examined the nature of the neural representation of temporal fine structure using three CV syllables (/ba/, /da/, and /ga/) in normal-hearing individuals and individuals with mild-moderate sensorineural hearing loss. They found that for all three stimuli, phase-locked activity in the normal group tracked the second formant transition in a robust fashion but not in the hearing-impaired group. Specifically, the phase-locked activity in the hearing-impaired group was fragmentary and not able to follow the frequency change over the duration of the transition (see Figure 8–22). Interestingly, their data suggested that lower speech recognition scores were associated with greater degradation in the representation of the formant change. Based on these results, the authors concluded that cochlear hearing loss likely degrades the representation of both time-varying and steady-state segments of speech sounds by disrupting the temporal pattern of phase-locked neural activity. Anderson, Parbery-Clark, et al. (2013), only observed an enhancement of the EFR but no changes in the FFRs elicited by a 40-ms CV /da/ in older individuals with a mild to moderate hearing loss. However, the ratio of the envelope to temporal fine-structure representation was greater in their hearing-impaired group compared to the normal group, suggesting SNHL induced alteration in neural encoding. This relative deficit of TFS encoding (enhanced EFR and normal FFR), also observed by Kale and Heinz (2010) in chinchillas with noise-induced SNHL, is likely due to the enhanced envelope encoding obscuring the much smaller TFS representation—an effect that gets worse in noise where the TFS cue is important for speech perception. Recently, Ananthakrishnan et al. (2016) examined the effects of mild-to-moderate SNHL on the neural representation of envelope periodicity and TFS using FFRs elicited by the English vowel /u/. Results showed that neural representation of both envelope periodicity (F0) and TFS (F1) was stronger in NH listeners compared to listeners with SNHL at both equal SPLs and equal SLs, suggesting that audibility is not a factor in accounting for the difference (Figures 8–27 and 8–28). Comparison at equal SPLs showed the growth of F1 was significantly steeper for the normal group compared to the relatively shallower slope of the F1 amplitude growth function (Figure 8–29). When comparisons were made at equal SLs, a robust linear growth in F1 amplitude for the normal-hearing listeners was observed while the F1 amplitude showed little or no change the SNHL group (Figure 8–30). Overall, they observed a relatively greater degradation in the neural representation of TFS compared to envelope periodicity in individuals with SNHL. The degradation of envelope representation in SNHL at lower sensation levels may be due to, at least in part, reduced audibility in higher-frequency regions that are necessary for the neural representation of F0 derived from modulations of unresolved harmonics. In contrast,

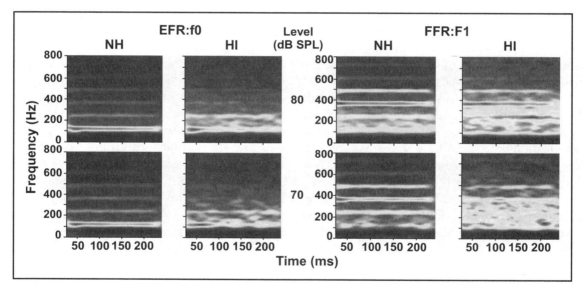

Figure 8–27. Grand averaged spectrograms for the EFR (*left*) and the FFR (*right*) at 80 dB SPL (*top row*) and 70 dB SPL (*bottom row*). In each row and panel, the plots on the left are for the normal-hearing groups (NH), and the plots on the right are for the hearing-impaired group (HI). at equal SPLs. Both the EFR data (showing the neural representation of f0) and the FFR data (showing the neural representation of the first formant, F1) show a robust neural representation of these features for the NH group with clear spectral bands of phase-locked neural activity. The representations for the HI group, particularly the temporal fine structure (including F1), is degraded with spectral bands smeared. Results suggest that a sensorineural loss degraded the neural representation of the temporal fine structure more severely than the envelope periodicity. f0 = 120 Hz; F1-related harmonic = 360 Hz. Reprinted with permission from "Human Frequency Following Response: Neural Representation of Envelope and Temporal Fine Structure in Listeners With Normal Hearing and Sensorineural Hearing Loss," by S. Ananthakrishnan, A. Krishnan, and E. Bartlett, 2016, *Ear and Hearing*, *37*(2), pp. e91–e103.

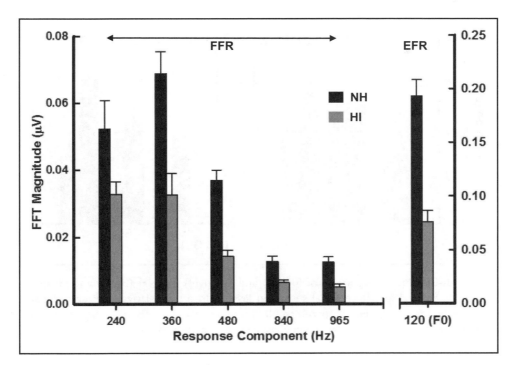

Figure 8–28. Mean response magnitude of the phase-locked neural activity at the formant-related harmonics in the FFR (*left*), and the f0 (120 Hz) in the EFR (*right*) in response to the vowel /u/ in NH (*black*) and HI (*gray*) at 80 dB SPL. In all conditions, both the FFR components and the EFR components are significantly larger in the NH group. Reprinted with permission from Ananthakrishnan, Krishnan, and Bartlett, 2016, *Ear and Hearing, 37*(2), pp. e91–e103.

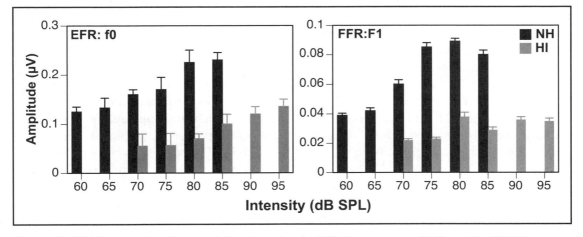

Figure 8–29. Mean amplitude growth functions for the EFR f0 component (*left*) and the FFR F1 component (*right*) for the normal-hearing (NH, *black bars*) and the hearing-impaired groups (*gray bars*). For both responses, the NH group shows greater magnitude across all levels with the HI group showing shallower growth functions suggesting that increasing audibility may not appreciably improve the degraded representation, particularly for the temporal fine-structure component. Created using data from Ananthakrishnan, Krishnan, and Bartlett, 2016 *Ear and Hearing, 37*(2), pp. e91–e103.

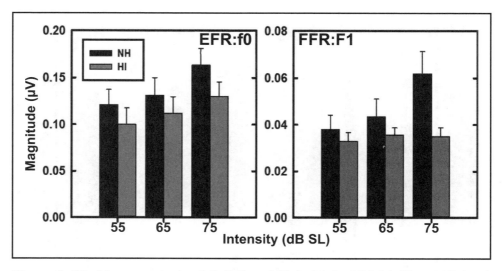

Figure 8–30. Mean magnitude of f0 (*left*) and F1 (*right*) for NH (black) and HI (gray) individuals plotted for three equal sensation levels. Note the relatively larger reduction in F1 magnitude for the HI compared to NH listeners relative to f0 magnitude. Reprinted with permission from Ananthakrishnan, Krishnan, and Bartlett, 2016, *Ear and Hearing, 37*(2), pp. e91–e103.

the persistence of degraded neural phase-locking of TFS even when audibility is restored may be due to a combination of impaired temporal synchrony due to altered tonotopicity, and loss of frequency selectivity. That is, the wider auditory filter bandwidths, which may disrupt the temporal pattern of phase-locked neural activity arising from altered tonotopic maps. Several observations related to changes in neural encoding at the AN level consequent to cochlear hearing loss may be invoked to explain these FFR results. Henry and Heinz (2013) found that phase-locking in neural fibers with CFs greater than 2.5 kHz encoded both the high-frequency envelope information and much low-frequency (between 0.5 and 1.5 kHz) TFS in mild-moderate hearing loss. That is, low-frequency TFS is encoded by all fibers irrespective of CF, but the encoding of high-frequency TFS information between 2.5 and 5 kHz is severely degraded. The combination of robust envelope information in the presence of diminished high-frequency TFS information at the single-unit level may account for the differential effects of SNHL on envelope and TFS observed in the FFR. In addition, Miller, Schilling, Franck, and Young (1997) observed that cats with noise-induced SNHL had reduced or absent *synchrony capture*—the ability of the ANFs to selectively enhance neural phase-locking synchrony to formant-related harmonics and diminish phase-locking synchrony to other non-formant-related harmonics, while phase-locking to other harmonic components located further away from the formants is diminished. Similarly, Palmer and Moorjani (1993) found reduced synchrony capture for F1 and F2 in guinea pigs with kanamycin-induced hearing loss, with a well-preserved robust encoding of the lower-frequency F0. This synchrony capture may also be present in the ensemble FFR to steady-state speech in normal-hearing listeners (Krishnan, 2002). Consistent with the previous findings, strong formant-related harmonic encoding, or "synchrony capture," was present in normal-hearing individuals but reduced or absent in the SNHL FFR in the present study, again suggesting reduced precision in brainstem neural phase-locking consequent to SNHL.

These results taken together suggest that the FFR offers a potentially robust analytic window that could be applied in objective clinical assessment to understand the nature of changes in the neural encoding of complex sounds so individual-specific recommendations can be made regarding the optimal amplification requirements to improve speech intelligibility, outcome measures of auditory training, and benefits from conventional amplification/cochlear implants. Clearly more concerted research efforts are needed to realize this potential. It will also be potentially worthwhile to pursue research utilizing a parametric evaluation of neural representation of acoustic features of speech to understand the relationship between neural representation and auditory perceptual ability.

XI. RECORDING AND ANALYSIS OF EFR AND FFR

EFR and FFR can be recorded using essentially the same procedures used in recording ABR in terms of electrode configurations and response averaging. However, given the typically longer stimuli used to elicit these responses and the sustained complex waveform, the recording epoch and the analysis methods are necessarily different. The parameters for recording FFR are summarized in Table 8–2.

Electrode Montage

These sustained responses can be recorded using similar electrode configurations utilized in the acquisition of ABR and ASSR. Responses can be recorded differentially using a vertical montage where the electrode serving as the noninverting input is placed on the high forehead (at the hairline) in the midline (alternatively, the vertex location [Cz] may be used as the noninverting electrode), and the electrode serving as the noninverting input can be placed either over the prominence of the seventh cervical vertebra (C7) location and/or on the ipsilateral mastoid. (It is also not uncommon to use a linked mastoid approach for binaural stimulation.) Another electrode placed on the mid-forehead at the midline (Fpz—approximately an inch below the noninverting electrode) serves as the common ground. For the horizontal electrode, configuration responses are recorded differentially between electrodes placed on each mastoid. There is some evidence to suggest that the vertical configuration may be picking up neural activity from more rostral generators, while the horizontal electrodes may be picking up neural activity from more caudal generators (Galbraith et al., 2001; King et al., 2016). King et al. (2016) used group delay measures to compare the EFRs and FFRs elicited by five multifrequency component amplitude-modulated tones (centered at 576 Hz, but each with a different modulation rate that produced different sideband frequencies across stimuli) using a vertical (high forehead to C7) and a horizontal montage (mastoid-to-mastoid). They estimated the response latency for both EFR and FFR by evaluating response phase changes across modulation- and sideband frequency (group delay). They found shorter latencies (shorter group delay) for the FFRs in the horizontal derivation compared to the vertical derivation suggesting a more caudal source generator for the former. The EFRs were longer in latency compared to the FFRs and did not differ across the two response montages. The authors caution that the FFR reflects activity from multiple sources (including the receptor potential CM) and thus complicates the interpretation of the group delay estimates.

As described earlier, this differential sensitivity may enable recording of higher-frequency FFRs since the upper-frequency limit for phase-locking is higher at caudal levels of the auditory system. More systematic evaluation is needed to test this hypothesis. Interelectrode impedances should preferably be well below 3 kilo-ohms to improve the SNR. More recently, the use of high-density EEG acquisition allows averaging responses across several electrodes to improve response SNR.

Stimulus Characteristics

Both responses can be recorded using tone bursts (tone burst repeating with a certain periodicity for the EFR) and more commonly using steady-state or time-varying complex sounds, including speech sounds. Complex sounds by virtue of their envelope periodicity and temporal fine structure will elicit both EFR and FFR. Care should be taken to select stimuli that have sufficient frequency components that fall below an upper-frequency limit of about 2000 Hz. It should be noted here that the response components above about 800 to 1000 Hz are significantly smaller in amplitude and will require a greater number of averages to isolate them from the noise baseline. This poses a challenge to elicit robust phase-locked activity for speech stimuli

Table 8–2. Summary of the Choice of Stimuli and Their Parameters, Transducer Types, Recording Parameters, and the Types of Time- and Frequency-Domain Analyses That Can Be Utilized to Characterize the EFR and the FFR

Parameter	Suggestion	Rationale, Comment
STIMULUS		
Type	Tone burst (below 2 kHz)	For optimal amplitude, use frequencies below 1000-Hz complex tones For recording DT (ASSR) and distortion product at 2f1-f2
	Steady-state vowels	Neural encoding of speech sounds
	Tonal sweeps	Neural encoding of time-variant stimuli
	CV syllables	Neural encoding of time-variant speech sounds
	Complex tones	Neural encoding of complex harmonic or inharmonic sounds
	Iterated rippled noise (IRN)	Neural encoding of complex sound with little or no envelope
Duration	15–250 ms	Longer for speech stimuli
Rise/fall time	5–10 ms	To reduce spectral splatter and reduce onset response component
Rate	3.1–7.1/s	Slower for longer stimuli
Polarity	Alternating phase	If interested in only the response locked to the envelope polarity
	Fixed phase	For recording responses phase-locked to spectral components level
	45–80 dB nHL	More robust responses at moderate level
Number of sweeps	1000–3000	Varies with size of response and background noise; may need closer to 4,000 sweeps to extract high-frequency TFS information
Presentation		
Ear(s)	Binaural, monaural, free-field	Typically binaural to obtain more robust responses; monaural if ear-specific information is required; free-field is required for unaided/aided comparisons
Mode	Air conduction/bone conduction	BC mostly in EFR clinical applications to rule out conductive loss
Transducer	Insert earphone/bone vibrator	Magnetically shielded earphones to avoid stimulus artifact; masking only if stimulus level exceeds 70 dB nHL; choice of ER-2 over ER 3-A since the former has output out of 10–13 kHz
ACQUISITION		
Amplification	100,000–200,000	
Analysis time	20 ms greater than stimulus duration	
Sampling frequency	10,000–25,000 Hz	Depends on the frequency components in the stimulus filters
Band-pass	30–3000 Hz	Recommend use of postaveraging digital filtering
Notch	None	Never indicated
Electrodes[a]		
Channel 1	High forehead-A1/A2	Will improve recording of higher-frequency components
Channel 2	High forehead-C7	Midline recording and biased toward more rostral generators
Channel 3	A1-A2 (horizontal)	Presumably favors caudal generators and therefore is able to detect higher-frequency components compared to the vertical montage (Channels 1 and 2).

Table 8–2. *continued*

Parameter	Suggestion	Rationale, Comment
Cap electrodes	32–64 channels	Averaging of responses from multiple electrodes will improve SNR and may reduce the number of averages required, therefore test time
Ground	Fpz (mid-forehead)	
RESPONSE ANALYSIS (see main text for description of each method)		
Time-domain		
RMS amplitude		Provides only a gross overall amplitude, limited use
Response latency		Can provide information about generator and cochlear place
S-R correlation		Good overall measure of response fidelity and consistency
Autocorrelation/autocorrelogram		Spectrotemporal periodicity strength information
Phase coherence/phase-locking value		Goodness of phase-locking
Frequency domain		
FFT		Quantitative index of magnitude of spectral components
Joint time frequency		Spectrogram allows analysis of time-variant signals
Spectral correlation		Response fidelity measure in the frequency domain

with formants above 1000 Hz due to the 6-dB/octave decrease in spectral energy above 500 Hz. If one is primarily interested in the sustained phase-locked components without contamination (at least in the initial portion of the response) from the onset responses, then the use of stimuli with gradual rise-fall times (greater than 5 ms) is recommended. This will reduce or eliminate the onset components and also increase the frequency specificity of the stimulus. However, the onset component, when present, serves as a useful reference for the onset of FFR components and also will serve as another measure to evaluate brainstem function. Longer rise and fall times will reduce the number of phase-locked cycles in the response because the smaller amplitude of stimulus cycles at the onset and offset will not be sufficient to elicit a response. EFRs are commonly recorded using alternating onset polarity to extract phase-locking to just the envelope periodicity, which is mostly unaltered by a change in the onset phase. For FFR, a single polarity is used typically when using tone bursts or tonal glides, since there is no concern of the envelope response overlapping the TFS response. However, when using complex sounds with the pronounced envelope, it is best to record responses to both condensation and rarefaction onset polarities separately, which can then be used to derive the EFR and FFR components. Using alternating onset polarity stimuli and split buffer averaging (implemented in several of the commercially available systems) will allow responses to each onset polarity to be stored in separate buffers, which then can be added or subtracted to extract EFR and FFR, respectively. Alternating polarity minimizes stimulus artifact and CM and doubles the frequency of the neural FFR that is discernible at least for single-frequency tone burst stimuli.

Choice of Earphones

The use of longer-duration stimuli to record FFRs creates a potential for the stimulus artifact to overlap and contaminate the true neural FFR. Both supra-aural and insert earphones can be used to record the FFR, but it is critical that these transducers be magnetically shielded. Alternatively, the recording electrodes and the transducer can be separated by using an insert earphone with a longer tube to couple the sound to the ear. However, this latter method does not ensure the elimination of the stimulus artifact. Both Etymōtic ER 3-A and ER-2 insert earphones have been used to record these responses, with the latter able to present higher-frequency components in the stimulus. Free-field testing has also been employed using the speaker(s) placed about a meter from the ear to evaluate unaided and aided responses. Finally, bone vibrators can be used to compare EFR elicited by bone- and air-conduction stimulation to assess middle ear status. Given the differences in the output and frequency response characteristics of these transducers, it is important to accurately calibrate their outputs.

Response Evaluation

Given the spectrotemporal complexity of the response, time-domain and frequency-domain measures are necessary to completely characterize the nature of stimulus features preserved in these responses. Like any complex signals, EFR and FFR lend themselves well to several time- and frequency-domain measures (Figure 8–31). However, the small magnitude of these responses poses a challenge to accurately measure their spectrotemporal attributes, particularly at high frequencies. In this section, we describe several commonly used measures ranging from a simple measure of the magnitude of the waveform of the response using its root-mean-square (RMS) amplitude to more complex measures like extracting instant spectral slices using joint time-frequency analysis.

Time-Domain Measures

RMS Amplitude

The overall amplitude of the response provides a gross index of how robust the phase-locked activity is. The root-mean-squared (RMS) amplitude of the entire response waveform (for steady-state sounds) or selected time windows (for time-variant sounds) is used. As the name implies, RMS is defined operationally as the square root of the mean of the squared instantaneous peak amplitudes. RMS for a true sinusoid is equal to approximately 0.707 times the peak amplitude. This amplitude measure can also be expressed as a SNR by expressing the RMS amplitude of the signal compared to the RMS amplitude of residual noise extracted by the prestimulus baseline or subtracting contents of two replicated buffers using a single polarity. It is somewhat easier to express the magnitude of the response relative to the noise using the fast Fourier transform (FFT) (i.e., from the spectrum).

Response Latency

This measure is largely limited to the clearly discernible onset components. It is difficult to accurately measure the latency of the FFR by visual observation, since it is difficult to identify the onset of the first effective response cycle. There are a couple of methods that are used to estimate the response latency of the phase-locked neural activity. One is to simply cross-correlate the stimulus waveform and the response by temporally shifting one relative to the other until the correlation between the two signals reaches a maximum value. Response latency will correspond to the shift in time to achieve maximal correlation. The latency of a sustained quasiperiodic complex response with multiple frequency components can also be estimated from the response group delays (i.e., negative slopes of the phase versus frequency function). That is, the phase angles of the complex are unwrapped for each frequency region (King et al., 2016) that produces a robust phase-locked activity after accounting for the acoustic delay of the tubal insert earphone. Ideally, unwrapping should be focused on group delays between 0 and 15 to 20 ms for the FFR. The latency of the phase-locked response, unlike the latency of the onset response, is primarily used to assess if neural timing (related to the index of neural synchronization) information is intact or disrupted. The estimated latency of the FFR is about 8 to 10 ms. The latency of each peak in the sustained EFR/FFR can be picked manually by experienced personnel, or automatic peak picking may be implemented, particularly for longer-duration stimuli with multiple cycles of the sustained response. Likewise, two responses can be compared (response-to-response auto- or cross-correlation) to see how well they are correlated in time. Thus, both measures can provide information about the fidelity of the response tracking of the temporal characteristics of the stimulus waveform or how response timing changes with stimulus conditions and/or pathology.

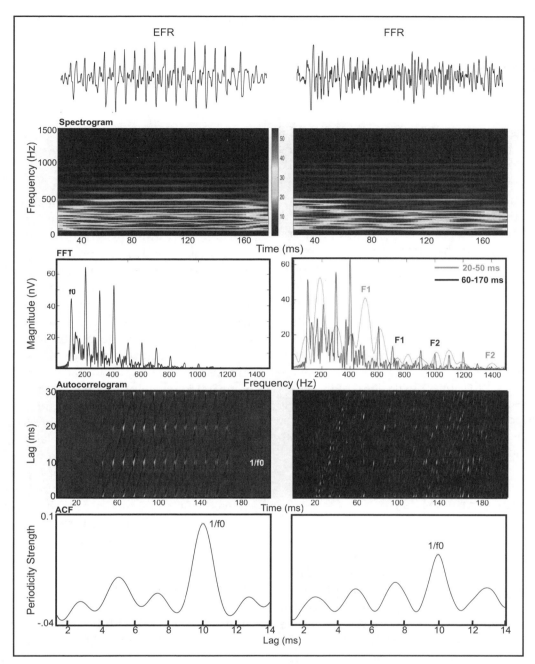

Figure 8–31. The time- and frequency-domain analysis methods for EFRs (*left*) and FFRs (*right*), including response waveforms (*top*), spectrograms (*second row*), FFT (*third row*), autocorrelogram (*fourth row*), and the autocorrelation function at the bottom (see text in the following sections for more details about each measure). The top traces show the response waveforms for the EFR (*left*) and FFR (*right*) elicited by the CV syllable /da/. Only the EFR shows a clear periodicity at f0. For all measures, responses are generally more robust for the EFR compared to the FFR. Interestingly, a comparison of the instant spectra representing the first 40 ms of formant transition (*gray spectrum*) and the instant spectra representing the steady-state segment clearly shows the earlier lower frequency of F1 during the transition, and the higher steady-steady F1 peak (*black trace*). The autocorrelogram (*row three*) plots the periodicities (over the entire duration of the stimulus) for which neurons phase-lock. Note the dotted bright line across the 10- and 20-ms delay values. Thus, there is a band of phase-locked activity that follows the fundamental periodicity of the stimulus (in this case, 100 Hz = 1/10 ms). The autocorrelation function simply measures the temporal correlation between the original response waveform and several time-shifted versions of this original response. The correlation will be maximal at a delay corresponding to the fundamental periodicity and its integer multiples—10 ms in this figure.

Autocorrelation

Autocorrelation Function (ACF)

Periodicities and periodicity strength in the EFR and FFR to complex sounds can be extracted using a periodicity detection short-term autocorrelation algorithm. Essentially, this analysis performs autocorrelation on several successive small frames taken from the response to obtain estimates of both pitch periodicity and pitch strength. The temporal correlation between the original response waveform and several time-shifted versions of this original response is determined. The correlation will be maximal at a delay corresponding to the fundamental periodicity. For example, a complex sound like /da/ with a fundamental frequency of 100 Hz will show a robust peak in the autocorrelation function at 10 ms—the period of 100 Hz (Figure 8–31, bottom panel). Pitch periodicity is defined as the time lag associated with the autocorrelation maximum; periodicity strength is the magnitude of the normalized autocorrelation peak expressed as harmonic/noise ratio ranging from 0 to 1.

Autocorrelogram (ACG)

The ACG represents the short-term autocorrelation function of windowed frames of a compound signal—that is, $ACG(\tau,t) = X(t) \times X(t-\tau)$ for each time t and time-lag τ. It is a three-dimensional plot quantifying the variations in periodicity and "neural periodicity strength" (i.e., degree of phase-locking) as a function of time (Figure 8–31, fourth row). The horizontal axis represents the time at which single ACF "slices" are computed, while the vertical axis represents their corresponding time lags (i.e., periods). The intensity of each point in the image represents the instantaneous ACF magnitude computed at a given time within the response. Mathematically, the running ACG is the time-domain analog to the frequency-domain spectrogram. In terms of neurophysiology, it represents the running distribution of all-order interspike intervals present in the population neural activity (Cariani & Delgutte, 1996a; Sayles & Winter, 2008). As such, running ACGs may be used to evaluate the distribution of phase-locked intervals in the EFR/FFR to a complex sound to extract steady-state and time-variant pitch-relevant periodicities (Swaminathan et al., 2008).

Pitch Tracking Accuracy Using Autocorrelation

A periodicity detection short-term autocorrelation algorithm is used (Boersma, 1993). Essentially, this algorithm performs a short-term autocorrelation analysis on a number of small segments (40-msec frames) taken from the signal (stimuli and FFR). The analysis window is shifted incrementally in 10-msec steps. The autocorrelation function is computed for each 40-msec frame after successive shifts. The time lag corresponding to the maximum autocorrelation value for each frame is recorded for both the stimulus and the FFR. Candidates below 75 Hz and above 200 Hz are not retained. Subsequently, the lag times associated with autocorrelation peaks in each frame are concatenated together to give a continuous f_0 contour. The cross-correlation coefficient between the f_0 contour extracted from the FFRs and the stimuli provides a measure of the accuracy of pitch tracking. Pitch-tracking accuracy can also be achieved using a frequency domain measure, since both FFT and autocorrelation are related and essentially two sides of the same coin.

Phase Coherence

Another special case of time-domain measure that can be applied to both EFR and FFR is to evaluate the distribution of phase-locking by examining the *coherence of the phase values* (i.e., the temporal similarity of the phase of the response on repeated trials) at the target periodicity (frequency) across repeated stimulus presentations. It is a special case of time, because timing information is obtained by using the phase information contained in the frequency-domain FFT. Other variants of this measure are magnitude square coherence (where both the phase and magnitude of the vector are used), intertrial phase-locking value (IPLV; a measure similar to synchronization index), and phase-locking factor (PLF). In this measure, the phase portion of the FFT analysis is used showing the vector plot of the individual trial phases and their relative magnitudes. The rationale is that for the small phase-locked responses from the brainstem to be detected, the trial-to-trial phase of neural phase-locking to the stimulus waveform should be about the same. The distribution of the individual vector in the polar plot will provide a measure of the temporal accuracy of phase-locking or phase coherence. If the vectors are closer together and show smaller standard deviation ellipses at their tip, then phase coherence is said to be high; if they are randomly distributed, then they more likely represent noise since they do not have many phase-locked responses to the stimulus (Figure 8–32). Phase coherence ranges from 0 to 1, where 1 indicates perfect agreement between phase angles obtained across sweeps. Phase coherence measures are influenced by the SNR of the signal being evaluated, performing better at higher SNRs. A variation of this measure implemented in several ASSR (EFR) modules includes both magnitude and phase angle of the vectors to magnitude squared coherence. Statistical analysis, like the Hotelling T^2, of the range of phase angles and their magnitude, can be used to determine if the response is statistically significant. Essentially, this test estimates the distribution of responses using both magnitude and phase and determines if zero is within the confidence interval of the mean (Picton et al., 1987).

Frequency-Domain Measures

Spectrum Analysis Using the Fast Fourier Transform (FFT)

For EFR and FFR recorded to tone bursts and steady-state complex sounds, response amplitude for the components forming the FFR is commonly measured from the magnitude spectrum derived by performing a Fourier transform of the time-domain response (Aiken & Picton, 2008; Ananthakrishnan,

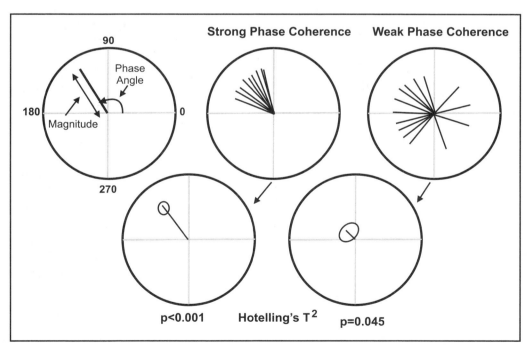

Figure 8–32. Polar plots illustrating phase coherence. The top left defines the vector's phase angle and the magnitude of the phase vector. The top middle plot shows intertrial response phases that are close to each other (so producing a strong coherence and a significant response [*bottom left*] with very little variability). The plot to the top and bottom right shows an intertrial phase that is almost randomly distributed, resulting in weak phase coherence and response (*bottom right*) that does not reach significance and therefore should be considered no response.

Krishnan, & Bartlett, 2016; Ananthakrishnan & Krishnan, 2018; Greenberg et al., 1987; Krishnan, 1999, 2002; Krishnan & McDaniel, 1998; Krishnan, Suresh, & Gandour, 2019; Pandya & Krishnan, 2004; Suresh & Krishnan, 2020; Suresh et al., 2020). However, for FFRs elicited by time-variant complex sounds, a joint time-frequency (similar to narrowband spectrograms) analysis is essential to determine not only the magnitude of the response but, more importantly, whether the FFR-related phase-locked activity can follow the time-varying features of the stimulus (Basu, Krishnan, & Weber-Fox, 2009; Krishnan & Parkinson, 2000; Krishnan et al., 2004; Plyer & Ananthanarayan, 2001; Suresh & Krishnan, 2020; Swaminathan et al., 2008). This spectral analysis typically uses short, windowed segments (about 40–50 ms long segments with minimal overlap) with zero padding (to ensure that spectral resolution is between 1 and 3 Hz), utilizing optimal windowing functions (e.g., Hanning or Gaussian window) to enhance the sensitivity of the spectral measure by reducing spectral splatter (leakage), particularly for short signal samples that have an abrupt onset and offset. The magnitudes of the spectral peaks of interest are measured and commonly expressed relative to an average noise floor estimate obtained from frequency bins on either side of the signal's spectral peaks. For steady-state stimuli, an *average FFT* (Figure 8–32, third row) can be performed over the entire duration of the response. However, for FFRs elicited by time-variant complex sounds, a joint time-frequency (similar to narrowband spectrograms) analysis is essential to determine not only the magnitude of the response but, more importantly, whether the FFR-related phase-locked activity can follow the time-varying features of the stimulus (Suresh & Krishnan, 2020). Essentially, *the joint time-frequency analysis* is a series of short-term discrete FFTs using a sliding time window that represents short response segments over the duration of the response. The result is a spectrogram that captures the magnitude and frequency of spectral components as a function of time. It is then possible to extract spectral slices from successive time windows (typically 40–50 ms in duration) over the duration of the response from this spectrogram to determine the representation of dynamic spectrotemporal properties of time-varying complex sounds. For example, the spectrotemporal properties of the formant transitions in the CV syllable /da/ can be examined (see Figure 8–31). Another useful measure in the frequency domain is the *spectral correlation* between the response spectrum and the stimulus spectrum (Krishnan et al., 2010; Suresh & Krishnan, 2020). This measurement involves the calculation of the correlation coefficient between the FFT of the EFR/FFR and the FFT of the stimulus eliciting the response. Like the joint time-frequency analysis, spectral correlations can also be performed on different temporal spectral slices representing a time-varying signal. For example, the instant response spectra representing the vowel /a/ and vowel /u/ in the diphthong can be compared with their respective stimulus spectra. The resulting correlation coefficient ranges between −1 and 1, where 1 represents a strong correlation, and −1 represents a weak correlation. This spectral correlation analysis provides the ability to examine the fidelity of the neural representation of the spectral components of the stimulus.

XII. SUMMARY

- Unlike the ABR that reflects neural activity synchronized to the onset of the stimulus, EFR reflects sustained neural phase-locking to the *envelope periodicity* of the stimulus waveform, and FFR reflects sustained neural phase-locking, primarily in the IC, to the *temporal fine structure* of complex sounds for frequencies below about 1700 Hz. A conventional clinical ASSR measure using amplitude-modulated stimuli is essentially an EFR. Neurons in the brainstem can phase-lock to both the modulation frequency to produce the EFR (ASSR in this case) and to the spectral components.

- Like tone burst ABR, EFRs also provide reliable, repeatable, accurate, and place-specific estimates of air-conduction and bone-conduction thresholds in both normal-hearing and hearing-impaired individuals. These estimates are within 5 to 15 dB (for the multifrequency EFR) and 15 to 25 dB (for the single-frequency EFR) of behavioral thresholds in normal-hearing adults. EFR thresholds in infants and young children are about 10 to 15 dB higher across frequencies compared to adults. It is generally agreed that simultaneous binaural multifrequency EFRs could provide a faster and reliable objective estimate of thresholds.

- EFRs have been used to describe the disruption in neural timing and neural encoding at the brainstem level in populations with a variety of language-based learning problems, including specific language impairment, dyslexia, autism spectrum disorders, the influence of bilingualism, sensorineural hearing loss, monitoring auditory training gains, and as a metric to evaluate benefits from amplification. EFRs are capable of measuring changes in both audibility and aided audible bandwidth.

- The scalp-recorded FFR has also been shown to preserve spectral and pitch relevant periodicity and temporal fine-structure information contained in steady-state and time-variant speech and nonspeech complex stimuli. Time-domain (e.g., waveform amplitude, ACF, ACG, and phase coherence), frequency-domain measures (spectrum analysis), and joint time-frequency analysis (spectrogram) can be performed on these responses to quantify the magnitude and neural timing strength of the EFR and FFR components.

- FFR representation of spectra and periodicity appears to be degraded in individuals with sensorineural loss and thus could provide a metric to assess the nature of the degradation of neural encoding of acoustic features important for speech perception. Thus, there is the potential to make individual-specific recommendations regarding the optimal amplification requirements to improve speech intelligibility, outcome measures of auditory training, and benefits from conventional amplification/cochlear implants. However, more concerted research efforts are needed to realize this potential. It will also be potentially worthwhile to pursue parametric research aimed at evaluating the relationship between neural representation and auditory perceptual ability.

- EFR and FFR can be used as an electrophysiologic metric to characterize the degradation of neural representation consequent to peripheral and/or central auditory pathologies. They could also be used to monitor treatment outcomes with amplification, evaluate effects of auditory retraining, and test and evaluate optimal signal processing strategies for hearing prosthetic devices.

REFERENCES

Aiken, S. J., & Picton, T. W. (2006). Envelope following responses to natural vowels. *Audiology Neurootology*, 11, 213–232.

Aiken, S. J., & Picton, T. W. (2008). Envelope and spectral frequency-following responses to vowel sounds. *Hearing Research, 245*, 35–47.

Aiken, S. J., & Purcell, D. W. (2013). Sensitivity to stimulus polarity in speech-evoked frequency-following responses. *Proceedings of Meetings on Acoustics, 19*, 050121. https://doi.org/10.1121/1.4800244

Aimoni, C., Crema, L., Savini, S., Negossi, L., Rosignoli, M., Sacchetto, L., . . . & Ciorba, A. (2018). Hearing threshold estimation by auditory steady state responses (ASSR) in children. *Acta Otorhinolaryngologica Italica, 38*(4), 361.

Aizawa, N., & Eggermont, J. J. (2006). Effects of noise-induced hearing loss at young age on voice onset time and gap-in-noise representations in adult cat primary auditory cortex. *Journal of the Association of Research in Otolaryngology, 7*(1), 71–81.

Akhoun, I., Gallégo, S., Moulin, A., Ménard, M., Veuillet, E., Berger-Vachon, C., . . . Thai-Van, H. (2008). The temporal relationship between speech auditory brainstem responses and the acoustic pattern of the phoneme /ba/ in normal-hearing adults. *Clinical Neurophysiology, 119*, 922–933.

Ananthakrishnan, S., & Krishnan, A. (2018). Human frequency following responses to iterated rippled noise with positive and negative gain: Differential sensitivity to waveform envelope and temporal fine structure. *Hearing Research, 367*, 113–123.

Ananthakrishnan, S., Krishnan, A., & Bartlett, E. (2016). Human frequency following response: Neural representation of envelope and temporal fine structure in listeners with normal hearing and sensorineural hearing loss. *Ear and Hearing, 37*(2), e91–e103.

Ananthakrishnan, S., Luo, X., & Krishnan, A. (2017). Human frequency following responses to vocoded speech. *Ear and Hearing, 38*(5), e256–e267.

Ananthanarayan, A. K., & Durrant, J. D. (1992). The frequency following response and the onset response: Evaluation of frequency specificity using a forward-masking paradigm. *Ear and Hearing, 13,* 228–233.

Anderson, D. J., Rose, J. E., Hind, J. E., & Brugge, J. F. (1971). Temporal position of discharges in single auditory nerve fibers within the cycle of a sine-wave stimulus: Frequency and intensity effects. *Journal of the Acoustical Society of America, 49,* 1131–1139. https://doi.org/10.1121/1.1912474

Anderson, S., & Kraus, N. (2013). The potential role of the cABR in assessment and management of hearing impairment. *International Journal of Otolaryngology, 2013.*

Anderson, S., Parbery-Clark, A., White-Schwoch, T., Drehobl, S., & Kraus, N. (2013). Effects of hearing loss on the subcortical representation of speech cues. *Journal of the Acoustical Society of America, 133*(5), 3030–3038.

Anderson, S., White-Schwoch, T., Parbery-Clark, A., & Kraus, N. (2013). Reversal of age-related neural timing delays with training. *Proceedings of the National Academy of Sciences, U.S.A., 110,* 4357–4362.

Arthur, R. M., Pffeifer, R. R., & Suga, N. (1971). Properties of two-tone inhibition in primary auditory neurons. *Journal of Physiology, 212,* 593–609.

Bacon, S. P., & Gleitman, R. M. (1992). Modulation detection in subjects with relatively flat hearing losses. *Journal of Speech, Language and Hearing Research, 35*(3), 642.

Bacon, S. P., & Viemeister, N. F. (1985). Temporal modulation transfer function in normal hearing and hearing-impaired subjects. *Audiology, 24,* 117–134.

Baillet, S. (2017). Magnetoencephalography for brain electrophysiology and imaging. *Nature Neuroscience, 20,* 327–339.

Baillet, S., Mosher, J. C., & Leahy, R. M. (2001). Electromagnetic brain mapping. *IEEE Signal Processing Magazine, 18,* 14–30.

Banai, K., Hornickel, J., Skoe, E., Nicol, T., Zecker, S., & Kraus, N. (2009). Reading and subcortical auditory function. *Cerebral Cortex, 19,* 2699–2707.

Banai, K., & Kraus, N. (2008). *The dynamic brainstem: Implications for APD.* San Diego, CA: Plural Publishing.

Banai, K., Nicol, T., Zecker, S. G., & Kraus, N. (2005). Brainstem timing: Implications for cortical processing and literacy. *Journal of Neuroscience, 25,* 9850–9857.

Basu, M., Krishnan, A., & Weber-Fox, C. (2010). Brainstem correlates of temporal auditory processing in children with specific language impairment. *Developmental science, 13*(1), 77-91.

Bidelman, G. M. (2015). Multichannel recordings of the human brainstem frequency-following response: Scalp topography, source generators, and distinctions from the transient ABR. *Hearing Research, 323,* 68–80.

Bidelman, G. M. (2018). Subcortical sources dominate the neuroelectric auditory frequency-following response to speech. *NeuroImage, 175,* 56–69.

Bidelman, G. M, Gandour, J., & Krishnan, A. (2011). Musicians and tone-language speakers share enhanced brainstem encoding but not perceptual benefits for musical pitch. *Brain and Cognition, 77*(1), 1–10.

Bidelman, G. M., & Krishnan, A. (2009). Neural correlates of consonance, dissonance, and the hierarchy of musical pitch in the human brainstem. *Journal of Neuroscience, 29*(42), 13165–13171.

Bidelman, G. M., & Krishnan, A. (2011). Brainstem correlates of behavioral and compositional preferences of musical harmony. *NeuroReport, 22*(5), 212–216.

Bidelman, G. M., & Momtaz, S. (2021). Subcortical rather than cortical sources of the frequency-following response (FFR) relate to speech-in-noise perception in normal-hearing listeners. *Neuroscience Letters, 746,* 135664.

Bidelman, G. M., Pousson, M., Dugas, C., & Fehrenbach, A. (2018). Test-retest reliability of dual-recorded brainstem versus cortical auditory-evoked potentials to speech. *Journal of the American Academy of Audiology, 29*(2), 164–174.

Bidelman, G. M., & Powers, L. (2018). Response properties of the human frequency-following response (FFR) to speech and nonspeech sounds: Level dependence, adaptation, and phase-locking limits. *International Journal of Audiology, 57*(9), 665–672.

Billings, C. J., Bologna, W. J., Muralimanohar, R. K., Madsen, B., & Molis, M. R. (2019). Frequency following responses to tone glides: Effects of frequency extent, direction, and electrode montage. *Hearing Research, 375,* 25–33.

Blackburn, C. C., & Sachs, M. B. (1990). The representations of the steady-state vowel sound /e/ in the discharge patterns of cat anteroventral cochlear nucleus neurons. *Journal of Neurophysiology, 63,* 1191–1212.

Bledsoe, J. S. C., & Moushegian, G. (1980). The 500 Hz frequency-following potential in kangaroo rat: An evaluation with noise masking. *Electroencephalography and Clinical Neurophysiology, 48,* 654–663.

Boersma, P. (1993). Accurate short-term analysis of the fundamental frequency and the harmonics-to-noise ratio of a sampled sound. *Proceedings of the Institute of Phonetic Science, 17,* 97–110.

Brown, R. (1958). *Words and things* (pp. 36–42). Glencoe, IL: Free Press.

Brugge, J. F., Nourski, K. V., Oya, H., Reale, R. A., Kawasaki, H., Steinschneider, M., & Howard 3rd, M. A. (2009). Coding of repetitive transients by auditory cortex on Heschl's gyrus. *Journal of Neurophysiology, 102*, 2358–2374.

Campbell, F. W., Atkinson, J., Francis, M. R., & Green, D. M. (1977). Estimation of auditory thresholds using evoked potentials. In J. E. Desmedt (Ed.), *Auditory evoked potentials in man. Psychopharmacology correlates of evoked potentials. Progress in Clinical Neurophysiology* (Vol. 2, pp. 68–78). Basel: Karger.

Cariani, P. (1998). *Neural computations in the time domain.* Poster session presented at the midwinter meeting of the Association for Research in Otolaryngology, Midwinter Meeting.

Cariani, P. A., & Delgutte, B. (1996a). Neural correlates of the pitch of complex tones. I. Pitch and pitch salience. *Journal of Neurophysiology, 76*, 1698–1716.

Cariani, P. A., & Delgutte, B. (1996b). Neural correlates of the pitch of complex tones. II. Pitch shift, pitch ambiguity, phase invariance, pitch circularity, rate pitch, and the dominance region for pitch. *Journal of Neurophysiology, 76*, 1717–1734.

Carlson, R., Fant, G., & Granstrom, B. T. (1975). Two-formant models, pitch and vowel perception. In G. Fant & M. A. A. Tatham (Eds.), *Auditory analysis and perception of speech* (pp. 55–82). London, UK: Academic Press.

Casey, K. A., & Small, S. A. (2014). Comparisons of auditory steady state response and behavioral air conduction and bone conduction thresholds for infants and adults with normal hearing. *Ear and Hearing, 35*, 423–439.

Caspary, D. M., Rupert, A. L., & Moushegian, G. (1977). Neuronal coding of vowel sounds in the cochlear nuclei. *Experimental Neurology, 54*, 414–431.

Chandrasekaran, B., Hornickel, J., Skoe, E., Nicol, T., & Kraus, N. (2009). Context-dependent encoding in the human auditory brainstem relates to hearing speech in noise: implications for developmental dyslexia. *Neuron, 64*(3), 311-319.

Chandrasekaran, B., & Kraus, N. (2010). The scalp-recorded brainstem response to speech: Neural origins and plasticity. *Psychophysiology, 47*(2), 236–246.

Chertoff, M. E., & Hecox, K. E. (1990). Auditory non-linearities measured with auditory-evoked potentials. *Journal of the Acoustical Society of America, 87*, 1248–1254.

Chertoff, M. E., Hecox, K. E., & Goldstein, R. (1992). Auditory distortion products measured with averaged auditory evoked potentials. *Journal of Speech and Hearing Research, 35*, 157–166.

Clinard, C. G., & Cotter, C. M. (2015). Neural representation of dynamic frequency is degraded in older adults. *Hearing Research, 323*, 91–98.

Coffey, E. B., Herholz, S. C., Chepesiuk, A. M., Baillet, S., & Zatorre, R. J. (2016). Cortical contributions to the auditory frequency-following response revealed by MEG. *Nature and Communication, 7*, 11070.

Cohen, D., & Cuffin, B. N. (1983). Demonstration of useful differences between magnetoencephalogram and electroencephalogram. *Electroencephalography and Clinical Neurophysiology, 56*, 38–51.

Cone-Wesson, B., & Dimitrijevic, A. (2009). The auditory steady-state response. In J. Katz, L. Medwetsky, R. F. Burkard, & L. Hood (Eds.), *Handbook of clinical audiology* (6th ed., pp. 322–350). Philadelphia, PA: Lippincott Williams & Wilkins.

Cone-Wesson, B., Dowell, R. C., Tomlin, D., Rance, G., & Ming, W.-J. (2002). The auditory steady-state response: Comparisons with the auditory brainstem response. *Journal of American Academy of Audiology, 13*, 173–187.

Cunningham, J., Nicol, T., Zecker, S. G., Bradlow, A., & Kraus N. (2001). Neurobiologic responses to speech in noise in children with learning problems: Deficits and strategies for improvement. *Clinical Neurophysiology, 112*, 758–767.

Dau, T. (2003). The importance of cochlear processing for the formation of auditory brainstem and frequency following responses. *Journal of the Acoustical Society of America, 113*, 936–950.

Davis, H., & Hirsh, S. K. (1976). The audiometric utility of brain stem responses to low-frequency sounds. *Audiology, 15*, 181–195.

Davis, R. L., & Britt, R. H. (1984). Analysis of the frequency following response in the cat. *Hearing Research, 15*, 29–37.

De Boer, E., Machiels, M. B., & Kruidenier, C. (1977). Low-level frequency-following response. *Audiology, 16*, 29–240.

Dong, S., Mulders, W. H., Rodger, J., Woo, S., & Robertson, D. (2010). Acoustic trauma evokes hyperactivity and changes in gene expression in guinea-pig auditory brainstem. *European Journal of Neuroscience, 31*(9), 1616-1628.

D'Haenens, W., Vinck, B. M., De Vel, E., Maes, L., Bockstael, A., Keppler, H., . . . Dhooge, I. (2008). Auditory steady-state responses in normal hearing adults: A test-retest reliability study. *International Journal of Audiology, 47*(8), 489–498.

Dimitrijevic, A., John, M. S., Van Roon, P., Purcell, D. W., Adamonis, J., Ostroff, J., . . . Picton, T. W. (2002). Estimating the audiogram using multiple auditory steady-state responses. *Journal of American Academy Audiology, 13*, 205–224.

Easwar, V., Beamish, L., Aiken, S., Choi, J. M., Scollie, S., & Purcell, D. (2015). Sensitivity of envelope following responses to vowel polarity. *Hearing Research, 320,* 38–50.

Easwar, V., Purcell, D. W., Aiken, S. J., Parsa, V., & Scollie, S. D. (2015a). Effect of stimulus level and bandwidth on speech-evoked envelope following responses in adults with normal hearing. *Ear and Hearing, 36*(6), 619–634.

Easwar, V., Purcell, D. W., Aiken, S. J., Parsa, V., & Scollie, S. D. (2015b). Evaluation of speech-evoked envelope following responses as an objective aided outcome measure: Effect of stimulus level, bandwidth, and amplification in adults with hearing loss. *Ear and Hearing, 36*(6), 635–652.

Easwar, V., Purcell, D. W., & Scollie, S. D. (2012). Electroacoustic comparison of hearing aid output of phonemes in running speech versus isolation: Implications for aided cortical auditory evoked potentials testing. *International Journal of Otolaryngology, 2012,* 518202. https://doi.org/10.1155/2012/518202.

Easwar, V., Scollie, S., & Purcell, D. (2019). Investigating potential interactions between envelope following responses elicited simultaneously by different vowel formants. *Hearing Research, 380,* 35–45.

Easwar, V., Scollie, S., Aiken, S., & Purcell, D. (2020). Test-retest variability in the characteristics of envelope following responses evoked by speech stimuli. *Ear and Hearing, 41*(1), 150–164.

Elsisy, H., & Krishnan, A. (2008). Comparison of response characteristics of acoustical and neural distortion product at 2f1-f2 in normal hearing adults. *International Journal of Audiology, 47,* 431–438.

Elberling, C., Don, M., Cebulla, M., & Stürzebecher, E. (2007). Auditory steady-state responses to chirp stimuli based on cochlear traveling wave delay. *The Journal of the Acoustical Society of America, 122*(5), 2772-2785.

Galbraith, G., Bagasan, B., & Sulahian, J. (2001). Brainstem frequency-following response recorded from one vertical and three horizontal electrode derivations. *Perception Motor Skills, 921,* 99–106.

Galbraith, G., Jhaveri, S. P., & Kuo, J. (1997). Speech-evoked brainstem frequency-following responses during verbal transformations due to word repetition. *Electroencephalography and Clinical Neurophysiology, 102,* 46–53.

Garcia, M. V., de Azevedo, M. F., Biaggio, E. P. V., Didone, D. D., & Gurgel Testa, J. R. (2014). Auditory steady-state responses air and bone conducted in children from zero to six months with and without conductive impairments. *Revista CEFAC, 16*(3), 699–706.

Gardi, J., & Merzenich, M. (1979). The effect of high-pass noise on the scalp-recorded frequency following response (FFR) in humans and cats. *Journal of the Acoustical Society of America, 65,* 14–91.

Gardi, J., Salamy, A., & Mendelson, T. (1979). Scalp-recorded frequency-following responses in neonates. *Audiology, 18,* 494–506.

Geisler, C. D., Rhode, W. S., & Kennedy, D. T. (1974). Responses to tonal stimuli of single auditory nerve fibers and their relationship to basilar membrane motion in the squirrel monkey. *Journal of Neurophysiology, 37,* 1156–1172.

Gerken, G. M., Moushegian, G., Stillman, R. D., & Rupert, A. L. (1975). Human frequency-following responses to monaural and binaural stimuli. *Electroencephalography and Clinical Neurophysiology, 38,* 379–386.

Glaser, E. M., Suter, C. M., Dasheiff, R., & Goldberg, A. (1976). The human frequency-following response: Its behavior during continuous tone and tone burst stimulation. *Electroencephalography and Clinical Neurophysiology, 40,* 25–32.

Goblick, T. J., & Pffeifer, R. R. (1969). Time-domain measurements of the cochlear nonlinearities using combination click stimuli. *Journal of the Acoustical Society of America, 46,* 924–938.

Goldstein, J. L. (1967). Auditory nonlinearity. *Journal of the Acoustical Society of America, 41,* 676–689.

Goldstein, J. L., & Kiang, N. Y. (1968). Neural correlates of the aural combination tone 2F1–F2. *Journal of the Acoustical Society of America, 44,* 362.

Greenberg, S. (1980). *Neural temporal coding of pitch and vowel quality: Human frequency-following response studies of complex signals* (Doctoral dissertation). Phonetics Laboratory, Department of Linguistics, UCLA.

Greenberg, S., Marsh, J. T., Brown, W. S., & Smith, J. C. (1987). Neural temporal coding of low pitch: I. Human frequency-following responses to complex tones. *Hearing Research, 25,* 91–114.

Grose, J. H., Mamo, S. K., & Hall, J. W., III. (2009). Age effects in temporal envelope processing: Speech unmasking and auditory steady state responses. *Ear and Hearing, 30,* 568–575.

Hall, J. W., III. (1979). Auditory brainstem frequency following responses to waveform envelope periodicity. *Science, 205,* 1297–1299.

Han, D., Mo, L., Liu, H., Chen, J., & Huang, L. (2006). Threshold estimation in children using auditory steady-state responses to multiple simultaneous stimuli. *ORL: Journal for Oto-Rhino-Laryngology and Its Related Specialties, 68,* 64–68.

Hao, W., Wang, Q., Li, L., Qiao, Y., Gao, Z., Ni, D., & Shang, Y. (2018). Effects of phase-locking deficits on speech recognition in older adults with presbycusis. *Frontiers in Aging Neuroscience, 10,* 397. https://doi.org/10.3389/fnagi.2018.00397

Harris, F. (1990). Distortion-product otoacoustic emissions in humans with high frequency sensorineural hearing loss. *Journal of Speech and Hearing Research, 33,* 594–600.

He, N., & Schmiedt, R. A. (1993). Fine structure of the 2f1-f2 acoustic distortion product: Changes with primary level. *Journal of the Acoustical Society of America, 94,* 2659–2669.

He, N., & Schmiedt, R. A. (1997). Fine structure of the 2f1-f2 acoustic distortion products: Effects of primary level and frequency ratios. *Journal of the Acoustical Society of America, 101,* 3554–3565.

Henry, K. S., & Heinz, M. G. (2013). Effects of sensorineural hearing loss on temporal coding of narrowband and broadband signals in the auditory periphery. *Hearing Research, 303,* 39–47.

Herdman, A. T., Lins, O., Van Roon, P., Stapells, D. R., Scherg, M., & Picton, T. W. (2002). Intracerebral sources of human auditory steady-state responses. *Brain Topography, 15,* 69–86.

Herdman, A. T., Picton, T. W., & Stapells, D. R. (2002). Place specificity of multiple auditory steady-state responses. *Journal of the Acoustical Society of America, 112,* 1569–1582.

Herdman, A. T., & Stapells, D. R. (2001). Thresholds determined using the monotic and dichotic multiple auditory steady-state response technique in normal-hearing subjects. *Scandinavian Audiology, 30,* 41–49.

Herdman, A. T., & Stapells, D. R. (2003). Auditory steady-state response thresholds of adults with sensorineural hearing impairments. *International Journal of Audiology, 42,* 237–248.

Hillebrand, A., & Barnes, G. R. (2002). A quantitative assessment of the sensitivity of whole-head MEG to activity in the adult human cortex. *Neuroimage, 16,* 638–650.

Holstein, S. B., Buchwald, J. S., & Schwafel, J. A. (1969). Tone response patterns of the auditory nuclei during normal wakefulness, paralysis, and anesthesia. *Brain Research, 15,* 483–499.

Hornickel, J., & Kraus, N. (2013). Unstable representation of sound: A biological marker of dyslexia. *Journal of Neuroscience, 33,* 3500–3504.

Hornickel, J., Skoe, E., Nicol, T., Zecker, S., & Krau, N. (2009). Subcortical differentiation of stop consonants relates to reading and speech-in-noise perception. *PNAS, 106*(31), 13022–13027.

Huis in't Veld, F., Osterhammel, P., & Terkildsen, K. (1977). The frequency selectivity of the 500 Hz frequency following response. *Scandinavian Audiology, 6,* 35–42.

Ishida, I. M., Cuthbert, B. P., & Stapells, D. R. (2011). Multiple auditory steady state response thresholds to bone conduction stimuli in adults with normal and elevated thresholds. *Ear and Hearing, 32,* 373–381.

Ismaila, N., El-Saiid, E., El-Sebaii, A., & Fadel, H. (2016). Reliability of auditory steady-state response to bone conduction stimuli in assessing hearing loss in children. *Egyptian Journal of Otolaryngology, 32,* 196–201.

Jacobson, R., Fant, G., & Halle, M. (1991). *Preliminaries to speech analysis.* Cambridge, MA: MIT.

Janssen, T., Steinhoff, H. J., & Bohnke, F. (1991). Zum Entstchungs Mechanismus der Frequenzfolgepotentiale. *Otorhinolaryngology Nova, 1,* 16–25.

Jeng, F. C., Brownt, C. J., Johnson, T. A., & Vander Werff, K. R. (2004). Estimating air–bone gaps using auditory steady-state responses. *Journal of the American Academy of Audiology, 15,* 67–78.

Jenkins, K. A., Fodor, C., Presacco, A., & Anderson, S. (2018). Effects of amplification on neural phase locking, amplitude, and latency to a speech syllable. *Ear and Hearing, 39*(4), 810–824.

John, M. S., Brown, D. K., Muir, P. J., & Picton, T. W. (2004). Recording auditory steady-state responses in young infants. *Ear and Hearing, 25,* 539–553.

John, M. S., Lins, O. G., Boucher, B. L., & Picton, T. W. (1998). Multiple auditory steady-state responses (MASTER): Stimulus and recording parameters. *Audiology, 37,* 59–82.

John, M. S., & Picton, T. W. (2000a). MASTER: A windows program for recording multiple auditory steady-state responses. *Computer Methods Programs Biomedicine, 61,* 125–150.

John, M. S., & Picton, T. W. (2000b). Human auditory steady-state responses to amplitude-modulated tones: Phase and latency measurements. *Hearing Research, 141,* 57–79.

Johnson, K. L., Nicol, T., Zecker, S. G., Bradlow, A. R., Skoe, E., & Kraus, N. (2008a). Brainstem encoding of voiced consonant-vowel stop syllables. *Clinical Neurophysiology, 119,* 2623–2635.

Jones, M., Kraus, N., Bonacina, S., Nicol, T., Otto-Meyer, S., & Roberts, M. Y. (2020). Auditory processing differences in toddlers with autism spectrum disorder. *Journal of Speech, Language, and Hearing Research, 63*(5), 1608–1617.

Joris, P. X., Schreiner, C. E., & Rees, A. (2004). Neural processing of amplitude-modulated sounds. *Physiological Reviews, 84,* 541–577.

Kale, S., & Heinz, M. G. (2010). Envelope coding in auditory nerve fibers following noise-induced hearing loss. *Journal of the Association for Research in Otolaryngology, 11*(4), 657–673.

Kim, D. O., Molnar, C. E., & Matthews, J. W. (1980). Cochlear mechanics: Nonlinear behavior in two-tone responses as reflected in cochlear-nerve-fiber responses and in ear-canal sound pressure. *Journal of the Acoustical Society of America, 67,* 1704–1721.

Kimberley, B. P., & Nelson, D. A. (1989). Distortion product emissions and sensorineural hearing loss. *Journal of Otolaryngology, 18,* 365–369.

King, A., Hopkins, K., & Plack, C. J. (2016). Differential group delay of the frequency Following response measured vertically and horizontally. *Journal of the Association for Research in Otolaryngology, 17,* 133–143.

Korczak, P., Smart, J., Delgado, R., Strobel, T., & Bradford, C. (2012). Auditory steady state responses. *Journal of the American Academy of Audiology, 23,* 146–170.

Kraus, N., & Nicol, T. (2018). Brainstem encoding of speech music sounds in humans. In K. Kandler (Ed.), *The Oxford handbook of the auditory brainstem* (Online). Oxford, UK: Oxford University Press.

Krishnan, A. (1999). Human frequency following responses to two-tone approximations of steady-state vowels. *Audiology and Neuro-Otology, 4,* 95–103.

Krishnan, A. (2002). Human frequency following response: Representation of steady-state vowels. *Hearing Research, 166,* 192–201.

Krishnan, A. (2007). Frequency following response. In R. F. Burkard, M. Don, & J. J. Eggermont (Eds.), *Auditory evoked potentials: Basic principles and clinical application* (pp. 313–333). Baltimore, MD: Lippincott Williams & Wilkins.

Krishnan, A., & Agrawal, S. (2010). Human frequency-following response to speech-like sounds: Correlates of off-frequency masking. *Audiology and Neuro-Otology, 15,* 221–228.

Krishnan, A., Bidelman, G. M., & Gandour, J. T. (2010). Neural representation of pitch salience in the human brainstem revealed by psychophysical and electrophysiological indices. *Hearing Research, 268,* 60–66.

Krishnan, A., & Gandour, J. T. (2014). Language experience shapes processing of pitch relevant information in the human brainstem and auditory cortex: Electrophysiological evidence. *Acoustics Australia, 42*(3), 187–199.

Krishnan, A., Gandour, J. T., & Suresh, C. (2016). Language-experience plasticity in neural representation of changes in pitch salience. *Brain Research, 1637,* 102–117.

Krishnan, A., & McDaniel, S. (1998). Binaural interaction in the human frequency following response: Effects of interaural intensity difference. *Audiology and Neurotology, 3,* 291–299.

Krishnan, A., & Parkinson, J. (2000). Human frequency-following response: Representation of tonal sweeps. *Audiology and Neuro-otology, 5,* 312–321.

Krishnan, A., & Plack, C. (2011). Neural encoding in the human brainstem relevant to the pitch of complex tones. *Hearing Research, 275*(1–2), 110–119.

Krishnan, A., Suresh, C., & Gandour, J. T. (2019). Tone language experience-dependent advantage in pitch representation in brainstem and auditory cortex is maintained under reverberation. *Hearing Research, 177,* 63–71.

Krishnan, A., Xu, Y., Gandour, J. T., & Cariani, P. A. (2004). Human frequency-following response: Representation of pitch contours in Chinese tones. *Hearing Research, 189*(1–2), 1–12.

Krishnan, A., Xu, Y., Gandour, J. T., & Cariani, P. (2005). Encoding of pitch in the human brainstem is sensitive to language experience. *Cognitive Brain Research, 25,* 161–168.

Krizman, J., Skoe, E., Marian, V., & Kraus, N. (2014). Bilingualism increases neural response consistency and attentional control: Evidence for sensory and cognitive coupling. *Brain and Language, 128,* 34–40.

Krizman, J., Slater, J., Skoe, E., Marian, V., & Kraus, N. (2015). Neural processing of speech in children is influenced by extent of bilingual experience. *Neuroscience Letters, 5,* 48–53.

Kumar, K., Bhat, J. S., D'Costa, P. E., Srivastava, M., & Kalaiah, M. K. (2013). Effect of stimulus polarity on speech evoked auditory brainstem response. *Audiology Research, 3,* 52–56.

Kuwada, S., Anderson, J. S., Batra, R., Fitzpatrick, D. C., Teissier, N., & D'Angelo, W. R. (2002). Sources of the scalp-recorded amplitude-modulation following response. *Journal of the American Academy of Audiology, 13,* 188–204.

Leek, M., & Summers, V. (1996). Reduced frequency selectivity and the preservation of spectral contrast in noise. *Journal of the Acoustical Society of America, 100*(3), 1796–1806.

Liberman, A. M., Delattre, P., Cooper, F., & Gerstman, L. (1954). The role of consonant-vowel transitions in the perception of the stop and nasal consonants. *Psychological Monographs: General and Applied, 68*(8), 1–13.

Lin, Y. H., Ho, H. C., & Wu, H. P. (2009). Comparison of auditory steady-state responses and auditory brainstem responses in audiometric assessment of adults with sensorineural hearing loss. *Auris Nasus Larynx, 36*(2), 140-145.

Lins, O. G., & Picton, T. W. (1995). Auditory steady-state responses to multiple simultaneous stimuli. *Electroencephalography and Clinical Neurophysiology, 96*, 420–432.

Lins, O. G., Picton, T. W., Boucher, B. L., Durieux-Smith, A., Champagne, S. C., Moran, L. M., . . . Savio, G. (1996). Frequency-specific audiometry using steady-state responses. *Ear and Hearing, 17*, 81–96.

Lonsbury-Martin, B. L., Harris, F. P., Stagner, B. B., Hawkins, M. D., & Martin, G. K. (1990). Distortion product emissions in humans: I. Basic properties in normally hearing subjects. *Annals of Otology, Rhinology and Laryngology (Supplement), 147*, 3–14.

Lu, T., Liang, L., & Wang, X. (2001). Temporal and rate representations of time-varying signals in the auditory cortex of awake primates. *Nature Neuroscience, 4*, 1131–1138.

Luts, H., Desloovere, C., Kumar, A., Vandermeersch, E., & Wouters, J. (2004). Objective assessment of frequency-specific hearing thresholds in babies. *International Journal of Pediatric Otorhinolaryngology, 68*, 915–926.

Luts, H., Desloovere, C., & Wouters, J. (2006). Clinical application of dichotic multiple-stimulus auditory steady-state responses in high-risk newborns and young children. *Audiology and Neuro-otology, 11*, 24–37.

Luts, H., & Wouters, J. (2005). Comparison of MASTER and AUDERA for measurement of auditory steady-state responses. *International Journal of Audiology, 44*, 244–253.

Madhavi, B., Krishnan, A., & Weber-Fox, C. (2009). Brainstem correlates of temporal auditory processing in children with specific language impairment. *Developmental Neuroscience, 13*(1), 77–91.

Mair, I. W. S., & Laukli, E. (1984). Frequency-following responses in the cat. *Hearing Research, 15*(1), 1–10.

Manley, G. A., Koppl, C., & Johnstone, B. M. (1990). Components of the 2F1–F2 distortion product in the ear canal of the Bobtail lizard. In P. Dallos, J. W. Matthews, M. A. Ruggero, & C. R. Steele (Eds.), *The mechanics and biophysics of hearing* (pp. 210–218). Berlin, Germany: Springer-Verlag.

Marsh, J. T., Brown, W. S., & Smith, J. C. (1975). Far-field recorded frequency-following responses: Correlates of low pitch auditory perception in humans. *Electroencephalography and Clinical Neurophysiology, 38*, 113–119.

Marsh, J. T., Smith, J. C., & Worden, F. G. (1972). Receptor and neural responses in auditory masking of low frequency tones. *Electroencephalography and Clinical Neurophysiology, 32*, 63–74.

Marsh, J. T., Worden, F. G., & Smith, J. C. (1970). Auditory frequency-following response: Neural or artifact? *Science, 169*, 1222–1223.

Meddis, R., & O'Mard, L. (1997). A unitary model of pitch perception. *Journal of the Acoustical Society of America, 102*(3), 1811–1820.

Ménard, M., Gallégo, S., Berger-Vachon, C., Collet, L., & Thai-Van, H. (2008). Relationship between loudness growth function and auditory steady-state response in normal-hearing subjects. *Hearing Research, 235*, 105–113.

Miller, R. L., Schilling, J. R., Franck, K. R., & Young, E. D. (1997). Effects of acoustic trauma on the representation of the vowel /ɛ/ in cat auditory nerve fibers. *Journal of the Acoustical Society of America, 101*, 3602–3616.

Mo, L., & Stapells, D. R. (2008). The effect of brief-tone stimulus duration on the brain stem auditory steady-state response. *Ear and Hearing, 29*, 121–133.

Moushegian, G., & Rupert, A. L. (1970). Response diversity of neurons in ventral cochlear nucleus of kangaroo rat to low-frequency tones. *Journal of Neurophysiology, 33*, 351–364.

Moushegian, G., Rupert, A. L., & Stillman, R. D. (1973). Scalp-recorded early responses in man to frequencies in the speech range. *Electroencephalography and Clinical Neurophysiology, 35*, 665–667.

Moushegian, G., Rupert, A. L., & Stillman, R. D. (1978). Evaluation of frequency-following potentials in man: Masking and clinical studies. *Electroencephalography and Clinical Neurophysiology, 45*, 711–718.

Nelson, D. A., & Kimberley, B. P. (1992). Distortion-product emissions and auditory sensitivity in human ears with normal hearing and cochlear hearing loss. *Journal of Speech and Hearing Research, 35*, 1142–1159.

Norton, S. J., & Rubel, E. W. (1990). Active and passive ADP components in mammalian and avian ears. In P. Dallos, J. W. Matthews, M. A. Ruggero, & C. R.

Steele (Eds.), *The mechanics and biophysics of hearing* (pp. 199–226). Berlin, Germany: Springer-Verlag.

Otto-Meyer, S., Krizman, J., White-Schwoch, T., & Kraus, N. (2018). Children with autism spectrum disorder have unstable neural responses to sound. *Experimental Brain Research, 236*(3), 733–743.

Palmer, A. R., & Moorjani, P. A. (1993). Responses to speech signals in the normal and pathological peripheral auditory system. *Progress in Brain Research, 97,* 107–115.

Palmer, A. R., & Russell, I. J. (1986). Phase-locking in the cochlear nerve of the guinea-pig and its relation to the receptor potential of inner hair-cells. *Hearing Research, 24*(1), 1–15.

Palmer, A. R., Winter, I. M., & Darwin, C. J. (1986). The representation of steady-state vowel sounds in the temporal discharge patterns of the guinea pig cochlear nerve and primary-like cochlear nucleus neurons. *Journal of the Acoustical Society of America, 79,* 100–113.

Pandya, P. K., & Krishnan, A. (2004). Human frequency-following response correlates of the distortion product at 2F1–F2. *Journal of the American Academy of Audiology, 15*(3), 184–197.

Peterson, G. E., & Barney, H. L. (1952). Control methods used in a study of vowels. *Journal of the Acoustical Society of America, 24,* 175–184.

Pethe, J., Mühler, R., Siewert, K., & von Specht, H. (2004). Near-threshold recordings of amplitude modulation following responses (AMFR) in children of different ages. *International Journal of Audiology, 43,* 339–345.

Picton, T. W. (2011). *Human auditory evoked potentials*. San Diego, CA: Plural Publishing.

Picton, T. W., & John, M. S. (2004). Avoiding electromagnetic artifacts when recording auditory steady-state responses. *Journal of the American Academy of Audiology, 15,* 541–554.

Picton, T. W., Dimitrijevic, A., Perez-Abalo, M. C., & Van Roon, P. (2005). Estimating audiometric thresholds using auditory steady-state responses. *Journal of the American Academy of Audiology, 16*(3), 140-156.

Picton, T. W., John, M., Dimitrijevic, A., & Purcell, D. (2003). Human auditory steady-state responses. *International Journal of Audiology, 42,* 177–219.

Picton, T. W., Skinner, C. R., Champagne, S. C., Kellett, A. J., & Maiste, A. C. (1987). Potentials evoked by the sinusoidal modulation of the amplitude or frequency of a tone. *Journal of the Acoustical Society of America, 82,* 165–178.

Picton, T. W., Vajsar, J., Rodriguez, R., & Campbell, K. B. (1987). Reliability estimates for steady state evoked potentials. *Electroencephalography and Clinical Neurophysiology, 68,* 119–131.

Picton, T. W., van Roon, P., & Sasha John, M. (2007). Human auditory steady-state responses during sweeps of intensity. *Ear and Hearing, 28*(4), 542–557.

Picton, T. W., van Roon, P., & Sasha John, M. (2009). Multiple auditory steady state responses (80–101 Hz): Effects of ear, gender, handedness, intensity and modulation rate. *Ear and Hearing, 30,* 100–109.

Plyler, P. N., & Ananthanarayan, A. K. (2001). Human frequency following responses: Representation of second formant transitions in normal-hearing and hearing-impaired listeners. *Journal of the American Academy of Audiology, 12,* 423–533.

Popelka, G. R., Osterhammel, P. A., Nielsen, L. H., & Rasmussen, A. (1993). Growth of distortion product otoacoustic emissions with primary tone level in humans. *Hearing Research, 71,* 12–22.

Poulsen, C., Picton, T. W., & Paus, T. (2009). Age-related changes in transient and oscillatory brain responses to auditory stimulation during early adolescence. *Developmental Science, 12,* 220–235.

Purcell, D. W., John, S. M., Schneider, B. A., & Picton, T. W. (2004). Human temporal auditory acuity as assessed by envelope following responses. *Journal of the Acoustical Society of America, 116,* 3581–3593.

Rance, G., & Briggs, R. J. (2002). Assessment of hearing in infants with moderate to profound impairment: The Melbourne experience with auditory steady-state evoked potential testing. *Annals of Otology, Rhinology and Laryngology, Supplement, 189,* 22–28.

Rance, G., & Rickards, F. (2002). Prediction of hearing threshold in infants using auditory steady-state evoked potentials. *Journal of the American Academy of Audiology, 13,* 236–245.

Rance, G., Rickards, F. W., Cohen, L. T., DeVidi, S., & Clarke, G. M. (1995). The automated prediction of hearing thresholds in sleeping subjects using auditory steady-state evoked potentials. *Ear and Hearing, 16,* 499–507.

Rance, G., & Tomlin, D. (2006). Maturation of auditory steady-state responses in normal babies. *Ear and hearing, 27*(1), 20–29.

Rance, G., Tomlin, D., & Rickards, F. W. (2006). Comparison of auditory steady-state responses and tone-burst auditory brainstem responses in normal babies. *Ear and Hearing, 27,* 751–762.

Recio, A., & Rhode, W. S. (2000). Representation of vowel stimuli in the ventral cochlear nucleus of the chinchilla. *Hearing Research, 146*(1–2), 167–184.

Rees, A., & Moller, A. R. (1983). Responses of neurons in the inferior colliculus of the rat to AM and FM tones. *Hearing Research, 10,* 301–330.

Rhode, W. (1978). Some observations on cochlear mechanics. *Journal of the Acoustical Society of America, 64,* 158–176.

Ribeiro, F. M., Carvallo, R. M., & Marcoux, A. M. (2010). Auditory steady-state evoked responses for preterm and term neonates. *Audiology and Neuro otology, 15,* 97–110.

Rickman, M. D., Chertoff, M. E., & Hecox, K. E. (1991). Electrophysiological evidence of nonlinear distortion products to two-tone stimuli. *Journal of the Acoustical Society of America, 89,* 2818–2826.

Robertson, D., & Johnstone, B. M. (1981). Primary auditory neurons: Nonlinear responses altered without changes in sharp tuning. *Journal of the Acoustical Society of America, 69,* 1096–1098.

Rodrigues, G. R., & Lewis, D. R. (2010). Threshold prediction in children with sensorineural hearing loss using the auditory steady-state responses and tone-evoked auditory brain stem response. *International Journal of Pediatric Otorhinolaryngology, 74,* 540–546.

Rose, J. E., Brugge, J. F., Anderson, D. J., & Hind, J. E. (1967). Phase-locked response to low-frequency tones in single auditory nerve fibers of the squirrel monkey. *Journal of Neurophysiology, 30,* 769–793.

Rose, J. E., Hind, J. E., Anderson, D. J., & Brugge, J. F. (1971). Some effects of stimulus intensity on response of auditory nerve fibers in the squirrel monkey. *Journal of Neurophysiology, 34,* 685–699.

Russo, N., Nicol, T., Trommer, B., Zecker, S., & Kraus, N. (2009). Brainstem transcription of speech is disrupted in children with autism spectrum disorders. *Developmental Science, 12,* 557–567.

Salvi, R., Perry, J., Hamernik, R. P., & Henderson, D. (1982). Relationships between cochlear pathologies and auditory nerve and behavioral responses following acoustic trauma. In R. P. Hamernik, D.Henderson, & R. Salvi (Eds.), *New perspectives on noise-induced hearing loss* (pp. 165–188). New York, NY: Raven.

Savio, G., Cárdenas, J., Pérez Abalo, M., González, A., & Valdés, J. (2001). The low and high frequency auditory steady state responses mature at different rates. *Audiology and Neuro-otology, 6,* 279–287.

Sayles, M., & Winter, I. M. (2008). Reverberation challenges the temporal representation of the pitch of complex sounds. *Neuron, 58*(5), 789–801.

Scherg, M., & Brinkmann, R. D. (1979). Least-square-fit technique applied to the frequency following potential: A method to determine components, latencies and amplitudes. *Scandinavian Audiology, Supplementum,* (9), 197–203.

Shinn-Cunningham, B., Varghese, L., Wang, L., & Bharadwaj, H. (2017). Individual differences in temporal perception and their implications for everyday listening. In N. Kraus, S. Anderson, T. White-Schwoch, R. R. Fay, & A. N. Popper (Eds.), *The frequency-following response: A window into human communication* (pp. 159–192). Cham, Switzerland: ASA Press and Springer.

Small, S. A., Hatton, J. L., & Stapells, D. R. (2007). Effects of bone oscillator coupling method, placement location, and occlusion on bone-conduction auditory steady-state responses in infants. *Ear and Hearing, 28,* 83–98.

Small, S. A., & Stapells, D. R. (2004). Artifactual responses when recording auditory steady-state responses. *Ear and Hearing, 25,* 611–623.

Small, S. A., & Stapells, D. R. (2006). Multiple auditory steady-state response thresholds to bone-conduction stimuli in young infants with normal hearing. *Ear and Hearing, 27,* 219–228.

Small, S. A., & Stapells, D. R. (2008a). Maturation of bone conduction multiple auditory steady-state responses. *International Journal of Audiology, 47,* 476–488.

Small, S. A., & Stapells, D. R. (2008b). Normal ipsilateral/contralateral asymmetries in infant multiple auditory steady-state responses to air- and bone-conduction stimuli. *Ear and Hearing, 29,* 185–198.

Smalt, C. J., Krishnan, A., Bidelman, G. M., Ananthakrishnan, S., & Gandour, J. T. (2012). Neural correlates of cochlear distortion products and their influence on representation of pitch relevant information in the human brainstem. *Hearing Research, 292,* 26–34.

Smith, J. C., Marsh, J. T., & Brown, W. S. (1975). Far-field recorded frequency-following responses: Evidence for the locus of brain-stem sources. *Electroencephalography and Clinical Neurophysiology, 39,* 465–472.

Sohmer, H., & Pratt, H. (1976). Recording of the cochlear microphonic potential with surface electrodes. *Electroencephalography and Clinical Neurophysiology, 40,* 253–260.

Sohmer, H., & Pratt, H. (1977). Identification and separation of acoustic frequency following responses (FFR) in man. *Electroencephalography and Clinical Neurophysiology, 42,* 493–500.

Sohmer, H., Pratt, H., & Kinarti, R. (1977). Sources of frequency following responses (FFR) in man. *Electroencephalography and Clinical Neurophysiology, 42,* 656–664.

Song, J. H., Nicol, T., & Kraus, N. (2011). Test–retest reliability of the speech-evoked auditory brainstem response. *Clinical Neurophysiology, 122*(2), 346–355.

Song, J., Skoe, E., Wong, P., & Kraus, N. (2008). Plasticity in the adult human auditory brainstem following short-term linguistic training. *Journal of Cognitive Neuroscience, 20,* 1892–1902.

Stapells, D., Herdman, A., Small, S., Dimitrijevic, A., & Hatton, J. (2005). Current status of the auditory steady-state responses for estimating an infant's audiogram. In R. Seewald & J. Bamford (Eds.), *A sound foundation through early amplification: Proceedings of an international conference* (Chapter 3, pp. 43–59). Stafa, Switzerland: Phonak AG.

Starr, A., & Hellerstein, D. (1971). Distribution of frequency following responses in cat cochlear nucleus to sinusoidal acoustic signals. *Brain Research, 33,* 367–377.

Stillman, R. D., Crow, G., & Moushegian, G. (1978). Components of the frequency-following potential in man. *Electroencephalography and Clinical Neurophysiology, 44,* 438–446.

Stillman, R. D., Moushegian, G., & Rupert, A. L. (1976). Early tone-evoked responses in normal and hearing-impaired subjects. *Audiology and Neurootology, 15,* 10–22.

Stover, L. J., Neely, S. T., & Gorga, M. P. (1996). Latency and multiple sources of distortion product otoacoustic emissions. *Journal of the Acoustical Society of America, 99,* 1016–1024.

Stover, L. J., & Norton, S. J. (1993). The effects of aging on otoacoustic emissions. *Journal of the Acoustical Society of America, 94,* 2670–2681.

Strait, D. L., Hornickel, J., & Kraus, N. (2011). Subcortical processing of speech regularities predicts reading and music aptitude in children. *Behavioral and Brain Functions, 7,* 44.

Strickland, E., & Viemeister, N. H. (1996). Cues for discrimination of envelopes. *Journal of the Acoustical Society of America, 99*(6), 3638–3646.

Stroebel, D., Swanepoel, D. W., & Groenewald, E. (2007). Aided auditory steady-state responses in infants. *International Journal of Audiology, 46,* 287–292.

Suresh, C. H., & Krishnan, A. (2020). Search for electrophysiological indices of hidden hearing loss in humans: Click auditory brainstem response across sound levels and in background noise. *Ear and Hearing, 42*(1), 53–67.

Suresh, C. H., Krishnan, A., & Luo, X. (2020). Human frequency following responses to vocoded speech: Amplitude modulation versus amplitude plus frequency modulation. *Ear and Hearing, 41*(2), 300–311.

Swaminathan, J., Krishnan, A., & Gandour, J. T. (2008). Pitch encoding in speech and nonspeech contexts in the human auditory brainstem. *Neuroreport, 19*(11), 1163–1167.

Swanepoel, D. W., Ebrahim, S., Friedland, P., Swanepoel, A., & Pottas, L. (2008). Auditory steady-state responses to bone conduction stimuli in children with hearing loss. *International Journal of Pediatric Otorhinolaryngology, 72*(12), 1861–1871.

Swanepoel, D. W., & Steyn, K. (2005). Short report: Establishing normal hearing for infants with the auditory steady-state response. *South African Journal of Communication Disorders, 52,* 36–39.

Tlumak, A. I., Durrant, J. D., & Collet, L. (2007). 80 Hz auditory steady-state responses (ASSR) at 250 Hz and 12,000 Hz: Respuestas Auditivas de Estado Estable de 80 Hz (ASSR) a 250 Hz y 12 kHz. *International Journal of Audiology, 46*(1), 26–30.

Vale, C., & Sanes, D. H. (2002). The effect of bilateral deafness on excitatory and inhibitory synaptic strength in the inferior colliculus. *European Journal of Neuroscience, 16*(12), 2394–2404.

Van Maanen, A., & Stapells, D. R. (2005). Comparison of multiple auditory steady-state responses (80 versus 40 Hz) and slow cortical potentials for threshold estimation in hearing-impaired adults: Comparación de las respuestas auditivas múltiples de estado estable (80 vs 40 Hz) y de los potenciales corticales lentos en la estimación de umbrales en adultos con hipoacusia. *International Journal of Audiology, 44*(11), 613–624

Van Maanen, A., & Stapells, D. R. (2009). Normal multiple auditory steady-state response thresholds to air-conducted stimuli in infants. *Journal of the American Academy of Audiology, 20,* 196–207.

Van Maanen, A., & Stapells, D. R. (2010). Multiple-ASSR thresholds in infants and young children with hearing loss. *Journal of American Academy of Audiology, 21,* 535–545.

Vander Werff, K. R., & Brown, C. J. (2005). Effect of audiometric configuration on threshold and suprathreshold auditory steady-state responses. *Ear and Hearing, 26*(3), 10–26.

Vargas Garcia, M., Frasson de Azevedo, M., Pinto Vieira Biaggio, E., Domeneghini Didoné, D., & Gurgel Testa, J. R. (2014). Auditory steady-state responses air and bone conducted in children from zero to six months with and without conductive impairments. *Revista CEFAC, 16*(3), 699–706.

Wallace, M. N., Rutkowski, R. G., Shackleton, T. M., & Palmer, A. R. (2000). Phase-locked responses to pure tones in Guinea pig auditory cortex. *NeuroReport, 11,* 3989–3993.

White-Schwoch, T., Anderson, S., Krizman, J., Nicol, T., & Kraus, N. (2019). Case studies in neuroscience: Subcortical origins of the frequency-following response. *Journal of Neurophysiology, 122*(2), 844–848.

White-Schwoch, T., Woodruff Carr, K., Thompson, E. C., Anderson, S., Nicol, T., Bradlow, A. R., . . . Kraus, N. (2015). Auditory processing in noise: A preschool biomarker for literacy. *PLOS Biology, 13,* e1002196.

Willott, J. F. (1991). *Aging and the auditory system: Anatomy, physiology, and psychophysics.* San Diego, CA: Singular Publishing.

Worden, F. G., & Marsh, J. T. (1968). Frequency-following (microphonic-like) neural responses evoked by sound. *Electroencephalography and Clinical Neurophysiology, 25,* 42–52.

Yamada, O., Kodera, K., Hink, R. F., & Suzuki, J. I. (1979). Cochlear distribution of frequency-following response initiation: A high-pass masking noise study. *Audiology, 18,* 381–387.

Yamada, O., Kodera, K., Hink, R. F., & Yamane, H. (1978). Cochlear initiation site of the frequency-following response: A study of patients with sensorineural hearing loss. *Audiology, 17,* 489–499.

Yamada, O., Marsh, R., & Potsic, W. (1980). Generators of the frequency-following response in the guinea pig. *Otolaryngology-Head and Neck Surgery, 88,* 613–618.

Year 2019 Position Statement: Principles and guidelines for early hearing detection and intervention programs (2019). *Journal of Early Hearing Detection and Intervention, 4*(2), 1–44.

Yin, T. C. T, & Kuwada, S. (1983). Binaural interaction in low-frequency neurons in inferior colliculus of the cat. III. Effects of changing frequency. *Journal of Neurophysiology, 50,* 1020–1042.

Young, E. D., & Sachs, M. B. (1979). Representation of steady-state vowels in the temporal aspects of the discharge patterns of populations of auditory-nerve fibers. *Journal of the Acoustical Society of America, 66,* 1381–1403.

9

Research Applications of the Frequency Following Response

SCOPE

In the previous chapter, we provided evidence that the sustained phase-locked neural activity generating the brainstem frequency following response (FFR), preserves spectrotemporal information of certain acoustic features of steady-state and time-variant complex sounds. Thus, the scalp-recorded human FFR provides an effective physiologic window to examine the early stages of subcortical processing of complex sounds. This review is deliberately limited to studies examining several aspects of neural encoding of complex sounds, including the pitch of steady-state and time-variant speech and nonspeech complex sounds, effects of language experience on the neural representation of pitch, binaural processing, effects of adverse listening conditions, and structural versus functional asymmetry. Most of the content in this chapter reflects research done in the author's laboratory over the last 17 years. The intent here is to introduce the reader to several basic science research applications of the FFR to mainly highlight its potential promise as a neural metric to understand the processing of complex sounds in the brainstem and how they could be applied to assess aspects of temporal auditory processing in different clinical populations. The level of presentation is directed at doctoral students and researchers to encourage further consideration of these measures in their research. However, any curious student of the auditory system is welcome. For a more comprehensive and diverse account of the envelope following response (EFR)/FFR and its potential applications in different clinical populations, the reader is strongly encouraged to consider the FFR book by Kraus et al. (2017).

I. PITCH: AN IMPORTANT PERCEPTUAL ATTRIBUTE

Pitch is a robust perceptual attribute that plays an important role in the processing of speech, language, and music, and in the segregation of concurrent sounds in complex auditory scenes (Oxenham, 2012). Voice pitch in speech contains information about taker identity, prosody, and semantic information in tonal languages. Pitch variations in music are associated with melody, and pitch differences provide a robust cue for sound segregation. Therefore, the sustained research efforts in understanding the neural mechanisms underlying pitch provide general insights into the neural basis of auditory information processing. Pitch perception has been studied extensively through psychophysical and physiological approaches. Most periodic complex sounds evoke low pitches associated with their fundamental frequency (f0), sometimes termed *periodicity pitch* (De Boer, 1976; Evans, 1978; Moore, 1989). Energy may or may not be present at the f0. Pitch salience (perceived pitch strength) for these complex sounds has been shown to decrease as the lowest present harmonic number is increased (Bernstein & Oxenham, 2003; Houtsma & Smurzynski, 1990).

The neural bases of pitch perception are still a matter of considerable debate, as reflected in the extant literature. While the specific neural mechanisms mediating pitch at different levels in the auditory system are not known, studies evaluating neural encoding of the pitch of harmonic complex tones in the auditory nerve (AN) and cochlear nucleus (CN) have shown that pitch cues are available in both the temporal patterns of neural activity (*temporal pitch* based on neural phase locking) and the spatial distribution of activity along the tonotopic axis (*spectral pitch* based on neural discharge rate). In the *spectral* scheme, pitch-relevant information is extracted from discharge rate–based spectral profile resulting from frequency-specific auditory input, followed by harmonic template matching mechanisms to derive pitch (Cohen, Grossberg, & Wyse, 1995). In the *temporal pitch* scheme, pitch-relevant information is extracted from the timing of auditory nerve fiber activity irrespective of frequency organization (i.e., frequency for place cochlear map). These temporal models are based solely on the timing information available in the interspike intervals represented in simulated (Meddis & O'Mard, 1997; Patterson, Allerhand, & Giguere, 1995) or actual (Cariani & Delgutte, 1996a, 1996b) auditory nerve activity. It is believed that these periodicity cues are extracted by an autocorrelation-type mechanism (Licklider, 1951; Meddis & Hewitt, 1991; Yost, 1996), equivalent to an all-order interspike interval distribution for neural spike trains. While this interval-based representation can predict the pitch of both resolved and unresolved harmonics (Cariani & Delgutte, 1996a; Cedolin & Delgutte, 2005; Meddis & Hewitt, 1991), it does not appear to be able to differentiate the stronger pitch salience for resolved harmonics from the weaker pitch salience for unresolved harmonics (Bernstein & Oxenham, 2005; Carlyon, 1998). A hybrid pitch-encoding mechanism using both spectral and temporal information has also been proposed (Cedolin & Delgutte, 2005). Thus, neural phase-locking related to voice fundamental frequency (f0) plays a dominant role in the encoding of low pitch associated with complex sounds. Temporal encoding schemes are favored because they provide a unified and parsimonious explanation of a diverse range of pitch phenomena observed at or below the level of the inferior colliculus (IC) (Meddis & O'Mard, 1997).

For any neural code of pitch to be useful, it should be available, at least in some form, at all levels of the processing hierarchy. While neurons in the primary auditory cortex have been shown to exhibit temporal and spectral response properties that could enable these pitch-encoding schemes (Lu, Liang, & Wang, 2001; Steinschneider, Reser, Fishman, Schroeder, & Arezzo, 1998), it is not clear if a network consisting of pitch-selective neurons would mediate this process. In subcortical auditory structures, periodicity and pitch are often represented by regular temporal patterns of action potentials that are phase-locked to the sound waveform. However, in the auditory cortex, neural phase-locking is largely limited to frequencies below about 100 to 150 Hz. Thus, the most commonly observed code for periodicity and pitch within cortical neurons is a modulation of spike rates as a function of f0. The wider temporal integration window at the cortical level may likely render the auditory cortical neurons too sluggish to provide phase-locked representations of periodicity within the pitch range (Walker, Bizley, King, & Schnupp, 2011). Therefore, it is not yet clear how cortical neurons transform the autocorrelation-like temporal analysis in the brainstem to a spike-rate code to extract pitch-relevant information. One possibility is that the temporal code is transformed into a response discharge rate–based synchrony code, where temporally coherent activity from the subcortical stages will produce a greater spike rate, yielding a larger response amplitude at the cortical level. Micheyl, Schrater, and Oxenham (2013) have shown that there is sufficient statistical information present in the population spike rate to account for small differences in frequency (pitch) and intensity (loudness).

Hierarchical Nature of Pitch Processing

There is growing evidence to indicate that a complex series of distributed processing stages are essential to transform speech sounds into meaning at the level of the cerebral cortex (Hickok & Poeppel, 2007; Poeppel, Isdsardi, & van Wassenhove, 2008). Functional brain-imaging studies provide strong evidence for hierarchical processing of pitch at the cortical level (Kumar, Stephan, Warren, Friston, & Griffiths, 2007). However, the encoding of temporal regularities relevant to pitch in subcortical structures begins as early as the cochlear nucleus (Griffiths, Uppenkamp, Johnsrude, Josephs, & Patterson, 2001) and continues up through Heschl's gyrus, planum polare, and planum temporale (Gutschalk, Patterson, Scherg, Uppenkamp, & Rupp, 2007). The IC is reported to be more sensitive to changes in temporal regularity than the cochlear nucleus. The spread of pitch-related neural activity from the primary auditory cortex for simpler complex tones to regions beyond the primary auditory cortex for melodies, with relatively more activity in the right hemisphere, provides further support for hierarchical processing of pitch (Patterson, Uppenkamp, Johnsrude, & Griffiths, 2002). Scalp-recorded evoked responses (FFRs and the cortical pitch response) that preserve pitch-relevant information provide an effective analytic physiologic window to examine the organization of this pitch-processing hierarchy at both cortical and subcortical levels and the interaction between the two levels (Krishnan & Gandour, 2014, 2017; Krishnan, Gandour, & Suresh, 2015; Krishnan, Suresh, & Gandour, 2017a, 2017b; Krishnan, Gandour, Xu, & Suresh, 2016; Krishnan, Suresh, & Gandour, 2019; Suresh, Krishnan, & Gandour, 2017). The focus on language and pitch in the brainstem is consistent with the view that a complete understanding of the processing of linguistically relevant dimensions of the auditory signal can only be achieved within a framework involving a series of computations that apply to representations at different stages of processing (Hickok & Poeppel, 2004, p. 69). Thus, within this framework, early processing stages (e.g., brainstem) may not only provide a more fine-grained representation of stimulus acoustic features but also perform transformations on the acoustic data that are relevant to linguistic as well as nonlinguistic auditory perception, presumably processed in a distributed hierarchical processing network at the cortical level, with the brainstem serving an important functional role in this network.

II. NEURAL REPRESENTATION OF PITCH-RELEVANT INFORMATION OF COMPLEX SOUNDS

Neural Correlates of Pitch of Harmonic, Inharmonic, and Frequency-Shifted Sounds

For a range of harmonic complex sounds that produce a low pitch percept, the dominant interval interspike interval present in the population of auditory nerve fibers always corresponds to the pitch heard in perceptual experiments (Cariani & Delgutte, 1996a)—the dominant interval hypothesis. Psychoacoustic studies have demonstrated that inharmonic and frequency-shifted complex tones (de Boer, 1956; Shouten, 1940) produce pitches that differ from that suggested by the envelope periodicity/harmonic spacing (pitch shift and/or pitch ambiguity). Consistent with this auditory nerve physiological data, similar stimuli indicate that these pitch shifts also have direct correlates in the population interspike interval distribution of the auditory nerve (Cariani & Delgutte, 1996b). That is, pooled interval distributions in response to inharmonic stimulus segments show multiple maxima corresponding to the multiple pitches heard by human listeners (pitch ambiguity). Similarly, for frequency-shifted complex sounds where octave drops in pitch are expected, there are corresponding patterns of peaks in the pooled interspike interval distribution.

Given that FFR reflects sustained phase-locked activity in a population of neural elements in the brainstem, Krishnan and Plack (2011) reasoned that the temporal pattern of phase-locked activity generating the FFR may preserve information consistent with pitch ambiguity of inharmonic complex sounds, and pitch shifts of frequency-shifted complex sound similar to what has been demonstrated in the pooled interval distribution at the auditory nerve level (Cariani & Delgutte, 1996a, 1996b). To evaluate pitch ambiguity, FFRs were recorded to amplitude modulated (AM) tones with fixed modulation frequency (Fm = 125 Hz) and different carrier frequencies (625 and 750 Hz: *harmonic*, since Fc/Fm is an integer; 687 and 733 Hz: inharmonic and aperiodic since Fc/Fm is not an integer) (Figure 9–1).

To evaluate pitch shift, FFRs were recorded using a three-component *harmonic* complex composed of the second (488 Hz), third (732 Hz), and fourth (976 Hz) harmonic of a 244 f0, and another three-component complex where the three components were shifted downward in frequency by 122 Hz (that is, 366, 610, and 854 Hz) (Figure 9–3, first two panels on the left). For all stimuli (harmonic, inharmonic,

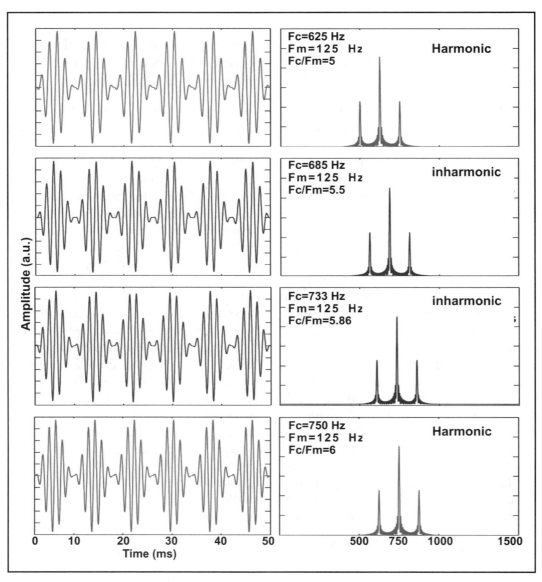

Figure 9–1. Waveforms (*left*) and corresponding spectra (*right*) of amplitude-modulated harmonic (*light traces*) and inharmonic (*dark traces*) tones, each with a modulation frequency (Fm) of 125 Hz. Note the rightward shift in the spectral components as a carrier frequency (Fc) is changed from 622 to 750 Hz. From A. Krishnan and C. J. Plack (2011), unpublished data presented at the 2011 midwinter meeting of the Association for Research in Otolaryngology.

and frequency shifted), EFRs showed autocorrelation function (ACF) peaks that corresponded to the invariant envelope periodicity (Figure 9–2, left panel; Figure 9–3, third panel from the left). Consistent with this, the EFR spectral data showed peaks at the harmonic spacing and at integer multiples of this value (Figure 9–2, second panel; Figure 9–3, left panel, light traces). In contrast, FFR (remember, reflects phase-locking to the fine-structure components) showed ACF peaks corresponding to the F0 for the harmonic stimuli, and single or multiple ACF peaks (which did not correspond to f0) for inharmonic/frequency-shifted stimuli (Figure 9–2 left panel; Figure 9–3, fourth panel, dark traces). FFR ACF peaks corresponding to pitch(es) for harmonic and inharmonic AM tones (Figure 9–2) are identical to the peaks in the pooled interspike interval distribution for the auditory nerve (Cariani & Delgutte, 1996b) (Figure 9–2, third panel). The pitches estimated from the population-interval

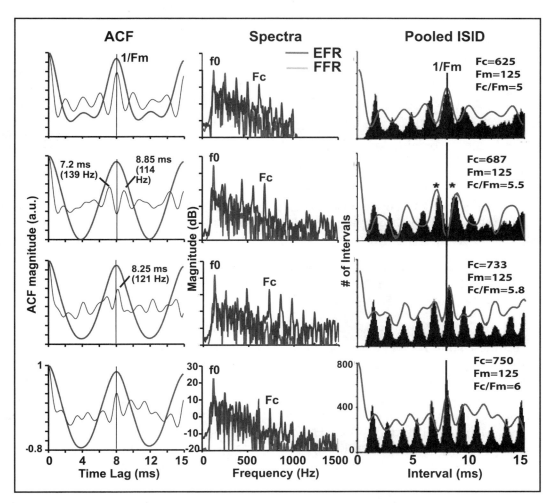

Figure 9–2. Autocorrelation functions (ACFs) (*left column*) and spectra (*middle column*) of the envelope following responses (EFRs; *dark*) and frequency following responses (FFRs; *light*) plotted for stimuli described in Figure 9–1. EFR ACFs show a robust peak at 1/Fm for all stimuli, and correspondingly, the spectral data show peaks at f0 and a few higher harmonics. FFR ACFs show a clear peak at 1/Fm only for the harmonic stimuli (rows 1 and 4) and shifted or multiple peaks for the inharmonic stimuli (the pitch periods are identified). The FFR spectra show clear peaks at Fc, its sidebands, and cubic difference tones. EFR ACFs overlaid on the auditory nerve pooled interspike intervals are remarkably similar across stimuli. From A. Krishnan and C. J. Plack (2011), unpublished data presented at the 2011 midwinter meeting of the Association for Research in Otolaryngology.

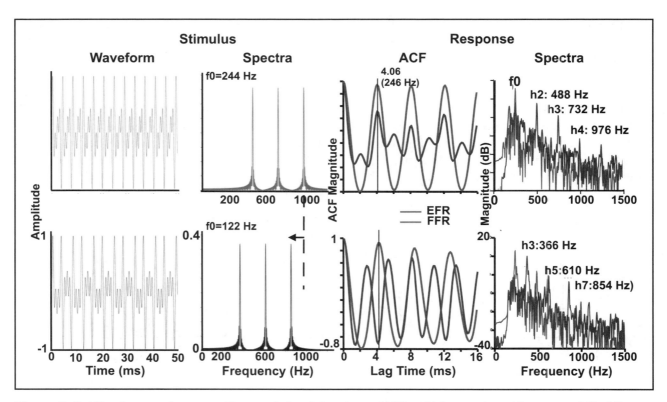

Figure 9–3. Waveforms and spectra of harmonic (*top left and top middle*) and inharmonic and frequency-shifted (*bottom left and bottom middle*) complex tones. Columns three and four illustrate the autocorrelation functions (ACFs) and spectra of the envelope following response (EFR; larger responses) and frequency following response (FFR; smaller responses). No clear peak proximal to perceived pitch is discernible in the FFR spectral data (lighter traces) for the frequency-shifted stimulus. Also, note that the multiple peaks of the FFR ACF for the frequency-shifted tone surround the dominant EFR ACF peak at 4 ms. From A. Krishnan and C. J. Plack (2011), unpublished data presented at the 2011 midwinter meeting of the Association for Research in Otolaryngology.

distribution for these stimuli closely correspond to the pitch shifts (the first period effect of pitch shift) that have been observed for human listeners and are in close agreement with de Boer's rule (de Boer, 1976). For inharmonic conditions, estimated pitch was 121 Hz for AM 733 and 114.5 Hz and 139 Hz for AM 687. For the frequency-shifted conditions, estimated pitches were 203 and 305 Hz—all approximating with de Boer's rule ($p = Fc/n$), where n is an integer near Fc/Fm) values. Although the spectral data for the FFR showed peaks (spectral data in Figures 9–2 and 9–3) at the frequency components and lower harmonics (presumably cubic difference distortion products) as expected, no clear peaks corresponding to the pitch were observed for the inharmonic/shifted stimuli. Based on these results, the authors concluded that FFR (fine structure) results are consistent with the auditory nerve response to AM tones (Cariani & Delgutte, 1996b) and with the FFRs to frequency-shifted complex sounds (Greenberg, Marsh, Brown, & Smith, 1987). These authors suggest that the multiple maxima in the ACFs for inharmonic/frequency shift stimuli correspond to the multiple pitches heard by human listeners (pitch shift/ambiguity). Consistent with these views, the results presented here suggest that the FFR does not merely reflect neural phase-locking to waveform envelope (Hall, 1979). Rather, information relevant to pitch shift and pitch ambiguity is preserved in the temporal distribution of neural activity in the midbrain phase-locked to the fine structure. Similar results for frequency-shifted complex tones have been reported by Gockel, Carlyon, Mehta, and Plack (2011). The similarity of these FFR results with auditory nerve data raises the question of whether the phase-locked activity in the midbrain, as reflected in the FFR, represents local pitch encoding or merely a passive reflection of pitch-relevant information preserved in the neural activity that has been transmitted from the auditory nerve. Based on their failure to observe any pitch-relevant information in the FFRs to three-tone harmonic stimuli presented dichotically, Gockel et al. (2011) concluded that there was no additional pitch-relevant processing at the level of the brainstem. Several arguments may be presented to counter this inference. First, if the temporal code for pitch available at the brainstem level also utilizes autocorrelation-like analysis to determine the global distribution of interspike intervals from the temporal pattern of neural activity across a population of neurons, it would necessarily share certain fundamental attributes of the same temporal code operating at the level of the auditory nerve. Second, it is not clear that their dichotic stimuli produced the same pitch as when all harmonics are presented to the same ear. Notwithstanding, the pitch salience of their stimuli would be weak. The neural activity underlying the FFR may not be sufficiently robust to preserve the less salient pitch for their stimuli. In our own experience, we failed to measure FFR correlates of the less salient dichotic Huggins pitch. Finally, the inference by Gockel et al. (2011) cannot adequately account for the experience-dependent effects reflected in the FFR that are sensitive to specific attributes of dynamic pitch contours without the assumption of solely top-down effects producing the experience-dependent effects.

Neural Correlates of Resolved Versus Unresolved Complex Sounds

Psychoacoustic studies have also shown that complex tones containing resolved harmonics evoke stronger pitches than complex tones with only unresolved harmonics (e.g., Carlyon & Shackleton, 1994; Houtsma & Smurzynski, 1990). Also, unresolved harmonics presented in the alternating sine and cosine (ALT) phase produce a doubling of pitch, presumably the result of harmonic interaction in the basilar membrane (Shackleton & Carlyon, 1994). Physiological studies show a consistent correlate of the pitch doubling for ALT stimuli as harmonic resolution decreases. That is, the interspike interval distributions (ISIDs) not only show peaks at F0 and 2F0, but also, the interval-based measure of pitch strength is almost as large at the envelope frequency 2F0 as at the F0 for alternating phase stimuli with unresolved harmonics based on both period histograms and ACGs (Cedolin & Delgutte, 2005; Horst, Javel, & Farley, 1990; Palmer & Winter, 1992, 1993; Shackleton, Liu, & Palmer, 2009). Krishnan and Plack (2011) examined whether the temporal pattern of phase-locked neural activity reflected in the scalp-recorded human FFR preserves information relevant to pitch strength and pitch doubling for ALT stimuli. FFR and behavioral discrimination measures were obtained for complex tone burst stimuli with harmonics added in either the sine (SIN) or alternating (ALT) phase. SIN-phase complexes had an F0 of 90 Hz (SIN 90) or 180 Hz (SIN 180). ALT phase complexes had an F0 of 90 Hz (ALT 90). For each of the complexes, harmonics were filtered into one of four spectral regions: 360 to 900 Hz, 720 to 1260 Hz, 1080 to 1620 Hz, and 1440 to 1980 Hz. These spectral regions were chosen to include stimuli with low-order harmonics that are completely resolved, and stimuli with higher-order harmonics that are completely unresolved, in the cochlea. A low-pass Gaussian noise with cutoff frequencies set 180 Hz below the start of the complex passband (180 Hz, 540 Hz, 900 Hz, and 1260 Hz for the four spectral regions) was used to mask combination tones. Their results showed that FFR periodicity strength decreased as harmonic resolution decreased, qualitatively consistent with previous behavioral measures but appreciably smaller compared to the large changes in f0 difference limen (F0DL) observed in behavioral measures (Figure 9–4 and Figure 9–5). Also, autocorrelation-based periodicity strength measure and FFR spectra (Figure 9–6) indicated a different pattern of phase-locked neural activity for ALT stimuli with resolved and unresolved harmonics consistent with the doubling of pitch observed in their behavioral estimates. Specifically, the shift in the relative prominence of the autocorrelation peaks in their FFR data for ALT 90 stimuli, and the clear shift in the spectral pattern (from one

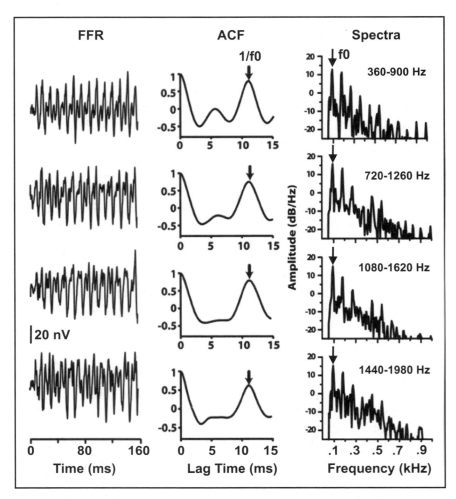

Figure 9–4. Grand averaged frequency following response (FFR) waveforms, autocorrelation function (ACF), and spectra across spectral regions (identified on the right) for SIN 90 stimulus. Only a small decrease in magnitude of the ACF peak is observed for the highest unresolved spectral band. Adapted from "Neural Encoding in the Human Brainstem Relevant to the Pitch of Complex Tones," by A. Krishnan and C. J. Plack, 2011, *Hearing Research, 275*(1–2), pp. 110–119. Copyright 2011, with permission from Elsevier.

consistent with a 90-Hz f0 for the resolved ALT 90 stimuli to one more consistent with a 180-Hz f0 for unresolved ALT 90 stimuli) clearly suggest that the temporal pattern of neural activity relevant to the perceptual doubling of pitch is preserved in the neural activity underlying the FFR. Furthermore, the similarity between the autocorrelation analyses performed at the level of the auditory nerve (model response) and the level of the IC (FFR) appears to suggest that a temporal representation of pitch based on pooled neural ISIDs is still potentially available at the level of the midbrain. Finally, the correlation between their FFR data and behavioral estimates of pitch suggests that the phase-locked neural activity reflected in the scalp-recorded FFR preserves sensory-level pitch-relevant information that may contribute to pitch perception. Thus, the scalp-recorded FFR may provide for a noninvasive analytic tool to evaluate neural encoding of complex sounds in humans.

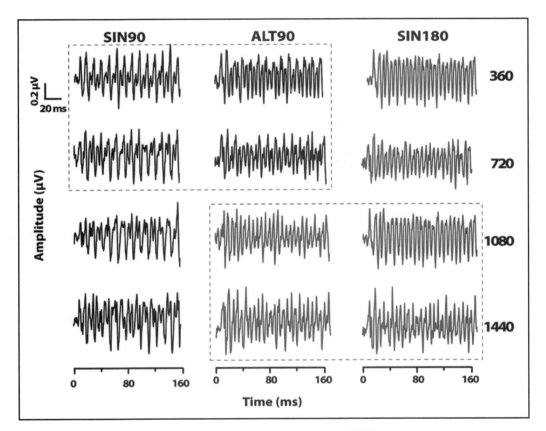

Figure 9–5. Grand averaged frequency following response (FFR) waveforms across spectral regions (identified on the right) for SIN 90, ALT 90, and SIN 180 stimuli. For the resolved conditions (720 Hz), the response waveform periodicity for the sin 90 and ALT 90 appear similar. However, for the higher unresolved (1080 and 1440 Hz) conditions, the ALT 90 waveform periodicity is more similar to the SIN 180 response periodicity consistent with doubling of pitch. Adapted from "Neural Encoding in the Human Brainstem Relevant to the Pitch of Complex Tones," by A. Krishnan and C. J. Plack, 2011, *Hearing Research, 275*(1–2), pp. 110–119. Copyright 2011, with permission from Elsevier.

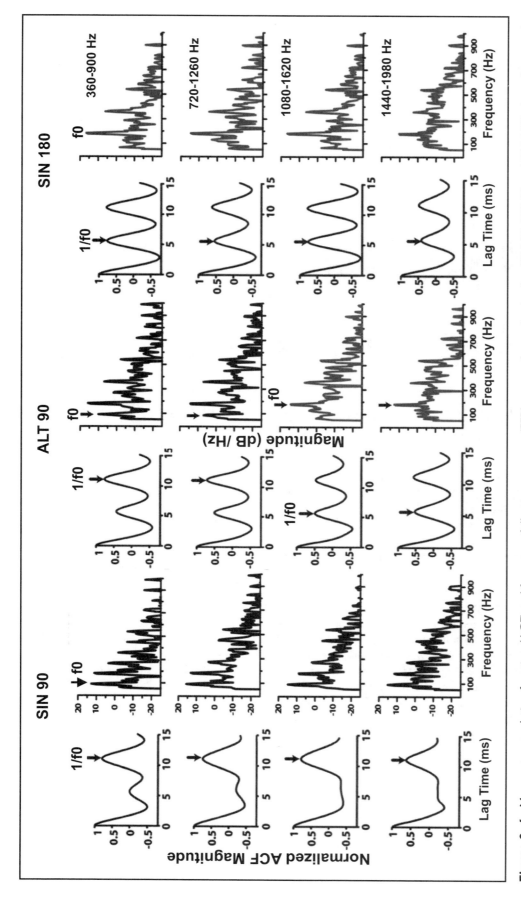

Figure 9–6. Mean autocorrelation function (ACF) and frequency following response (FFR) spectra for each stimulus (SIN 90, ALT 90, and SIN 180) plotted across the four spectral regions. The spectral regions are identified on the right of each row of plots. For resolved conditions, both SIN 90 all conditions show ACF and spectral peaks that correspond to a fundamental frequency of 90 Hz with no appreciable change in magnitude. For ALT 90, ACF peaks and spectral peaks correspond to a fundamental of 90 Hz for the resolved conditions (360 and 720 Hz). However, for the ALT unresolved conditions (1080 and 1440 Hz), both the ACF and the spectral peaks shift to a 180-Hz fundamental frequency (similar to the SIN 180 ACF peak and spectral pattern) consistent with doubling of pitch. Reprinted from "Neural Encoding in the Human Brainstem Relevant to the Pitch of Complex Tones," by A. Krishnan and C. J. Plack, 2011, *Hearing Research, 275*(1–2), pp. 110–119. Copyright 2011, with permission from Elsevier.

Relative Roles of Envelope and Temporal Fine Structure in Pitch

Periodic complex sounds (e.g., amplitude-modulated tones, complex tones, synthetic vowels) that are commonly used to evaluate the temporal representation of pitch-relevant information in the auditory system contain strong envelope (ENV) modulation in addition to the waveform temporal fine structure (TFS). The relative roles of ENV and TFS in the temporal encoding of stimulus features relevant to pitch have been evaluated in the cochlear nucleus using iterated rippled noise (IRN) with positive (IRNp) and negative (IRNn) gain (Neuert, Verhey, & Winter, 2005; Sayles & Winter 2008a; Shofner, 1991, 1999; Verhey & Winter, 2006). IRN is generated using wideband noise (WBN) that is delayed, attenuated, and then added/subtracted to the original WBN in an iterative manner. Unlike other pitch-producing periodic complex sounds, IRN stimuli do not have highly modulated envelopes but impart a temporal regularity in the TFS. The ACFs for IRNp and IRNn are identical for waveform ENV (peak at time lag corresponding to the delay [d ms]) but are different for the TFS (Neuert et al., 2005; Shofner, 1991, 1999). For TFS, the ACF of IRNp shows a peak at time lag corresponding to the delay, and the ACF of IRNn shows a peak at twice the delay (2*d). The pitch of IRNp corresponds to the reciprocal of the delay (Bilsen & Ritsma, 1970; Sayles & Winter, 2008a; Yost, 1996), and for IRNn, the pitch corresponds to 1/(2*d) Hz (Shofner, 1999; Yost, 1996). That is, the perceived pitch of IRNn is an octave lower than that of IRNp. IRNp and IRNn have the same ENV but different TFS, which likely accounts for this perceived pitch difference.

Shofner (1999) showed that the neural autocorrelograms in response to IRNp and IRNn indicated that the temporal discharge of primary-like units in the CN reflected the TFS of the stimulus, whereas the temporal discharge patterns of chopper units reflected the stimulus ENV.

Shofner (1999) concluded that the primary-like neurons are more likely to preserve temporal information relevant to pitch. These findings have been corroborated by both Verhey and Winter (2006) and Sayles and Winter (2008a). Robust FFRs preserving pitch-relevant information have been recorded using IRN stimuli with both constant and dynamic pitch (Krishnan, Gandour, & Bidelman, 2010, 2012; Krishnan, Gandour, Bidelman, & Swaminathan, 2009; Krishnan, Suresh, & Gandour, 2017a, 2017b; Krishnan et al., 2016; Krishnan, Swaminathan, & Gandour, 2009; Swaminathan, Krishnan, & Gandour, 2008). Ananthakrishnan and Krishnan (2018) examined whether the differential sensitivity to ENV and TFS in response to differences in pitch produced by IRNp and IRNn stimuli is preserved in the temporal pattern of ensemble phase-locked neural activity at more rostral levels in the brainstem as reflected in the human FFR. They reasoned that if FFRs simply reflect neural phase-locking to the waveform envelope and not pitch per se, then the FFRs to both IRNp and IRNn should be nearly identical. However, if the temporal pattern of activity reflected in the FFR aligns with the TFS for IRNp and IRNn, it would support the view that the temporal pattern of FFR neural activity phase-locked to the TFS does indeed contain temporal information relevant to pitch. FFRs were obtained in response to IRNp and IRNn stimuli with 2 and 4 ms delays.

Comparison of the independent analysis of the phase-locked activity to ENV and TFS revealed that only the phase-locked activity to the TFS showed differences in both spectra and ACF that closely matched the pitch difference between the two stimuli (Figure 9–8) but not the phase-locked responses to the envelope periodicity (Figure 9–7). That is, both the ACF peak locations and the spectral patterns were consistent with the behaviorally observed pitch for both IRNp and IRNn stimuli (Figure 9–8). The temporal pattern of phase-locking to the envelope likely preserves information relevant to pitch change due to changes in delay (2 versus 4 ms) (see Figure 9–7). This is consistent with previous results from Shofner (1999) that indicate that the envelope responses to IRNp and IRNn for a given delay are identical and therefore cannot index pitch change. Only the temporal pattern of phase-locked neural activity to the TFS accounts for the behaviorally observed pitch and pitch lowering for all stimuli. Shofner (1991, 1999) showed that the ACFs for IRNp and IRNn were identical for waveform ENV (with a peak corresponding to the delay), but for TFS, IRNp showed a peak at the delay (similar to the envelope ACF) and IRNn showed a peak at twice the delay (Neuert et al.,

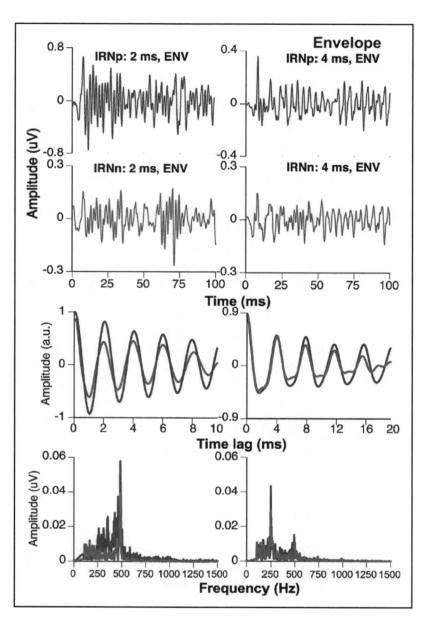

Figure 9–7. Grand average frequency following response (FFR) envelope (ENV) waveform segments (*top*), autocorrelation functions (ACFs) (*middle*), and spectra (*bottom*) representing neural phase-locking to ENV for the 2-ms delay (*left*) and 4-ms delay (*right*) stimuli. Positive gain iterated rippled noise (IRNp) is indicated by the darker traces and negative gain IRN (IRNn) by the lighter traces. For both delays, the ACF peak remains unchanged for both IRNp and IRNn stimuli (although the IRNn responses appear smaller in magnitude compared to the IRNp responses), suggesting that the envelope periodicity is not affected by change from positive to negative gain. However, note the change in periodicity of the response and a shift in the ACF peak from 2 to 4 ms as the delay is changed, suggesting a change in periodicity pitch. Adapted from "Human Frequency Following Responses to Iterated Rippled Noise With Positive and Negative Gain: Differential Sensitivity to Waveform Envelope and Temporal Fine Structure," by S. Ananthakrishnan and A. Krishnan, 2018, *Hearing Research, 367,* pp. 113–123. Copyright 2018, with permission from Elsevier.

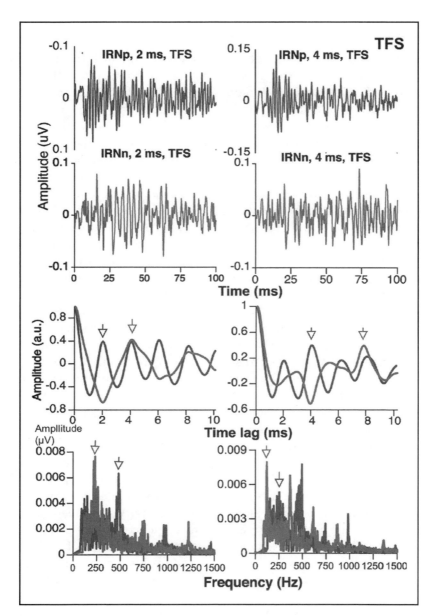

Figure 9–8. Grand average frequency following response (FFR) temporal fine structure (TFS) waveform segments (*top*), autocorrelation functions (ACFs) (*middle*), and spectra (*bottom*) representing neural phase-locking to TFS for the 2-ms delay (*left*) and 4-ms delay (*right*) stimuli. Positive gain iterated rippled noise (IRNp) is indicated by the darker traces and negative gain IRN (IRNn) by the lighter traces. For both IRNn stimuli, waveform periodicity is halved and, correspondingly, ACF peak shifts to 4 ms (250 Hz) for the 2 ms (500 Hz), and from 4 ms (250 Hz) to 8 ms (125 Hz), suggesting that TFS-related phase-locked activity represents the perceived pitch shift associated with change in positive to negative gain in the IRN stimulus. Adapted from "Human Frequency Following Responses to Iterated Rippled Noise With Positive and Negative Gain: Differential Sensitivity to Waveform Envelope and Temporal Fine Structure," by S. Ananthakrishnan and A. Krishnan, 2018, *Hearing Research, 367*, pp. 113–123. Copyright 2018, with permission from Elsevier.

2005; Shofner, 1991, 1999). Also, for IRNp, behavioral measures of pitch correspond to the reciprocal of the delay (Bilsen & Ritsma, 1970; Sayles & Winter, 2008; Yost, 1996), and for IRNn, pitch corresponds to 1/(2*d) Hz (Shofner, 1999; Yost, 1996). Shofner (1999), based on a comparison of the neural autocorrelograms in response to IRNp and IRNn, concluded that the primary-like neurons in the cochlear nucleus reflecting responses to the waveform TFS are more likely to preserve temporal information relevant to pitch, whereas envelope-related activity is preserved in chopper neurons more involved in encoding the envelope modulation. These findings have been corroborated by both Verhey and Winter (2006), and Sayles and Winter (2008a). In addition, current models that explain pitch encoding of IRN stimuli rely on the temporal processing of waveform fine-structure information (Patterson, Handel, Yost, & Datta, 1996; Yost, 1996; Yost, Patterson, & Sheft, 1996). Taking the results from these physiologic studies and the results of the FFR study described in this section (Ananthakrishnan & Krishnan, 2018), it is clear that the temporal pattern of neural activity encoding "pitch change" is primarily driven by the waveform fine structure and appears to be available in the phase-locked neural activity in the midbrain. Finally, these results also suggest that the use of alternating polarity alone will not be optimal to evaluate the neural representation of pitch, since they represent phase-locking to only the envelope periodicity.

Neural Correlates of Pitch Salience

For a variety of complex sounds, including speech or music, perceived pitch and its salience are closely related to the periodicity strength of the stimulus waveform (Fastl & Stoll, 1979; Shofner & Selas, 2002; Yost, 1996). We have already described that pitch salience is weaker for complex sounds with only unresolved components. IRN stimuli allow systematic manipulation of the waveform temporal regularity and TFS, and therefore pitch salience. Perceptually, IRN produces a pitch corresponding to the reciprocal of the delay, and its pitch salience grows with the increasing number of iterations (Patterson et al., 1996; Yost, 1978, 1996; Yost & Hill, 1979). Physiologically, recordings of responses to static (i.e., single pitch) and time-varying (i.e., dynamic pitch) IRN stimuli from auditory nerve fibers (Fay, Yost, & Coombs, 1983; ten Kate & van Bekkum, 1988) and cochlear nucleus neurons (Bilsen, ten Kate, Buunen, & Raatgever, 1975; Sayles & Winter, 2008a; Shofner, 1991, 1999; Winter, Wiegrebe, & Patterson, 2001) show that the pitch of harmonic IRN is represented in the firing patterns of action potentials locked to either the TFS or envelope periodicity. Krishnan, Bidelman, and Gandour (2010) sought to demonstrate that the pitch-relevant information preserved in the phase-locked neural activity generating the FFR is sensitive to changes in pitch salience and is correlated with corresponding changes in perceptual pitch salience. They recorded FFRs using an IRN version of lexical tone with time-varying pitch that varied only in degree of pitch salience (the number of iterations of the IRN stimulus was systematically [Figure 9–9, stimulus panels] varied to produce a continuum from no pitch to very strong pitch). They also measured behavioral frequency difference limens (F0DLs) to obtain a perceptual estimate related to pitch salience. Their results showed that neural periodicity strength increased systematically with an increase in temporal regularity in stimulus periodicity, suggesting that the FFR pitch-relevant neural activity is indeed sensitive to changes in pitch salience (Figure 9–9, response panels). Consistent with this, F0DLs decreased with increasing stimulus temporal regularity (Figure 9–10). The negative correlation between neural periodicity strength and behavioral F0DL suggests that increasing strength in the representation of pitch salience may, at least in part, contribute to improvement in the perceptual ability to discriminate pitch with increasing temporal regularity in the stimulus periodicity. This finding is consistent with electrophysiological studies that show a predictable relationship between neural and behavioral measures of pitch salience. For example, the latency and amplitude of the pitch-onset response (a cortical pitch-specific response) vary systematically with the pitch salience of an IRN stimulus (Krumbholz, Patterson, Seither-Preisler, Lammertmann, & Lütkenhoner, 2003; Soeta, Nakagawa, & Tonoike, 2005), suggesting that the neural activity underlying the generation of the pitch-onset response is involved in extracting an initial estimate of the pitch salience

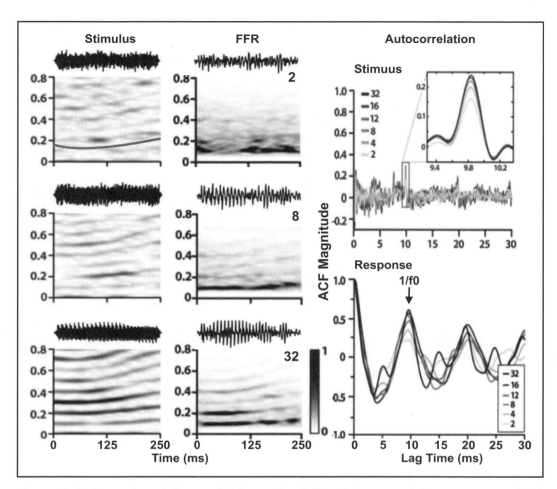

Figure 9–9. Iterated rippled noise (IRN) stimulus (*left*) and frequency following response (FFR) (*middle*) waveforms (plotted at the top of the spectrogram for each stimulus), stimulus autocorrelation functions (*top right*), and the FFR autocorrelation functions (ACFs) (*bottom right*) are all plotted as a function of iteration steps (2, 8, 32). The pitch contour is shown in the stimulus spectrogram for iteration 2. Consistent with the stimulus, the response spectrograms and the ACFs show clearly the steady growth of the response at the pitch period as the temporal regularity of the stimulus improves with an increase in iteration steps. Replotted from "Neural Representation of Pitch Salience in the Human Brainstem Revealed by Psychophysical and Electrophysiological Indices," by A. Krishnan, G. M. Bidelman, and J. T. Gandour, 2010, *Hearing Research, 268*, pp. 60–66. Copyright 2010, with permission from Elsevier.

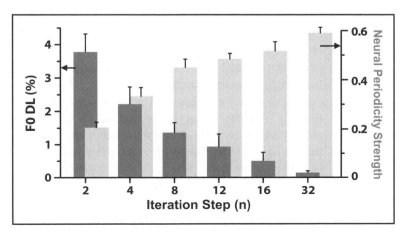

Figure 9–10. Comparison of the changes in the fundamental frequency difference limen (F0DL) and the neural periodicity strength as a function of IRN iteration steps. Note the inverse relationship between F0DL and neural periodicity strength. That is, as F0DL improves with iteration steps (when pitch salience is increasing), the neural pitch strength increases. Recreated using data from Krishnan, Bidelman, and Grandour (2010).

of the sound; the strong correspondence between neural pitch strength of complex sounds and their pitch salience in auditory nerve responses (Cariani & Delgutte, 1996a, 1996b); and the more robust neural periodicity strength in the FFR for consonant intervals compared to dissonant pitch intervals in music (Bidelman & Krishnan, 2009). Overall, these results showing growth in FFR neural periodicity strength with increasing iteration steps likely reflect an improvement in neural encoding of pitch-relevant periodicities in the brainstem. Thus, neural information relevant to pitch salience may already be emerging in preattentive, early sensory-level processing in the midbrain.

Neural Representation of Speech in Adverse Listening Conditions

Speech communication almost always occurs in the presence of competing background sounds and/or in a less than optimal acoustical environment. These adverse listening conditions challenge the auditory system's ability to extract certain acoustic features of sounds that are important for speech perception. While background noise effects are usually explained in terms of masking of the target, in reverberant conditions, the original sound waves are reflected from walls, floors, and ceilings. Reflected sound waves arrive at the listener's ear delayed relative to the original. The temporal overlap between them results in a noisier signal compromised by multiple delays, attenuation, and spectrotemporal distortions. With its ability to preserve f0 and formant information, the FFR serves as an effective analytic tool to study the neural representation of certain acoustic features in quiet and how they may be degraded in adverse listening conditions like noise and reverberation.

Effects of Reverberation

Psychophysical studies have shown that reverberation-induced spectrotemporal distortion can have deleterious effects on an individual's ability to identify and discriminate acoustic features of consonants (Gelfand & Silman, 1979), vowels (Drgas & Blaszak, 2009; Nabelek & Letowski, 1988), and time-varying formant cues (Nabelek & Dagenias, 1986). The consequent reduction in identification and discrimination reflects both forward masking, where preceding segments mask subsequent segments, and self-masking, where temporal smearing occurs within each phoneme (Nabelek, Letowski, & Tucker, 1989; Wang & Brown, 2006). Physiological data from single neurons in the ventral cochlear nucleus (Sayles, Stasiak, & Winter, 2015, 2016; Sayles & Winter, 2008b) and the scalp-recorded brainstem FFR data (Krishnan et al., 2019; Bidelman, 2017; Bidelman & Krishnan, 2011b) show that neural representation of pitch-relevant fine-structure information based on neural phase-locking is degraded in the presence of reverberation. Bidelman and Krishnan (2011b) using the vowel /i/ with time-varying f0, observed that speech-evoked FFRs show an overall reduction in response magnitude due to reverberation-induced desynchronization—Figure 9–11, left and middle panels showing disruption of phase-locking in both the autocorrelogram (left) and the spectrogram (middle), particularly pronounced at the higher frequencies (formant-related harmonics), while maintaining the representation of f0 with only a gradual decrease in magnitude until at least the most severe reverberation condition (Figure 9–11, right top). However, they did show a progressively decreasing correlation between the response in the dry condition (no reverberation) and the responses in reverberant conditions (Figure 9–11, right bottom). In contrast, Bidelman, Davis, and Pridgen (2018) showed little or no change in the f0 component of the FFR elicited by a vCv speech token in the presence of mild and medium levels of reverberation. Sayles et al. (2016) showed a significant degradation in the periodicity tagged discharge for only stimuli with a time-varying pitch with little or no change for stimuli with steady-state pitch. It is possible that the absence of an appreciable reverberation-induced degradation in Bidelman, Davis, and Pridgen (2018) may be due to the very gradual change in pitch over time in their stimulus. More recently, Krishnan et al. (2019), using a lexical tone with time-varying pitch (Mandarin tone 2 with a curvilinear rising pitch contour) preceded by a long noise segment, showed that the neural representation of pitch-relevant information (as reflected in the ability to follow the f0 changes) progressively deteriorated

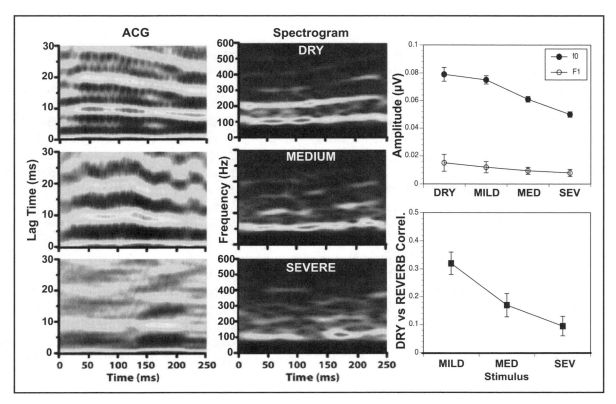

Figure 9–11. Autocorrelograms (*left*), spectrograms (*middle*), mean degradation in f0 and F1 amplitude (*right, top*), and change in f0 amplitude (*bottom right*) plotted as change relative to the DRY condition. Both the autocorrelogram and the spectrogram show progressive degradation in the neural representation of pitch-relevant periodicities and spectral harmonics. Note the reverberation-related degradation in f0 appears to be relatively greater than the F1 representation, particularly at the medium and severe degrees of reverberation. Recreated using data from Bidelman and Krishnan (2011b).

with increasing reverberation (slight to moderate levels) with greater disruption of the later rapidly accelerating pitch segment. This latter result is consistent with animal studies that show the neural encoding of pitch based on timing information is severely degraded in the presence of reverberation in the caudal brainstem (Sayles et al., 2015, 2016; Sayles & Winter, 2008b—ventral cochlear nucleus). Reverberation likely degrades the sustained fine-grained, phase-locked temporal discharge pattern of brainstem neural responses following the pitch contour. This degradation is likely due to the loss of robust periodicity and the smearing of dynamic changes over time in the fine structure of the stimulus (Houtgast & Steeneken, 1973, 1985).

Another possible explanation for the relative resilience of f0 is that the FFR is dominated by phase-locking to low-frequency resolved components rather than phase-locking to the envelope modulation resulting from the interaction of unresolved higher harmonics. This latter, weaker, pitch-relevant cue has been shown to degrade markedly with increasing reverberation, due to the breakdown of temporal envelope modulation caused by randomization of phase relationships between unresolved harmonics (Sayles & Winter, 2008b); therefore, pitch of complex sounds with only unresolved harmonics will be severely degraded by reverberation. In contrast, for complex sounds containing both resolved and unresolved harmonics, pitch encoding in the presence of reverberation relies solely on the temporally smeared fine-structure information in resolved regions. The observation of smaller change in FFR phase-locking to F0 with increasing reverberation compared to F1 (Bidelman & Krishnan, 2011b) is consistent with the observation of lack of degradation in low-frequency phase-locked units in the cochlear nucleus encoding spectrally resolved pitch (Sayles & Winter, 2008b; Stasiak, Winter, & Sayles, 2010). Sayles and Winter (2008b) suggest that both the more robust neural phase-locking in the low-frequency channels in general and the more salient responses to resolved components increase their resistance to temporal smearing resulting from reverberation. It is also plausible that the slower rate of F0 change in our stimuli reduced the smearing effects of reverberation on the neural encoding of F0. However, it is not entirely clear why the encoding of the resolved first formant (F1) related harmonics in our FFR data showed greater degradation with increased reverberation. This differential effect of reverberation on encoding may be due to the relatively greater spectrotemporal smearing of the formant related higher frequency harmonics in our stimuli than the F0 component.

Effects of Background Noise

Reduced amplitude and/or latency prolongations have been observed in the presence of noise for cortical-evoked potentials (Billings, Tremblay, Stecker, & Tolin, 2009; Kaplan-Neeman, Kishon-Rabin, Henkin, & Muchnik, 2006; Suresh et al., 2017 [cortical pitch response]; Whiting, Martin, & Stapells, 1998), MEG (Chait, Poeppel, & Simon, 2006; Hughes et al., 2014; Sasaki et al., 2005), and brainstem EFR/FFR (Bidelman et al., 2018; Li & Jeng, 2011; Parbery-Clark, Skoe, & Kraus, 2009; Prevost, Laroche, Marcoux, & Dajani, 2013; Russo, Nicol, Musacchia, & Kraus, 2004; Smalt, Krishnan, Bidelman, Ananthakrishnan, & Gandour, 2012; Song, Skoe, Banai, & Kraus, 2011). Smalt et al. (2012), using a complex tone with unresolved harmonics (12th–17th) of a 90-Hz f0 and low-pass masking to eliminate distortion products in the lower frequencies, observed robust peaks at f0 (envelope) and lower harmonics (EFR due to modulation at 90 Hz resulting from the periodicity of the complex stimulus and the distortion produced by the interaction of the unresolved harmonics). While the cubic distortion component showed a systematic decrease in amplitude with the increasing noise level, f0 remained largely unaltered even at high noise levels (Figure 9–12). However, as the noise level was increased, phase-locked components at higher harmonics (2f0-to-8f0-overlapping the F1 and F2 harmonics of English back vowels) reduced in magnitude, which in turn may contribute to difficulties in speech perception in noise. There is also some evidence showing enhancement of f0 in the presence of noise (Bidelman et al., 2018; Prevost et al., 2013; Smalt et al., 2012). One possible explanation for this enhancement is the presence of stochastic resonance in the auditory system (Cunningham, Nicol, King, Zecker, & Kraus, 2002; Henry, 1999). That is, the addition of noise presumably improves (the underlying neural mechanism is not known) the neural entrainment of a weak periodic signal. Given the high stimulus presentation levels used to elicit these responses, it is more likely that low-frequency tails of higher-frequency neurons are recruited at higher intensities so that a broad array of fibers are phase-locking to the f0 and consequently reducing the effects of noise. Another possible explanation is that the FFR is dominated by phase-locking to low-frequency resolved components rather than the weaker cue resulting from phase-locking to the envelope modulation resulting from the interaction of unresolved higher harmonics that would be more suspectable to noise degradation due to increased susceptibility to masking (Laroche, Dajani, Prevost, & Marcoux, 2013; Sayles et al., 2015, 2016; Sayles & Winter, 2008b). Thus, it appears that the neural representation of the source-related component (f0) is more resilient to degradation in adverse listening conditions. In contrast, vocal tract filter-related components (formant-related harmonics) are relatively more susceptible to degradation (Bidelman & Krishnan, 2011b; Russo et al., 2004). Interestingly, this differential effect of reverberation may enhance the music experience but degrade speech intelligibility.

The resilience of at least the f0 component of the FFR to degradative effects of noise and reverberation suggests that neural synchronization to f0 is robust (at least for steady-state pitch where enough cycles of pitch information may be preserved to extract pitch) and not readily susceptible to degradation by noise or reverberation. This resilience to degradation by noise or reverberation is fortuitous, since f0 plays a critical role in the perception of speech, music, and the ability to seg-

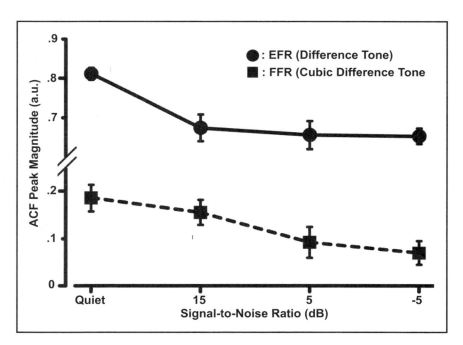

Figure 9–12. Mean periodicity strength plotted for the envelope following response (EFR; *solid circle*) and the frequency following response (FFR; cubic difference tone) for the quiet and increasing levels of noise. Both show a decrease in periodicity strength as the signal-to-noise ratio decreases. Recreated using data from "Neural Correlates of Cochlear Distortion Products and Their Influence on the Representation of Pitch Relevant Information in the Human Brainstem," by C. J. Smalt, A. Krishnan, G. M. Bidelman, S. Ananthakrishnan, and J. T. Gandour, 2012, *Hearing Research, 292*, pp. 26–34.

regate concurrent sounds, all of which invariably occur in the presence of other sounds (Assmann & Sumerfield, 1990). In sharp contrast to the sustained phase-locked response, the onset brainstem components show both latency prolongation and amplitude reduction (Burkard & Hecox, 1983) in the presence of noise, suggesting a reduction in cochlear regional contributions and disruption in neural synchrony. However, it should be noted here that the higher formant-related components in the FFR are indeed degraded by noise and reverberation, much like what is observed perceptually (Liu & Kewley-Port, 2004). For example, difference limens (f0 discrimination ability) for speech F0 are not appreciably altered with increasing reverberation, while formant discrimination deteriorates even at low levels of reverberation (Bidelman & Krishnan, 2011b).

Noise and reverberation are fundamentally different in terms of how they distort the spectrotemporal attributes of complex stimuli; therefore, it follows that their effects could also manifest differently in the phase-locked neural activity. Bidelman et al. (2018) demonstrated that speech-evoked brainstem FFR (f0) and early cortical responses were degraded more by noise than reverberation. Previous physiological studies (Al Osman et al., 2017; Bidelman & Krishnan, 2011b; Sayles et al., 2016; Sayles & Winter 2008b) have also shown better preservation of neural representation in reverberation compared to noise (Bidelman, 2017, review). A qualitative comparison of changes in cortical pitch response (CPR) due to reverberation (Krishnan et al., 2019) and background noise (Suresh et al., 2017) reveals that both types of adverse listening conditions result in degradation of CPR neural activity. In reverberation, language-dependent enhancement is maintained across conditions; in background noise, it is maintained only for the most favorable signal-to-noise ratio (SNR; +5 dB) condition. Behavioral measures have also shown different patterns of vowel confusions in noise and reverberation (Nabelek & Dagenais, 1986). Taken together, these results are consistent with Bidelman et al. (2018), suggesting differential effects of noise and reverberation. Sayles et al. (2016) also observed differential effects for noise and reverberation. Specifically, reverberation significantly impaired segregation of concurrent vowels that had a pitch contour but not vowels with steady-state pitch. In contrast, noise impaired segregation of vowels with both steady-state and time-variant pitch contour. Vowels with changing pitch will have a dramatic effect on template contrast in reverberation, due to spectral smearing. Noise impairs neural segregation of concurrent vowels independent of intonation pattern, but in a best frequency-dependent manner due to increased effective masking within the higher best frequency filters—that is, the within-band SNR is lower in the higher-frequency filters. It remains unclear if these differences simply reflect fundamental differences in the extent to which spectrotemporal pitch-relevant acoustic features are disrupted and/or the relative effectiveness of masking mechanisms under both noise and reverberation. Surprisingly, the differential effects of noise and reverberation on speech representations are not observed at the cortical level (Mesgarani, David, Fritz, & Shamma, 2014), suggesting the operation of central compensatory mechanisms to mitigate the effects of reverberation on the encoding of time-varying periodicity at the subcortical levels. We cannot rule out the interplay between bottom-up and top-down mechanisms (Suga et al., 2000; Suga, Ma, Gao, Sakai, & Chowdhury, 2003) to aid signal selection in adverse listening conditions. Such interplay, however, does not explain why signal selection would be selectively aided in reverberation but not noise. Consequently, it may be that reverberation is a more effective masker of acoustic features over the entire duration of the stimulus. In reverberation, acoustic cues relevant to pitch are likely to remain available for at least some portions of the signal. Clearly, more research is needed to provide a more complete, quantitative characterization of how noise and reverberation differentially affect the neural encoding of complex sounds. Development of optimal signal processing strategies implemented in conventional amplification devices will have to consider appropriate strategies to mitigate the deleterious effects of noise and reverberation on the neural representation of certain acoustic features of speech important for speech perception.

III. NEURAL REPRESENTATION OF LINGUISTIC PITCH-RELEVANT INFORMATION IN THE BRAINSTEM

Perceptual Attributes of Pitch in Tonal Languages

Tone languages, like Mandarin, exploit phonologically contrastive pitch at the word or syllable level (Gandour, 1994; Yip, 2002). In Mandarin, for example, four words may comprise a minimal quadruplet, minimally distinguished by variations in pitch, but otherwise identical in terms of consonant and vowel segments. Mandarin has four lexical tones (Howie, 1976): yi^1 "clothing" high level [T1]; yi^2 "aunt" high rising [T2]; yi^3 "chair" low falling-rising [T3]; yi^4 "easy" high falling [T4] (see Figure 9–13, panel B). Such languages are to be distinguished from those in which pitch variations are usually not contrastive at the syllable or word level (e.g., English). In nontonal languages, like English for example, variations in pitch may be used to signal stress and intonation patterns at postlexical levels of representation. The crucial feature that differentiates between these two types of languages is whether or not pitch variations are contrastive in the lexicon. The relative importance of these pitch attributes varies depending on listeners' familiarity with specific types of pitch patterns that occur in their native language. For example, the long-term experience of tonal language speakers enhances their attention to perceptual saliency of the contour dimension, whereas English listeners give greater weight to the height dimension.

Thus, tone languages not only provide a physiologic window to evaluate how neural representations of linguistically relevant pitch attributes emerge along the early stages of sensory processing in the hierarchy, but they may also shed light on the nature of the interaction between early sensory levels and later higher levels of cognitive processing in the human brain. Pitch also provides an excellent window for studying experience-dependent effects on both cortical and brainstem components of a well-coordinated, hierarchical processing network. In the brainstem, computations are applied to representations, which, in turn, are shaped by experience within a specific domain (e.g., language). Recent empirical data show that these neural representations of pitch, at both the brainstem and cortical level, are shaped by one's experience with language and music (Besson, Chobert, & Marie, 2011; Krishnan & Gandour, 2014, 2017; Zatorre & Baum, 2012). While it is not known how language experience shapes subcortical and cortical stages of pitch processing, it is likely that the neural processes underlying such experience-dependent plasticity at each stage along the processing hierarchy are modulated by a coordinated interplay between ascending, descending, and local neural pathways that involve both sensory and cognitive components (Chandrasekaran & Kraus, 2010; Krishnan, Suresh, & Gandour 2017a, 2017b; Krishnan et al., 2016). That is, feedback from language-dependent cortical processes shapes early sensory-level processing at both the brainstem and cortical level to extract outputs that transform, later functionally more salient cortical representations that drive processes mediating linguistic performance.

Tone languages are especially advantageous for isolating effects of encoding of voice pitch at the level of the auditory brainstem. In Mandarin, for example, all four tones exhibit voice F0 trajectories and harmonics that lie within the range of easily recordable FFRs (below 2 kHz). The relatively long duration of citation forms of lexical tones (200–350 ms) necessitates the use of slower stimulus repetition rates. This, in turn, enables the recording of robust FFRs with little or no neural adaptation.

Language Experience–Dependent Plasticity in Pitch Processing in the Brainstem

Historically, the role of the brainstem in the processing of speech/language has not been considered seriously. Until recently, the prevailing wisdom was that the processing in the brainstem and thalamus was general to all sounds, and speech-specific operations emerged only in the cerebral cortex (Scott & Johnsrude, 2003, p. 100). Although operations specific to speech perception are largely confined to the cortex, evidence of experience-dependent modulation of pitch-relevant neural activity in the brainstem suggests that early sensory processing involves more than a simple transmission of pitch information from the ear to the cerebral cortex.

The neural substrates of pitch perception in the processing of lexical tones are shaped by language experience in both the auditory cortex (Gandour & Krishnan, 2014; Zatorre & Gandour, 2008) and the early sensory processing of pitch-relevant information in the brainstem (Krishnan & Gandour, 2009, 2014, 2017; Krishnan, Gandour, & Bidelman, 2010, 2012; Krishnan, Xu, Gandour, & Cariani, 2005). Indeed, the neural representation of pitch-relevant attributes, as reflected in the FFR, may emerge as early as 8 to 10 ms after stimulus onset (Krishnan & Gandour, 2009). In contrast, the pitch-related neural activity in the auditory cortex emerges at about 140 to 170 ms after stimulus onset (Griffiths & Hall, 2012; Krumbholz et al., 2003). Additional evidence supporting experience-dependent plasticity in the brainstem includes improvement in phase-locked activity post auditory training in children with learning impairments (Russo, Nicol, Zecker, Hayes, & Kraus, 2005), better pitch tracking accuracy of Mandarin tones in nonnative musicians than nonmusicians (Wong, Skoe, Russo, Dees, & Kraus, 2007), and improved pitch-tracking accuracy in native English-speaking adults after undergoing short-term training on using Mandarin tones in word identification (Song, Skoe, Wong, & Kraus, 2008). Also relevant is the consequence of a disruption in the normal interaction between local processes and the corticofugal modulation of subcortical function, which contributes to plasticity. The deficits in brainstem encoding in children with a variety of language-based learning problems could very well reflect such a disruption in the ability of the corticofugal system to fine-tune subcortical processes (Russo et al., 2008; Song, Banai, & Kraus, 2008). That this neural plasticity is not limited to the cortex is already well-established in animal research that has shown that response properties and frequency maps in the IC of bats change after auditory conditioning or focal electrical stimulation of the auditory cortex (Suga, 1990, 1994). Also, the auditory experience of altered interaural cues for localization in young owls leads to frequency-dependent changes in interaural time difference tuning and frequency tuning in IC neurons (Gold & Knudsen, 2000).

Preattentive stages of pitch processing in the brainstem are also influenced by language experience. In a cross-language study using Mandarin and English speakers, Krishnan et al. (2005) sought to determine if native speakers' long-term exposure and experience using pitch patterns in a tonal language influenced the properties of FFRs elicited by four prototypical Mandarin lexical tones (Krishnan et al., 2005) (Figure 9–13A and B). Their results showed that both neural periodicity strength (Figure 9–13C, top) and pitch-tracking accuracy (Figure 9–13C, bottom) were significantly greater for the Chinese group than for the English group across

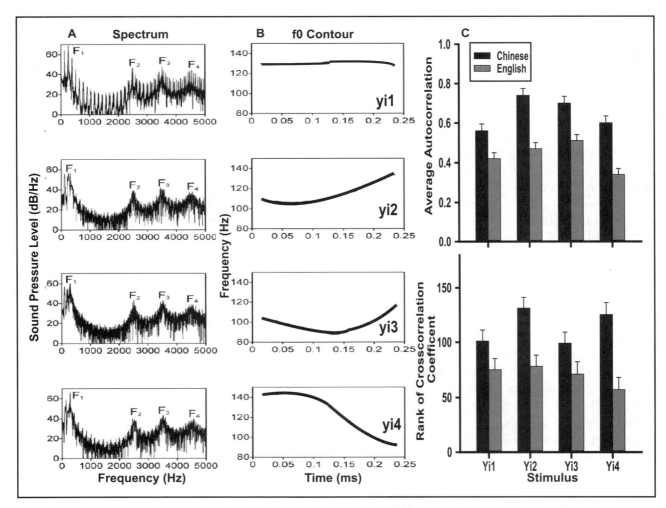

Figure 9–13. Stimulus spectrum (**A**) corresponding F0 contours of the four Mandarin Chinese synthetic speech stimuli (**B**), frequency following response (FFR) periodicity strength (**C**, *top*), and FFR pitch-tracking accuracy (**C**, *bottom*) of the four Mandarin lexical tones. Note the invariant spectra of the speech stimuli across the four tones. The syllable is identified in the bottom right of each panel (**B**). Comparison of pitch strength (**C**, *top*) and pitch-tracking accuracy (**C**, *bottom*) for Chinese and English listeners per lexical tone. Chinese listeners show better tracking accuracy and greater periodicity strength across the four stimuli compared to English listeners. Recreated using data from "Encoding of Pitch in the Human Brainstem Is Sensitive to Language Experience," by A. Krishnan, Y. Xu, J. T. Gandour, and P. A. Cariani, 2005, *Cognitive Brain Research*, 25(1), pp. 161–168.

all four Mandarin tones. These results suggest that experience-driven adaptive neural mechanisms (via top-down modulation and/or local experience shaped) sharpen response properties of neurons tuned for processing pitch contours that are sensitive to the prosodic needs of a particular language. That is, language-dependent plasticity enhances or primes temporal intervals that carry linguistically relevant features of pitch contours. Auditory processing in the brainstem is not limited to a simple representation of acoustic features of speech stimuli but may also perform language-dependent operations well before the signal reaches the cerebral cortex.

Language Experience–Dependent Effects in the Brainstem Are Feature Specific

There is compelling evidence that language experience shaped pitch processing is largely limited to temporal attributes of the stimulus that produce pitch percepts that are native to the listeners' experience. The question is, to what extent can a stimulus deviate from natural speech exemplars before exceeding the upper or the lower limit of linguistically shaped sensitivity of brainstem neurons? By examining FFRs elicited by linear approximations of the normally curvilinear Mandarin T2 and T4 (Xu, Krishnan, and Grandour, 2006), it was possible to assess the tolerance limits for priming linguistically relevant features of the auditory signal involved in pitch extraction at the level of the brainstem (Figure 9–14, left and right panels). Results show no language-dependent effects in FFR periodicity strength or pitch-tracking accuracy (Figure 9–14, right panel, top and bottom, respectively) for both the rising and falling contours, because these linear variants are not part of native Chinese listeners' experience. The fact that Mandarin and English FFRs are homogeneous in response to dynamic linear trajectories suggests that representations of pitch-relevant information in the brainstem are acutely sensitive to dynamic, curvilinear changes in trajectory throughout a pitch contour. In the auditory brainstem, neural mechanisms respond to specific dimensions of pitch contours to which native speakers have been exposed. Language-dependent neuroplasticity occurs only when salient dimensions

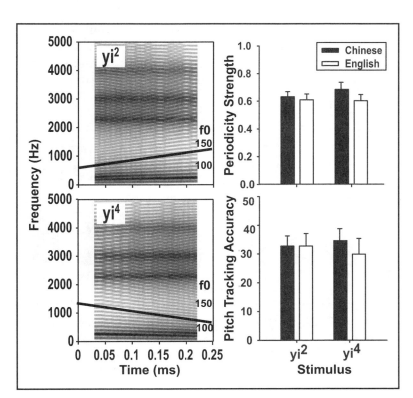

Figure 9–14. Stimulus spectrograms (*left*) of Chinese synthetic speech stimuli (yi^2 "aunt" and yi^4 "easy") with the linear version of the rising (*top*) and falling (*bottom*) F0 contours. Frequency following response (FFR) periodicity strength (*top, right*), and FFR pitch-tracking accuracy (*bottom, right*). FFR pitch-tracking accuracy revealed no significant main effects for either language group (Chinese, English) or pitch direction (rising, falling). Adapted with permission from "Specificity of Experience-Dependent Pitch Representation in the Brainstem," by Y. Xu, A. Krishnan, and J. Gandour, 2006, *NeuroReport, 17*(15), pp. 1601–1605.

of pitch-relevant to speech perception are present in the auditory signal.

Further support for feature specificity comes from FFRs recorded from Chinese and English participants in response to IRN homologs of pitch contours. IRN stimuli preserve the perception of the pitch but do not have a prominent waveform periodicity or highly modulated stimulus envelopes that are characteristic of speech stimuli. An IRN stimulus is generated using a broadband noise, which is delayed and added to itself repeatedly, and therefore, does not have a prominent modulated envelope (Patterson et al., 1996; Yost, 1996). The perceived pitch corresponds to the reciprocal of the delay, and the pitch salience increases with the number of iterations of the delay-and-add process. Increases in temporal regularity of steady-state IRN stimuli lead to better temporally locked neural activity in auditory structures from the cochlear nucleus to the cortex (Griffiths, Büchel, Frackowiak, & Patterson, 1998; Shofner, 1999). Importantly, a novel generalization of the IRN algorithm makes it possible to generate time-variant, dynamic curvilinear pitch contours representative of those that occur in natural speech (Swaminathan et al., 2008). IRN homologs of a prototypical T2 were presented in contrast to three F0 variants (two linear, one curvilinear) that do not occur in the Mandarin tonal space (Krishnan, Gandour, et al., 2009). Of the two linear variants (Figure 9–15, left panel), one represented a linear ascending ramp; the other, a trilinear approximation of T2, preserving the major points of inflection besides onset and offset. The curvilinear variant was an inverted version of T2. No group differences in either neural periodicity strength or neural pitch-tracking accuracy were observed for any of these variants (Figure 9–15, middle and right panels). The absence of language group effects in response to curvilinear as well as linear variants of T2 emphasizes that language-dependent neuroplasticity in the brainstem extends only to native Mandarin pitch contours.

Domain Specificity of the Experience-Dependent Effects in the Brainstem

Speech Versus Nonspeech

To address the question of domain specificity of experience-dependent effects on the processing of pitch-relevant information in the brainstem, FFRs were recorded from native speakers of Mandarin and English speakers using speech and IRN version (nonspeech) homologs of the four Mandarin tones (Swaminathan et al., 2008). The Chinese group showed stronger periodicity strength than the English group in three (T2-4) out of the four tones for both speech (Figure 9–16, left column) and nonspeech (Figure 9–16, right column) sounds. Segmental evaluation of FFR periodicity strength reveals that the Chinese group exhibits a more robust pitch

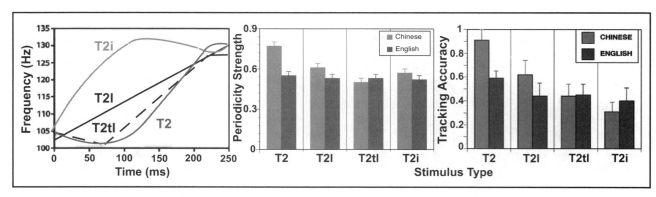

Figure 9–15. Native Mandarin (T2) and nonnative linear (T2l-T2 linear), T2tl-T2 trilinear, and curvilinear pitch contours (T2i-T2 inverted) incorporated in iterated rippled noise (IRN) stimuli are shown on the left. The middle and the right panels show the comparison of periodicity strength and pitch-tracking accuracy in Chinese and English speakers across the four pitch contours. Only the native T2 pitch contour shows a significant group difference. Replotted from Krishnan, Grandour, Bidelman, and Swaminathan (2009).

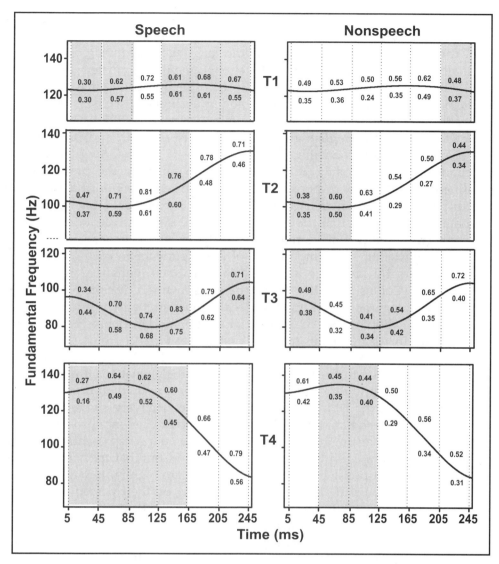

Figure 9–16. Segmental (six 40-ms segments) comparison of neural periodicity strength across for the four Mandarin pitch contours (T1, T2, T3, and T4) presented in a speech context (*left*) and in a nonspeech context (*right*) in Chinese and English speakers. In each panel, the periodicity strength for each segment is noted above the contour for the Chinese and below the contour for the English. The unshaded segments represent regions where the periodicity strengths were significantly different for the two groups. Note that group differences tend to occur in segments with rapid change in pitch. Adapted with permission from "Pitch Encoding in Speech and Nonspeech Contexts in the Human Auditory Brainstem," by J. Swaminathan, A. Krishnan, and J.T. Gandour, 2008, *Neuroreport, 19*(11), pp. 1163–1167.

representation of those segments containing rapidly changing pitch movements across all four tones for both speech and nonspeech sounds. However, given the relatively less robust temporal periodicity in the IRN waveform, pitch strength was observed to be greater for speech than nonspeech stimuli across language groups. These findings suggest that neural mechanisms underlying pitch representation are shaped by particular dimensions of the auditory stream rather than speech, per se.

A discriminant analysis was used to determine the extent to which individual subjects can be classified into their respective language groups based on a weighted linear combination of their pitch strength of three 40-ms temporal intervals that were maximally differentiated in terms of slope (flat, rising, falling). About 83% of subjects were correctly classified into their respective language groups. The group centroid of the Chinese group was larger than that of the English group. Univariate tests of pitch strength confirmed that more dynamic changes in pitch (rising, falling) had a greater influence on the FFR responses of the Chinese group relative to the English group, whereas less dynamic changes in pitch (flat) did not yield a language group effect. Pitch strength of the rising F0 trajectory was the most important in discriminating listeners by language affiliation. Both psychoacoustic (Collins & Cullen, 1978; Schouten, 1985) and physiologic studies (Krishnan & Parkinson, 2000; Shore, Clopton, & Au, 1987) indicate better sensitivity for rising versus falling tones. Multidimensional scaling analyses show that the perceptual dimension related to the direction of pitch change is spatially distributed primarily in terms of rising versus nonrising F0 movements (Gandour, 1983; Gandour & Harshman, 1978). This response asymmetry in FFRs presumably reflects greater neural synchrony (Shore & Nuttall, 1985) and more coherent temporal response patterns to rising than to falling tones (Shore et al., 1987).

In summary, these experimental findings support the view that at early stages of processing in the brain, particular features or dimensions of pitch patterns—regardless of the stimulus context in which they are embedded—shape neural mechanisms underlying speech perception. The role of the brainstem is to facilitate cortical-level processing of pitch-relevant information by optimally capturing those dimensions of the auditory signal that are of linguistic relevance. By focusing on tonal sections instead of the whole tone, it is possible to assess whether language-dependent effects are better conceptualized as applying to sections that exhibit certain acoustic features irrespective of tonal category.

Speech Versus Music

Neural encoding of pitch in the auditory brainstem is known to be shaped by long-term experience with language or music, implying that early sensory processing is subject to experience-dependent neural plasticity. The comparisons between the language and music domains reveal overall enhancement in brainstem FFRs elicited by either musical or linguistic pitch patterns in musicians and tone language speakers alike (Bidelman, Gandour, & Krishnan, 2011b, 2011c) both in terms of periodicity strength and pitch-tracking accuracy (Figure 9–17). Thus, long-term pitch experience seems to improve the brain's ability to represent pitch-relevant information regardless of the domain of expertise. However, subtle differences in these sensory representations suggest a domain-specific sensitivity to acoustic features that are part of the experience in each domain. Musicians, for example, show enhanced responses when pitch patterns intersect discrete notes along the musical scale; tone language speakers, on the other hand, show enhanced responses during rapidly changing portions of tonal contours (Bidelman, Gandour, & Krishnan, 2011a, 2011b). Such cue weighting is consistent with the relative importance of these perceptual dimensions in their respective domains. These findings collectively suggest that both language and musical experience provide some mutual benefit to the neural representation of pitch-relevant information, but that specific features of the acoustic signal are highlighted in subcortical responses depending on their perceptual salience and function within a listener's domain of expertise.

Experience-Dependent Effects Are More Resilient to Signal Degradation

Most human communication occurs against a background of noise. The auditory system must have mechanism(s) in place to encode behaviorally relevant acoustic features of pitch that may be degraded in the presence of noise. By using IRN homologs of pitch contours associated with lexical tones, it is possible to systematically vary their degree of temporal regularity and, therefore, their pitch salience. The question then arises whether pitch representation in the brainstem is less vulnerable to systematic degradation in the temporal regularity of an IRN stimulus that represents a native pitch contour (Krishnan, Gandour, & Bidelman, 2010; Krishnan, Gandour, & Suresh, 2016;). FFRs were elicited by

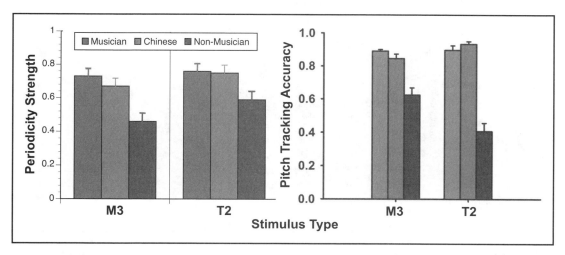

Figure 9–17. Mean periodicity strength (*left*) and mean pitch-tracking accuracy (*right*) plotted for the musical stimulus (M3) and the tonal stimulus (T2) for English musicians (*dark gray*), Chinese-Mandarin speakers (*light gray*), and English nonmusicians (*black*). Both measures show that both the musicians and Chinese are superior compared to the nonmusicians and are equally good for music and tone stimuli. Adapted from Bidelman, Gandour, and Krishnan (2011b).

IRN homologs of Mandarin T2 systematically varying in pitch salience along a six-step continuum ranging from low to high FFR neural periodicity strength. Grand average FFRs and their corresponding spectra appear to show that response magnitude increases with an increase in temporal regularity of the stimulus for both groups but with the Chinese responses relatively larger than the English (Figure 9–18, left and middle panels). Neural periodicity strength is higher in the Chinese group relative to the English group except for the two lowest steps along the continuum (Figure 9–18, right panel). FFR periodicity strength was greater in the Chinese group even in severely degraded stimuli for sections of the response that exhibit rapid changes in pitch. Exponential time constants reveal that pitch strength growth emerges two to three times faster in Chinese than in English listeners as a function of increasing temporal regularity of the stimulus. Collectively, these findings suggest that experience-dependent brainstem mechanisms for pitch are especially sensitive to those dimensions of tonal contours that provide cues of high perceptual saliency in degraded as well as normal listening conditions.

Another way to degrade pitch-relevant information in the stimulus is to systematically increase the rate of pitch change in the dynamic portions of the stimulus. The question then arises whether language-related expertise in pitch encoding of linguistically relevant stimuli can transfer to pitch encoding of stimuli that are characterized by acceleration rates that do not occur in natural speech. Four click-train homologs of Mandarin T2 (Figure 9–19, left panels) with maximum rates of pitch acceleration ranging from low (0.3 Hz/ms; Mandarin Tone 2) to high (2.7 Hz/ms; two octaves) were presented to Chinese and English listeners (Krishnan, Gandour, Smalt, & Bidelman, 2010). Regardless of language group, neural periodicity strength is greater in response to acceleration rates within or proximal to natural speech relative to those beyond its range (Figure 9–19, right panel). Though both groups show decreasing neural periodicity strength with increasing acceleration rates, representations of pitch-relevant information in the Chinese group are more resistant to degradation. These findings indicate that perceptually salient pitch cues associated with lexical tone influence brainstem pitch extraction not only in the speech domain but also in auditory signals that clearly fall outside the range of dynamic pitch that a native listener is exposed to.

The most common adverse listening condition encountered in communication is background noise and reverberation. We already described the effects of noise and reverberation on the neural

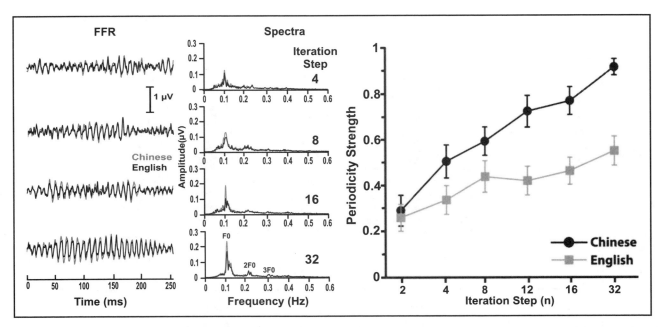

Figure 9–18. Grand average frequency following responses (FFRs) (*left*) and corresponding spectra (*middle*), overlaid for the Chinese (*lighter traces*) and English (*darker traces*) speakers, are plotted as a function of iteration steps (4, 8, and 32). Mean periodicity strength is plotted as a function of the iteration step for the Chinese (*black*) and English (*gray*) speakers on the right. Note that even at a low iteration step (where pitch salience is weak), the Chinese show stronger periodicity strength compared to the English. Left panel showing FFR waveform and spectra adapted with permission from "Language-Experience Plasticity in Neural Representation of Changes in Pitch Salience," by A. Krishnan, J. T. Gandour, and C. H. Suresh, 2016, *Brain Research*, *1637*, pp. 102–117. Copyright 2016, with permission from Elsevier; Right panel adapted with permission from "Neural Representation of Pitch Salience in the Human Brainstem Revealed by Psychophysical and Electrophysiological Indices," by A. Krishnan, G. M. Bidelman, and J. T. Gandour, 2010, *Hearing Research*, *268*, pp. 60–66.

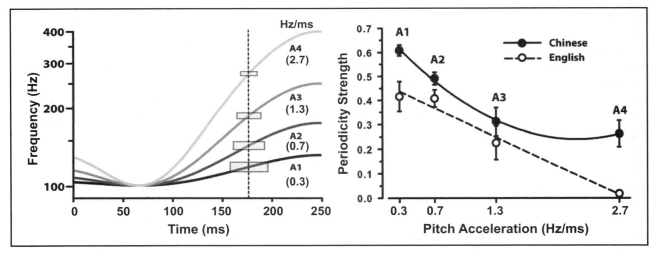

Figure 9–19. Click-train stimuli that are differentiated by varying degrees of rising acceleration. F0 contours of all four stimuli are displayed on a logarithmic scale spanning two octaves—from 100.8 Hz, the minimum stimulus frequency, to 400 Hz (*left, top*). These stimuli represent a continuum of rates of acceleration from an exemplary Tone 2 (A1) rate in a natural speech to an F0 rate that falls well beyond the normal voice range (A4). The vertical dotted line at 177 ms (represents maximum pitch acceleration) defines the center of the analysis window for each stimulus (*left, bottom*). Group comparisons of periodicity strength are shown within the region of maximum acceleration of the stimulus derived from FFR responses to click-train stimuli as a function of pitch acceleration (*right*). FFR periodicity strength of the Chinese group is greater than that of the English group in response to Mandarin Tone 2 (A1, 0.3 Hz/ms) as well as to a pitch pattern that does not occur in natural speech (A4, 2.7 Hz/ms). From Krishnan, Grandour, Smalt, and Bidelman (2010).

representation of speech sounds in an earlier section. The question arises whether experience-dependent pitch mechanisms are more resilient to the degradative effects of reverberation and noise. Krishnan, Suresh, and Gandour (2019) examined whether brainstem and cortical pitch mechanisms shaped by long-term language experience are more resilient to reverberation-induced degradation in pitch representation. They evaluated the concurrently recorded brainstem FFR and the cortical pitch responses (CPRs) from Chinese and English speakers using a Mandarin word exhibiting a high rising pitch (/yi2/) in quiet (dry) and different degrees of reverberation (slight, mild, and moderate). Their results found that both groups showed that both the FFR f0 magnitude and the CPR response amplitude decreased with increasing reverberation, but the responses were larger for the Chinese in all reverberant conditions (Figure 9–20). Comparison of the responses from the two levels revealed a similar magnitude of change with increasing reverberation for both groups. These findings suggest that experience-dependent brainstem and cortical pitch mechanisms provide an enhanced and stable neural representation of pitch-relevant information that is maintained even in the presence of reverberation. Relatively greater degradative effects of reverberation on the brainstem (FFR) compared to CPR suggest relatively stronger top-down influences on CPRs. Similar findings have been reported for the CPR in the presence of noise (Suresh et al., 2017).

Structural Versus Functional Asymmetries in Neural Representation

Hemispheric functional asymmetries in the cerebral cortex are predictable based on low-level,

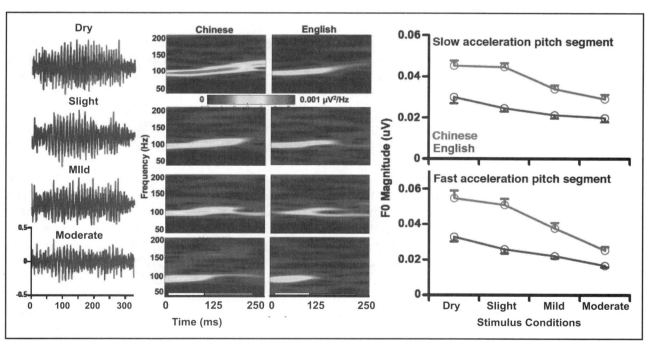

Figure 9–20. Grand average overlaid frequency following response (FFR) waveforms (Chinese, lighter trace; English, darker trace), spectrograms (Chinese, English), mean F0 magnitude for the slow accelerating pitch segment (*top, right*), and mean F0 magnitude for the fast accelerating pitch segment (*bottom, right*) plotted as a function of increasing reverberation. Note that in each panel the responses for the Chinese are more robust in dry and all reverberant conditions, although both groups show a decrease in response magnitude with an increase in reverberation. Adapted from "Tone Language Experience-Dependent Advantage in Pitch Representation in Brainstem and Auditory Cortex Is Maintained Under Reverberation," by A. Krishnan, C. Suresh, and J. T. Gandour, 2019, *Hearing Research*, 177, pp. 63–71. Copyright 2019, with permission from Elsevier.

spectrotemporal features of stimuli, but they can also be modulated by their linguistic function (Meyer, 2008; Poeppel et al., 2008; Wildgruber, Ackermann, Kreifelts, & Ethofer, 2006; Zatorre & Gandour, 2008, reviews). It is also well established that there are structural (anatomical) asymmetries in the nuclei and tracts along the auditory pathway. More recently, language experience has been shown to produce a robust functional right hemispheric preference for pitch processing of certain linguistically relevant temporal attributes of pitch (e.g., Krishnan, Gandour, & Suresh, 2016; Krishnan, Suresh, & Gandour, 2017b, 2019; Suresh, Krishnan & Gandour, 2017) suggesting a language experience–induced selective recruitment of the pitch-processing mechanism in the right auditory cortex. Whether ear asymmetries at the level of the brainstem can be modulated by functional changes in pitch processing is an open question. Using two synthetic speech stimuli (native M2; nonnative flipped variant of M2), the magnitude of the f0 component in the FFR (amplitude of the spectral component at f0) was obtained from a perceptually salient portion of M2 that exhibits rapidly changing pitch (Krishnan, Gandour, Ananthakrishnan, Bidelman, et al., 2011). The native tone (M2) evoked a comparatively larger degree of rightward ear asymmetry in pitch encoding than the nonnative pitch pattern. In response to left-ear and right-ear stimulation, the FFR evoked by M2 was larger than its flipped variant with right ear stimulation only. On an absolute scale, asymmetry favoring left ear stimulation was evoked by the nonnative pitch contour. These differences in ear asymmetry may reflect an emerging functional separation of periodicity and spectral representations at the midbrain level. More recently, Krishnan, Gandour, and Suresh (in press) reported differences in the pattern of ear asymmetries in the brainstem FFRs elicited by a native lexical high rising tone presented to the right or the left ear in Chinese and English listeners. They recorded both brainstem FFR and cortical CPR concurrently. For the FFR response, the English group showed a modest left ear advantage in the response to the slow accelerating segment only (Figure 9–21), while the Chinese group showed no significant ear asymmetry. In contrast, for the "fast accelerating segment, the Chinese show a robust left ear advantage (Figure 9–21; seen both in the spectrograms and the mean f0 plot in panel C), while the English group showed no ear asymmetry. At the cortical level, the hemispheric preference of the CPR response in the English group was in line with the structural dominance of the contralateral pathway. That is, the English group showed a larger response in the hemisphere contralateral to the ear stimulated. However, in the Chinese, left ear stimulation produced a clear right hemisphere dominance, but with right ear stimulation, no hemispheric differences were observed. The experience-dependent effects were limited to the right hemisphere, which is primarily driven by left ear stimulation. The fact that the FFR at the brainstem level also showed a left ear advantage for the Chinese group suggests that experience-dependent recruitment of optimal resources in the right hemisphere for pitch processing is already emerging in the brainstem and likely contributing, at least in part, to the cortical right hemispheric preference for pitch processing in the Chinese.

While the focus of this review is on the influence of long-term language experience on the neural representation of pitch-relevant information in the auditory brainstem, there is growing empirical evidence suggesting it also shapes pitch mechanisms at early sensory levels of processing in the auditory cortex, and that the hemispheric preference for processing pitch information may vary depending on the relative linguistic importance of specific temporal attributes of dynamic pitch (Krishnan, Gandour, Ananthakrishnan, & Vijayaraghavan, 2015; Krishnan & Gandour, 2014; Krishnan, Gandour & Suresh, 2014, 2015a, 2015b, 2016; Krishnan, Suresh, & Gandour, 2017a, 2017b, 2019; Krishnan, Gandour, et al., 2016; Suresh et al., 2017). As in the brainstem, cortical responses sharpen the properties of neural elements to enable the optimal representation of temporal attributes of native pitch contours. However, differences in the pattern of responses at the brainstem and early sensory-level processing in the auditory cortex with manipulation of pitch salience, pitch acceleration, and pitch height have been observed, suggesting differential sensitivity to temporal attributes of pitch and/or a fundamental transformation from the brainstem to the auditory cortex in the neural mechanisms encoding pitch (Krishnan & Gandour, 2014; Krishnan,

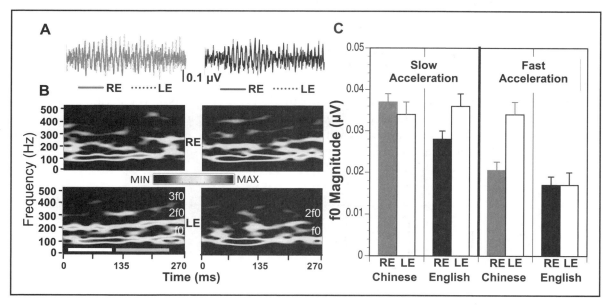

Figure 9–21. Grand average frequency following response (FFR) waveforms for the Chinese (*light trace on the left*) and English (*dark trace*) listeners overlapped for the right ear (*solid*) and left ear (*dotted*) monaural stimulation (**A**), corresponding spectrograms (**B**), and mean f0 magnitude plotted for each ear group, and the slow (*left*) and fast (*right*) pitch accelerating segments (**C**). It is clear from the spectrogram and means f0 data that the Chinese and the English groups show different patterns of ear asymmetry. For the slow accelerating segment, only the English show a modest left ear advantage with the Chinese showing no significant ear asymmetry. In contrast, for the fast accelerating segment, the Chinese show a robust left ear advantage that can also be seen clearly in the spectrogram. Unpublished data from Krishnan et al. (2020).

Gandour, & Suresh, 2015a, 2015b, 2016; Krishnan, Suresh, and Gandour, 2017a, 2017b; Krishnan, Smalt, Bidelman, & Gandour, 2010). Krishnan, Gandour, and Suresh (2016) showed that a direct comparison of cortical and brainstem pitch-related neural activity responses for the Chinese group revealed different patterns of relative changes in magnitude along the pitch salience continuum. (FFR showed a monotonic amplitude growth, while the cortical-pitch response showed a nonmonotonic amplitude growth behavior.) Similarly, Krishnan, Gandour, and Suresh (2015b) demonstrated that the experience-dependent enhancement of cortical-pitch responses was limited to native pitch acceleration rates with no group differences observed at faster rates. An earlier study (Krishnan, Smalt, et al., 2010) using the same stimuli but evaluating the brainstem FFR revealed the persistence of the experience-dependent advantage at all acceleration rates. These differences in the response properties at the brainstem and cortical levels likely reflect a greater selectivity of the neural mechanisms at the cortical level to native contours and/or a transformation in pitch processing at the cortical level presumably mediated by local sensory and/or extrasensory influence overlaid on the brainstem output.

Hierarchical Processing as a Basis of Experience-Dependent Pitch Processing

Empirical evidence suggests that pitch-relevant information is processed in multiple brain regions including the primary auditory cortex as well as nonprimary areas well beyond Heschl's gyrus (HG) anteriorly and posteriorly (Griffiths & Hall, 2012; Griffiths et al., 2010; Patterson et al., 2002; Puschmann, Uppenkamp, Kollmeier, & Thiel, 2010; Zatorre & Belin, 2001). In addition, higher language areas along the posterior-anterior axis of STG and inferior/middle frontal areas are engaged for processing lexical tones (Gandour et al., 2002; Li et al., 2003, 2010; Wang, Jongman, & Sereno, 2003). Thus, the question arises of how these areas interact in a coordinated manner during pitch processing. We propose an empirically driven, physiologically plausible theoretical framework using predictive coding for experience-dependent pitch processing (Kumar & Schönwiesner, 2012; Rao & Ballard, 1999) including cortical and brainstem areas in a well-coordinated, hierarchical, distributed processing network (Figure 9–22). Operationally, higher-level areas in the pitch hierarchy (lateral Heschl's gyrus [HG]; planum temporale [PT], anterior superior temporal gyrus [STGa], posterior superior temporal gyrus [STGp], and inferior frontal gyrus [IFG]) use stored pitch representations to make a pitch prediction. Top-down connections pass this prediction to lower levels in the processing hierarchy (medial/middle HG, IC, MGB). The prediction error is then passed to a higher level via bottom-up

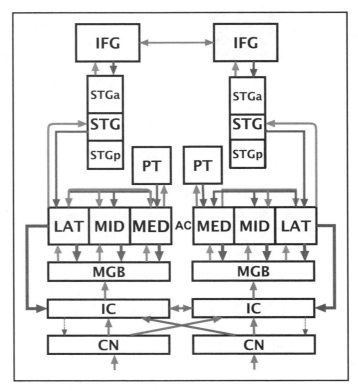

Figure 9–22. Block diagram of the proposed theoretical framework for hierarchical processing of pitch at both subcortical and cortical levels. Operationally, higher-level areas in the hierarchy contributing to pitch (lateral AC) use *stored representations* of pitch to make a pitch prediction. This prediction is passed to the lower areas in the processing hierarchy (medial and middle AC) via the *top-down connection(s)* (*darker downward arrows*). The lower areas then compute a prediction error (the difference between the higher-level prediction and the lower-level representation), which is passed to the higher level via *bottom-up connections* (*light upward arrows*). The *lateral connections* (same level in the hierarchy) between middle and medial AC (*bidirectional arrows*) are also subject to modulation and presumably play a role in reducing redundancy and making representations more efficient. Inputs from subcortical (*bottom-up*) structures (IC and MGB) that are themselves subject to experience-dependent plasticity are presumably mediated by *top-down* connections (AC to MGB; and AC to IC). These top-down connections in the hierarchy likely provide feedback to adjust the effective time scales of processing at each stage to optimally control the temporal dynamics of pitch processing. Language-dependent changes at the early sensory level of processing in the auditory cortex may reflect the interplay between sensory and cognitive processing in language-related areas beyond the auditory cortex (STG, superior temporal gyrus; IFG, inferior frontal gyrus). CN: cochlear nucleus; IC, inferior colliculus; AC, auditory cortex (MED, medial; MID, middle; and LAT, lateral); MGB, medial geniculate body; PT, planum temporale; STG, superior temporal gyrus (STGp, STG posterior; STGa, STG anterior).

connections. Also relevant are connections across hemispheres at cortical (IFG) and subcortical (CN, IC) levels. The strength of these connections is continually adjusted recursively in order to minimize predictive error and to optimize representation at a higher level. Inputs from subcortical, bottom-up structures are themselves subject to experience-dependent plasticity mediated by top-down connections (corticothalamic and corticocollicular). These top-down connections in the hierarchy provide feedback to adjust the effective time scales of processing to optimally control the temporal dynamics of pitch processing (Balaguer-Ballester, Clark, Coath, Krumbholz, & Denham, 2009). Our previous results and current preliminary results are consistent with the hierarchical and distributed nature of cortical and subcortical regions contributing to pitch processing as well as the experience-dependent effects predicted by our hierarchical pitch-processing network. We hypothesize that language-dependent changes at early sensory levels of pitch processing in the auditory cortex may reflect the interplay between sensory and higher-level cognitive processes beyond the auditory cortex (PT, STGa, STGp, and IFG).

Dynamic causal modeling essentially tries to determine how the activity of one brain area changes the dynamics and/or responses of other areas. Using Bayesian model comparisons to determine the configuration(s) that best explain the data, they showed that the lateral part of HG is at a higher level of hierarchy compared to middle and medial HG, with the latter two at the same level. This is in agreement with evidence from depth-electrode recording along the stretch of the HG. It confirms that middle and medial electrode contacts are in the primary auditory cortex, whereas the lateral contacts are in the nonprimary auditory cortex (Brugge et al., 2009). Consistent with the predictions of the model, they also show that strength of connectivity varies with pitch salience such that the strength of the top-down connection from lateral HG to medial and middle HG increases with pitch salience, whereas the strength of the bottom-up connection from middle HG to lateral HG decreases. This distributed view of pitch processing, however, is not necessarily at odds with a single specialized pitch center. It is likely that lateral HG has more pitch-specific mechanisms and therefore plays a relatively greater role in pitch perception.

In this case, the predictive coding of the pitch model provides a framework to explain the language-dependent (cognitive) and language-universal (sensory) effects on pitch-related neural activity in the brainstem and auditory cortex. Changes at different stages of processing attributable wholly to acoustic properties of the stimulus implicate the recursive process (initial pitch prediction, error generation, error correction) in the representation of pitch. At this fundamental level of pitch processing, the hierarchical flow of processing, and the connectivity strengths along the HG are essentially the same regardless of one's language background. For changes that are dependent on language experience, the initial pitch prediction at the level of the lateral HG is more precise for Chinese because of their access to stored information about lexical tones with a smaller error term. Consequently, the top-down connections from lateral HG to medial and middle HG and the brainstem are stronger than the bottom-up connections from the medial and middle HG to the lateral HG and the brainstem. The opposite would be true for English because of their less precise initial prediction. In addition, the recursive process would be expected to take a longer time for English relative to Chinese in determining pitch. Language experience, therefore, alters the nature of the interaction between levels along the hierarchy of pitch processing by modulating connection strengths.

It is clear that pitch processing in the auditory cortex is influenced by inputs from subcortical structures that are themselves subject to experience-dependent plasticity, presumably mediated by top-down connections. These top-down connections in the hierarchy likely provide feedback to adjust the effective time scales of processing at each stage to optimally control the temporal dynamics of pitch processing (Balaguer-Ballester et al., 2009). Language-dependent changes at the early sensory level of processing in the auditory cortex may reflect the interplay between sensory and cognitive processing. This model represents a unified, physiologically plausible, theoretical framework that includes both cortical and subcortical components in the hierarchical processing of pitch.

IV. FFR CORRELATES OF BINAURAL PROCESSING

It is well established that the auditory system makes use of interaural differences in time (ITD) and intensity (IID) at each ear to localize low- and high-frequency sounds, respectively. These cues are also utilized to improve signal detection in noise, like in improvement of signal threshold when the interaural phase of dichotically presented signal and noise are varied, producing the well-established phenomenon of binaural masking level difference (BMLD). A related phenomenon is the improvement in detectability of a signal when the noise location is changed from spatially converging to spatially separated from the tone using the interaural cues, termed listening in spatialized noise. Physiological studies aimed at determining the neural bases of these binaural phenomena have implicated binaural neurons (sensitive to ITD and IID) in the brainstem that exhibit coincidence detection. Evidence of binaural interaction mediating sound localization has also been presented in the surface-recorded ABR.

FFR Correlates of Binaural Interaction

A binaural interaction component (BIC) can be derived from the ABR by subtracting the potential evoked by binaural stimulation from the summed responses to monaural stimulation, and it is thought to reflect the binaural processing of neural outputs from both ears converging on the binaural neurons in the brainstem (Dobie & Berlin, 1979; Furst, Levine, & McGaffigan, 1985; McPherson & Starr, 1995). The systematic change in the BIC component resulting from parametric manipulation of both interaural cues (ITD and IID) has been interpreted to suggest that this component may be indexing the binaural processing of cues relevant to certain binaural phenomena. Furst, Levine, and McGaffin (1985) demonstrated that ABR-BIC was present only when binaural stimuli were perceived as a fused image and that the BIC latency exhibited a positive correlation with the location of the fused image suggests this component may reflect neural processes mediating sound fusion and lateralization.

There are a few published reports that have attempted to evaluate if the FFR-BIC reflects binaural processing underlying lateralization and improved signal detection in noise. Clark, Moushegian, and Rupert (1997) reported that the FFR amplitude to a binaurally presented 450-Hz tone burst was greater for an ITD value of 0 ms than for an ITD equal to 0.66 ms. Extending this work, Ballachanda and Moushegian (2000) confirmed these initial findings and also showed that FFR amplitude decreased when ITD and IID were increased in concert and was relatively unaltered when the cues were in opposition. However, the FFR-BIC was unaltered by changes in either the IID or ITD. These authors interpret these findings to suggest that the scalp-recorded FFR likely reflects brainstem binaural processes relevant to lateralization. Krishnan and McDaniel (l998) demonstrated that the 500-Hz FFR-BIC decreased in amplitude progressively as the IID was increased (Figure 9–23, left, middle, and right panels), with no clear component present for IIDs greater than 20 dB.

These results taken together suggest that the binaural neurons in the brainstem can use IID cues presented in both low-frequency (FFR) and high-frequency (click) sounds. Thus, the FFR to binaural stimulation reflects the output of nonlinear interactive active processes within the brainstem and does not simply reflect a passive linear sum of neural activity from two independent generators (Gerken, Moushegian, Stillman, & Rupert, 1975). The neural basis for this interaction component is explained using binaural interaction models that assume that monaural inputs are initially processed in each cochlea before the outputs from the cochlea converge on a central binaural processor (Colburn & Latimer, 1978). The processor acts either as a correlation device or a coincidence detector. It is likely that binaural neurons in the medial superior olive and the IC contribute to the BIC described in this section (Caird, Sontheimer, & Klinke, 1985; Sontheimer, Caird, & Klinke, 1985).

FFR Correlates of Binaural Masking Level Difference (BMLD)

BMLD is a binaural phenomenon that is characterized by an improvement in signal threshold in dich-

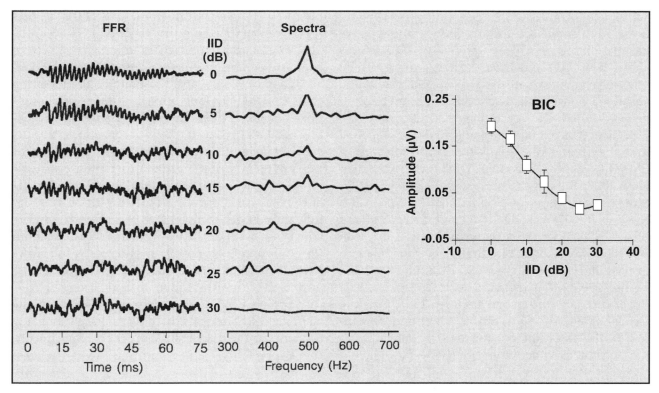

Figure 9–23. Frequency following response (FFR)–binaural interaction component (BIC) waveforms (*left*), BIC-spectra (*middle*), and mean BIC amplitude (*right*) are plotted as a function of interaural level difference (ILD). Both the spectral data and the mean amplitude data show a progressive decrease in the BIC amplitude as ILD is increased. Note that no discernible response component is present for IIDs greater than about 20 dB. Adapted with permission from "Binaural Interaction in the Human Frequency-Following Response: Effects of Interaural Intensity Difference," by A. Krishnan and S. McDaniel, 1998, *Audiology and Neuro-otology, 3*, 291–299. Copyright 1998, Karger Publishers, Basel, Switzerland.

otic antiphasic masked conditions where either the signal is out of phase at the ears with the maskers in phase difference (SπNo) or the reverse (SoNπ), relative to the signal threshold obtained in a homophasic diotic masked condition (SoNo). Psychoacoustic studies have shown that maximum BMLD occurs when using low-frequency pure tones below 2000 Hz with an interaural phase difference (IPD) of 180° (Egan, 1965; Hirsch, 1948; Jeffress, Blodgett, & Deatherage, 1952; Robinson & Jeffress, 1963). At 500 Hz, the BMLD with an inverted signal starting phase (SπNo) is 12 to 15 dB and is greater than the 9 to 12 dB BMLD with an inverted masked (SoNπ). This perceptual release from masking reflected in BMLD presumably reflects brainstem binaural processing in the medial superior olivary (MSO) neurons (Jenkins & Masterton, 1982). Many units in this nucleus have low characteristic frequencies and receive bilateral excitatory inputs. Single-unit responses show many ITD (interaural time difference) sensitive units in which the maximum discharge rate occurs with a specific interaural delay, the characteristic delay (Brand, Behrend, Marquardt, McAlpine, & Grothe, 2002; Crow, Rupert, & Moushegian, 1978; Fitzpatrick, Batra, Stanford, & Kuwada, 1997; Goldberg & Brown, 1968). Threshold disparity is partially related to these coincidence-detecting units in the medial superior olive that are sensitive to low-frequency binaural stimuli with interaural phase differences.

A couple of electrophysiologic studies using low-frequency tones in a BMLD paradigm have reported changes in amplitude and latency changes consistent with BMLD for the cortical potentials (P1, N1, P2) but not for the ABR (Kevanishvili & Lagidze, 1987; Tanis & Teas, 1974). The absence of BMLD in the low-frequency elicited ABR was interpreted to suggest that the synchronized neural activity to stimulus onset generating the ABR to these high-intensity, low-frequency tones were basally biased (cochlear activity at frequencies above 2000 Hz) and thus do not show a robust release from masking. It is more likely that the sustained phase-locked activity, in a population of neurons tuned to lower frequencies, reflected in the FFR elicited by a moderate-intensity, low-frequency tone may better preserve information relevant to BMLD (Ananthanarayan & Durrant, 1992; Krishnan, 2007; Suresh, Krishnan, & Gandour, 2017; Moushegian, Rupert, & Stillman, 1973). Wilson and Krishnan (2005) reasoned that since the FFR reflects phase-locked neural activity in brainstem nuclei and tracts involved in binaural processing relevant to BMLD (Ehret & Merzenich, 1988; Lavine, 1971; Møller, 2000; Moushegian, Rupert, & Gidda, 1975; Rose, Brugge, Anderson, & Hind, 1967; Sinex & Geisler, 1981; Young & Sachs, 1979) and perceptual BMLD is prominent for low-frequency tones, the phase-locked activity underlying FFR elicited by a low-frequency tone burst (500 Hz) may preserve information relevant to BMLD. That is, the FFR might be a more effective analytical tool to examine binaural processes underlying BMLD. To this end, Wilson and Krishnan (2005) recorded FFRs to a 500-Hz tone burst in unmasked, homophasic masked diotic (SoNo) and antiphasic dichotic masked (SπNo, and SoNπ) conditions. Results showed a significant FFR amplitude reduction for the SoNo condition, with masker intensities near the psychoacoustic SoNo masking level. For the antiphasic conditions the FFR amplitude was significantly larger compared to the SoNo condition, consistent with a release from masking, for both the SoNπ and SπNo conditions (Figure 9–24). However, using a tone in noise and a threshold detection approach, Clinard, Hodgson, and Scherer (2017) did not observe a release from masking in the 500-Hz FFR. Differences in methodology may likely account for the discrepancy in results. Specifically, the appreciably higher stimulus level (increas-

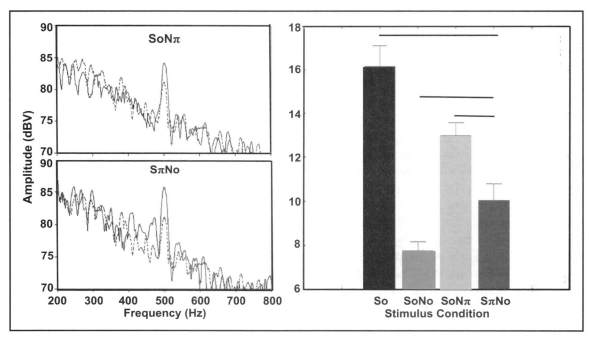

Figure 9–24. Frequency following response (FFR) spectra (*left*) for the binaural masking level difference (BMLD) antiphasic conditions showing enhancement of the 500-Hz FFR relative to the homophasic condition. Mean FFR spectral amplitude is plotted for the binaural tone alone condition (So), for the homophasic condition (SoNo), and the two antiphasic conditions (*right*). Note the improvement in response amplitude for the antiphasic conditions consistent with BMLD. From "Human Frequency Following Response to Stimuli Producing Masking Level Difference," by J. Wilson and A. Krishnan, 2005, *Journal of the American Academy of Audiology, 16*, pp. 184–195. Copyright 2005, Georg Thieme Verlag KG.

ing the possibility of contamination by cross-talk, acoustic reflexes, and increasing the possibility of a broader cochlear region contributing to the FFR) used by Clinard et al. (2017) may, at least in part, account for the differences in the results observed compared to Wilson and Krishnan (2005).

The demonstration of FFR amplitude recovery in antiphasic dichotic masking conditions suggests that the phase-locked neural activity reflected in the FFR may indeed preserve the temporal pattern of neural activity relevant to BMLD. Similar BMLD has been observed in binaural neurons in the medial superior olive (Langford, 1984) and the IC (Caird, Palmer, & Rees, 1991; Jiang, McAlpine, & Palmer, 1997; McAlpine, Jiang, & Palmer, 1996; Palmer, Jiang, & McAlpine, 1999, 2000). The results of these physiologic studies are consistent with cross-correlation models of BMLD that involve coincidence detectors (Colburn, 1977; Jiang et al., 1997; Jeffress, 1948). For the SπNo condition, the No noise generates a peak of activation in neurons with best delays close to zero ITD, and the addition of So tone at masked threshold produces only a small increase in the amplitude of this peak. In contrast, at the same SNR, the introduction of the Sπ signal produces a larger decrease in the peak amplitude. Since increases and decreases in discharge are equally detectable to achieve the same detectability, the Sπ signal can be reduced in level, giving a substantial BMLD. Also, the reduction in activity caused by the Sπ signal is believed to disrupt or desynchronize the response to the No noise (Palmer et al., 1999), thereby making it a less effective masker. Now for the SoNπ condition, Nπ noise is an ineffective masker because it produces a minimum or trough in activation centered on zero ITD. The addition of the So signal at zero ITD raises the discharge rate of neurons with the best delays near-zero ITD. This represents a desynchronization effect of the noise in the SoNπ condition. The net effect is an increase in the number of coincident spikes delivered to the coincidence detector. That is, the So signal produces a larger change to the Nπ noise response than to the No noise response. However, this change in neural activity level for the SoNπ condition is still smaller than that observed for the SπNo condition. The result is a smaller BMLD for NπSo than for the NoSπ condition (Palmer et al., 2000).

FFR Correlates of Spatial Release From Masking

Another related binaural phenomenon is the spatial release from masking. Auditory stream segregation is the process by which a listener can differentiate the various auditory signals that arrive simultaneously at the ears to form a meaningful representation of the incoming acoustic signals (Sussman, Ritter, & Vaughan, 1999). Auditory cues, such as the perceived spatial location of sounds or the pitch of speakers' voices, help this process of segregating the total stream of sound (Bregman, 1990). Spatial release from masking (the improvement in the detection or reception threshold of a signal when spatially separated from competing sounds relative to when the target is colocated with the competing sounds) may, in part, account for this spatial auditory stream segregation. Based on the results of the Listening in Spatialized Noise (LiSN) test in children with central auditory processing disorders (CAPDs) that revealed auditory streaming deficits in these children, Cameron and Dillon (2008) suggested that the LiSN test was sensitive enough to differentiate not only an auditory versus language disorder but also a spatial versus vocal streaming segregation disorder. They observed that spatial release from masking was reduced in these kids, suggesting that they may have difficulty using the binaural cues to improve detection of a target present with a competing sound even when the target and the competing sound were spatially separated. Krishnan et al (2012), reasoned that binaural processes, similar to the ones mediating BMLD, may be at play to account for spatial release from masking. Further, since the scalp-recorded FFR reflects activity from a population of brainstem neurons that include binaural neurons involved in binaural processing, it may preserve information relevant to spatial release from masking. They recorded FFRs from normal-hearing individuals to a target (vowel /i/) in quiet and in conditions masked by colocated speech babble (0 degrees) and spatially separated speech babble (±90 degrees). For the masked conditions, SNR was set at +10 dB. They also obtained FFRs for the binaural ±90 condition (separated), and monaural presentation of the same stimuli to either the left or the right ear to evaluate binaural interaction. Results showed that the mean spectral magnitude at f0 was significantly greater for the BIN separated condition compared to the spatially colocated target + noise condition. That is, f0 magnitude for the BIN separated condition showed a significant release from masking even though the objective SNR at each ear is relatively poorer in the separated condition (Figure 9–25). When the sum of the monaural responses was compared with the binaural responses for both the colocated and separated conditions, only the separated condition showed significantly larger amplitude for the binaural response compared to the sum of the monaural responses (Figure 9–26). Taken together, these results suggest that binaural processing relevant to spatial release from masking (as opposed to a simple linear sum of monaural responses) may be reflected in the phase-locked neural activity in the brainstem. That brainstem binaural unmasking processes, as described earlier for the BMLD, mediate this release is also suggested by the objectively poorer SNR in the separated compared to the colocated condition. FFR in this spatial paradigm shows promise as an objective analytic tool to evaluate spatial processing in children with CAPD and peripheral hearing loss.

Neural Representation of Vocoded Speech Sounds

The commonly employed speech processing strategies in cochlear implants (CIs) using only amplitude modulation (AM) in a limited number of frequency channels (Wilson et al., 1991) works well in quiet conditions, but performance in noise is severely degraded (e.g., Wilson & Dorman, 2008). Zeng et al. (2005), using a novel speech processing strategy that encodes both frequency and amplitude modulation (AM + FM), reported significantly better speech, speaker, and tone recognition, particularly in noise, compared to the AM-alone strategy. Suresh, Krishnan, and Luo (2020) extracted EFR and FFR to examine the differences in the neural representation of a sine vocoded speech sound

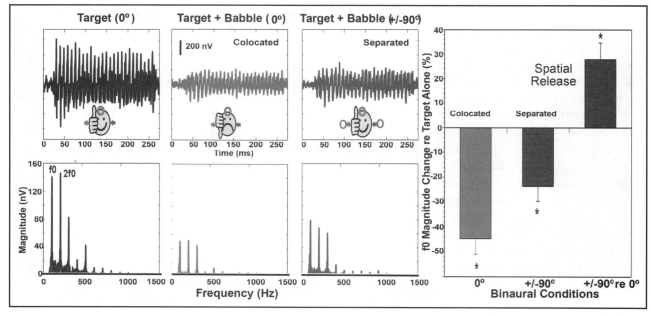

Figure 9–25. Grand averaged frequency following responses (FFRs) (*top*) and spectra (*bottom*) for the Target alone (black), colocated Target + Babble (*light gray*), and separated Target + Babble conditions (*dark gray*). The target was a 250-ms-long steady-state English back vowel /u/, and the noise was a four-talker babble with a different speaker in each ear. Target was presented at +10 dB SNR. Both the FFR waveform amplitude and its spectra for the separated condition show a relatively larger amplitude compared to the collocated conditions. However, both show a much smaller amplitude compared to when the target is presented alone. The mean f0 magnitude change shown in the right panel confirms this observation. From Krishnan, Van Dun, et al. (2012).

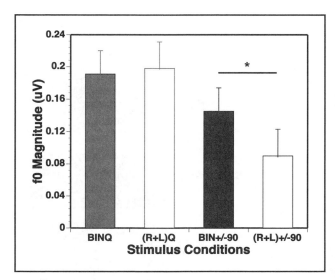

Figure 9–26. Mean f0 magnitude plotted for the binaural quiet (BINQ), the sum of monaural responses in quiet (R + L)$_Q$, binaural separated condition (BIN ±90), and the sum of monaural responses for the separated condition (R + L)$_{±90}$. While the f0 magnitude for the BINQ and (R + L)$_Q$ are not significantly different, the f0 magnitude in the binaural separated condition is significantly larger than its equivalent summed monaural condition, suggesting improvement of signal capture, presumably due to binaural processing underlying spatial separation of the target and the noise.

(diphthong /au/, see Figure 9–27) with AM alone and AM + FM as the number of spectral bands were varied (2, 4, 8, and 16 channels) to determine if neural representation improved in the AM + FM condition. Their results showed that the periodicity strength for the EFR decreased more for the AM stimulus compared to the AM + FM stimulus as the number of channels was increased (Figure 9–28A and C). Also, independent of the number of channels, spectral peak always corresponded to the f0 only for the AM + FM stimulus (Figure 9–28D). Similarly, FFR (representing TFS) showed a better neural representation of the stimulus spectrum for the AM + FM condition (Figure 9–29C). Furthermore, the neural representation of the time-varying formant-related harmonics, as revealed by spectral correlation, was also better for the AM + FM stimulus (Figure 9-30C) compared to the AM only stimulus (Figure 9-30C). In general, the FFR spectral components for the AM + FM stimuli corresponded well with those of the unprocessed stimulus and the FFR (Figure 9-30A). In contrast, the FFR spectral components for the AM stimulus were more aligned with the center and sideband frequencies of individual channels and not with the spectral components of the unprocessed stimulus. Consequently, there was a better neural representation of the original formant-related harmonics for AM + FM than for AM across all channel numbers. The decreased spectral correlation between FFR for the unprocessed and AM stimuli with the increasing number of channels clearly suggests that the spectral components in the FFR to AM stimuli reflect phase-locking to the different channel center frequencies and prominent sidebands rather than formant-related harmonics. Results of the segmental spectral analysis of FFR to the AM (Figure 9-30B), and the AM + FM (Figure 9–30C) stimulus confirmed that spectral correlation increased only for the segments representing steady-state vowels /a/ and /u/ but not for the time-varying segment representing the /au/ segment for the AM stimulus (Figure 9–30B). The results for the AM stimulus in this study are mostly consistent with the observations of Ananthakrishnan, Luo, and Krishnan (2017), who examined the neural representation of a vocoded steady-state vowel /u/ using only AM. They also showed improvement in the neural representation of periodicity and TFS encoding with the increase in the number of channels but that the TFS encoding, like in this study, represented phase-locking to the center frequencies and the sidebands generated around the center frequencies of the vocoder channel. Collectively, these results suggest that the significantly better neural representation of envelope periodicity, TFS, and time-varying spectrotemporal features for the AM + FM strategy likely account for the superior performance on speech, speaker, and tone recognition observed by Zeng et al. (2005).

While these results are promising, an extension of these results to the CI is not straightforward given the differences in auditory and electrical stimulation of the auditory system. While cochlear processes in the normal ear introduce temporal inaccuracies in TFS transmission to the brain (Middlebrooks & Snyder, 2010), electrical stimulation bypassing the cochlea does not. However, CI users show poorer sensitivity to TFS compared to normal-hearing individuals even though electrically driven auditory nerve fibers can phase-lock

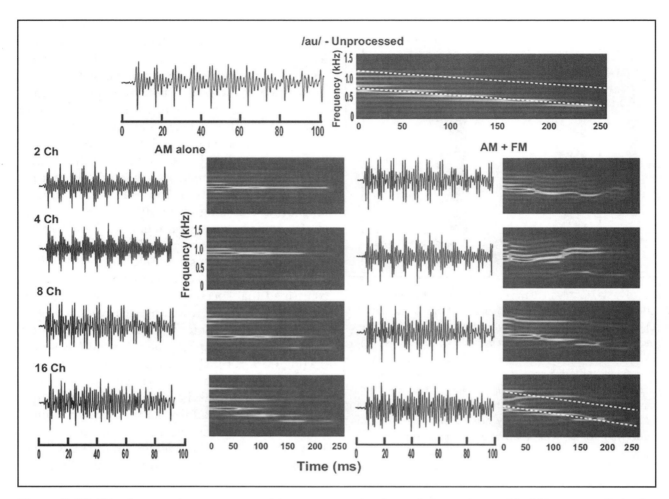

Figure 9–27. Waveforms and spectrograms of the unprocessed and vocoded speech sound /au/. Unprocessed stimulus waveform (*top*) shows robust periodicity, and spectrogram shows clear formant transitions. The white dotted line overlaid on F1 and F2 follows the changes in formant frequency over the duration of the stimulus. Both the AM + FM (*right*) and AM (*left*) waveforms show a decrease in periodicity with the increasing number of channels from 2 to 16 with the degradation more pronounced for the AM stimuli at 8 and 16 channels. Overall, spectrograms show a better representation of the formant transitions for AM + FM compared to AM across all channel numbers except 16 channels. Reprinted with permission from "Human Frequency Following Responses to Vocoded Speech: Amplitude Modulation Versus Amplitude Plus Frequency Modulation," by C. H. Suresh, A. Krishnan, and X. Luo, 2020, *Ear and Hearing*, *41*(2), pp. 300–311.

to higher frequencies compared to acoustic stimulation (Hartmann & Klinke, 1990; Javel, 1990). Nevertheless, electrical stimulation using the AM + FM processing strategy shows promise since auditory nerve and brainstem neurons could extract and encode the FM presented in AM + FM stimuli to improve performance, particularly in adverse listening conditions. The use of TFS information to modulate frequency may also improve encoding of pitch-relevant information, which is not possible with the current AM alone strategy utilized in CIs. Other confounding factors like the hearing experience before implantation, anatomical changes consequent to auditory deprivation, neural survival, and electrode placement may affect the optimal use of AM and FM cues in CI users.

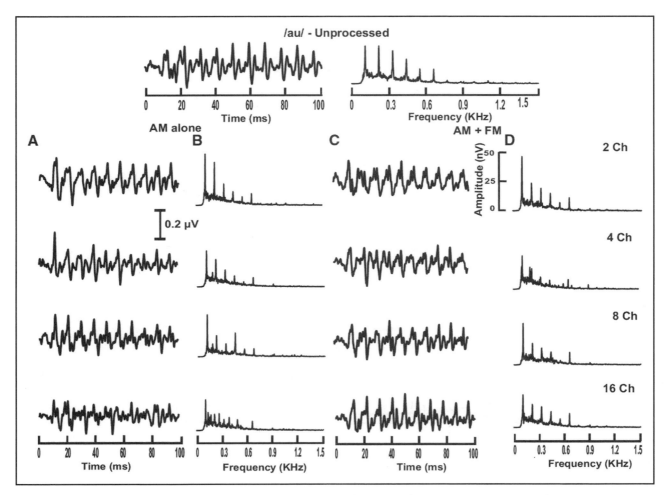

Figure 9–28. Grand average envelope following response (EFR) waveforms and their spectra for the unprocessed stimulus (*top*), the processed 2-, 4-, 8-, and 16-channel AM stimuli (**A** and **B**, respectively), and the processed 2-, 4-, 8-, and 16-channel AM + FM stimuli (**C** and **D**, respectively). AM, amplitude modulation; FFR, frequency following response; FFRENV, envelope periodicity; FM, frequency modulation. In general, the AM + FM stimuli elicit EFRs with more robust periodicity compared to the responses elicited by the AM alone stimuli. Reprinted with permission from "Human Frequency Following Responses to Vocoded Speech: Amplitude Modulation Versus Amplitude Plus Frequency Modulation," by C. H. Suresh, A. Krishnan, and X. Luo, 2020, *Ear and Hearing, 41*(2), pp. 300–311.

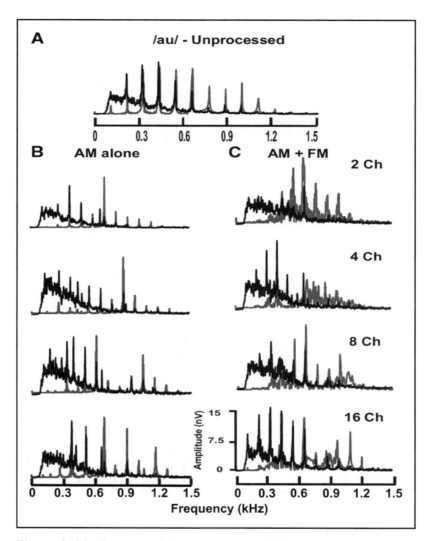

Figure 9–29. Frequency following response (FFR) spectra for the unprocessed (**A**), the processed (2-, 4-, 8-, and 16-channel) AM (**B**) and AM + FM stimuli (**C**). Stimulus spectra (*gray*) are superimposed on the FFR spectra (*black*) for better comparison. For the AM stimuli, the largest spectral component corresponds to the channel center frequencies. The spectral components in the FFRs generated by the AM + FM stimuli are more robust and well correlated with stimulus spectral peaks for 2-, 8-, and 16-channel stimulus conditions. AM, amplitude modulation; FFRTFS, temporal fine structure; FM, frequency modulation. Reprinted with permission from "Human Frequency Following Responses to Vocoded Speech: Amplitude Modulation Versus Amplitude Plus Frequency Modulation," by C. H. Suresh, A. Krishnan, and X. Luo, 2020, *Ear and Hearing, 41*(2), pp. 300–311.

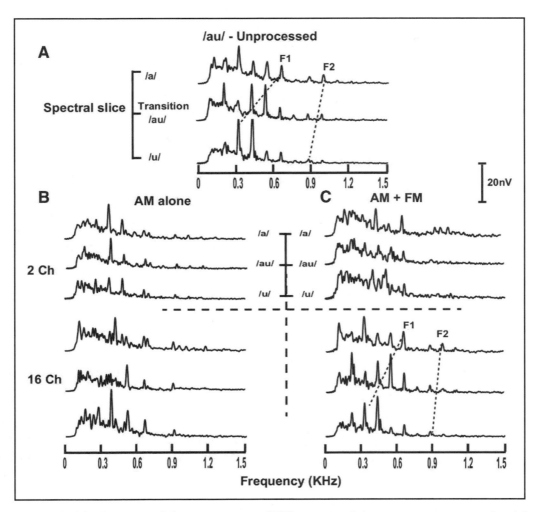

Figure 9–30. Frequency following response (FFR) spectra of time segments representing /a/ (*top*), /au/ (*middle*), and /u/ (*bottom*) for the unprocessed stimulus (**A**), AM (2 and 16 channels; **B**), and AM + FM stimuli (2 and 16 channels; **C**). For the unprocessed stimulus, F1- and F2-related spectral peaks shift downward in frequency (indicated by the diagonal dashed line) over the three time segments representing a transition from /a/ to /au/ then to /u/. A similar pattern is observed for FFR to the 16-channel AM + FM stimulus but not for the 2-channel condition. In contrast, the EFR to the AM stimuli did not show a downward shift of the formant-related peaks across the transition from /a/ to /u/ for both the 2- and 16-channel conditions. Note that the vertical scale marker applies to all panels. AM, amplitude modulation; AM, amplitude modulation; FFR, frequency following response; FFRTFS, temporal fine structure; FM, frequency modulation. Reprinted with permission from "Human Frequency Following Responses to Vocoded Speech: Amplitude Modulation Versus Amplitude Plus Frequency Modulation," by C. H. Suresh, A. Krishnan, and X. Luo, 2020, *Ear and Hearing, 41*(2), pp. 300–311.

EFR/FFR Applications in Different Populations—Potential for Development of Clinical Measures

While not covered here, it should be noted that there has been a rather prolific growth in the use of EFR/FFR to examine neural encoding deficits of speech (most of these studies focusing on the nature of speech f0 representation) in a variety of populations, including individuals with language-based learning problems, auditory processing disorders, speech understanding in noise, mild cognitive impairment in the elderly, bilingualism, traumatic brain injury, reading disability, autism, and aging-related changes. Examples of findings from these studies include the following: there are reports of delayed timing of the V/A complex of speech EFR masked by noise in children with diagnosed reading disability (Banai et al., 2009; Cunningham et al., 2001) and auditory processing disorders (Rocha-Muniz, Befi-Lopes, & Schochat, 2012, 2014; White-Schwoch et al., 2015); variability in speech understanding in noise is reflected in changes in f0 amplitude to speech stimuli (Anderson, Parbery-Clark, Yi, & Kraus, 2011; Anderson, Skoe, Chandrasekaran, Zecker, & Kraus, 2010; Coffey, Chepesiuk, Herholz, Baillet, & Zatorre, 2017; Song et al., 2011); bilinguals show stronger neural representation of speech f0 (Krizman, Marian, Shook, Skoe, & Kraus, 2012); positive correlation is found between strength of f0 phase-locking to speech sound of a foreign language and the ability to learn that language (Omote, Jasmin, & Tierney, 2017); increased f0 amplitude has been observed in older adults with mild cognitive impairment suggesting operation of a compensatory sensory processing mechanism to mitigate cognitive processing deficits (Bidelman, Lowther, Tak, & Alain, 2017); and reduced amplitude of f0 representation was found in children with brain trauma resulting from sports-related concussions (Kraus et al., 2017). Thus, it is clear from these results that the FFR elicited by complex sounds provides a potentially promising physiologic window to evaluate temporal auditory processing in normal and impaired auditory systems. More imaginative quantitative studies using a parametric approach are needed to explore the relationship between the neural representation of stimulus features (keeping in mind that the representation is limited to low frequencies) and measures of perception. It may be a daunting task given that the neural representation of limited acoustic features in the midbrain is not isomorphic with the complex cortical networks mediating perception. Rather than a thundering herd approach, a more cautious approach that clearly understands the strengths and limitations of the FFR is needed to effectively translate several of these research ideas into effective clinical measures of auditory processing. Several published EFR/FFR studies in different populations claim that small changes in just the periodicity strength (reflected in f0 from EFR measures) and/or latency of the onset component as "biological markers" of deficits in auditory processing and/or language learning. Caution should also be exercised in the overinterpretation and generalization of FFR indices.

V. SUMMARY

- From the evidence presented here, it is clear that the temporal pattern of phase-locked activity in the brainstem, as reflected in the scalp-recorded human FFR, preserves information relevant to pitch of complex sounds (including speech and nonspeech sounds) and binaural processes relevant to BMLD and spatial release from masking. For stimuli that elicit either a shift in the pitch percept or ambiguous pitch, the phase-locked activity to the TFS rather than just the envelope appears to be critical. The pitch-relevant neural activity reflected in the FFR also correlates well with perceptual measures, suggesting the emergence of neural representations in the brainstem that may contribute to the development of percept downstream.

- Pitch-relevant information in the FFR shows a robust tonal language experience-dependent enhancement. By focusing on specific properties of the auditory signal, irrespective of a speech or nonspeech context, it is argued that the neural representation of acoustic–phonetic features relevant to speech perception is already emerging in the brainstem and, importantly, can be shaped by experience. These sensory-level auditory processes are tuned differentially to such features depending on their linguistic relevance. The focus on pitch processing in tonal languages notwithstanding, these findings should be contextualized within the broader framework of language experience shaping subcortical processing.

- Experience-dependent shaped pitch processing is more resilient to the distinct degradative effects of noise and reverberation.

- While it is not known how language experience shapes subcortical and cortical stages of pitch processing, it appears that long-term language experience shapes adaptive, hierarchical pitch processing. Top-down connections provide selective gating of inputs to both cortical and subcortical structures to enhance the neural representation of behaviorally relevant attributes of the stimulus and instantiate local mechanisms that exhibit an enhanced representation of behaviorally relevant pitch attributes.

- With respect to speech perception, each pitch feature is defined by an auditory pattern that triggers its detection (Poeppel et al., 2008, p. 1082, review). Their precise definition, however, varies depending on the level of brain structure, time window, and functional representation in speech perception.

- Concurrent recordings of the brainstem and cortical pitch-relevant responses may provide a new window to evaluate the online interplay between feedforward and feedback components in the processing of complex sounds at the level of the brainstem and the auditory cortex. What is needed are more studies that parametrically manipulate behaviorally relevant stimulus attributes or features in order to gain insights on the functional organization of the hierarchical processing network and the relative contributions of the brainstem and cortical components. The results of these experiments are essential to further our understanding of both the nature of the interplay between levels of processing and interactions between sensory and cognitive processes influencing pitch representation and how experience or training can shape these processes. Complementary functional imaging studies are crucial to accurately identify the component anatomical sources and the functional connections between the components along the hierarchical stages.

REFERENCES

Abrams, D. A., Nicol, T., Zecker, S. G., & Kraus, N. (2006). Auditory brainstem timing predicts cerebral asymmetry for speech. *Journal of Neuroscience*, 26(43), 11131–11137.

Akhoun, I., Gallégo, S., Moulin, A., Ménard, M., Veuillet, E., Berger-Vachon, C., . . . Thai-Van, H. (2008). The temporal relationship between speech auditory brainstem responses and the acoustic pattern of the phoneme /ba/ in normal-hearing adults. *Clinical Neurophysiology*, 119, 922–933.

Ananthakrishnan, S., & Krishnan, A. (2018). Human frequency following responses to iterated rippled noise with positive and negative gain: Differential sensitivity to waveform envelope and temporal fine structure. *Hearing Research*, 367, 113–123.

Ananthakrishnan, S., Luo, X., & Krishnan, A. (2017). Human frequency following responses to vocoded speech. *Ear and Hearing*, 38, e256–e267.

Ananthanarayan, A. K., & Durrant, J. D. (1992). The frequency-following response and the onset response: Evaluation of frequency specificity using a forward masking paradigm. *Ear and Hearing*, 13, 228–232.

Anderson, S., Parbery-Clark, A., Yi, H. G., & Kraus, N. (2011). A neural basis of speech-in-noise perception in older adults. *Ear and Hearing*, 32(6), 750–757.

Anderson, S., Skoe, E., Chandrasekaran, B., Zecker, S., & Kraus, N. (2010). Brainstem correlates of speech-in-noise perception in children. *Hearing Research*, 270(1–2), 151–157.

Assmann, P. F., & Summerfield, Q. (1990). Modeling the perception of concurrent vowels: Vowels with different fundamental frequencies. *Journal of the Acoustical Society of America*, 88(2), 680–697.

Balaguer-Ballester, E., Clark, N. R., Coath, M., Krumbholz, K., & Denham, S. L. (2009). Understanding pitch perception as a hierarchical process with top-down modulation. *PLOS Computational Biology*, 5(3), e1000301. https://doi.org/10.1371/journal.pcbi.1000301

Ballachanda, B. B., & Moushegian, G. (2000). Frequency following response: Effects of interaural time and differences. *Journal of the American Academy of Audiology, 11*, 1–11

Banai, K., Abrams, D., & Kraus, N. (2007). Sensory-based learning disability: Insights from brainstem processing of speech sounds. *International Journal of Audiology, 46*(9), 524–532.

Banai, K., Hornickel, J., Skoe, E., Nicol, T., Zecker, S., & Kraus, N. (2009). Reading and subcortical auditory function. *Cerebral Cortex, 19*(11), 2699–2707.

Bernstein, J. G., & Oxenham, A. J. (2003). Pitch discrimination of diotic and dichotic tone complexes: Harmonic resolvability or harmonic number? *Journal of the Acoustical Society of America, 113*, 3323–3334.

Besson, M., Chobert, J., & Marie, C. (2011). Language and music in the musician brain. *Language and Linguistics Compass, 5*(9), 617–634.

Bidelman, G. M. (2017). Communicating in challenging environments: Noise and reverberation. In N. Kraus, S. Anderson, T. White-Schwoch, R. R. Fay, & A. N. Popper (Eds.), *Springer handbook of auditory research: The frequency-following response: A window into human communication* (pp. 193–224). Cham, Switzerland: Springer International.

Bidelman, G. M., Davis, M. K., & Pridgen, M. H. (2018). Brainstem-cortical connectivity for speech is differentially challenged by noise and reverberation. *Hearing Research, 367*, 149–160.

Bidelman, G. M., Gandour, J. T., & Krishnan, A. (2011a). Musicians demonstrate experience-dependent brainstem enhancement of musical scale features within continuously gliding pitch. *Neuroscience Letters, 503*(3), 203–207.

Bidelman, G. M., Gandour, J. T., & Krishnan, A. (2011b). Cross-domain effects of music and language experience on the representation of pitch in the human auditory brainstem. *Journal of Cognitive Neuroscience, 23*(2), 425–434.

Bidelman, G. M., Gandour, J. T., & Krishnan, A. (2011c). Musicians and tone-language speakers share enhanced brainstem encoding but not perceptual benefits for musical pitch. *Brain and Cognition, 77*(1), 1–10.

Bidelman, G. M., & Krishnan, A. (2009). Neural correlates of consonance, dissonance, and the hierarchy of musical pitch in the human brainstem. *Journal of Neuroscience, 29*(42), 13165–13171.

Bidelman, G. M., & Krishnan, A. (2011a). Brainstem correlates of behavioral and compositional preferences of musical harmony. *Neuroreport, 22*(5), 212–216.

Bidelman, G. M., & Krishnan, A. (2011b). Effects of reverberation on brainstem representation of speech in musicians and non-musicians. *Brain Research, 1355*, 112–125.

Bidelman, G. M., Lowther, J. E., Tak, S. H., & Alain, C. (2017). Mild cognitive impairment is characterized by deficient brainstem and cortical representations of speech. *Journal of Neuroscience, 37*(13), 3610–3620.

Billings, C. J., Tremblay, K. L., Stecker, G. C., & Tolin, W. M. (2009). Human evoked cortical activity to signal-to-noise ratio and absolute signal level. *Hearing Research, 254*(1–2), 15–24.

Bilsen, F. A., & Ritsma, R. J. (1970). Some parameters influencing the perceptibility of pitch. *Journal of the Acoustical Society of America, 47*(28), 469–475.

Bilsen, F. A., ten Kate, J. H., Buunen, T. J. F., & Raatgever, J. (1975). Responses of single units in the cochlear nucleus of the cat to cosine noise. *Journal of the Acoustical Society of America, 58*, 858–866.

Brand, A., Behrend, O., Marquardt, T., McAlpine, D., & Grothe, B. (2002). Precise inhibition is essential for microsecond interaural time difference encoding. *Nature, 417*, 543–547.

Bregman, A. S. (1990). *Auditory scene analysis: The perceptual organisation of sound.* Cambridge, MA: MIT Press.

Brugge, J. F., Nourski, K. V., Oya, H., Reale, R. A., Kawasaki, H., Steinschneider, M., & Howard, M. A., 3rd. (2009). Coding of repetitive transients by auditory cortex on Heschl's gyrus. *Journal of Neurophysiology, 102*(4), 2358–2374.

Burkard, R., & Hecox, K. (1983). The effect of broadband noise on the human brainstem auditory evoked response. I. Rate and intensity effects. *Journal of the Acoustical Society of America, 74*(4), 1204–1213.

Caird, D., Sontheimer, D., & Klinke, R. (1985). Intra- and extracranially recorded auditory evoked potentials in the cat: I. Source location and binaural interaction. *Electroencephalography and Clinical Neurophysiology, 61*, 50–60.

Caird, D. M., Palmer, A. R., & Rees, A. (1991). Binaural masking level difference effects in single units of the guinea pig inferior colliculus. *Hearing Research, 57*, 91–106.

Cameron, S., & Dillon, H. (2008). The listening in spatialized noise-sentences test (LISN-S): Comparison to the prototype LiSN and results from children with either a suspected (central) auditory processing disorder or a confirmed language disorder. *Journal of the American Academy of Audiology, 19*, 377–391.

Cariani, P. A., & Delgutte, B. (1996a). Neural correlates of the pitch of complex tones. I. Pitch and pitch salience. *Journal of Neurophysiology, 76*(3), 1698–1716.

Cariani, P. A., & Delgutte, B. (1996b). Neural correlates of the pitch of complex tones. II. Pitch shift, pitch ambiguity, phase invariance, pitch circularity, rate pitch, and the dominance region for pitch. *Journal of Neurophysiology, 76*(3), 1717–1734.

Carlyon, R. P., & Shackleton, T. M. (1994). Comparing the fundamental frequencies of resolved and unresolved harmonics: Evidence for two pitch mechanisms. *Journal of the Acoustical Society of America, 95*, 3541–3554.

Cedolin, L., & Delgutte, B. (2005). Pitch of complex tones: Rate-place and interspike interval representations in the auditory nerve. *Journal of Neurophysiology, 94*(1), 347–362.

Chait, M., Poeppel, D., & Simon, J. Z. (2006). Neural response correlates of detection of monaurally and binaurally created pitches in humans. *Cerebral Cortex, 16*(6), 835–848.

Chandrasekaran, B., & Kraus, N. (2010). The scalp-recorded brainstem response to speech: Neural origins and plasticity. *Psychophysiology, 47*(2), 236–246.

Clark, J. L., Moushegian, G., & Rupert, A. L. (1997). Interaural time effects on the frequency-following response. *Journal of the American Academy of Audiology, 8*, 308–313.

Clinard, C., Hodgson, S. L., & Scherer, M. L. (2017). Neural correlates of the binaural masking level difference in human frequency-following responses. *Journal of the Association for Research in Otolaryngology, 18*, 355–369.

Coffey, E. B. J., Chepesiuk, A. M. P., Herholz, S. C., Baillet, S., & Zatorre, R. J. (2017). Neural correlates of early sound encoding and their relationship to speech-in-noise perception. *Frontiers in Neuroscience, 11*, 479.

Cohen, M. A., Grossberg, S., & Wyse, L. L. (1995). A spectral network model of pitch perception. *Journal of the Acoustical Society of America, 98*(2), 862–879.

Colburn, H. S. (1977). Theory of binaural interaction based on auditory nerve data. II. Detection of tones in noise. *Journal of the Acoustical Society of America, 61*, 525–533.

Colburn, H. S., & Latimer, J. S. (1978). Theory of binaural interaction based on auditory-nerve data: III. Joint dependence on interaural time and amplitude differences in discrimination and detection. *Journal of the Acoustical Society of America, 64*, 95–106.

Collins, M. J., & Cullen, J. K., Jr. (1978). Temporal integration of tone glides. *Journal of the Acoustical Society of America, 63*(2), 469–473.

Crow, G., Rupert, A. L., & Moushegian, G. (1978). Phase locking in monaural and binaural medullary neurons: Implications for binaural phenomena. *Journal of the Acoustical Society of America, 64*, 493–501.

Cunningham, J., Nicol, T., King, C., Zecker, S. G., & Kraus, N. (2002). Effects of noise and cue enhancement on neural responses to speech in auditory midbrain, thalamus, and cortex. *Hearing Research, 169*, 97–111.

Cunningham, J., Nicol, T., Zecker, S. G., Bradlow, A., & Kraus, N. (2001). Neurobiologic responses to speech in noise in children with learning problems: Deficits and strategies for improvement. *Clinical Neurophysiology, 112*(5), 758–767.

De Boer, E. (1956). *On the "residue" in hearing* (Doctoral thesis). University of Amsterdam, the Netherlands.

De Boer, E. (1976). On the "residue" and auditory pitch perception. In W. D. Keidel & W. D. Neff (Eds.), *Auditory system. Handbook of Sensory Physiology* (Vol. 5, pp. 479–583). Berlin, Germany: Springer.

Dobie, R. A., & Berlin, C. I. (1979). Binaural interaction in brainstem-evoked responses. *Archives of Otolaryngology, 105*, 391–398.

Drgas, S., & Blaszak, M. A. (2009). Perceptual consequences of changes in vocoded speech parameters in various reverberation conditions. *Journal of Speech, Language, and Hearing Research, 52*(4), 945–955.

Egan, J. P. (1965). Masking-level differences as a function of interaural disparities in intensity of signal and of noise. *Journal of the Acoustical Society of America, 38*, 1043–1049.

Ehret, G., & Merzenich, M. M. (1988). Complex sound analysis (frequency resolution, filtering, and spectral integration) by single units of the inferior colliculus of the cat. *Brain Research Review, 13*, 139–163.

Evans, E. F. (1978). Place and time coding of frequency in the peripheral auditory system: Some physiological pros and cons. *International Journal of Audiology, 17*(5), 369–420.

Fastl, H., & Stoll, G. (1979). Scaling of pitch strength. *Hearing Research, 1*, 293–301.

Fay, R. R., Yost, W. A., & Coombs, S. (1983). Psychophysics and neurophysiology of repetition noise processing in a vertebrate auditory system. *Hearing Research, 12*, 31–55.

Fitzpatrick, D. C., Batra, R., Stanford, T. R., & Kuwada, S. (1997). A neuronal population code for sound localization. *Nature, 388*, 871–874.

Furst, M., Levine, R. A., & McGaffigan, P. M. (1985). Click lateralization is related to the beta component of the dichotic brainstem auditory evoked potentials of human subjects. *Journal of the Acoustical Society of America, 78*, 1644–1651.

Galbraith, G. C. (2008). Deficient brainstem encoding in autism. *Clinical Neurophysiology, 119*(8), 1697–1700.

Galbraith, G. C., Amaya, E. M., Diaz de Rivera, J. M., Donan, N. M., Duong, M. T., Hsu, J. N., . . . Tsang, L. P. (2004). Brain stem evoked response to forward and reversed speech in humans. *Neuroreport, 15*(13), 2057–2060.

Gandour, J. T. (1983). Tone perception in Far Eastern languages. *Journal of Phonetics, 11*, 149–175.

Gandour, J. T. (1994). Phonetics of tone. In R. Asher & J. Simpson (Eds.), *The encyclopedia of language and linguistics* (Vol. 6, pp. 3116–3123). New York, NY: Pergamon Press.

Gandour, J. T., & Harshman, R. A. (1978). Cross-language differences in tone perception: A multi-dimensional scaling investigation. *Language and Speech, 21*(1), 1–33.

Gandour, J. T., & Krishnan, A. (2014). Neural bases of lexical tone. In H. Winskel & P. Padakannaya (Eds.), *South and Southeast Asian psycholinguistics* (pp. 339–349). Cambridge, UK: Cambridge University Press.

Gelfand, S. A., & Silman, S. (1979). Effects of small room reverberation upon the recognition of some consonant features. *Journal of the Acoustical Society of America, 66*(1), 22–29.

Gerken, G. M., Moushegian, G., Stillman, R. D., & Rupert, A. L. (1975). Human frequency-following responses to monaural and binaural stimuli. *Electroencephalography and Clinical Neurophysiology, 38*, 379–386.

Gockel, H. E., Carlyon, R. P., Mehta, A., & Plack, C. J. (2011). The frequency following response (FFR) may reflect pitch-bearing information but is not a direct representation of pitch. *Journal of the Association for Research in Otolaryngology, 12*(6), 767–782.

Gold, J. I., & Knudsen, E. I. (2000). A site of auditory experience-dependent plasticity in the neural representation of auditory space in the barn owl's inferior colliculus. *Journal of Neuroscience, 20*(9), 3469–3486.

Goldberg, J. M., & Brown, P. B. (1968). Functional organization of the superior olivary complex of the dog: An anatomical and electrophysiological study. *Journal of Neurophysiology, 31*, 639–656.

Greenberg, S., Marsh, J. T., Brown, W. S., & Smith, J. C. (1987). Neural temporal coding of low pitch. I. Human frequency-following responses to complex tones. *Hearing Research, 25*(2–3), 91–114.

Griffiths, T. D., Büchel, C., Frackowiak, R. S., & Patterson, R. D. (1998). Analysis of temporal structure in sound by the human brain. *Nature Neuroscience, 1*(5), 422–427.

Griffiths, T. D., & Hall, D. A. (2012). Mapping pitch representation in neural ensembles with fMRI. *Journal of Neuroscience, 32*(39), 13343–13347.

Griffiths, T. D., Kumar, S., Sedley, W., Nourski, K. V., Kawasaki, H., Oya, H., . . . Howard, M. A. (2010). Direct recordings of pitch responses from human auditory cortex. *Current Biology, 20*(12), 1128–1132.

Griffiths, T. D., Uppenkamp, S., Johnsrude, I., Josephs, O., & Patterson, R. D. (2001). Encoding of the temporal regularity of sound in the human brainstem. *Nature Neuroscience, 4*(6), 633–637.

Gutschalk, A., Patterson, R. D., Scherg, M., Uppenkamp, S., & Rupp, A. (2004). Temporal dynamics of pitch in human auditory cortex. *Neuroimage, 22*(2), 755–766.

Gutschalk, A., Patterson, R. D., Scherg, M., Uppenkamp, S., & Rupp, A. (2007). The effect of temporal context on the sustained pitch response in the human auditory cortex. *Cerebral Cortex, 17*(3), 552–561.

Hall, J. W., III (1979). Auditory brainstem frequency following responses to waveform envelope periodicity. *Science, 205*, 1297–1299.

Hartmann, R., & Klinke, R. (1990). Response characteristics of nerve fibers to patterned electrical stimulation. In J. M. Miller & F. A. Spelman (Eds.), *Cochlear implants, models of the electrically stimulated ear* (pp. 136–160). New York, NY: Springer-Verlag.

Henry, K. R. (1999). Noise improves transfer of near-threshold, phase-locked activity of the cochlear nerve: Evidence for stochastic resonance? *Journal of Comparative Physiology A: Sensory, Neural, and Behavioral Physiology, 184*(6), 577–584.

Hickok, G., & Poeppel, D. (2004). Dorsal and ventral streams: A framework for understanding aspects of the functional anatomy of language. *Cognition, 92*(1–2), 67–99.

Hickok, G., & Poeppel, D. (2007). The cortical organization of speech processing. *Nature Reviews Neuroscience, 8*(5), 393–402.

Hirsch, I. (1948). The influence of interaural phase on interaural summation and inhibition. *Journal of the Acoustical Society of America, 20*, 536–544.

Horst, W., Javel, E., & Farley, G. R. (1990). Coding of spectral fine structure in the auditory nerve. II. Level-dependent nonlinear responses. *Journal of the Acoustical Society of America, 88*, 2656–2681.

Houtgast, T., & Steeneken, H. J. M. (1973). The modulation transfer function in room acoustics as a predictor of speech intelligibility. *Journal of the Acoustical Society of America, 54,* 557.

Houtgast, T., & Steeneken, H. J. M. (1985). A review of the MTF-concept in room acoustics, *Journal of the Acoustical Society of America, 77,* 1069–1077.

Houtsma, A., & Smurzynski, J. (1990). Pitch identification n and discrimination for complex tones with many harmonics. *Journal of the Acoustical Society of America, 87,* 304–310.

Howie, J. M., & Howie, J. M. (1976). *Acoustical studies of Mandarin vowels and tones* (Vol. 18). Cambridge University Press.

Hughes, L. E., Rowe, J. B., Ghosh, B. C. P., Carlyon, R. P., Plack, C. J., & Gockel, H. E. (2014). The binaural masking level difference: Cortical correlates persist despite severe brain stem atrophy in progressive supranuclear palsy. *Journal of Neurophysiology, 112*(12), 3086–3094.

Javel, E. (1990). Acoustical and electrical encoding of temporal information. In J. M. Miller & F. A. Spelman (Eds.), *Cochlear implants, models of the electrically stimulated ear* (pp. 247–291). New York, NY: Springer-Verlag.

Jeffress, L. A. (1948). A place theory of sound localization. *Journal of Comparative Physiological Psychology, 41,* 35–39.

Jeffress, L. A., Blodgett, H. C., & Deatherage, B. H. (1952). The masking of tones by white noise as a function of the interaural phases of both components. I. 500 cycles. *Journal of the Acoustical Society of America, 24,* 523–527.

Jenkins, W. M., & Masterton, R. B. (1982). Sound localization: Effects of unilateral lesions in the central auditory system. *Journal of Neurophysiology, 47,* 987–1016.

Jiang, D., McAlpine, D., & Palmer, A. R. (1997). Responses of neurons in the inferior colliculus to binaural masking level difference stimuli measured by rate-versus-level functions. *Journal of Neurophysiology, 77,* 3085–3106.

Kaplan-Neeman, R., Kishon-Rabin, L., Henkin, Y., & Muchnik, C. (2006). Identification of syllables in noise: Electrophysiological and behavioral correlates. *Journal of the Acoustical Society of America, 120*(2), 926–933.

Kevanishvili, Z., & Lagidze, Z. (1987). Masking level difference: An electrophysiologic approach. *Scandinavian Audiology, 16,* 3–11.

Kraus, N., Lindley, T., Colegrove, D., Krizman, J., Otto-Meyer, S., Thompson, E. C., & White-Schwoch, T. (2017). The neural legacy of a single concussion. *Neuroscience Letters, 646,* 21–23.

Kraus, N., & Nicol, T. (2005). Brainstem origins for cortical "what" and "where" pathways in the auditory system. *Trends in Neurosciences, 28*(4), 176–181.

Krishnan, A. (1999). Human frequency-following responses to two-tone approximations of steady-state vowels. *Audiology and Neuro-Otology, 4*(2), 95–103.

Krishnan, A. (2002). Human frequency-following responses: Representation of steady-state synthetic vowels. *Hearing Research, 166*(1–2), 192–201.

Krishnan, A. (2007). Human frequency following response. In R. F. Burkard, M. Don, & J. J. Eggermont (Eds.), *Auditory evoked potentials: Basic principles and clinical application* (pp. 313–335). Baltimore, MD: Lippincott Williams & Wilkins.

Krishnan, A., Bidelman, G. M., & Gandour, J. T. (2010). Neural representation of pitch salience in the human brainstem revealed by psychophysical and electrophysiological indices. *Hearing Research, 268,* 60–66.

Krishnan, A., Bidelman, G. M., Smalt, C. J., Ananthakrishnan, S., & Gandour, J. T. (2012). Relationship between brainstem, cortical and behavioral measures relevant to pitch salience in humans. *Neuropsychologia, 50,* 2849–2859.

Krishnan, A., & Gandour, J. T. (2009). The role of the auditory brainstem in processing linguistically-relevant pitch patterns. *Brain and Language, 110,* 135–148.

Krishnan, A., & Gandour, J. T. (2014). Language experience shapes processing of pitch relevant information in the human brainstem and auditory cortex: Electrophysiological evidence. *Acoustics Australia, 42*(3), 187–199.

Krishnan, A., & Gandour, J. T. (2017). Brainstem representation of pitch relevant information is shaped by language experience. In N. Kraus, S. Anderson, T. White-Schwoch, R. R. Fay, & A. N. Popper (Eds.), *Springer handbook of auditory research: The frequency-following response: A window into human communication* (pp. 45–73). Cham, Switzerland: Springer International.

Krishnan, A., Gandour, J. T., Ananthakrishnan, S., Bidelman, G. M., & Smalt, C. J. (2011). Functional ear (a) symmetry in brainstem neural activity relevant to encoding of voice pitch: A precursor for hemispheric specialization?. *Brain and language, 119*(3), 226-231.

Krishnan, A., Gandour, J. T., Ananthakrishnan, S., & Vijayaraghavan, V. (2015). Language experience enhances early cortical pitch-dependent responses. *Journal of neurolinguistics, 33,* 128-148.

Krishnan, A., Gandour, J., & Bidelman, G. (2010). Brainstem pitch representation in native speakers of Mandarin is less susceptible to degradation of stimulus temporal regularity. *Brain Research, 1313,* 124–133.

Krishnan, A., Gandour, J. T., & Bidelman, G. M. (2012). Experience-dependent plasticity in pitch encoding: From brainstem to auditory cortex. *Neuroreport, 23,* 498–502.

Krishnan, A., Gandour, J. T., Bidelman, G. M., & Swaminathan, J. (2009). Experience-dependent neural representation of dynamic pitch in the brainstem. *Neuroreport, 20*(4), 408–413.

Krishnan, A., Gandour, J. T., Smalt, C. J., & Bidelman, G. M. (2010). Language-dependent pitch encoding advantage in the brainstem is not limited to acceleration rates that occur in natural speech. *Brain and Language, 114*(3), 193-198.

Krishnan, A., Gandour, J. T., & Suresh, C. (2014). Cortical pitch response components show differential sensitivity to native and nonnative pitch contours. *Brain and Language, 138,* 51–60.

Krishnan, A., Gandour, J. T., & Suresh, C. H. (2015a). Pitch processing of dynamic lexical tones in the auditory cortex is influenced by sensory and extrasensory processes. *European Journal of Neuroscience, 41*(11), 1496-1504.

Krishnan, A., Gandour, J. T., & Suresh, C. (2015b). Experience-dependent enhancement of pitch-specific responses in the auditory cortex is limited to acceleration rates in normal voice range. *Neuroscience, 303*(10), 433–455.

Krishnan, A., Gandour, J. T., & Suresh, C. H. (2016). Language-experience plasticity in neural representation of changes in pitch salience. *Brain research, 1637,* 102–117.

Krishnan, A., Gandour, J.T., & Suresh (in press). Cortical hemisphere preference and brainstem ear asymmetry reflect experience-dependent functional modulation of pitch. *Brain & Language* (paper accepted).

Krishnan, A., Gandour, J. T., Xu, Y., & Suresh, C. H. (2016). Language-dependent changes in pitch-relevant neural activity in the auditory cortex reflect differential weighting of temporal attributes of pitch contours. *Journal of Neurolinguistics, 41,* 38–49.

Krishnan, A., & McDaniel, S. (1998). Binaural interaction in the human frequency-following response: Effects of interaural intensity difference. *Audiology and Neuro-otology, 3,* 291–299.

Krishnan, A., & Parkinson, J. (2000). Human frequency-following response: Representation of tonal sweeps. *Audiology and Neuro-Otology, 5*(6), 312–321.

Krishnan, A., & Plack, C. J. (2011). Neural encoding in the human brainstem relevant to the pitch of complex tones. *Hearing Research, 275*(1–2), 110–119.

Krishnan, A., Smalt, C., Bidelman, G., & Gandour, J. (2010). Language-dependent pitch encoding advantage in the brainstem is not limited to acceleration rates that occur in natural speech. *Brain and Language, 114*(3), 193–198.

Krishnan, A., Suresh, C. H., & Gandour, J. T. (2017a). Changes in pitch height elicit both language-universal and language-dependent changes in neural representation of pitch in the brainstem and auditory cortex. *Neuroscience, 346,* 52–63.

Krishnan, A., Suresh, C. H., & Gandour, J. T. (2017b). Differential sensitivity to changes in pitch acceleration in the auditory brainstem and cortex. *Brain and Language, 169,* 22–27.

Krishnan, A., Suresh, C., & Gandour, J. T. (2019). Tone language experience-dependent advantage in pitch representation in brainstem and auditory cortex is maintained under reverberation. *Hearing Research, 177,* 63–71.

Krishnan, A., Swaminathan, J., & Gandour, J. T. (2009). Experience-dependent enhancement of linguistic pitch representation in the brainstem is not specific to a speech context. *Journal of Cognitive Neuroscience, 21*(6), 1092–1105.

Krishnan, A., Van Dun, B., Dillon, H., Smalt, C., Buchholz, J., & Ananthakrishnan, S. (2012). *Human frequency following response: Correlates of spatial release from masking.* Paper presented at the annual meeting of the American Auditory Society, Scottsdale, AZ.

Krishnan, A., Xu, Y., Gandour, J. T., & Cariani, P. A. (2004). Human frequency-following response: Representation of pitch contours in Chinese tones. *Hearing Research, 189*(1–2), 1–12.

Krishnan, A., Xu, Y., Gandour, J. T., & Cariani, P. A. (2005). Encoding of pitch in the human brainstem is sensitive to language experience. *Cognitive Brain Research, 25*(1), 161–168.

Krizman, J., Marian, V., Shook, A., Skoe, E., & Kraus, N. (2012). Subcortical encoding of sound is enhanced in bilinguals and relates to executive function advantages. *Proceedings of the National Academy of Sciences USA, 109*(20), 7877–7881.

Krumbholz, K., Patterson, R. D., Seither-Preisler, A., Lammertmann, C., & Lütkenhoner, B. (2003). Neuromagnetic evidence for a pitch processing center in Heschl's gyrus. *Cerebral Cortex, 13*(7), 765–772.

Kumar, S., & Schönwiesner, M. (2012). Mapping human pitch representation in a distributed system using depth-electrode recordings and modeling (Review). *Journal of Neuroscience, 32*(39), 13348–13351.

Kumar, S., Stephan, K. E., Warren, J. D., Friston, K. J., & Griffiths, T. D. (2007). Hierarchical processing of auditory objects in humans. *PLOS Computational Biology, 3*(6), e100.

Langford, T. L. (1984). Responses elicited from medial superior olivary neurons by stimuli associated with binaural masking and unmasking. *Hearing Research, 15*(1), 39–50.

Laroche, M., Dajani, H. R., Prevost, F., & Marcoux, A. M. (2013). Brainstem auditory responses to resolved and unresolved harmonics of a synthetic vowel in quiet and noise. *Ear and Hearing, 34*(1), 63–74.

Lavine, R. A. (1971). Phase-locking in cochlear nuclear complex of the cat to low-frequency tonal stimuli. *Journal of Neurophysiology, 34*, 467–483.

Li, X., Gandour, J. T., Talavage, T., Wong, D., Dzemidzic, M., Lowe, M., & Tong, Y. (2003). Selective attention to lexical tones recruits left dorsal frontoparietal network. *Neuroreport, 14*(17), 2263–2266.

Li, X., Gandour, J. T., Talavage, T., Wong D., Hoffa, A., Lowe, M., & Dzemidzic, M. (2010). Hemispheric asymmetries in phonological processing of tones versus segmental units. *Neuroreport, 21*(10), 690–694.

Li, X., & Jeng, F.-C. (2011). Noise tolerance in human frequency-following responses to voice pitch. *Journal of the Acoustical Society of America, 129*, 21–26.

Licklider, J. C. R. (1951). A duplex theory of pitch perception. *Experientia, 7*(4), 128–134.

Liu, C., & Kewley-Port, D. (2004). Formant discrimination in noise for isolated vowels. *Journal of the Acoustical Society of America, 116*(5), 3119–3129.

Lu, T., Liang, L., & Wang, X. (2001). Temporal and rate representations of time-varying signals in the auditory cortex of awake primates. *Nature Neuroscience, 4*(11), 1131–1138.

McAlpine, D., Jiang, D., & Palmer, A. R. (1996). Binaural masking level differences in the inferior colliculus of the guinea pig. *Journal of the Acoustical Society of America, 100*, 490–503.

McPherson, D. L., & Starr, A. (1995). Auditory time-intensity cues in the binaural interaction component of the auditory evoked potentials. *Hearing Research, 89*(1–2), 162–171.

Meddis, R., & Hewitt, M. J. (1991). Virtual pitch and phase-sensitivity of a computer model of the auditory periphery. I: Pitch identification. *Journal of the Acoustical Society of America, 89*(6), 2866–2882.

Meddis, R., & O'Mard, L. (1997). A unitary model of pitch perception. *Journal of the Acoustical Society of America, 102*(3), 1811–1820.

Mesgarani, N., David, S. V., Fritz, J. B., & Shamma, S. A. (2014). Mechanisms of noise robust representation of speech in primary auditory cortex. *Proceedings of the National Academy of Science, USA, 111*(18), 6792–6797.

Meyer, M. (2008). Functions of the left and right posterior temporal lobes during segmental and suprasegmental speech perception. *Zeitshcrift fur Neuropsycholgie, 19*(2), 101–115.

Micheyl, C., Schrater, P. R., & Oxenham, A. J. (2013). Auditory frequency and intensity discrimination explained using a cortical population rate code. *PLOS Computational Biology, 9*(11), e1003336.

Middlebrooks, J. C., & Snyder, R. L. (2010). Selective electrical stimulation of the auditory nerve activates a pathway specialized for high temporal acuity. *Journal of Neuroscience, 30*, 1937–1946.

Møller, A. R. (2000). Electrical potentials in the auditory nervous system. In A. R. Møller (Ed.), *Hearing: Its physiology and pathophysiology.* San Diego, CA: Academic Press.

Moore, B. C. J. (1989). *An introduction to the psychology of hearing* (3rd ed.). London, UK: Academic Press.

Moushegian, G., Rupert, A. L., & Gidda, J. S. (1975). Functional characteristics of superior olivary neurons to binaural stimuli. *Journal of Neurophysiology, 38*, 1037–1048.

Moushegian, G., Rupert, A. L., & Stillman, R. D. (1973). Scalp recorded early responses in man to frequencies in the speech range. *Electroencephalography and Clinical Neurophysiology, 35*, 665–667.

Nabelek, A. K., & Dagenais, P. A. (1986). Vowel errors in noise and in reverberation by hearing-impaired listeners. *Journal of the Acoustical Society of America, 80*(3), 741–748.

Nabelek, A. K., & Letowski, T. R. (1988). Similarities of vowels in nonreverberant and reverberant fields. *Journal of the Acoustical Society of America, 83*(5), 1891–1899.

Nabelek, A. K., Letowski, T. R., & Tucker, F. M. (1989). Reverberant overlap- and self-masking in consonant identification. *Journal of the Acoustical Society of America, 86*(4), 1259–1265.

Neuert, V., Verhey, J. L., & Winter, I. M. (2005). Temporal representation of the delay of iterated rippled noise in the dorsal cochlear nucleus. *Journal of Neurophysiology, 93*(5), 2766–2776.

Omote, A., Jasmin, K., & Tierney, A. (2017). Successful non-native speech perception is linked to frequency following response phase consistency. *Cortex, 93*, 146–154.

Oxenham, A. J. (2012). Pitch perception. *Journal of Neuroscience, 32*(39), 13335–13338.

Palmer, A. R., Jiang, D., & McAlpine, D. (1999). Desynchronizing responses to correlated noise: A mechanism for binaural masking level differences at the inferior colliculus. *Journal of Neurophysiology, 81,* 722–734.

Palmer, A. R., Jiang, D., & McAlpine, D. (2000). Neural responses in the inferior colliculus to binaural masking level differences created by inverting the noise in one ear. *Journal of Neurophysiology, 84,* 844–852.

Palmer, A. R., & Winter, I. M. (1992). Cochlear nerve and cochlear nucleus responses to the fundamental frequency of voiced speech sounds and harmonic complex tones. In Y. Cazals, K. Horner, & L. Demany (Eds.), *Auditory Physiology and Perception, Proceedings of the 9th International Symposium on Hearing, Carcens, France* (pp. 231–239). Oxford, UK: Pergamon Press.

Palmer, A. R., & Winter, I. M. (1993). Coding of the fundamental frequency of voiced speech sounds and harmonic complexes in the cochlear nerve and ventral cochlear nucleus. In M. A. Merchán, J. M. Juiz, D. A. Godfrey, & E. Mugnaini (Eds.), *The mammalian cochlear nuclei: Organization and function* (pp. 373–384). New York, NY: Plenum Press.

Parbery-Clark, A., Skoe, E., & Kraus, N. (2009). Musical experience limits the degradative effects of background noise on the neural processing of sound. *Journal of Neuroscience, 29*(45), 14100–14107.

Patterson, R. D., Allerhand, M. H., & Giguere, C. (1995). Time-domain modeling of peripheral auditory processing: A modular architecture and a software platform. *Journal of the Acoustical Society of America, 98*(4), 1890–1894.

Patterson, R. D., Handel, S., Yost, W. A., & Datta, A. J. (1996). The relative strength of the tone and noise components in iterated ripple noise. *Journal of the Acoustical Society of America, 100,* 3286–3294.

Patterson, R. D., Uppenkamp, S., Johnsrude, I. S., & Griffiths, T. D. (2002). The processing of temporal pitch and melody information in the auditory cortex. *Neuron, 36*(4), 767–776.

Penagos, H., Melcher, J. R., & Oxenham, A. J. (2004). A neural representation of pitch salience in nonprimary human auditory cortex revealed with functional magnetic resonance imaging. *Journal of Neuroscience, 24*(30), 6810–6815.

Plyler, P. N., & Ananthanarayan, A. K. (2001). Human frequency-following responses: Representation of second formant transitions in normal-hearing and hearing-impaired listeners. *Journal of the American Academy of Audiology, 12*(10), 523–533.

Poeppel, D., Idsardi, W. J., & van Wassenhove, V. (2008). Speech perception at the interface of neurobiology and linguistics. *Philosophical Transactions of the Royal Society of London. Series B: Biological Sciences, 363*(1493), 1071–1086.

Prevost, F., Laroche, M., Marcoux, A. M., & Dajani, H. R. (2013). Objective measurement of physiological signal-to-noise gain in the brainstem response to a synthetic vowel. *Clinical Neurophysiology, 124*(1), 52–60.

Puschmann, S., Uppenkamp, S., Kollmeier, B., & Thiel, C. M. (2010). Dichotic pitch activates pitch processing centre in Heschl's gyrus. *Neuroimage, 49*(2), 1641–1649.

Rao, R. P., & Ballard, D. H. (1999). Predictive coding in the visual cortex: A functional interpretation of some extra-classical receptive-field effects. *Nature Neuroscience, 2*(1), 79–87.

Robinson, D. E., & Jeffress, L. A. (1963). Effect of varying the interaural noise correlation on the detectability of tonal signals. *Journal of the Acoustical Society of America, 35,* 1947–1952.

Rocha-Muniz, C. N., Befi-Lopes, D. M., & Schochat, E. (2012). Investigation of auditory processing disorder and language impairment using the speech-evoked auditory brainstem response. *Hearing Research, 294*(1), 143–152.

Rocha-Muniz, C. N., Befi-Lopes, D. M., & Schochat, E. (2014). Sensitivity, specificity and efficiency of speech-evoked ABR. *Hearing Research, 317,* 15–22.

Rose, J. E., Brugge, J. F., Anderson, J. D., & Hind, J. E. (1967). Phase-locked responses to low-frequency tones in single auditory nerve fibers of the squirrel monkey. *Journal of Neurophysiology, 30,* 769–793.

Russo, N., Nicol, T., Musacchia, G., & Kraus, N. (2004). Brainstem responses to speech syllables. *Clinical Neurophysiology, 115*(9), 2021–2030.

Russo, N. M., Nicol, T. G., Zecker, S. G., Hayes, E. A., & Kraus, N. (2005). Auditory training improves neural timing in the human brainstem. *Behavioral Brain Research, 156*(1), 95–103.

Russo, N. M., Skoe, E., Trommer, B., Nicol, T., Zecker, S., Bradlow, A., & Kraus, N. (2008). Deficient brainstem encoding of pitch in children with Autism Spectrum Disorders. *Clinical Neurophysiology, 119*(8), 1720–1731.

Sasaki, T., Kawase, T., Nakasato, N., Kanno, A., Ogura, M., Tominaga, T., & Kobayashi, T. (2005). Neuromagnetic evaluation of binaural unmasking. *NeuroImage, 25*(3), 684–689.

Sayles, M., Stasiak, A., & Winter, I. M. (2015). Reverberation impairs brainstem temporal representations of voiced vowel sounds: Challenging "periodicity-tagged" segregation of competing speech in rooms. *Frontiers in Systems Neuroscience, 8,* 248. https://doi.org/10.3389/fnsys.2014.00248

Sayles, M., Stasiak, A., & Winter, I. M. (2016). Neural segregation of concurrent speech: Effects of background noise and reverberation on auditory scene analysis in the ventral cochlear nucleus. *Advances in Experimental Medicine and Biology, 894,* 389–397.

Sayles, M., & Winter, I. M. (2008a). Ambiguous pitch and the temporal representation of inharmonic iterated rippled noise in the ventral cochlear nucleus. *Journal of Neuroscience, 28*(46), 11925–11938.

Sayles, M., & Winter, I. M. (2008b). Reverberation challenges the temporal representation of the pitch of complex sounds. *Neuron, 58*(5), 789–801.

Schönwiesner, M., Rubsamen, R., & von Cramon, D. Y. (2005). Hemispheric asymmetry for spectral and temporal processing in the human antero-lateral auditory belt cortex. *European Journal of Neuroscience, 22*(6), 1521–1528.

Schouten. J. F. (1940). The residue: A new component in subjective sound analysis. *Proceedings. Koninklijke Nederlandsche Akademie van Wetenschappen, 43,* 356–365.

Schouten, M. E. (1985). Identification and discrimination of sweep tones. *Perception and Psychophysics, 37*(4), 369–376.

Scott, S. K., & Johnsrude, I. S. (2003). The neuroanatomical and functional organization of speech perception. *Trends in Neurosciences, 26*(2), 100–107.

Shackleton, T. M., & Carlyon, R. P. (1994). The role of resolved and unresolved harmonics in pitch perception and frequency modulation discrimination. *Journal of the Acoustical Society of America, 95,* 3529–3540.

Shackleton, T. M., Liu, L. F., & Palmer, A. R. (2009). Responses to diotic, dichotic, and alternating phase harmonic stimuli in the inferior colliculus of guinea pigs. *Journal of the Association for Research in Otolaryngology, 10*(1), 76–90.

Shofner, W. P. (1991). Temporal representation of rippled noise in the anteroventral cochlear nucleus of the chinchilla. *Journal of the Acoustical Society of America, 90,* 2450–2466.

Shofner, W. P. (1999). Responses of cochlear nucleus units in the chinchilla to iterated rippled noises: Analysis of neural autocorrelograms. *Journal of Neurophysiology, 81*(6), 2662–2674.

Shofner, W. P., & Selas, G. (2002). Pitch strength and Stevens's power law. *Perception Psychophysics, 64,* 437–450.

Shore, S. E., Clopton, B. M., & Au, Y. N. (1987). Unit responses in ventral cochlear nucleus reflect cochlear coding of rapid frequency sweeps. *Journal of the Acoustical Society of America, 82*(2), 471–478.

Shore, S. E., & Nuttall, A. L. (1985). High-synchrony cochlear compound action potentials evoked by rising frequency-swept tone bursts. *Journal of the Acoustical Society of America, 78*(4), 1286–1295.

Sinex, D. G., & Geisler, C. D. (1981). Auditory nerve fiber responses to frequency-modulated tones. *Hearing Research, 4,* 127–148.

Smalt, C. J., Krishnan, A., Bidelman, G. M., Ananthakrishnan, S., & Gandour, J. T. (2012). Neural correlates of cochlear distortion products and their influence on the representation of pitch relevant information in the human brainstem. *Hearing Research, 292,* 26–34.

Soeta, Y., Nakagawa, S., & Tonoike, M. (2005). Auditory evoked magnetic fields in relation to iterated rippled noise. *Hearing Research, 205,* 256–261.

Song, J. H., Banai, K., & Kraus, N. (2008). Brainstem timing deficits in children with learning impairment may result from corticofugal origins. *Audiology and Neuro-otology, 13,* 335–344.

Song, J., Skoe, E., Banai, K., & Kraus, N. (2011). Perception of speech in noise: Neural correlates. *Journal of Cognitive Neuroscience, 23*(9), 2268–2279.

Song, J. H., Skoe, E., Wong, P. C., & Kraus, N. (2008). Plasticity in the adult human auditory brainstem following short-term linguistic training. *Journal of Cognitive Neuroscience, 20*(10), 1892–1902.

Sontheimer, D., Caird, D., & Klinke, R. (1985). Intra- and extracranially recorded auditory evoked potentials in the cat: II. Effects of interaural time and intensity differences. *Electroencephalography and Clinical Neurophysiology, 61,* 539–547.

Stasiak, A., Winter, I., & Sayles, M. (2010). *The effect of reverberation on the representation of single vowels, double vowels, and consonant-vowel syllables.* Poster session conducted at the 33rd Midwinter Meeting of the Association for Research in Otolaryngology. 2010. Single Units in the Ventral Cochlear Nucleus, Abstract 231, retrieved from http://www.aro.org/abstracts/abstracts.html

Steinschneider, M., Reser, D. H., Fishman, Y. I., Schroeder, C. E., & Arezzo, J. C. (1998). Click train encoding in primary auditory cortex of the awake monkey: Evidence for two mechanisms subserving pitch perception. *Journal of the Acoustical Society of America, 104*(5), 2935–2955.

Suga, N. (1990). Biosonar and neural computation in bats. *Scientific American, 262*(6), 60–68.

Suga, N. (1994). Processing of auditory information carried by complex species specific sounds. In M. S. Gazzaniga & E. Bizzi (Eds.), *The cognitive neurosciences* (pp. 295–318). Cambridge, MA: MIT Press.

Suga, N., Gao, E., Zhang, Y., Ma, X., & Olsen, J. F. (2000). The corticofugal system for hearing: recent progress. *Proceedings of the National Academy of Sciences, 97*(22), 11807–11814.

Suga, N., & Ma, X. (2003). Multiparametric corticofugal modulation and plasticity in the auditory system. *Nature Reviews Neuroscience, 4*(10), 783–794.

Suga, N., Ma, X., Gao, E., Sakai, M., & Chowdhury, S. A. (2003). Descending system and plasticity for auditory signal processing: Neuroethological data for speech scientists. [Review]. *Speech Communication, 41*(1), 189–200.

Suresh, C., Krishnan, A., & Gandour, J. T. (2017). Language experience-dependent advantage in pitch representation in the auditory cortex is limited to favorable signal-to-noise ratios *Hearing Research, 35*, 42–53.

Suresh, C. H., Krishnan, A., & Luo, X. (2020). Human frequency following responses to vocoded speech: Amplitude modulation versus amplitude plus frequency modulation. *Ear and Hearing, 41*(2), 300–311.

Sussman, E., Ritter, E. W., & Vaughan, H. G., Jr. (1999). An investigation of the auditory streaming effect using event-related brain potentials. *Psychophysiology, 36*, 22–34.

Swaminathan, J., Krishnan, A., & Gandour, J. T. (2008). Pitch encoding in speech and nonspeech contexts in the human auditory brainstem. *Neuroreport, 19*(11), 1163–1167.

Tanis, D. C., & Teas, D. C. (1974). Evoked potential correlates of interaural phase reversals. *Audiology, 13*, 357–365.

ten Kate, J. H., & van Bekkum, M. F. (1988). Synchrony-dependent autocorrelation in eighth-nerve-fiber response to rippled noise. *Journal of the Acoustical Society of America, 84*, 2092–2102.

Verhey, J. L., & Winter, I. M., (2006). The temporal representation of the delay of iterated rippled noise with positive or negative gain by chopper units in the cochlear nucleus. *Hearing Research, 216*(217), 43–51.

Walker, K. M., Bizley, J. K., King, A. J., & Schnupp, J. W. (2011). Cortical encoding of pitch: Recent results and open questions. *Hearing Research, 271*(1–2), 74–87.

Wang, D., & Brown, G. J. (2006). *Computational auditory scene analysis: Principles, algorithms, and applications.* New York, NY: Wiley/IEEE Press.

Wang, Y., Jongman, A., & Sereno, J. A. (2003). Acoustic and perceptual evaluation of Mandarin tone productions before and after perceptual training. *Journal of the Acoustical Society of America, 113*(2), 1033–1043.

White-Schwoch, T., Woodruff Carr, K., Thompson, E. C., Anderson, S., Nicol, T., Bradlow, A. R., . . . Kraus, N. (2015). Auditory processing in noise: A preschool biomarker for literacy. *PLOS Biology, 13*(7), e1002196.

Whiting, K. A., Martin, B. A., & Stapells, D. R. (1998). The effects of broadband noise masking on cortical event-related potentials to speech sounds /ba/ and /da/. *Ear and Hearing, 19*(3), 218–231.

Wildgruber, D., Ackermann, H., Kreifelts, B., & Ethofer, T. (2006). Cerebral processing of linguistic and emotional prosody: fMRI studies. *Progress in Brain Research, 156*, 249–268.

Wilson, B. S., & Dorman, M. F. (2008). Cochlear implants: A remarkable past and a brilliant future. *Hearing Research, 242*, 3–21.

Wilson, B. S., Finley, C. C., Lawson, D. T., Wolford, R. D., Eddington, D. K., & Rabinowitz, W. M. (1991). Better speech recognition with cochlear implants. *Nature, 352*, 236–238.

Wilson, J., & Krishnan, A. (2005). Human frequency following response to stimuli producing masking level difference. *Journal of the American Academy of Audiology, 16*, 184–195.

Winter, I. M., Wiegrebe, L., & Patterson, R. D. (2001). The temporal representation of the delay of iterated rippled noise in the ventral cochlear nucleus of the guinea-pig. *Journal of Physiology, 537*, 553–566.

Wong, P. C., Skoe, E., Russo, N. M., Dees, T., & Kraus, N. (2007). Musical experience shapes human brainstem encoding of linguistic pitch patterns. *Nature Neuroscience, 10*(4), 420–422.

Xu, Y., Krishnan, A., & Gandour, J. T. (2006). Specificity of experience-dependent pitch representation in the brainstem. *Neuroreport, 17*(15), 1601–1605.

Yip, M. (2002). *Tone.* New York, NY: Cambridge University Press.

Yost, W. A. (1978). Strength of the pitches associated with ripple noise. *Journal of the Acoustical Society of America, 64*, 485–492.

Yost, W. A. (1996). Pitch of iterated rippled noise. *Journal of the Acoustical Society of America, 100*, 511–518.

Yost, W. A., & Hill, R. (1979). Models of the pitch and pitch strength of rippled noise. *Journal of the Acoustical Society of America, 66*, 400–411.

Yost, W. A., Patterson, R., & Sheft, S. (1996). A time domain description for the pitch strength of iterated rippled noise. *Journal of the Acoustical Society of America, 99*(2), 1066–1078.

Young, E. D., & Sachs, M. B. (1979). Representation of steady state vowels in the temporal aspects of the discharge patterns of populations of auditory-nerve fibers. *Journal of the Acoustical Society of America, 66*, 1381–1403.

Zatorre, R. J., & Baum, S. R. (2012). Musical melody and speech intonation: Singing a different tune. *PLOS Biology, 10*(7), e1001372.

Zatorre, R. J., & Belin, P. (2001). Spectral and temporal processing in human auditory cortex. *Cerebral Cortex, 11*(10), 946–953.

Zatorre, R. J., & Gandour, J. T. (2008). Neural specializations for speech and pitch: Moving beyond the dichotomies. [Review]. *Philosophical Transactions of the Royal Society of London. Series B: Biological Sciences, 363*(1493), 1087–1104.

Zeng, F.-G., Nie, K., Stickney, G. S., Kong, Y.-Y., Vongphoe, M., Bhargave, A., . . . Cao, K. (2005). Speech recognition with amplitude and frequency modulations. *Proceedings of the National Academy of Sciences, USA, 102,* 2293–2298.

10

Auditory Brainstem Responses Laboratory Exercises

SCOPE

There is no substitute for sufficient hands-on experience to develop sound skills to record, analyze, and interpret the auditory brainstem responses (ABRs) from real people. This essential requirement not only reinforces the understanding of concepts presented in the classroom relevant to the effects of various stimulus and recording factors on the ABR components but also facilitates learning and reinforcing practical skills necessary to accurately record and interpret the responses for optimal clinical application. The clinician needs to know what a normal response looks like and its normal quantitative indices (latency and amplitude) and what specific response indices to focus on to answer a specific clinical question. The laboratory exercises also help the clinician to optimize the test strategy for each client in terms of the most appropriate choice of stimulus and recording parameters to answer a specific clinical question. Furthermore, it also helps the clinician to develop troubleshooting skills to solve common problems encountered while recording the response. Fortunately, most commercially available evoked potential systems provide easy-to-learn, intuitive, user-friendly, and interactive platforms that are not system-specific and can be mastered quickly with the aid of these laboratory exercises. The labs presented were developed for my graduate-level course in auditory electrophysiology using the Intelligent Hearing System's (IHS) SmartEP system; however, I am confident these labs can be performed using other comparable auditory evoked potential systems. I will leave it to the discretion of the instructor to adopt all or some of the most relevant labs presented here. The execution of the labs will no doubt require guidance and assistance, at least initially, from the course instructor and/or the teaching assistants assigned for the course.

PRELIMINARY CONSIDERATIONS FOR RECORDING AUDITORY BRAINSTEM RESPONSES

Students must get initial hands-on familiarity with a few essential features of the interactive signal generation and data acquisition software and hardware setup required to record the ABR. Continued use throughout the labs will enable students to expand on their ability to use other features of the system. Several important elements of subject preparation before data acquisition are as follows:

- Ideally, record the responses in an electrically and acoustically quiet room because both electrical interference and/or unacceptable noise levels will contaminate the response.

- Decide on the electrode configuration and test protocol to be used. The simplest and most commonly used electrode configuration to capture all ABR components is a high forehead to the ipsilateral mastoid. The proposed laboratory exercises will also include the effects of electrode montage on the ABR components.
- Ensure that the skin underneath the electrode locations is gently abraded to obtain low electrode impedances (less than 5000 ohms; the lower the interelectrode impedance the better the signal-to-noise ratio (SNR). Also, make sure that the electrodes are attached well so they do not come loose during testing. For the mastoid location, orient the electrode with the cable running down parallel to the pinna. For the forehead electrode, orient the electrode with the cable running at an angle oriented toward the amplifier (not down and over the eyes or the nose). For infants reclining on mother's lap, an upward orientation of the all electrode cables is preferable to facilitate connection to the preamplifier.
- Instruct the individual to be tested to relax and refrain from body movements.
- Perform an otoscopic examination to rule out excessive cerumen in the ear canal and/or other signs of ear infection that may contraindicate testing.
- Attach the foam tip to the insert earphone tube. Squeeze the foam tip and insert it into the ear canal deep enough so that the back end of the foam tip is in line with the opening of the ear canal. Improper insertion depth may affect the signal level.

It is recommended that the instructor demonstrate all of these preliminary steps and how to use the software to control stimulus and recording parameters, data acquisition, the procedure for preliminary peak picking, and latency and amplitude measurements. This will be sufficient for the students to start their lab exercises. However, the instructor or the teaching assistant should be available to assist students through the initial labs.

I. EFFECTS OF STIMULUS FACTORS ON THE ABR COMPONENTS

Lab 1. Effects of Stimulus Intensity of Click-Evoked ABR

Objectives: After this module, students will be able to:

1. Record multiple channel ABRs.
2. Understand the effects of signal intensity on the amplitude and latency of the ABR.
3. Understand the physiological bases of the changes in latency and amplitude with manipulation of stimulus intensity.

Stimulus and Recording Parameters

Electrode configuration: Two channels: High forehead-ipsilateral mastoid/high forehead-contralateral mastoid (Figure 10–1). Two channels are used to improve the accuracy of the detection of wave V, since the contralateral montage shows a clear separation of the IV–V complex.

Intensity: 80, 60, 40, 20, 0 dB nHL

Transducer: Insert earphones (ER-3A [now ER-3C] or ER-2)

Stimuli: Clicks (0.1-ms duration), 500-Hz tone burst (compare amplitude growth for basal and apical responses). For the tone burst use a 2-1-2 ramp approximated by a Blackman window.

Stimulus polarity: Alternating

Number of sweeps: 1500. Use 2,000 sweeps at 20 and 0 dB nHL to improve SNR and detectability.

Repetition rate: 26.6/sec (fast enough to save time but does not adapt the response)

Amplification: 150,000

Filter setting: 100–3000 Hz (30–3000 Hz at 20 and 0 dB nHL to capture the broader wave V waveform better) to improve detectability.

1. Record from six (3 × 2) ears with replication of each condition.
2. Identify and label the components and measure latency (absolute latency and interpeak latency [IPL]) and amplitude of each component.

Response Analysis and Laboratory Report

1. Summarize (for both channels) the effects of intensity on the amplitude and latency (again both absolute latency and IPLs) of response components using mean latency-intensity (L-I) plots and amplitude-intensity plots. Include a plot of exemplar waveform data (with replicates superimposed) as a function of intensity.

2. Compare your two-channel results with known literature (see normative data in Table 10–1). Specify if there were any problems encountered during testing and how they were overcome.

3. Include in your report an explanation for the observed changes in latency and amplitude in terms of underlying physiological

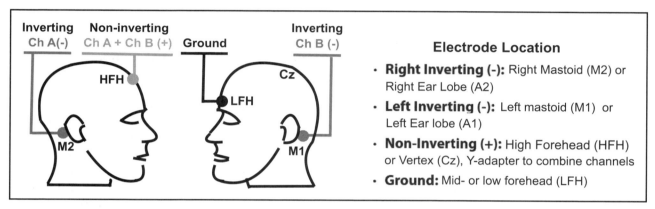

Figure 10–1. Schematic illustration of the inverting and non-inverting electrode locations and their connections to the pre-amplifier inputs from a two channel recording.

Table 10–1. Auditory Brainstem Response (ABR) Absolute Latency and Interpeak Latency (IPL) as a Function of Click-Level Normal Hearing

Intensity (dB nHL)	ABR Component I	ABR Component III	ABR Component V	IPL I–III	IPL III–V	IPL I–V
90	1.72 (0.11)	3.98 (0.17)	5.74 (0.17)	2.25 (0.15)	1.72 (0.12)	3.98 (0.15)
80	1.73 (0.11)	3.98 (0.16)	5.68 (0.18)	2.24 (0.12)	1.70 (0.11)	3.95 (0.12)
70	1.93 (0.11)	4.06 (0.17)	5.86 (0.19)	2.19 (0.16)	1.80 (0.15)	3.99 (0.24)
60	2.25 (0.30)	4.45 (0.30)	6.12 (0.19)	2.25 (0.21)	1.66 (0.31)	3.88 (0.31)
50			6.38 (0.20)			
40			6.74 (0.29)			
30			7.12 (0.32)			
20			7.89 (0.43)			

Note: Standard deviation values for adults are shown in parentheses. The 0.1-ms click stimuli were presented using Etymōtic ER2 insert earphone at 29.9/sec, alternating polarity, amplifier setting of 100–3000 Hz, 1,500 sweeps × 2, and a high-forehead to ipsilateral mastoid recording montage. These latency values are essentially similar to those obtained with an Etymōtic ER-3A insert earphone.

determinants of response latency and amplitude with changes in stimulus intensity.

Lab 2. Effects of Stimulus Intensity on the Broadband Chirp-Evoked ABR

Follow protocol as in Lab 1, except replace clicks with a broadband chirp. Also, compare your results for the chirp-evoked ABR with the click-evoked ABR. Summarize the differences in both latency and amplitude of these responses.

Lab 3. Effects of Stimulus Frequency on Tone Burst-Evoked ABR

Objectives: After this module, students will be able to:

1. Record multiple channel ABRs.
2. Understand the effects of stimulus frequency on the amplitude and latency of the ABR.
3. Understand the physiological bases of the changes in latency and amplitude with manipulation of stimulus frequency.

Stimulus and Recording Parameters

Electrode configuration: Two channels: High forehead-ipsilateral mastoid/high forehead-contralateral mastoid. Two-channels used to improve accuracy of detection of wave V since the contralateral montage shows a clear separation of the IV–V complex.

Intensity: 80 and 40 dB nHL

Transducer: Insert earphones (ER-3C or ER2)

Stimuli: Tone bursts: 500, 1000, 2000, and 4000 Hz with a 2-0-2 ramp using exact Blackman window.

Stimulus polarity: Alternating

Number of sweeps: 1,500. Use 2,000 sweeps at 40 dB nHL to improve SNR and detectability.

Repetition rate: 26.6/sec (fast enough to save time but does not adapt the response)

Amplification: 150,000

Filter setting: 100–3000 Hz (30–3000 Hz at 40 dB nHL to capture the broader wave V waveform better) to improve detectability.

1. Record from six (3 × 2) ears with replication of each condition.
2. Identify and label the components and measure the absolute latency and amplitude of each component across frequencies.

Response Analysis and Lab Report

1. Summarize (for both channels) the effects of frequency on the amplitude and absolute latency of response components using mean plots showing (a) how absolute latency changes with frequency, and level; and (b) how amplitude changes with frequency, and level. Include a plot of exemplar waveform data (with replicates superimposed) as a function of intensity.
2. Compare your two-channel results with known literature (see normative data in Table 10–2). Specify if there were any problems encountered during testing and how they were overcome.
3. Include in your report an explanation for the observed changes in latency and amplitude with changes in frequency and stimulus level in terms of underlying physiological determinants of response latency and amplitude with changes in stimulus frequency.

Normative ABR Tone Burst Data From Adults (Intelligent Hearing Systems Data)

Refer to Table 10–2.

ABR Thresholds and Wave V Normative Latency Values for Narrowband Chirps

Refer to Table 10–3.

Table 10–2. Normative Tone Burst Wave V Latency Data Plotted as a Function of Stimulus Intensity (dB nHL)

Intensity (dB nHL)	Tone Burst Frequency (Hz)			
	500 (SD)	1000 (SD)	2000 (SD)	4000 (SD)
80	9.2 (0.40)	7.7 (0.05)	7.1 (0.05)	6.2 (0.10)
70	9.8 (0.50)	7.9 (0.10)	7.4 (0.10)	6.5 (0.15)
60	10.2 (0.40)	8.0 (0.20)	7.8 (0.15)	6.9 (0.15)
50	10.8 (0.40)	8.9 (0.25)	8.3 (0.15)	7.4 (0.20)
40	11.8 (0.45)	9.7 (0.25)	8.9 (0.35)	7.7 (0.15)
30	13.2 (0.40)	10.9 (0.24)	9.4 (0.25)	8.1 (0.15)
20	14.8 (0.85)	11.9 (0.30)	10.2 (0.25)	8.6 (0.25)
10		12.9 (0.55)	11.1 (0.35)	9.3 (0.25)

Note: Standard deviation values are shown in parentheses. *Stimuli:* tone bursts, exact Blackman window (500 Hz: 8 ms; 1000 and 2000 Hz: 4 ms; 4000 Hz: 2 ms); *repetition rate:* 13.3/s; *filter:* 30–3000 Hz; *amplification:* 100,000.

Table 10–3. ABR Thresholds (dB nHL) and Wave V Latency (ms) Plotted as a Function of Stimulus Level (dB nHL) for Narrowband iChirps

Narrowband iChirps	Threshold (dB nHL)	Wave V Latency (ms) as a Function of Stimulus Intensity (dB nHL)			
		80	60	40	20
500 Hz	20 (4.7)	7.3 (0.1)	8.1 (0.2)	9.3 (0.3)	11.3 (0.4)
1000 Hz	20 (8.1)	7.0 (0.1)	7.7 (0.2)	8.6 (0.2)	10.4 (0.1)
2000 Hz	18 (8.8)	6.2 (0.1)	6.7 (0.1)	7.4 (0.1)	8.7 (0.3)
4000 Hz	21 (8.7)	6.0 (0.1)	6.4 (0.07)	7.2 (0.1)	8.0 (0.2)

Note: Standard deviations are shown in parentheses.
Source: Table data provided by Dr. Rafael Delgado, Intelligent Hearing Systems.

Lab 4. Effects of Stimulus Repetition Rate on the ABR

Objectives: After this module, students will be able to:

1. Record multiple channel ABRs.
2. Understand the effects of stimulus repetition rate on the amplitude and latency of the ABR.
3. Understand the physiological bases of the changes in latency and amplitude with manipulation of stimulus repetition rate.

Stimulus and Recording Parameters

Electrode configuration: Two channels: High forehead-ipsilateral mastoid/high forehead-contralateral mastoid. Two channels used to improve accuracy of detection of wave V since the contralateral montage shows a clear separation of the IV–V complex.

Intensity: 80 and 40 nHL

Transducer: Insert earphones (ER-3A or ER2)

Stimuli: Clicks (0.1-ms duration)

Stimulus polarity: Alternating

Number of sweeps: 1,500. Use 2,000 sweeps at 40 dB nHL to improve SNR and detectability.

Repetition rate: 19.9, 29.9, 49.9, 69.9, and 89.9/sec. Note that a 10-ms analysis window should be used to prevent waveform distortion due to more than one response occurring in a longer analysis window.

Amplification: 150,000

Filter setting: 100–3000 Hz (30–3000 Hz at 40 dB nHL to capture the broader wave V waveform better) to improve detectability.

1. Record from six (3 × 2) ears with replication of each condition.

2. Identify and label the components and measure latency (absolute latency and IPLs) and amplitude of each component.

Response Analysis and Lab Report

1. Summarize (for both channels) the effects of intensity on the amplitude and latency (both absolute latency and IPLs) of response components using mean latency as a function of repetition rate plots and amplitude-repetition rate plots for both levels. Include a plot of exemplar waveform data (with replicates superimposed) as a function of repetition rate.

2. Compare your two-channel results with known literature (see normative data in Table 10–4). Specify if there were any problems encountered during testing and how they were overcome.

3. Include in your report an explanation for the observed changes in latency and amplitude in terms of underlying physiological determinants of response latency and amplitude with stimulus rate manipulation.

Lab 5. Effects of Stimulus Rise-Fall Time

Objectives: After this module, students will be able to:

1. Record multiple channel ABRs.

2. Understand the effects of stimulus rise-fall time on the amplitude and latency of the ABR.

3. Understand the physiological bases of the changes in latency and amplitude with manipulation of stimulus rise-fall times.

Stimulus and Recording Parameters

Electrode configuration: Two channels: High forehead-ipsilateral mastoid/high forehead-

Table 10–4. Normative Latency Values of Auditory Brainstem Response (ABR) Components With Stimulus Rate Manipulation

Rate	ABR Components			IPL		
	I	III	V	I–III	III–V	I–V
23.1	1.73 (0.11)	3.98 (0.16)	5.67 (0.18)	2.24 (0.12)	1.70 (0.11)	3.95 (0.12)
43.1	1.77 (0.12)	4.02 (0.17)	5.87 (0.16)	2.25 (0.13)	1.85 (0.12)	4.10 (0.11)
63.1	1.76 (0.09)	4.10 (0.18)	6.01 (0.19)	2.33 (0.14)	1.92 (0.15)	4.25 (0.16)
83.1	1.83 (0.13)	4.15 (0.18)	6.09 (0.19)	2.36 (0.15)	1.99 (0.19)	4.36 (0.17)

Note: Standard deviation values are shown in parentheses. *Stimulus level:* 80 dB nHL; *transducer:* ER2; *polarity:* alternating; *electrode montage:* high forehead to ipsilateral mastoid; *analog filter setting:* 100–3000 Hz; and *sweeps:* 1,500 × 2.

contralateral mastoid. Two channels are used to improve the accuracy of the detection of wave V, since the contralateral montage shows a clear separation of the IV–V complex.

Intensity: 80 and 40 nHL

Transducer: Insert earphones (ER-3C or ER2)

Stimuli: 4000-Hz tone burst (20-ms long to accommodate the longer rise-fall times.

Stimulus polarity: Alternating

Number of sweeps: 1,500. Use 2,000 sweeps at 40 dB nHL to improve SNR and detectability.

Repetition rate: 29.9/sec

Rise-fall times: 1, 2, 4, 6, 8, and 10 ms

Amplification: 150,000

Filter setting: 100–3000 Hz (30–3000 Hz at 40 dB nHL to capture the broader wave V waveform better) to improve detectability.

1. Record from six (3 × 2) ears with replication of each condition.
2. Identify and label the components and measure absolute latency and IPLs (where possible) and amplitude of each component (where possible).

Response Analysis and Lab Report

1. Summarize (for both channels) the effects of intensity on the amplitude and latency (both absolute latency and IPLs) of response components using mean latency as a function of rise-fall time plots and amplitude–rise-fall time plots for both levels. Include a plot of exemplar waveform data (with replicates superimposed) as a function of rise-fall time.
2. Compare your two-channel results with known literature (see normative data in table). Specify if there were any problems encountered during testing and how they were overcome.
3. Include in your report an explanation for the observed changes in latency and amplitude in terms of underlying physiological determinants of response latency and amplitude with stimulus rise-fall time manipulation.

Lab 6. Effects of Stimulus Onset Polarity on the ABR

Objectives: After this module, students will be able to:

1. Record multiple channel ABRs.
2. Understand the effects of stimulus onset polarity on the amplitude and latency of the ABR.
3. Understand the physiological bases of the changes in latency and amplitude with manipulation of stimulus onset polarity.

Stimulus and Recording Parameters

Electrode configuration: Two channels: High forehead-ipsilateral mastoid/high forehead-contralateral mastoid. Two channels are used to improve the accuracy of the detection of wave V, since the contralateral montage shows a clear separation of the IV–V complex.

Intensity: 80 and 40 nHL

Transducer: Insert earphones (ER-3C or ER2)

Stimuli: Click (0.1 ms), 500 Hz, and 2000 Hz tone bursts with 2-0-2 exact Blackman ramp

Stimulus polarity: Rarefaction, condensation

Number of sweeps: 1,500. Use 2,000 sweeps at 40 dB nHL to improve SNR and detectability.

Repetition rate: 29.9/sec

Amplification: 150,000

Filter setting: 100–3000 Hz (30–3000 Hz at 40 dB nHL to capture the broader wave V waveform better) to improve detectability.

1. Record from six (3 × 2) ears with replication of each condition.
2. Identify and label the components and measure absolute latency and IPLs (where possible) and amplitude of each component (where possible).

Response Analysis and Lab Report

1. Summarize (for both channels) the effects of onset polarity on the amplitude and latency (both absolute latency and IPLs) of response components using mean latency as a function of stimulus onset polarity plots and mean amplitude as a function of onset polarity for both levels. Include a plot of exemplar waveform data (with replicates superimposed) as a function of stimulus polarity across the stimulus.

2. Compare your two-channel results with known literature (see normative data in table). Specify if there were any problems encountered during testing and how they were overcome.

3. Include in your report an explanation for the observed changes in latency and amplitude in terms of underlying physiological determinants of response latency and amplitude with stimulus onset polarity manipulation.

II. EFFECTS OF RECORDING PARAMETERS ON THE ABR

Lab 7. Effects of Number of Sweeps on Averaging the ABR

Objectives: After this module, students will be able to:

1. Record multiple channel ABRs.

2. Understand the effects of the number of sweeps used for averaging on detectability and SNR of the ABR components.

3. Understand the averaging principles that influence detectability and SNR of the recorded ABR components.

Stimulus and Recording Parameters

Electrode configuration: Two channels: High forehead-ipsilateral mastoid/high forehead-contralateral mastoid. Two channels are used to improve the accuracy of the detection of wave V, since the contralateral montage shows a clear separation of the IV–V complex.

Intensity: 80 and 40 dB nHL

Transducer: Insert earphones (ER-3C or ER2)

Stimuli: Click (0.1 ms) and 500-Hz tone bursts with 2-1-2 Blackman ramp.

Stimulus polarity: Alternating

Number of sweeps: 50, 100, 200, 400, 600, 800, 1,000, and 2,000 sweeps.

Repetition rate: 39.9/sec (little adaptation but will reduce test time)

Amplification: 150,000

Filter setting: 100–3000 Hz (30–3000 Hz at 40 dB nHL to capture the broader wave V waveform better) to improve detectability.

1. Record from six (3 × 2) ears with replication of each condition.

2. Identify and label the components and measure absolute latency and IPLs (where possible) and amplitude of each component (where possible).

Response Analysis and Lab Report

1. Summarize (for both channels) the effects of changing sweep numbers on the detectability and SNR of the ABR response components. Generate separate plots showing how the percentage detectability and mean SNR changes (use data from all six ears) with sweeps number for both levels and both channels. Include a plot of exemplar waveform data (with replicates superimposed) as a function of sweep number for both channels and both stimuli.

2. Compare your two-channel results with known literature. Specify if there were any problems encountered during testing and how they were overcome.

3. Include in your report an explanation for the observed changes in detectability and SNR terms of what is predicted by the principles of averaging.

Lab 8. Effects of Recording Electrode Montage

Objectives: After this module, students will be able to:

1. Record multiple channel ABRs.

2. Understand the effects of recording electrode montage on the morphology, response latency, and amplitude of the ABR components.

3. Understand the physiological and/or volume conduction bases of the changes in latency and amplitude with manipulation of electrode montage.

Stimulus and Recording Parameters

Electrode montage: Four-channel recording: High forehead-ipsilateral mastoid; high forehead-contralateral mastoid; contralateral mastoid-ipsilateral; and high forehead-C7. Note that the responses can record two channels at a time if a four-channel system is not available.

Intensity: 80 dB nHL

Transducer: Insert earphones (ER-3C or ER2)

Stimuli: Clicks (0.1 ms)

Stimulus polarity: Alternating

Number of sweeps: 1,500.

Repetition rate: 39.9/sec

Amplification: 150,000

Filter set: 100–3000 Hz

1. Record from six (3 × 2) ears with replication of each condition.

2. Identify and label the components and measure the absolute latency and amplitude of each component.

Response Analysis and Lab Report

1. Summarize (for all channels) the effects of recording montage on the amplitude and latency of response components. Plot mean latency and amplitude as a function of electrode montage. Include a plot of exemplar waveform data (with replicates superimposed) comparing the ABRs recorded using each electrode montage.

2. Compare your four-channel results with known literature. Specify if there were any problems encountered during testing and how they were overcome.

3. Include in your report an explanation for the observed changes in latency and amplitude in terms of underlying physiological and/or volume conduction determinants of response latency and amplitude.

Lab 9. Effects of High-Pass and Low-Pass Analog Filter Settings on the ABR

Objectives: After this module, students will be able to:

1. Record single-channel ABRs using different high-pass and low-pass analog filter settings.

2. Understand the effects of recording electrode montage on the latency and amplitude of the ABR components.

3. Understand that analog filter settings used to record have significant effects on the latency and amplitude of the ABR components.

Stimulus and Recording Parameters

Electrode configuration: Single channel: High forehead-ipsilateral mastoid

Intensity: 80 dB nHL

Transducer: Insert earphones (ER-3C or ER2)

Stimuli: Click (0.1 ms)

Stimulus polarity: Alternating

Number of sweeps: 1,500

Repetition rate: 29.9/sec

Amplification: 150,000

Filter setting:
A. *High-Pass settings: 30, 50, 100, 150, and 300 Hz with low-pass set at a constant 3000 Hz.*
B. *Low-pass settings: 5000, 3000, 1500, 1000, and 500 Hz with the constant high-pass setting of 100 Hz.*

1. Record from six (3 × 2) ears with replication of each filter condition.
2. Identify and label the components and measure absolute latency and amplitude of each component (where possible).

Response Analysis and Lab Report

1. Summarize (for both channels) the effects of analog filter setting on the amplitude and absolute latency of response components. Plot the mean latency and the amplitude of each component as a function of (a) high-pass settings and (b) low-pass settings. Include a plot of exemplar waveform data (with replicates superimposed) as a function of (a) high-pass filter settings and (b) low-pass filter settings.
2. Compare your two results with known literature (see normative data in table). Specify if there were any problems encountered during testing and how they were overcome.
3. Include in your report an explanation for the observed changes in latency and amplitude in terms of effects of phase shifts produced by analog filtering on the ABR latency and amplitude.

III. THRESHOLD ESTIMATION USING THE ABR

Lab 10. Estimation of Air-Conduction Threshold Using Simulated Conductive Hearing Loss

Objectives: After this module, students will be able to:

1. Record single-channel ABRs in individuals with simulated conductive loss.
2. Understand the effects of conductive hearing loss on the ABR components.
3. Understand the physical bases of latency and amplitude change resulting from a conductive hearing loss.

Preliminary Pure-Tone Air-Conduction Threshold Measurements

1. Record air-conduction thresholds at audiometric frequencies with and without earplug in one ear.
2. Record ABRs with replication from two (four ears) subjects under the following conditions:
   A. Obtain pure-tone audiograms without and with earplugs.
   B. Next, obtain ABRs with and without earplugs in place.

Note: **You will have to use oto-block to generate LI function for wave V for each condition.**

Stimulus and Recording Parameters

Electrode montage: Two-channel recording: High forehead-ipsilateral mastoid; and high forehead-contralateral mastoid

Intensity: 80, 70, 60, 50, 40, 30 dB nHL until response threshold.

Transducer: Supra-aural TDH-39 headphones. This transducer enables use of the oto-block to simulate a conductive loss. Note that this lab exercise may be repeated with a bone-conduction transducer to estimate the bone-conduction ABR threshold (BC-ABR), and later comparison with the AC-ABR threshold will provide an estimate of the air-bone gap or the magnitude of the conductive component.

Stimuli: Clicks (0.1 ms)

Stimulus polarity: Alternating

Number of sweeps: 1,500 × 2

Repetition rate: 39.9/sec

Amplification: 150,000

Filter setting: 50–3000 Hz

1. Record from six (3 × 2) ears with replication of each condition.
2. Identify and label the components and measure the absolute latency and amplitude of each component.

Response Analysis and Lab Report

1. Summarize (both channels) the effects of simulated conductive loss on the latency and amplitude of the response components. Plot the mean wave V latency-intensity functions for both the normal (responses obtained without the oto-block) and the simulated conductive loss conditions for both montages, and amplitude as a function of electrode montage.
2. Include a plot of the exemplar waveform data plotted as a function of stimulus intensity for both the unblocked and simulated conductive loss condition.
3. Interpret ABR waveforms and compare the ABR estimate of air-conduction threshold with the pure-tone air-conduction thresholds for the simulated conductive loss. Estimate the magnitude of the conductive loss from the ABR latency-intensity function using the methods described in Chapter 6.
4. Compare your results with known literature. Specify if there were any problems encountered during testing and how they were overcome.
5. Include in your report an explanation for the observed changes in latency and amplitude in terms of underlying physical determinants of response latency and amplitude.

IV. THRESHOLD ASSESSMENT IN BABIES (BIRTH TO SIX MONTHS)

Example of an ABR Protocol for Threshold Estimation in Babies

Preliminary Steps

1. Obtain a brief case history regarding the nature of pregnancy and delivery, other prenatal, and postnatal high-risk factors for hearing loss, family history of hearing loss, and newborn hearing screening results.
2. Perform an otoscopic examination whenever possible. Make note of the baby's movements.
3. Although the focus here is on an ABR protocol for threshold estimation, it is important to complete a comprehensive audiologic evaluation including assessment of middle ear function (immittance) and cochlear function using distortion product otoacoustic emission (DPOAE). DPOAE amplitudes are quite robust in babies and provide a quick frequency-specific functional status of the cochlea. While the presence of DPOAE likely suggests normal hearing, the absence could also result from a middle ear problem.
4. During testing, the baby is either in the mother's lap or resting on the car seat. Depending on how the baby is situated and the access to both ears, it may or may not be possible to place insert earphones in both ears. However, if inserts can be placed in both ears, an ear-switching test approach is possible.

Electrode montage: Single-channel recording using a vertical-ipsilateral montage. Noninverting electrode placed on the vertex or high forehead, inverting/ground electrodes on each mastoid (while testing each ear, the electrode on the contralateral mastoid will serve as the ground electrode). Make sure electrode impedances are below 7000 ohms —remember, the lower the electrode impedance, the better the SNR of the response, and this may reduce test time. It is also important that the impedances at each electrode site are similar (within 2–3 kilo-ohms of each other). Note: if BC-ABR is also planned, then a two-channel electrode montage (vertical-ipsilateral, and vertical contralateral, with the common ground electrode placed an inch below the high forehead electrode) is essential to obtain ear specific BC-ABR thresholds.

Stimulus and Recording Parameters

An appropriate test strategy will assess the functional integrity of the peripheral and brainstem structures and provides ear-specific hearing sensitivity information within a short test time. Make sure that the protocol can be completed in the 25- to 40-minute time window. Thus, it is important to make sure that the optimal stimulus and recording parameters are chosen.

Choice of stimuli: Both broadband clicks and frequency-specific tone bursts (500, 1000, 2000, and 4000 Hz) are chosen to provide optimal measures of functional integrity and frequency-specific threshold estimation, respectively (see Chapter 5 for more details about the frequency-specific tone bursts). Remember that the click stimulus can also provide information that correlates best with behavioral thresholds in the 2000 to 4000 Hz region. However, click ABRs are recorded only at a single high intensity to assess the functional integrity of the auditory nerve and the brainstem to primarily confirm or rule out Auditory Neuropathy Spectrum Disorders (ANSD). The prevalence of ANSD is higher in high-risk infants. This measure will also provide information about the neural maturation state.

Stimulus parameters: All stimuli are presented monaurally via an insert earphone using alternating polarity at a relatively rapid rate of 31.1/sec (to reduce test time). Click stimuli can be presented at 80 or 60 dB nHL. While the higher intensity is preferable for a most robust response, the softer level may prevent causing discomfort and the resulting movement artifacts.

Recording parameters: We recommend a *filter setting* of 30 to 3000 Hz. The lower high-pass filter setting is particularly useful while using tone burst threshold estimation given the broader wave V morphology at low intensities. For click-evoked ABRs at higher intensity, filters can be set to bandpass between 100 and 3000 Hz. If low-frequency electrical noise is distorting the response waveform morphology, then a higher high-pass cutoff should be considered. Unless necessary, the *60-Hz notch filter* should not be enabled. *Amplifier gain* between 100,000 and 150,000 is recommended. The *analysis epoch* for the click-evoked ABR could be as short as 12 to 15 ms. However, for the longer wave V latencies associated with the tone burst elicited ABRs, an *analysis epoch* of about 25 ms is optimal. The *number of sweeps averaged* at higher intensities could be between 1,000 and 2,000 sweeps. However, near the threshold where the SNR is poorer and the response more variable, it is recommended that a higher sweep count for averaging be used—between 2,000 and 2,500 sweeps. All recordings must be replicated to verify the repeatability of the response. The ongoing electroencephalograph (EEG) should be monitored during recording to minimize noisy time segments. *Artifact rejection* should be enabled, and the rejection threshold should be set to a voltage range that will reject about 10% of the total number of sweeps.

Test Procedure

While some clinicians adopt switching ears during testing to ensure that there are data from both ears, others use an approach of testing one ear at a time. Both are reasonable options, but the goal should be to try and obtain complete ear-specific data, which may not be always possible given the short time window for testing in infants. We present a single-ear approach here.

1. Obtain click responses at 80 or 60 dB nHL for each ear first.

2. If the baby is fully asleep, start threshold assessment using a 2000-Hz tone burst (as these high-frequency responses appear to be more affected by movements of an awake baby. If the baby is awake, start with a 500-Hz tone burst followed by 500 then 4000 Hz (to quickly determine if there is a high-frequency hearing loss) and last the 1000 Hz, if time permits. Two sessions may be needed to complete testing.

3. Start testing at 60 dB nHL. If a clear, repeatable response is present, decrease the level in 20-dB steps and obtain ABR at each level. This process will allow you to get to the threshold quickly. If no response, increase level by 20 dB.

4. When you reach a level where there is no response, obtain ABRs with intensity increased in 5-dB steps to approach the threshold. Find the lowest level where you can still identify a repeatable wave V well above the noise floor.

5. To ascertain this, increase the level in 5-dB steps and confirm that wave V amplitude grows and the latency decreases.

6. Repeat Steps 3 through 5 to obtain ABR threshold information at 500 and 4000 Hz next.

7. Repeat Steps 3 through 6 for the other ear.

8. Become familiar with the estimated hearing level (EHL) correction factors for each frequency, and express your results in EHL.

Lab II. Identification and AC-ABR Threshold Estimation From ABR Waveforms Recorded From Infants

ABR waveform data elicited by clicks and tone bursts as a function of intensity are provided from several infants for evaluation and determination of the AC-ABR threshold. A brief history and age at ABR evaluation are also provided.

Objectives: After this module, students will be able to identify the normal morphology of ABR in infants, identify response components, determine whether a response is present or not, and determine the AC-ABR threshold in terms of effective hearing level.

Response Analysis and Lab Report

1. Using the ABR data from each of the five infants, identify the repeatable components, identify the absolute latencies and IPLs (for the click response), and determine the wave V threshold (the lowest level where a repeatable and reliable response is present well above the noise floor). Using the estimated hearing levels, plot the thresholds on an audiogram. Speculate how these estimated auditory steady-state response (ASSR) thresholds will compare with the behavioral thresholds.

2. Compare the latencies with age-appropriate normative (see Table 10–5) to determine if the response latencies are normal and consistent with a normal maturational time course.

3. Write a short report to your referring ENT summarizing the test results and your recommendations.

Case 1 (Simon). History of normal pregnancy and delivery, familial childhood hearing loss, and failed newborn hearing screening. ABR obtained at the age of 4 weeks (Figure 10–2).

Case 2 (Ernie). History of normal pregnancy and delivery; failed newborn hearing screening in both ears. ABR obtained at the age of 6 weeks (Figure 10–3).

Case 3 (Simon). Normal pregnancy and delivery. Family history of hearing loss: older brother identified as an infant and wears hearing aids. Failed newborn hearing screening. ABR obtained at the age of 4 weeks (Figure 10–4).

Case 4 (Maria). Latino family. A baby diagnosed with Down syndrome. Failed newborn hearing screening in both ears. ABR obtained at the age of 4 weeks (Figure 10–5).

Case 5 (Nolan). Normal pregnancy and delivery. Failed newborn hearing screening in the right ear. Initial ABR obtained at age 5 weeks (not reported here) and identified with unilateral hearing loss. Fit with hearing aid in the right ear at age 3½ months but not using it consistently. Regular behavioral testing was attempted every 4–6 months, but Nolan did not condition the task and refused earphones. The left ear continues to be normal with DPOAE present at each assessment. Language development testing at the age of 2 years indicated that Nolan is at 9–12 months for expressive and receptive language. ABRs shown in Figure 10–6 were obtained during naptime at age 2 years and 2 months to reassess hearing status in the right ear.

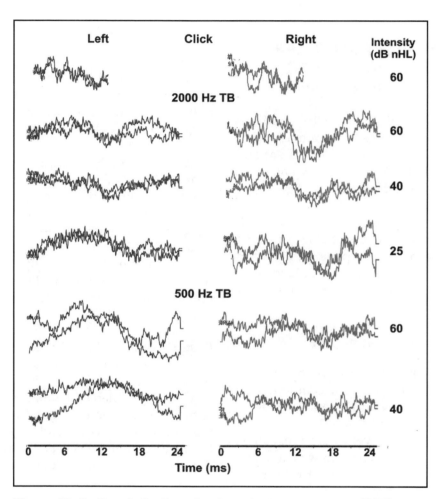

Figure 10–2. Case 1: Replicated auditory brainstem response (ABR) waveforms plotted as function of intensity for clicks (*top*), 2000 Hz tone burst (*middle*), and 500 Hz tone burst (*bottom pairs*) for the left (*black*) and the right ear (*gray*).

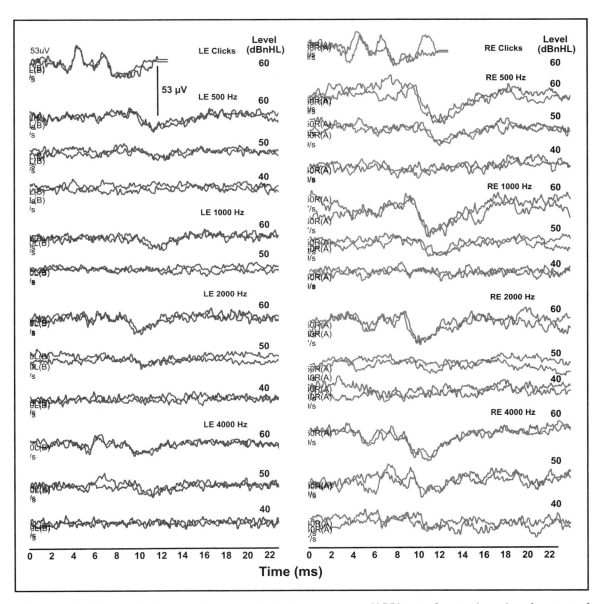

Figure 10–3. Case 2: Replicated auditory brainstem response (ABR) waveforms plotted as function of intensity for clicks (*top panel*), 500 Hz, (*second panel*), 1000 Hz (*third panel*) 2000 Hz (*fourth panel*), and 4000 Hz tone bursts (*bottom panel*) for the left (*black*) and the right ear (*gray*).

352 *Auditory Brainstem Evoked Potentials: Clinical and Research Applications*

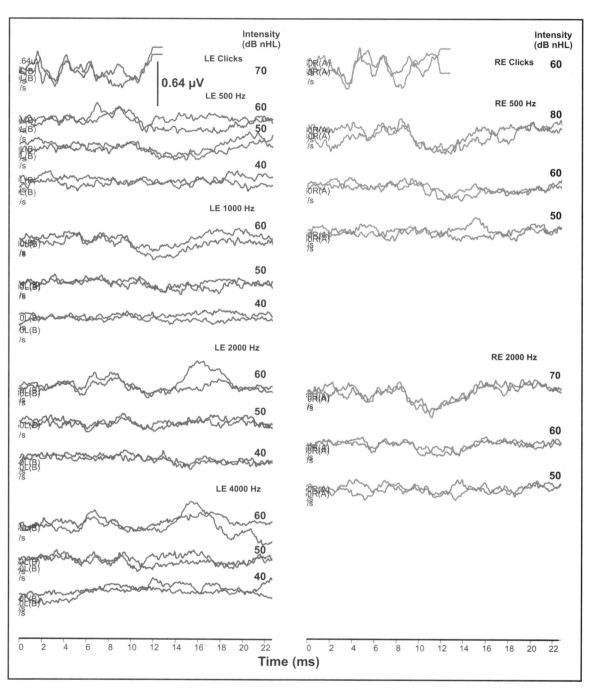

Figure 10–4. Case 3: Replicated auditory brainstem response (ABR) waveforms plotted as function of intensity for clicks (*top panel*), 500 Hz, (*second panel*), 1000 Hz (*third panel*) 2000 Hz (*fourth panel*), and 4000 Hz tone bursts (*bottom panel*) for the left (*black*) and the right ear (*gray*). Note that for the right ear, waveforms are shown for clicks (*top*), 500 Hz (*middle*) and 2000 Hz (*bottom*) tone bursts only.

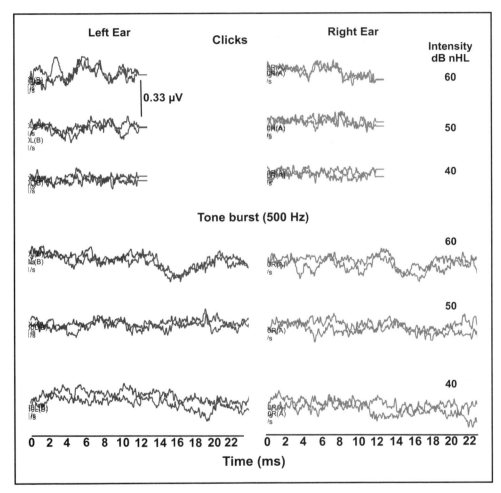

Figure 10–5. Case 4: Replicated auditory brainstem response (ABR) waveforms plotted as function of intensity for clicks (*top*), and 500 Hz tone burst (*bottom*) for the left (*black*) and the right ear (*gray*).

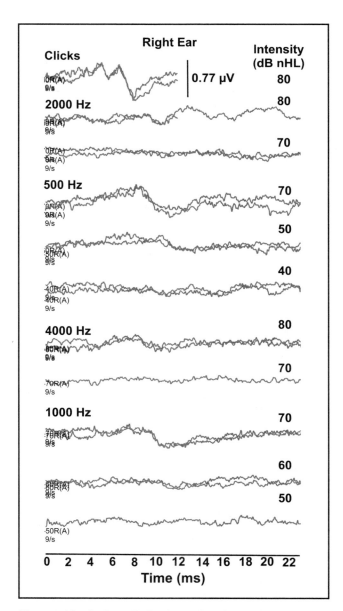

Figure 10–6. Case 5: Replicated auditory brainstem response (ABR) waveforms plotted as function of intensity for clicks (*top panel*), 2000 Hz, (*second panel*), 500 Hz (*third panel*), 4000 Hz (*fourth panel*), and 1000 Hz tone bursts (*bottom panel*) for the right ear only.

Table 10–5. Mean Absolute Latencies for Auditory Brainstem Response (ABR) Waves I, III, and V and Interpeak Latency (IPL) I–V Shown as a Function of Age (in Weeks) at 80, 50, and 30 dB nHL

Age (weeks)	80 I	80 III	80 V	80 I–V	50 I	50 III	50 V	50 I–V	30 I	30 III	30 V	30 I–V
33–34	2.36 (0.81)	5.01 (0.74)	7.38 (0.72)	5.13 (0.67)	3.21 (0.88)	5.79 (0.64)	8.19 (0.56)	4.98 (0.73)	4.17 (1.1)	6.46 (1.0)	8.88 (0.97)	4.71 (0.98)
35–36	2.13 (0.69)	4.47 (0.71)	7.19 (0.72)	5.06 (0.69)	3.18 (0.51)	5.72 (0.84)	8.11 (0.56)	4.93 (0.77)	4.06 (0.95)	6.58 (0.82)	8.77 (0.99)	4.72 (0.87)
37–38	2.02 (0.53)	4.61 (0.47)	7.01 (0.48)	4.99 (0.48)	2.94 (0.64)	5.43 (0.73)	7.65 (0.72)	4.71 (0.68)	3.78 (1.0)	6.31 (0.78)	8.39 (0.88)	4.61 (0.90)
39–40	1.79 (0.59)	4.26 (0.62)	6.72 (0.40)	4.93 (0.59)	2.65 (0.72)	5.01 (0.59)	7.31 (0.53)	4.66 (0.60)	3.59 (0.81)	5.79 (0.84)	8.03 (0.72)	4.44 (0.69)
2 Months	1.64 (0.43)	4.18 (0.32)	6.39 (0.29)	4.75 (0.36)	2.35 (0.44)	4.85 (0.37)	6.91 (0.34)	4.56 (0.37)	3.11 (0.62)	5.64 (0.39)	7.58 (0.48)	4.47 (0.52)
6 Months	1.60 (0.26)	4.10 (0.31)	6.27 (0.21)	4.67 (0.28)	2.28 (0.41)	4.75 (0.37)	6.68 (0.41)	4.40 (0.36)	2.86 (0.61)	5.08 (0.50)	7.20 (0.44)	4.34 (0.42)
12 Months	1.62 (0.24)	3.79 (0.18)	5.93 (0.17)	4.31 (0.19)	2.18 (0.26)	4.43 (0.32)	6.47 (0.21)	4.29 (0.27)	2.90 (0.44)	5.11 (0.51)	7.09 (0.39)	4.19 (0.30)
Adults	1.59 (0.24)	3.64 (0.17)	5.57 (0.16)	3.98 (0.25)	2.23 (0.34)	4.49 (0.18)	6.12 (0.22)	3.89 (0.24)	2.83 (0.36)	5.00 (0.31)	5.79 (0.29)	3.86 (0.30)

Note: The values in parentheses are standard deviations.

Source: Data from Cox. In *The Auditory Brainstem Response*, by J. T. Jacobson (Ed.), 1985. Copyright 1985 by College-Hill Press, San Diego, CA.

Table 10–6. Click Auditory Brainstem Response (ABR) Wave V Latency (ms) Plotted as a Function of Stimulus Intensity for Children Between 12 and 27 Months

Intensity (dB nHL)	12–15 (SD)	15–18 (SD)	18–21 (SD)	21–24 (SD)	24–27 (SD)
80	5.91 (0.27)	5.84 (0.27)	5.74 (0.19)	5.71 (0.26)	5.71 (0.19)
60	6.30 (0.33)	6.24 (0.24)	6.19 (0.18)	6.14 (0.29)	6.09 (0.22)
40	7.10 (0.45)	7.00 (0.38)	6.95 (0.36)	6.79 (0.33)	6.89 (0.29)
20	8.28 (0.60)	8.33 (0.61)	8.22 (0.62)	8.05 (0.58)	8.03 (0.58)

Note: Stimulus: 0.1 ms click; *repetition rate:* 13/s, Beyer DT-48 earphone with circumaural cushion, 0 dB nHL = 30 pe dB SPL; *filter:* 100–3000 Hz; *amplification:* 100,000; *electrode:* vertex to ipsilateral mastoid; *sweeps*; 1,024 × 2.

Source: Data extracted from Gorga et al., 1989.

V. INTERPRETATION OF ABRS TO DETERMINE THE SITE OF LESION

Lab 12. Unmarked ABR Waveform Data (audiograms in some cases)

Unmarked ABR waveform data (audiograms in some cases) elicited by clicks in individuals with the auditory nerve and/or brainstem lesions are provided below.

A brief history for each case is provided.

Objectives: After this module, students will be able to identify the normal morphology of ABR in infants, identify response components, and measure ABR absolute latency, IPLs, ILD, and V/I amplitude ratios. The specific objective of this lab exercise is to apply these response indices to determine if the ABRs are consistent with the normal functional integrity of the auditory nerve and brainstem structures, abnormal and consistent with an auditory nerve or a lower brainstem lesion, or abnormal and consistent with an upper brainstem lesion.

Response Analysis and Lab Report

1. Using the ABR data from each of these cases, identify the repeatable components. Then measure the absolute latency of waves I, III, and V; IPLs I–III, I–V, and III–V; interaural latency difference (ILDv); and the V/I amplitude ratio, where appropriate.

2. What other appropriate stimulus and/or recording parameters manipulation(s) or other tests would you consider to improve the sensitivity of your measure? Please provide a rationale for each choice of audiologic tests or parameters that you would consider for a site of lesion testing. What is the rationale for recommending an ABR (when information is available to address this)?

3. Using the well-established tolerance values for these measures, interpret the ABRs and write a short report to the referring physician (Table 10–7).

4. Write a short report to your referring ENT summarizing the test results and your recommendations.

Case 1. 36-year-old female with a history of tinnitus and occasional vertigo. Hearing sensitivity within normal limits for the right ear with a mild to moderate sloping sensorineural hearing loss in the left ear. Word recognition scores were excellent in the right ear and good in the left ear (Figure 10–7).

Case 2. 36-year-old female with a history of left-sided numbness, tingling in the face, arm, and leg. Also, occasional tinnitus and mild imbalance. Hearing sensitivity was essentially normal bilaterally with excellent word recognition scores. Adapted with permission from Pro-Ed Publishers (Figure 10–8).

Case 3. 12-year-old male. Severe bilateral sensorineural hearing loss. Poor word recognition scores. Adapted with permission from Pro-Ed Publishers (Figure 10–9).

Case 4. 50-year-old male with a history of sudden-onset headaches, slurred speech, and bilateral incoordination. Hearing sensitivity within normal limits bilaterally. Adapted with permission from Pro-Ed Publishers (Figure 10–10).

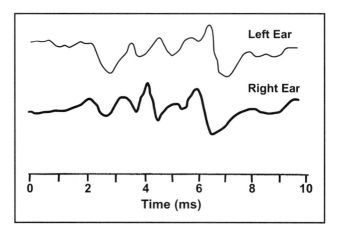

Figure 10–7. Case 1: Auditory brainstem responses (ABRs) elicited by clicks at 80 dB nHL in a 36-year-old female with a history of tinnitus and occasional vertigo. Hearing sensitivity was within normal limits for the right ear with a mild to moderate sloping sensorineural hearing loss in the left ear. Word recognition scores were excellent in the right ear and good in the left ear.

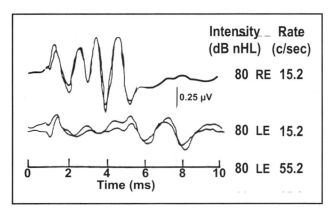

Figure 10–8. Case 2: Auditory brainstem responses (ABRs) elicited by clicks at 80 dB nHL in a 36-year-old female with a history of left-sided numbness, tingling in the face, arm, and leg; also, occasional tinnitus and mild imbalance. Hearing sensitivity was essentially normal bilaterally with excellent word recognition scores. For the left ear responses are also shown at a faster rate (55.2/s) and at a lower intensity (60 dB nHL).

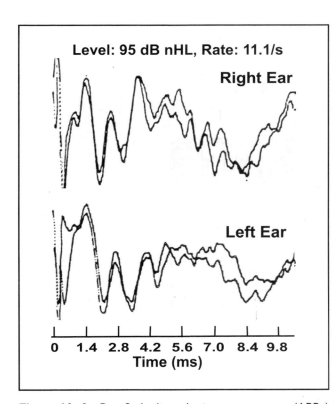

Figure 10–9. Case 3: Auditory brainstem responses (ABRs) elicited by clicks at 95 dB nHL in a 12-year-old male with severe bilateral sensorineural hearing loss. Word recognition scores were poor bilaterally.

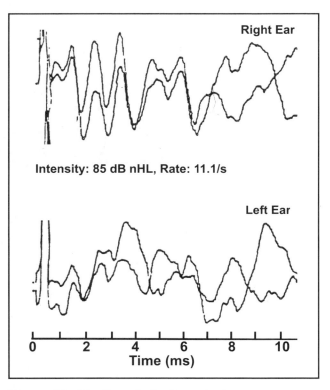

Figure 10–10. Case 4: Auditory brainstem responses (ABRs) elicited by clicks at 85 dB nHL in a 50-year-old male with a history of sudden-onset headaches, slurred speech, and bilateral incoordination. Hearing sensitivity was within normal limits bilaterally.

Case 5. 34-year-old female with a history of neurological symptoms including left extremity weakness, left eyelid twitch, and blurred vision. Hearing sensitivity was within normal limits with excellent word recognition scores. Adapted with permission from Pro-Ed Publishers (Figure 10–11).

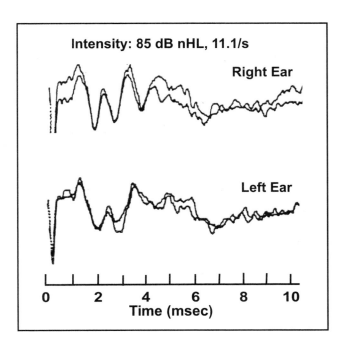

Figure 10–11. Case 5: Auditory brainstem responses (ABRs) elicited by clicks at 85 dB nHL usng a stimulus rate of 11.1/s.

Table 10–7. Tolerance Values for Auditory Brainstem Response (ABR) Indices Used in the Diagnosis of Auditory Nerve and Brainstem Pathology in Adults

ABR	Latency (ms) (SD)	Tolerance Values (2.5 SD)
Absolute		
Wave I	1.67 (0.16)	1.71
Wave III	3.83 (0.12)	4.13
Wave V	5.65 (0.14)	6.00
IPLs		
I–III	2.16 (0.12)	2.46
III–V	1.82 (0.20)	2.32
I–V	3.98 (0.23)	4.56
ILD		
Wave V	0.15 (0.10)	0.4
Amplitude ratio		
V/I	1.60 (0.34)	<0.75

Note: Measurement parameters: *stimulus:* 0.1 ms clicks, 19.9/sec, ER-3A insert earphone, level +80 db nHL, 0 dB nHL = 32 pe SPL acquisition; *filters:* 100–3000 Hz; *amplification:* 150,000; *sweeps:* 2 × 1,500; *analysis time:* 25 ms; *electrodes:* high-forehead to ipsilateral mastoid.

VI. RECORDING OF AUDITORY STEADY-STATE RESPONSE, ENVELOPE FOLLOWING RESPONSE, AND FREQUENCY FOLLOWING RESPONSE

Lab 13. Recording and Analysis of ASSR

Objectives: After this module, students will be able to:

1. Record single-channel ASSRs using single and multifrequency monaural and binaural stimulation at different modulation rates.
2. Analyze and interpret ASSR data for threshold estimation.
3. Understand the effects of mode of stimulation (monaural versus binaural) on the ASSR, and the effects of modulation frequency on the ASSR.

Stimulus and Recording Parameters

Electrode configuration: Single channel: high forehead-C7.

Intensity:
Single-frequency ASSR: 60 dB nHL, 80 dB nHL
Multifrequency ASSR: 60, 50, 40, and 30 dB nHL

Transducer: Insert earphones (ER-3C or ER2)

Stimuli:
1. Single-frequency ASSR: 500 Hz and 4000 Hz
   Modulation rates: Low (40–50 Hz), Mid (55–75 Hz), High (80–105 Hz)
   Stimulus mode: Monaural
2. Multifrequency ASSR: 500, 1000, 2000, and 4000 Hz with multiple modulation frequencies —use default
   Stimulus mode: Binaural

Filter setting: 30–1000 Hz

Stimulus polarity: Alternating

Number of sweeps: 1,500 × 2

Amplification: 100,000

Record from six individuals with normal hearing sensitivity ears with replication of each condition.

Response Analysis and Lab Report

1. Perform spectral analysis to determine the presence or absence of response at the modulation frequency, and a phasor analysis to determine the goodness of phase-locking (phase coherence).
2. Plot the ASSR thresholds (the lowest level at which a response peak was observed in the spectrum) on the audiogram to the estimated threshold.
3. Compare the results for the binaural and monaural ASSRs. Also, compare your results with the ASSR threshold literature.

Lab 14. Recording and Analysis of EFRs and FFRs

Objectives: After the conclusion of this module, students will be able to:

1. Record single-channel EFRs and FFRs using a speech syllable and a complex tone.
2. Analyze and interpret EFR and FFR data.
3. Understand the difference between EFRs and FFRs in terms of the auditory information they represent.

Stimulus and Recording Parameters

Electrode configuration: Two channels: high forehead-C7, and contralateral to ipsilateral mastoid

Intensity: 80 dB nHL

Transducer: Magnetically shielded insert earphones (ER-3A or 3C or ER2)

Stimuli: Speech syllables /ba/ and /da/; complex tone (f0 = 100 Hz) 160-ms duration, monaural presentation

Repetition rate: 4.3/sec

Filter setting: 50–3000 Hz

Stimulus polarity: Alternating

Number of sweeps: 1,000 × 2

Amplification: 100,000

1. Record from six individuals with normal hearing sensitivity ears with replication of each condition.

Response Analysis and Lab Report

1. Response Analysis
   i. Obtain the EFR using the average to the alternating polarity (response to condensation response to rarefaction onset polarity). Perform a spectrum analysis on each EFR, and measure the magnitude of the spectral peak at F0. Compare this measure across the three stimuli, montage, and between ears.
   ii. Obtain the FFR by subtracting the responses to the condensation and rarefaction polarities (split buffer averaging will save response to each polarity in different buffers). Perform a spectrum analysis on each FFR and measure the magnitude of the spectral peaks at F0 and F1 (harmonic close to the first formant frequency for the speech stimuli). Compare this measure across the three stimuli, montage, and between ears.
2. Plot the grand averaged response waveform of the EFR and the FFR and their spectra.
3. Compare and contrast the EFR and FFR results using the relevant literature for each.

Troubleshooting Common Problems Encountered During Data Acquisition

ABR recording in an electrically and acoustically quiet environment is relatively easy and quite straightforward and does not usually create problems if all the required steps and procedures are followed. However, from time to time, certain problems related to tester errors, test environment, and/or equipment malfunction may pose challenges to recording a clean, repeatable, and interpretable response. Some of the problems commonly experienced, their possible causal origin(s), and solutions are summarized in Table 10–8. It is important to become familiar with the origin of these problems and how they can be resolved so that ABRs can be recorded successfully in a test session.

VII. PROTOCOL CONSIDERATION FOR ELECTROCOCHLEOGRAPHY (ECochG)

Reliable and diagnostically useful information using the cochlear receptor potentials and the whole nerve action potential is limited to invasive approaches using the transtympanic needle electrode and therefore can only be performed by a physician. The noninvasive methods available for audiologists include the use of intrameatal TM electrode or the TIPtrode. While the TM electrode does produce a large action potential (AP) and robust cochlear receptor potentials, there is no reliable, easy way to position and stabilize (other than compression of the electrode cable by the foam tip of the insert earphone as the cable exits the ear canal) the position of the TM electrode. The response amplitude is also quite variable. The clinical validity of this approach is not confirmed. Last, the use of a TIPtrode, the least invasive method (not listed in Table 10–9), is not an effective method to evaluate cochlear potentials since it does not produce robust responses. See Chapter 7 for more details about ECochG. The stimulus and recording considerations for ECochG are summarized in Table 10–9.

VIII. SUMMARY

- It is very important to obtain hands-on experience in recording, analyzing, and interpreting these brainstem responses to not only reinforce the relevant theoretical concepts presented in the classroom but also to reinforce optimal recording skills to obtain reliable recordings to facilitate the interpretation of the results required for accurate clinical diagnosis.

- This experience should help the student to become familiar with the normal response morphology and how stimulus and recording factors alter the ABR response indices in individuals with normal hearing sensitivity.

- As part of the preliminary considerations, clinicians should know the operation and

Table 10–8. Commonly Encountered Auditory Brainstem Response (ABR) Recording Problems and Solutions

Problem	Cause(s)	Solution(s)
No response	No stimulus	Listening check to make sure stimulus is on. Select correct transducer.
	The amplifier is off	Turn amplifier on.
Noisy recording with poor signal-to-noise ratio of the ABR	High electrode impedance	Make sure all electrode impedances are less than 5000 ohms.
	High-frequency interference	Keep test room electrically isolated from other electrical equipment. Turn the light off in the test room. Use braided electrode cables to cancel interfering signals. Use odd stimulus rates to reduce entrainment.
	Degraded or faulty electrode	Check integrity of electrical continuity of the electrode cables.
	Movement artifact	Reinstruct to relax and refrain from extraneous movements.
	Electrode(s) displaced	Check and replace displaced electrode(s).
Periodic peaks with 2-ms interval in the first six milliseconds	500-Hz tone burst stimulus artifact Cochlear microphonic?	Use alternating stimulus polarity to cancel artifact/CM or use magnetically shielded earphones.
Large peak biphasic peaks in the first two milliseconds in the average	Click stimulus artifact	Same as above.
ABR waves I, III, and V are inverted	Inverting and noninverting electrode inputs switched	Check and correct this or simply invert the using software.
Wave I absent at high intensity in an individual with normal hearing	Response recorded with contralateral montage	Switch noninverting input electrode to ipsilateral mastoid.
Only delayed wave V (8 ms) present at 90 dB nHL in an ear with significant hearing loss	Brainstem lesion or contralateralized response	Need to repeat ABR with masking in the nontest ear to rule out contralateralization.
The average count remains unchanged	Artifact rejection threshold set too low	Reinstruct and set artifact rejection threshold to a higher level to achieve 10% rejection.
Only a large response component is visualized in the 12–14 ms time range	Dominant postauricular muscle response scaling down the ABR amplitude	Reinstruct to relax. Consider using earlobe, or preauricular, or C7 electrode as noninverting electrode. Set analysis window to 10 ms.
Large sine wave with a 16.67-period artifact	60 Hz power line	Electrical grounding issues should be resolved. Increase high-pass filter setting (100 Hz). 60-Hz notch filter—last resort.

Table 10–9. Stimulus and Recording Parameters for Electrocochleography (ECochG)

Choice of Stimuli and Parameters	
Clicks:	Best for eliciting onset responses. However, CM and SP are of very short duration and may not be a reliable clinical measure for diagnosing Ménière disease. Receptor potentials (CM and SP) are detectable only above about 55–60 dB nHL.
Tone bursts:	Use of longer-duration (2 ms rise-fall time and a 12-ms plateau duration) tone bursts of different frequencies (1000, 2000, 4000, and 8000 Hz) has been shown to provide quick, easy to record, reliable, and diagnostically reliable information to confirm the presence or absence of Ménière disease.
Transducer:	ER-3A or ER2. ER2 will enable recording of higher frequencies up to 12 kHz
Intensity:	60, 70, 80, and 90 dB nHL. The responses are more robust at higher levels.
Polarity:	Alternating
Rate:	7.1/s to 13.1/s for clicks. 30.1/s for tone bursts. Slower rates will generate more robust responses.
Recording Parameters	
Electrodes:	
Transtympanic needle electrode:	Invasive. Placed on the round-window niche or promontory (TT: ipsilateral mastoid; Fpz: ground). Most reliable approach. Largest amplitude because it is closer to the generators. Short acquisition time (100–200 sweeps).
Intrameatal tympanic membrane electrode:	Noninvasive. Electrode at TM (TM: ipsilateral mastoid; Fpz: ground). Large amplitude but not as large as TT approach. Not an easy task to place the electrode, and there is potential for TM perforation. Response amplitude quite variable. Diagnostic utility is not validated. Longer test time (500–1,500 sweeps).
Filter:	50–2500 Hz. Need higher low-frequency cutoff for higher-frequency tone bursts.
Amplification:	75,000–100,000×. Need more amplification as the electrode is farther away from the generator.
Analysis epoch:	5–15 ms, longer if ABR is also recorded simultaneously.

minor maintenance of their equipment, and the test protocol(s) to be used to address specific clinical questions. Most commercial systems are intuitive and user friendly and provide easy-to-use interactive software with easy control of the stimulus and recording properties. Ensure proper and stable placement of electrodes with impedances close to 1000 ohms.

- Follow all recommended procedures for ABR recording to obtain a response with good SNR. Always replicate recordings to ensure repeatability and validity of the measure.

- As a good practice, always set the equipment back to its default condition after each use to help other users of the equipment. Turn off the recording amplifiers after use so the battery is not drained, and clean the electrodes promptly after each use.

- While removing the electrodes, do not pull on the electrode cables to remove the electrode. Instead, gently peel the tape off with the electrode to avoid damaging the functional integrity of the cable, and therefore the electrode.
- Become familiar with the causes and remedies for commonly encountered problems while recording the ABR.

IX. RECOMMENDED READING

Burkard, R. F., (2007). Auditory evoked potential laboratory exercises. In R. F. Burkard, M. Don, & J. J. Eggermont (Eds.), *Auditory evoked potentials: Basic principles and clinical applications* (Chapter 32, pp. 672–693). Baltimore, MD: Lippincott Williams & Wilkins.

INDEX

Note: Page numbers in **bold** reference non-text material.

A

A-ABR. *See* Automated auditory brainstem response
ABR. *See* Auditory brainstem response
Absolute latency
  of auditory brainstem response
    changes in, **55**
    in conductive hearing loss, 126
    definition of, 52
    description of, 53
    determinants, 52
    frequency-induced, 58–59
    intensity-induced, 56–57
    onset polarity-induced differences, 61–63
    rise time-induced changes in, 63–64
    stimulus intensity effects on, **55**, 56–57, **339**
    stimulus rate-induced, 60–61
    wave V, **55**
  of auditory evoked potentials, 27
Absolute refractory period, 21
AC-EFR. *See* Air-conduction envelope following response
Acetylcholine, 23
Acoustic neuroma
  cochlear dysfunction caused by, 189
  cochlear hearing loss versus, **144**
  compound action potential findings in, 189
  description of, 140–141
  middle fossa surgical approach to, 199–200
Action potential
  definition of, 19
  depolarizing phase of, 21
  generation of, 21
  hyperpolarization, 21
  propagation of, 21–23, **22**
  repolarization phase of, 21
ADC. *See* Analog-to-digital converter
AEPs. *See* Auditory evoked potential(s)
Age
  conceptual, 70–71
  sinusoidally amplitude modulated tones affected by, 226–227
Aging, 73
Air-conduction envelope following response, 227–229
Air conduction thresholds
  behavioral threshold correction factors, **102**
  bone-conduction ABR threshold estimates affected by, 108–109
  estimation of, 106, 108–110, 349, **350–355**
  frequency-specific tone bursts for, 107
  high-pass filter settings, 107
  laboratory exercises, 346–347
  narrowband chirp stimuli to estimate, 111–112, **113**
  protocols, 106
  simulated conductive hearing loss for estimating of, 346–347
ALGO1, 88, **89**
ALGO2, 89
ALGO3, 89
ALGO5, 89–90
Aliasing, 41
AMLR. *See* Auditory middle latency response
Amplitude, of auditory brainstem response
  body temperature effects on, 74
  in conductive hearing loss, 126
  contributing factors to, 53–54
  description of, 53–54
  frequency-induced change in, 58–59
  physiological determinants, 53
  sex differences in, 73–74
  stimulus rate-induced change in, 60–61
Amplitude ratio, 53
Amplitude resolution, 42
AN-CAP. *See* Auditory nerve compound action potential
Analog filter, 41
Analog filtering, 67
Analog-to-digital conversion, 41–43, **42**
Analog-to-digital converter, 41

Analysis time, 43
ANF. *See* Auditory nerve fibers
ANOW. *See* Auditory nerve overlapped waveform
Anterior ventral cochlear nucleus
   description of, 5, 7, 9
   posterior portion of, 7
AP. *See* Action potential
Artifact rejection, 44
Audiometric zero, 37
Auditory brainstem, 130–132
Auditory brainstem response
   absolute latency of
      changes in, **55**
      in conductive hearing loss, 126
      definition of, 52
      description of, 53
      determinants, 52
      frequency-induced, 58–59
      intensity-induced, 56–57
      onset polarity-induced differences, 61–63
      rise time-induced changes in, 63–64
      stimulus intensity effects on, **55**, 56–57, **339**
      stimulus rate-induced, 60–61
      wave V, **55**
   age effects on, 70, 73
   air conduction
      description of, 34–35
      insert earphones for, 34–35
   air conduction thresholds
      behavioral threshold correction factors, **102**
      bone-conduction ABR threshold estimates affected by, 108–109
      estimation of, 106, 108–110, 349, **350–355**
      frequency-specific tone bursts for, 107
      high-pass filter settings, 107
      laboratory exercises, 346–347
      narrowband chirp stimuli to estimate, 111–112, **113**
      protocols, 106
      simulated conductive hearing loss for estimating of, 346–347
   alternating polarity, 62
   amplitude of
      body temperature effects on, 74
      in conductive hearing loss, 126
      contributing factors to, 53–54
      description of, 53–54
      frequency-induced change in, 58–59
      physiological determinants, 53
      sex differences in, 73–74
      stimulus rate-induced change in, 60–61
   analog filtering, 67

   in auditory nerve lesions/tumors. *See* Auditory nerve lesions/tumors, auditory brainstem response in
   in auditory neuropathy, 110–111, 153–155, **154**, 179
   auditory steady-state response and, 112–116, **115**
   automated, for hearing screening
      conventional approach, 87–88
      description of, 85, 87–88
      devices, 88
      efficacy of, 93
      frequency-domain algorithms, 90–92
      hearing loss in babies, 93–94
      otoacoustic emissions versus, 87, 92–93
      PASS-REFER criteria, **88**, 88–89
      stimulus intensity calibration issues, 94
      time-domain approach, 88–90
   averaging of, sweeps for, 344
   background noise in test environment, 70
   band-pass filter
      high-frequency cutoff of, 68, **68–69**
      low-frequency cutoff of, 67, **68–69**
   body temperature effects on, 74
   bone conduction
      bone vibrator for recording, 35
      description of, 35
   bone conduction thresholds
      air-conduction thresholds and, 108
      cochlear status assessments, 126
      estimation of, 103–110
      frequency-specific tone bursts, 103–107
      high-pass filter settings, 107
      limitations of, 110
      narrowband chirp stimuli to estimate, 111–112, **113**
      protocols, 106
   in brainstem lesions
      characteristics of, 139
      differential diagnosis uses of, 140, **144**
      interpeak latencies, 141–142
      laboratory exercises for, 356–358, **356–358**
      onset polarity, 163
      repetition rate, 163
      sensitivity of, 143–145, **144**
      stacked, 145–150
      stimulus, 162–163
      test strategy, 162–164
      transducer, 163
      tumor size and, 151
      V/I amplitude ratio, 152–153
   chirp-evoked
      acoustic waveforms for, **33**
      broadband, 32–34, 149–150, 340

narrowband, 111–112, **113**, **341**
chronic middle ear infection effects on, 129–130,
    130
click-evoked
    acoustic waveforms for, **33**
    auditory neuropathy identification using,
        110–111
    description of, 32, 110–111, 204
    narrowband responses using high-pass masking
        noise on, 96–98
    stacked ABR versus, **150**
    stimulus intensity of, 338–340
    tone burst ABR versus, **150**
clinical applications of
    auditory neuropathy, 110–111
    hearing screening. *See* Hearing screening
    neuro-otologic, 83
    overview of, 83
in cochlear hearing loss
    acoustic neuroma versus, **144**
    characteristics of, 133
    interpeak latencies, 138–139
    latency shift, 133–134
    wave V latency-intensity function, 135–138, **136**
in cochlear synaptopathy, **155**, 155–161, **157–158**,
    160
components of
    analog filter setting effects on, 67
    description of, 47–48
    neural generators of, 48–49
    wave I, 50, **62**
    wave II, 50
    wave III, 50, **62**
    wave IV, 51
    wave V, 51, **62**
conceptual age, 70–71
in conductive hearing loss, 125–132, **127**, **129**
description of, 3, 27
detection criteria for, 109–110
digital filtering, 68–70
electrical
    analysis of, 197–198
    artifacts, 198
    cochlear implant evaluation uses of, 194–198
    data acquisition methods, 198
    electrical stimulation methods for, 197–198
    recording montage for, 198
    recording of, 197–198
    response amplitude of, 196, **197**
    response analysis, 198
    response characteristics of, 195–196, **195–196**
    response latency of, 195–196
    thresholds, 196
    waveform morphology, 195, **195**
electrodes
    configuration of, 64–65, 345
    description of, 38–39, **39**
    montage, 64–65, 261–264
    placement of, **65**, 107
    10-20 placement system, **65**
envelope following response versus, 219
frequency following response versus, 241
frequency-specific threshold estimation
    air-conduction threshold, 100–103
    auditory steady-state response for, 112–116
    bone-conduction threshold, 103
    frequency-specific tone bursts, 100–103, **102**
    frequency specificity, 96
    narrowband responses using high-pass masking
        noise on clicked-evoked ABRs, 96–98, **97**
    notched noise masking for ensuring place
        specificity of, 98–100
    overview of, 95–96
    place specificity, 96
generators, 48–49, 51–52
high-pass filter settings, 107, 345–346
indices, 52–53
in infants, **71**, 112
interaural latency difference of
    in auditory nerve lesions, 142–143
    description of, 53
    stacked ABR technique, 149
    in wave V, 142–143
interpeak latencies of
    in acoustic neuroma, 141
    in auditory nerve lesions, 141–142
    cochlear hearing loss effects on, 138–139
    description of, 53
    stimulus intensity, **339**
intracranial, 50–51
laboratory exercises
    auditory nerve lesion/tumor site determination,
        356–358, **356–358**
    recording parameters, 344–346
    stimulus factors, 338–344
    threshold assessment in infants, 347–355,
        350–355
    threshold estimation, 346–347
latency-intensity function of, 54, **55**
latency of
    absolute. *See* Auditory brainstem response,
        absolute latency of
    body temperature effects on, 74
    description of, 53

Auditory brainstem response *(continued)*
  latency of *(continued)*
    frequency-induced changes in, 58–59
    intensity-induced changes in, **55**, 56–57
    interpeak. *See* Auditory brainstem response, interpeak latencies of
    onset polarity-induced differences in, 61–63
    physiological determinants, 53
    rise time-induced changes in, 63–64
    sex differences in, 73–74
  low-pass filter settings, 345–346
  middle ear infection effects on, 129–130, **130**
  in multiple sclerosis, **162**
  neural conduction time, 53
  neural generators, 48–49, 51–52
  neural maturation of, 70–73, **71–72**
  in older adults, 73
  onset polarity
    in auditory nerve lesion evaluation, 163
    description of, 61–63
    laboratory exercises involving, 343–344
  place specificity of, notched noise masking for ensuring, 98–100
  protocols, for threshold estimation, 106
  recording of
    in auditory nerve and brainstem lesion evaluations, 163–164
    electrodes, 38–39, **39**, 64–65, 163–164, 345
    horizontal, 66–67
    laboratory exercises involving, 344–346
    montage, 64–65, 107, 345
    preliminary considerations for, 337–338
    problems involving, **361**
    troubleshooting of, **361**
    vertical, 66–67
    vertical-contralateral, 65–66, **66**, 163
    vertical-ipsilateral, 65–66, **66**, 163
  response morphology of, 47–48
  scalp-recorded
    description of, 47, 175
    electrical auditory brainstem responses, 194
    latency correspondence, 50–51
  sex differences in, 73–74
  stacked derived narrowband
    acoustic tumor detection using, 145–150
    chirp stimuli for, 162
  stimulus
    absolute latency affected by intensity of, **55**, 56–57
    for auditory nerve and brainstem lesion detection, 162–163
    chirps. *See* Auditory brainstem response, chirp-evoked
    clicks. *See* Auditory brainstem response, click-evoked
    description of, 31–32
    frequency of, 57–59
    intensity of, 35–36, 54–56, 162–163
    laboratory exercises involving, 338–344
    onset polarity of, 61–62, **62**, 163, 343–344
    repetition rate, 59–60, **59–60**, 163, 341–342
    rise-fall time, 34, **34**, 63–64, 342–343
    tone bursts. *See* Auditory brainstem response, tone burst-evoked
  stimulus section, 31–38
  subject factors, 70–74
  tone burst-evoked
    air conduction threshold estimations using, 100–103
    bone conduction threshold estimations using, 103–106
    click-evoked ABR versus, **150**
    description of, 34, **34**
    frequency of, 57–58
    laboratory exercises, 340, **341**
    notched noise masking effects on, 99
    stacked ABR versus, **150**
    waveform for, **34**
  transducers
    for auditory nerve and brainstem lesion evaluations, 163
    types of, 34–35
  in upper brainstem lesions, 161–162
  V/I amplitude ratio, 152–153, 157
  waveform of, 74–75, **350–354**
    idealized, **48**, **50**
    in infants, **71**
    morphology of, 48
Auditory cortex, 310
Auditory evoked potential(s)
  classification of, **28**, 28–29
  differential amplification, 39–41, **40**
  embedded, 42
  envelope following response. *See* Envelope following response
  exogenous, 29
  filtering, 41
  frequency following response. *See* Frequency following response
  late, 28
  latency-based categories of, 28, **28**
  neural activity-based classification of, 29
  temporal sequence of, 27–28
Auditory evoked potential zero, 37
Auditory middle latency response, 28

Auditory nerve
  auditory brainstem responses generated by, 50–51
  bifurcation of, 7, **7**
  dysfunction/impairment of, 110
  formation of, 5, **6**
  Type I and II fibers of, 7
Auditory nerve compound action potential
  auditory nerve stretching effects on, **202**
  characteristics of, 201–202
  description of, 175
  intraoperative monitoring uses of, 206
  recording of, 200–201
  sequence of, **207–208**
  in vestibular schwannoma surgery, **203**, **207**
  waveform of, 201
Auditory nerve fibers, 61, 176, 185, 194, 220, 247
Auditory nerve lesions/tumors
  acoustic neuroma, 140
  auditory brainstem response in
    characteristics of, 139
    differential diagnosis uses of, 140, **144**
    interpeak latencies, 141–142
    laboratory exercises for, 356–358, **356–358**
    onset polarity, 163
    repetition rate, 163
    sensitivity of, 143–145, **144**
    stacked, 145–150
    stimulus, 162–163
    test strategy, 162–164
    transducer, 163
    tumor size and, 151
    V/I amplitude ratio, 152–153
  bilateral effects of, 151–152
  intraoperative monitoring of, 199–200, 209
  size of, 151
  surgical approaches for
    description of, 199–200
    middle fossa, 199, **199**
    retrosigmoidal, 200, **200**
    translabyrinthine, 199
  vestibular schwannoma, 140, **140**, **203**, **207**
Auditory nerve overlapped waveform, **188**, 188–189, 209
Auditory nerve stretching, 209
Auditory neuropathy
  auditory brainstem responses in, 110–111, 153–155, **154**, 179
  cochlear microphonic in, 179
  compound action potential in, 179
Auditory neuropathy spectrum disorders, 85
Auditory steady-state response
  amplitude of, **225**
  analysis of, 359
  auditory brainstem response and, 112–116, **115**
  auditory brainstem response versus, 112
  frequency-specific threshold estimation using, 112–116
  hearing screening uses of, 116
  laboratory exercises, 359
  recording of, 359
Auditory stream segregation, 317
Aural atresia, 126
Autocorrelation function, 266, **285**, **292–293**
Autocorrelogram, 266, **296**, **297**
Automated auditory brainstem response, for hearing screening
  conventional approach, 87–88
  description of, 85, 87–88, 228
  devices, 88
  efficacy of, 93
  frequency-domain algorithms, 90–92
  hearing loss in babies, 93–94
  otoacoustic emissions versus, 87, 92–93
  PASS-REFER criteria, **88**, 88–89
  stimulus intensity calibration issues, 94
  time-domain approach, 88–90
AVCN. *See* Anterior ventral cochlear nucleus
Axon(s)
  anatomy of, 19, **20**
  myelinated, **22**
  neural conduction in, **22**
  unmyelinated, **22**
Axon hillock, 24
Axonal action potential, 192

B

Background noise, 70, 296, 298–300, 307
Band-pass filter
  high-frequency cutoff of, 68, **68–69**
  low-frequency cutoff of, 67, **68–69**
Basilar membrane
  anatomy of, 2
  excitation of, 134
  functions of, 1
  stiffness of, **3**, 190
  width of, **3**
Bekesy traveling wave envelope, **3**
BERAphone, 90–91, 93
Binaural interaction, 314, **315**
Binaural masking level difference, 130, 314–317, **316**
Binaural neurons, 131
Binaural processing, 314–320
Bipolar neurons, 4

Blackman window, 34, **34**, 107
BMLD. *See* Binaural masking level difference
Body temperature, auditory brainstem response affected by, 74
Bone-conduction envelope following response, 231–232
Bone conduction thresholds
　air-conduction thresholds and, 108
　cochlear status assessments, 126
　estimation of, 103–110
　frequency-specific tone bursts, 103–107
　high-pass filter settings, 107
　limitations of, 110
　narrowband chirp stimuli to estimate, 111–112, **113**
　protocols, 106
Bone vibrators, 35
Brainstem
　auditory, conductive hearing loss effects on, 130–132
　experience-dependent effects in, 304–306
　language experience-dependent effects in, 303–304
　organization of, 5–7, **6**
　pathways of, 5–7, **6**
　pitch processing in, 302
　in speech/language processing, 301
　structures of, 5–7, **6**
Brainstem evoked responses
　envelope following response. *See* Envelope following response
　frequency following response. *See* Frequency following response
　overview of, 219–220
Brainstem lesions. *See also* Auditory nerve lesions/tumors
　auditory brainstem response in
　　characteristics of, 139
　　generators, 51–52
　　stimulus parameters for, 162–163
　bilateral effects of, 151–152
　upper, 161–162
Broadband chirp-evoked auditory brainstem response, 32–34, 149–150, 340

C

CAP. *See* Compound action potential
Carrier frequency, 224–225
Central auditory processing disorders, 317
Central nucleus of the inferior colliculus, 8, 10, 12–13, **14**
Cerebellopontine angle, 50, 139–140, 200, 295
Cerebellopontine angle tumors, 205

Cerebral cortex, 309
CHAMP. *See* Cochlear hydrops analysis masking procedure
Chirps
　auditory brainstem response evoked with
　　acoustic waveforms for, **33**
　　broadband, 32–34, 149–150, 340
　　narrowband, 111–112, **113**, 341
　stacked derived narrowband auditory brainstem response evoked with, 162
CHL. *See* Conductive hearing loss
CIs. *See* Cochlear implants
Clicks
　auditory brainstem response evoked with
　　acoustic waveforms for, **33**
　　auditory neuropathy identification using, 110–111
　　description of, 32, 110–111, 204
　　narrowband responses using high-pass masking noise on, 96–98
　　stacked ABR versus, **150**
　　stimulus intensity of, 338–340
　　tone burst ABR versus, **150**
　compound action potential evoked using, 185–186
　description of, 32, **33**
　notched noise masking with, 99–100
CM. *See* Cochlear microphonic
CMRR. *See* Common mode rejection ratio
CN-CAP. *See* Cochlear nucleus compound action potential
CNIC. *See* Central nucleus of the inferior colliculus
Cochlea
　afferent innervation of, 4–5
　dysfunction of, 189
　efferent innervation of, 14, **15**
　lesions of, hearing losses caused by, 189
　structure of, 1–4
Cochlear amplification, 3
Cochlear amplifier, 3
Cochlear hearing loss
　air-conduction and bone-conduction EFR uses in, 231
　auditory brainstem response in
　　acoustic neuroma versus, **144**
　　characteristics of, 133
　　interpeak latencies, 138–139
　　latency shift, 133–134
　　wave V latency-intensity function, 135–138, **136**
　cochlear microphonic in, 179, **180**
　compound action potential in, 179
Cochlear hydrops analysis masking procedure, 190–191

Cochlear impairment
 envelope encoding affected by, 237–238
 frequency following response evaluation of, 257
Cochlear implants
 auditory perception in, 193
 description of, 154–155
 electrical auditory brainstem response application in, 194–198
 electrically evoked compound action potential application in, 193–194
 spectral resolution in, 193
Cochlear microphonic. *See also* Electrocochleography
 amplitude of, 177
 in auditory neuropathy, 154, **154**, 179
 basal bias of, 208
 characteristics of, 177
 clinical applications of, 178–179
 in cochlear hearing loss, 179, **180**
 components of, 177
 definition of, 176
 electrode location effects on, 177
 frequency following response and, 241
 inner hair cells, 176–177
Cochlear nucleus
 auditory nerve termination in, **6**
 dorsal, 5
 inputs to, 7–8
 location of, 7
 outputs, 8
 projections of, to binaural neurons, 131
 subdivisions of, 7, **8**
 tonotopic organization of, 8
 ventral, 7
Cochlear nucleus compound action potential, 200–202, 207
Cochlear receptor potentials, 28, 175
Cochlear synaptopathy, **155**, 155–161, **157–158**, **160**
Common mode rejection ratio, 40–41
Compound action potential
 in acoustic neuroma, 189
 amplitude of, 184–185
 auditory nerve. *See* Auditory nerve compound action potential
 in auditory neuropathy, 179
 click-evoked, 185–186
 clinical applications of, 188–190
 in cochlear hearing loss, 179
 cochlear nucleus, 200–202, 207
 description of, 26
 differential diagnosis uses of, 189–190
 electrically evoked, 191–194, 209
 latency of, 184–185
 recording methods, 186
 response recording, 186–188
 summating potential and, **181**, 182
 threshold estimation using, 188–189
 tone burst-elicited, 185, **189**
 transtympanic electrodes for, 186, **187**, 209
 whole-nerve, 184–190
Conceptual age, 70–71
Conductive hearing loss
 air-conduction and bone-conduction EFR uses in, 231
 auditory brainstem changes caused by, 130–132
 auditory brainstem response in, 125–132, **127**, **129**
 characteristics of, 125–126
Congenital sensorineural hearing loss, 86
Cortical pitch response, 299
Corticocollicular fibers, 14, **15**
Cosine-squared gating window, 34, **34**
CPA. *See* Cerebellopontine angle
CPR. *See* Cortical pitch response
Cranial nerve VIII. *See* Auditory nerve
CV syllable /da/, 232–235, **234**

D

DAC. *See* Digital-to-analog converter
DAS. *See* Dorsal acoustic stria
dB eHL. *See* Decibel estimated hearing level
dB nHL. *See* Decibel normal hearing level
db SL. *See* Decibel sensation level
dB SPL. *See* Decibel sound pressure level
DCN. *See* Dorsal cochlear nucleus
Decibel estimated hearing level, 110
Decibel normal hearing level, 35–38
Decibel sensation level, 36
Decibel sound pressure level, 35
Deiters' cells, 3–4
Dendrites, 19, **20**
Dendritic action potential, 192
Differential amplification, 39–41, **40**
Digital filtering, 41, 68–70
Digital-to-analog converter, 41, **42**
Dipoles, 24–26, **25**
Distortion product otoacoustic emissions, 85, 87, 92, 154, 246
DNAPs. *See* Dorsal cochlear nucleus potentials
DNLL. *See* Dorsal nucleus of lateral lemniscus
Dorsal acoustic stria, **8**
Dorsal cochlear nucleus, 5
Dorsal cochlear nucleus potentials, 205
Dorsal nucleus of lateral lemniscus, **6**, 8, **8**
Dorsomedial nucleus, 13

DPOAEs. *See* Distortion product otoacoustic emissions
Dynamic causal modeling, 313

E

eABR. *See* Electrical auditory brainstem response
Early hearing detection and intervention, 84, 116
eCAP. *See* Electrically evoked compound action potential
ECochG. *See* Electrocochleography
Efferent pathways, 14–16, **15**
EFR. *See* Envelope following response
EHDI. *See* Early hearing detection and intervention
eHL. *See* Estimated hearing level
Electrical auditory brainstem response
    analysis of, 197–198
    artifacts, 198
    cochlear implant evaluation uses of, 194–198
    data acquisition methods, 198
    electrical stimulation methods for, 197–198
    recording montage for, 198
    recording of, 197–198
    response amplitude of, 196, **197**
    response analysis, 198
    response characteristics of, 195–196, **195–196**
    response latency of, 195–196
    thresholds, 196
    waveform morphology, 195, **195**
Electrically evoked compound action potential, 191–194, 209
Electrocochleography
    cochlear microphonic. *See* Cochlear microphonic
    definition of, 175–176
    description of, 28
    electrodes used in, 186, **187**, 205
    inner hair cell evaluations, 176
    intracochlear, 191–194
    laboratory exercises involving, 360
    outer hair cell evaluations, 176
    recording parameters for, **362**
    response recording, 186–188
    stimuli for, **362**
    summating potential. *See* Summating potential
    transtympanic, 200
Electrodes
    in auditory brainstem response. *See* Auditory brainstem response, electrodes
    in electrocochleography, 186, **187**
    transtympanic, 186, **187**, 209
    tympanic membrane, 186, **187**
Electromotility, 3
Embedded auditory evoked potentials, 42

Endolymphatic hydrops, 181, 184
Envelope encoding, cochlear impairment effects on, 237–238
Envelope following response
    accuracy of, 239
    auditory brainstem response versus, 219
    auditory threshold estimation uses of, 226–232
        air-conduction EFR, 227–229
        bone-conduction EFR, 231–232
        in sensorineural hearing loss, 229–231
    autocorrelation function, 266, **285**
    background noise effects on, **299**
    bandwidth effects on amplitude of, **240**
    bone-conduction, 231–232
    clinical applications of, 237
    definition of, 220
    description of, 29, 90
    in different populations, 324
    extraction of, **221**
    frequency-domain analysis of, **265**
    frequency following response versus, 241
    grand average, **321**
    in hearing aid outcome measure, 238–240
    in infants, 229
    neural encoding deficits in speech studied using, 324
    neural generators of, 254–257
    periodicities in, 266
    phase coherence, 266–267, **267**
    pitch periodicity in, 266
    recording of
        earphones, 263–264
        electrode montage, 261–264
        laboratory exercises involving, 359–360
        stimulus characteristics, 261–263, **262**
    scalp-recorded, 238
    sinusoidally amplitude modulated tones for elicitation of
        age effects on, 226–227
        amplitude, 223, **226**
        carrier frequency, 224–225
        creation of, 222
        description of, 221–222
        modulation rate, 225–226
        stimulus intensity effects, 223–224
        waveform for, **222**
    speech sounds for eliciting
        characteristics of, 232–234
        CV syllable /da/, 232–235, **234**
        description of, 232
        stimulus polarity effects on, 235
        stimulus specificity, 235–236
        test-retest reliability, 235

summary of, 268–269
terminology for, 219
waveforms for, **220**
Epoch, 43
EPSP. *See* Excitatory postsynaptic potential
Equivalent dipole, 26
ER-2, 35, **35**, **38**, 263
ER-3A, 35, **35**, **37–38**, 163
ER-3C, 35, **38**
Estimated hearing level, 110
Etymotic tubal insert phones, 35, **38**. *See also* ER-3A; ER-3C
Evoked potentials
   auditory. *See* Auditory evoked potential(s)
   definition of, 24
   myogenic, 29, **29**
   neural basis of, 19, 24
   time-domain averaging of, 43–45, **44**
Excitatory postsynaptic potentials, 19, 24, 56–57, 153
Exogenous potentials, 29
Experience-dependent effects
   in brainstem, 304–306
   signal degradation resiliency of, 306–309
Experience-dependent pitch processing, 311–313

F

Fast Fourier transform, 90, 264, 267–268
F0DL. *See* Fundamental frequency difference limens
FFR. *See* Frequency following response
FFR$_{DP}$, 246
FFT. *See* Fast Fourier transform
Filtering, 41
Forward masking, 60, 296
Frequency following response
   amplitude of, 264
   auditory brainstem response versus, 241
   autocorrelation function, 266, 285
   autocorrelogram, 266
   background noise effects on, **299**
   binaural interaction, 314, **315**
   binaural masking level difference, 314–317, **316**
   binaural processing, 314–320
   brainstem origin of, 254–255
   clinical applications of, 257–261, **258–260**
   cochlear impairment applications of, 257
   cochlear microphonic and, 241. *See also* Cochlear microphonic
   cochlear nonlinearity, 244, 246–249
   cochlear regions contributing to, 250–253
   complex sounds, 244–250
   definition of, 219
   description of, 29, 240–241
   in different populations, 324
   distortion product otoacoustic emissions and, 246
   envelope following response versus, 241
   extraction of, **221**
   frequency-domain analysis of, **265**
   grand averaged, **288–289**, **292–293**, **308**, **311**, **318**
   latencies of, 254
   low-frequency, place specificity of, 253
   medial superior olive, 254
   neural encoding deficits in speech studied using, 324
   neural generators of, 254–257
   periodicities in, 266
   periodicity strength in, 266
   phase coherence, 266–267, **267**
   phase-locking strength, 243–244, **245**
   pitch periodicity in, 266
   pitch-tracking accuracy, 266
   place specificity of, 252–253
   population response, 253
   recording of
      earphones, 263–264
      electrode montage, 261–264
      laboratory exercises involving, 359–360
      stimulus characteristics, 261–263, **262**
   scalp-recorded, 241, 243, 252, 254–255, 269, 281
   single-neuron activity and, 253
   spatial release from masking, 317–318
   speech-like sounds for eliciting
      steady-state, 246–249
      time-variant, 249–250
   speech sounds for eliciting
      CV syllables, 249–250, **250**
      steady-state, 246–249
      time-variant, 249–250
   stimulus
      amplitude of, 241–243, **242**
      frequency of, 243–244
      level of, 241–243, **242**
   summary of, 268–269
   to temporal fine structure, 244
   terminology for, 219
   time-domain measures, **263**, 264, **265**
   tone burst-elicited, 241, **242**
   waveforms for, **220**, **242**, **248**, **252**, **288**
Frequency-shifted sounds, 283–287, **286**
Frequency-specific threshold estimation
   auditory brainstem response for
      air-conduction threshold, 100–103
      bone-conduction threshold, 103
      frequency-specific tone bursts, 100–103, **102**
      frequency specificity, 96

Frequency-specific threshold estimation *(continued)*
   auditory brainstem response for *(continued)*
      narrowband responses using high-pass masking noise, 96–98, **97**
      notched noise masking for ensuring place specificity of, 98–100
      overview of, 95–96
      place specificity, 96
   auditory steady-state response for, 112–116
F_{sp} ratio, 45
Fundamental frequency difference limens, 294, **295**
Fusiform cells, 9

G

GABA. *See* Gamma aminobutyric acid
Gain, in signal-to-noise ratio, 44
Gamma aminobutyric acid, 24
Globular cells, 13–14
Glutamate, 24

H

Hair cells
   anatomy of, 1, **2**
   excitation of, 61
   inner. *See* Inner hair cells
   outer. *See* Outer hair cells
Hearing impairment
   early identification of, 84
   in infants, 84
Hearing loss
   cochlear. *See* Cochlear hearing loss
   conductive, auditory brainstem response in, 125–132, **127**, **129**
   congenital sensorineural, 86
   hidden, 155–156
   sensorineural
      auditory threshold estimation in, using envelope following response, 229–231
      peripheral, 257
Hearing preservation, in intraoperative monitoring, 206–207, 209–210
Hearing screening
   auditory steady-state response for, 116
   automated auditory brainstem response for
      conventional approach, 87–88
      description of, 85, 87–88, 228
      devices, 88
      efficacy of, 93
      frequency-domain algorithms, 90–92
      hearing loss in babies, 93–94
      otoacoustic emissions versus, 87, 92–93
      PASS-REFER criteria, **88**, 88–89
      stimulus intensity calibration issues, 94
      time-domain approach, 88–90
   factors that affect, 83–84
   hearing loss after passing of, 91
   JCIH protocol for, 94
   justification for, 84–85
   location of, 86
   loss to follow-up, 86
   mandatory universal newborn, 84
   measures used in, 85
   National Institutes of Health consensus statement on, 84
   in neonatal intensive care unit, 86
   newborn, 84–85
   otoacoustic emissions for
      automated auditory brainstem response versus, 87, 92–93
      description of, 85–87
      distortion production, 87
      efficacy of, 93
      transient evoked, 87
   postdischarge, 94
   prevalence of, 85
   protocols for, 86–94
   purpose of, 116
   stimulus intensity calibration issues in, 94
   timing of, 85–86
   two-stage, 94, **95**
Helicotrema, 2
Hensen's cells, 3
Heschl's gyrus, 311, 313
HFPTA. *See* High-frequency pure-tone average
HHL. *See* Hidden hearing loss
Hidden hearing loss, 155–156
High-frequency pure-tone average, 126, 128
High-pass filter, **41**, 107, 345–346
High-pass masking
   cochlear hydrops analysis masking procedure, 190–191
   description of, 186
   narrowband auditory brainstem responses derived using, 96–98, **97**
   wave V latency, **146**
Hotelling T^2, 267
Hyperpolarization, 21

I

IAS. *See* Intermediate acoustic stria
IHCs. *See* Inner hair cells

IID. *See* Interaural differences in intensity
ILD. *See* Interaural latency difference
ILPs. *See* Interpeak latencies
Infants
   auditory brainstem response in, 112
   hearing impairment in, 84
   sensorineural hearing loss in, threshold estimation in, 229–231
   threshold assessment in, 347–355, **350–355**
Inferior colliculus
   cell types of, 12–13
   central nucleus of, 8, 10, 12–13, **14**
   dorsal cortex of, 13
   efferent innervation of, 14–16, **15**
   inputs, 13
   location of, 12
   outputs, 13, **13**
   pitch phenomena at, 282
   subdivisions of, 12, **12**
   tonotopic organization of, 13–14
Inhibitory postsynaptic potential, 19
INLL. *See* Intermediate nucleus of lateral lemniscus
Inner hair cells
   anatomy of, 4
   auditory neuropathy and, 110
   cochlear microphonic generated by, 177
   description of, **2**
   efferent innervation of, **15**
   electrocochleography of, 176
   stereocilia pattern of, **4**
Inner radial fiber, 5
Inner spiral fibers, 14
Interaural amplitude difference in wave V, 147–148, **148–149**
Interaural differences in intensity, 314
Interaural differences in time, 314, 317
Interaural latency difference
   in auditory nerve lesions, 142–143
   description of, 53
   stacked ABR technique, 149
   in wave V, 142–143
Intermediate acoustic stria, **8**
Intermediate nucleus of lateral lemniscus, 11, **11**
Interpeak latencies
   in acoustic neuroma, 141
   in auditory nerve lesions, 141–142
   cochlear hearing loss effects on, 138–139
   description of, 53
   stimulus intensity, **339**
Interspike interval distributions, 287–288
Interstimulus interval, **59**, 59–60
Intertrial phase-locking value, 266

Intracanalicular tumors, 140
Intraoperative monitoring
   auditory nerve and brainstem responses in, 198–207
   auditory nerve compound action potential for, 200–201, 206
   in auditory nerve tumor surgery, 199–200
   definition of, 198–199, 209
   hearing preservation in, 206–207, 209–210
   measures for, 200–203
   preliminary considerations for, 204
   response interpretation and recording, 206
   response recording, 205
   stimulus, 204–205
IOM. *See* Intraoperative monitoring
IPLV. *See* Intertrial phase-locking value
IPSP. *See* Inhibitory postsynaptic potential
IRF. *See* Inner radial fiber
IRN. *See* Iterated rippled noise
ISI. *See* Interstimulus interval
ISIDs. *See* Interspike interval distributions
ITD. *See* Interaural differences in time
Iterated rippled noise, 236, 291, **292**, **295**, 304

J

JCIH. *See* Joint Committee on Infant Hearing
Joint Committee on Infant Hearing, 84, 94
Joint time-frequency analysis, 268

L

Labyrinth
   membranous, 1
   osseous, 1
LAEP. *See* Late auditory evoked potential
Late auditory evoked potential, 28
Latency
   absolute. *See* Absolute latency
   interpeak. *See* Interpeak latencies
   relative, 53
Latency-intensity function, 54, **55**
Lateral efferents, 14
Lateral lemniscus
   dorsal nucleus of, **6**, 8, **8**
   intermediate nucleus of, 11, **11**
   ventral nucleus of, **6**, 8, **8**, 11, **11**
Lateral superior olive
   cell types in, 9
   description of, 8
   inputs, **10**
LiSN test. *See* Listening in Spatialized Noise test

Listening in Spatialized Noise test, 317
Low-pass filter, **41**, 345–346
LSO. *See* Lateral superior olive

M

Magnetoencephalography, 255
Mandarin, 300–303, 307
Mandatory universal newborn hearing screening, 84
MAP curve. *See* Minimum audible pressure curve
Marginal cells, 9
MB11 BERAphone, 90–91, 93
Medial efferents, 14
Medial geniculate body, 13
Medial nucleus of the trapezoid body, 8–11
Medial superior olive
    cell types in, 9
    description of, 8
    frequency following response leaving, 254
    inputs, **10**
    marginal cells in, 9
MEG. *See* Magnetoencephalography
Membrane potential, 19
Membranous labyrinth, 1
Ménière disease, 181–184, **183–184**, 190, **191**
MGB. *See* Medial geniculate body
Middle ear infection, 129–130, **130**
Middle fossa surgical approach, for auditory nerve tumors, 199, **199**
Minimum audible pressure curve, 37
MNTB. *See* Medial nucleus of the trapezoid body
Modiolus, 4
MPZ. *See* Myelin protein zero
MSO. *See* Medial superior olive
Multiple sclerosis, **162**
Multipolar cells, 9
Music, 281, 306
Myelin protein zero, 153
Myelinization, 23
Myogenic evoked potentials, 29, **29**

N

Na^+/K^+ pump, 20
Narrowband chirp, 34
Neonatal intensive care unit, hearing screenings in, 86
Neural conduction time, 53
Neural phase-locking, 220–221, 241, 267, 296
Neural representation
    structural versus functional asymmetries in, 309–310
    of vocoded speech sounds, 318–319, **320**

Neurons
    potassium ions in, 20, **21**
    signaling by, 19
    sodium ions in, 20, **21**
    structure of, 19, **20**
NICU. *See* Neonatal intensive care unit
Nodes of Ranvier, **20**, **22**, 23
Noise
    background, 70, 296, 298–300, 307
    signal-to-noise ratio. *See* Signal-to-noise ratio
Notched noise masking
    with clicks, 99–100
    description of, 96
    illustration of, **98**
    place specificity of auditory brainstem response, 98–100
    with tone bursts, 100
Nuclei of lateral lemniscus, 11, **11**
Nyquist theorem of sampling, 43

O

OAEs. *See* Otoacoustic emissions
Octopus cells, **7**, 8, 11
OHCs. *See* Outer hair cells
Olivocochlear bundle, **15**
Onset polarity
    in auditory nerve lesion evaluation, 163
    description of, 61–63
    laboratory exercises involving, 343–344
Organ of Corti, 3–4
OSFs. *See* Outer spiral fibers
Osseous labyrinth, 1
Otitis media, 126
Otitis media with effusion
    auditory brainstem response affected by, 129, **130**
    conductive hearing loss caused by, 132
Otoacoustic emissions
    in auditory neuropathy evaluations, 111, 153
    definition of, 86
    distortion product, 85, 87, 92, 154
    hearing screening uses of, 85–87
    transient evoked, 85, 87, 154
Otoscopic evaluation, 204
Outer hair cells
    afferent innervation pattern of, **5**
    anatomy of, **2**, 2–3
    cochlear amplification from, 3
    efferent innervation of, **15**
    electrocochleography of, 176
    otoacoustic emissions of, 85
    stereocilia pattern of, **4**
Outer spiral fibers, 4

P

Peak sound pressure level, 36
Peak-to-peak equivalent sound pressure level, 36–37, **37**
Peak-to-trough, 52
peRETSPL. *See* Specific reference equivalent threshold sound pressure levels
Perilymph, 1
Periodicity pitch, 266, 282
Peripheral myelin protein 22, 153
peSPL. *See* Peak-to-peak equivalent sound pressure level
Phase coherence, 266–267, **267**
Phase-locking factor, 266
Phase-locking strength, 243–244, **245**
Physiologic threshold level, 38
Pitch
   description of, 281–282
   envelope modulation in, 291–294
   of frequency-shifted sounds, 283–287, **286**
   of harmonic sounds, 283–287
   of inharmonic sounds, 283–287
   language experience-dependent plasticity in processing of, 301–303
   in music, 281
   neural correlates of, 283–287
   neural encoding of, 297, 306
   spectral, 282
   temporal, 282
   temporal fine structure in, 291–294
   in tonal languages, 300–301
Pitch perception, 281–282, 301
Pitch periodicity, 266, 282
Pitch processing
   in auditory cortex, 313
   experience-dependent, 311–313
Pitch salience, 294–296
Pitch shift, 284
Pitch-tracking accuracy, 266
PLF. *See* Phase-locking factor
PMP22. *See* Peripheral myelin protein 22
Population neural response, 53
Postauricular muscle potential, 29
Posterior fossa tumors, 140
Posterior ventral cochlear nucleus
   description of, 5
   stellate cells in, 7
Postsynaptic neuron, 23, **23**
Postsynaptic potentials, 24, 26
Potassium ions, in neuron, 20, **21**
Prestimulus baseline, 43
Principal cells, 9, 12

pSPL. *See* Peak sound pressure level
PTL. *See* Physiologic threshold level
PVCN. *See* Posterior ventral cochlear nucleus

R

RadioEar B71, 35, **36**
RadioEar B81, 35, **36**
Rasmussen's bundle, 14
Reference equivalent threshold sound pressure levels, 104
Reissner's membrane, 1
Relative latency, 53
Relative refractory period, 21
Repetition rate, 59–60, **59–60**, 163, 341–342
Resolved complex sounds, 287–290
Resting membrane potential-polarized cells, 20–21, **22**
Retrosigmoidal surgical approach, for auditory nerve tumors, 200, **200**
RETSPL. *See* Reference equivalent threshold sound pressure levels
Reverberation, 296–300, 307, 309
Rise-fall time
   auditory brainstem response affected by, 342–343
   description of, 34, **34**
   laboratory exercises involving, 342–343
   latency affected by, 63–64
RMP. *See* Resting membrane potential
Root-mean-squared amplitude, 264

S

SABR. *See* Stacked derived narrowband auditory brainstem response
Saltatory conduction, **22**
SAM tones. *See* Sinusoidally amplitude modulated tones
Sampling frequency, 42
Sampling period, 42
Scala tympani, 1, **2**
Scala vestibuli, 1, **2**
Schwann cells, 19
Self-masking, 296
Sensorineural hearing loss
   auditory threshold estimation in, using envelope following response, 229–231
   peripheral, 257
Signal averaging, 43
Signal-to-noise ratio
   in averaging, 44, 344–345
   description of, 38–39
   gain in, 44

Signaling, neural, 19
Sink, 24
Sinusoidally amplitude modulated tones, for envelope following response elicitation
    age effects on, 226–227
    amplitude, 223, **226**
    carrier frequency, 224–225
    creation of, 222
    description of, 221–222
    modulation rate, 225–226
    stimulus intensity effects, 223–224
    waveform for, **222**
SπNo, 315–316
SNR. *See* Signal-to-noise ratio
SOC. *See* Superior olivary complex
Sodium ions, in neuron, 20, **21**
Soma, 19
Somatosensory evoked potentials, 24
SoNπ, 315–317
Sound level meters, 36
Source, 24
SP. *See* Summating potential
Spatial release from masking, 317–318
Spatial summation, 26–27
Specific reference equivalent threshold sound pressure levels, 37
Spectral pitch, 282
Spectral resolution, 193
Speech
    in adverse listening conditions, 296
    perception of, 158, 193
Speech sounds
    envelope following response elicited using
        characteristics of, 232–234
        CV syllable /da/, 232–235, **234**
        description of, 232
        stimulus polarity effects on, 235
        stimulus specificity, 235–236
        test-retest reliability, 235
    frequency following response elicited using, 246–249
    vocoded, 318–319, **320**
Spiral ganglion cells, 5
Split-buffered averaging, 45
Stacked derived narrowband auditory brainstem response
    acoustic tumor detection using, 145–150
    chirp stimuli for, 162
    interaural, 148
Stellate cells, 7
Stiffness gradient, 2, **3**
Stimulus
    absolute latency affected by intensity of, **55**, 56–57
    for auditory nerve and brainstem lesion detection, 162–163
    chirps. *See* Chirps
    clicks. *See* Clicks
    description of, 31–32
    frequency of, 57–59
    intensity of, 35–36, 54–56, 94, 162–163
    interstimulus interval, 59
    laboratory exercises involving, 338–344
    onset polarity, 61–62, **62**, 163, 343–344
    repetition rate, 59–60, **59–60**, 163, 341–342
    rise-fall time, 34, **34**, 63–64, 342–343
    tone bursts, 34, **34**
Stria vascularis, 4
Summating potential
    clinical applications of, 182–184
    compound action potential and, **181**, 182
    definition of, 180, 208
    in Ménière disease, 181–184, **183–184**
    tone burst, 184
    transtympanic, **181**
Superior olivary complex
    description of, 5, **6**, 50
    frequency following response leaving, 254
    generator source, 51
    inputs to, 9–10
    location of, 9
    outputs to, 10
    periolivary region of, **15**
    subdivisions of, 9
    tonotopic organization of, 10
Synapses
    definition of, 23
    description of, 19
    transmission, 23–24
Synaptic cleft, 23, **23**
Synchrony capture, 260

T

Temporal encoding, 282–283, 291
Temporal fine structure
    definition of, 219
    frequency following response to, 244
    neural phase-locking of, 260
    neural representation of, 258
    in pitch, 291–294
Temporal pitch, 282
Temporal resolution, 42
Temporal synchronization, 26–27
Temporal synchrony, 26, 53
TEOAEs. *See* Transient evoked otoacoustic emissions
TFS. *See* Temporal fine structure
Time-domain averaging, 43–45, **44**
Tonal languages, pitch in, 300–301

Tone bursts
  auditory brainstem response evoked with
    air conduction threshold estimations using, 100–103
    bone conduction threshold estimations using, 103–106
    click-evoked ABR versus, **150**
    description of, 34, **34**
    frequency of, 57–58
    laboratory exercises, 340, **341**
    notched noise masking effects on, 99
    stacked ABR versus, **150**
    waveform for, **34**
  description of, 34, **34**
  frequency-specific, 100–103
  notched noise masking with, 100
Transient evoked otoacoustic emissions, 85, 87, 154
Translabyrinthine surgical approach, for auditory nerve tumors, 199
Transmembranic current flow, 26
Transtympanic electrocochleography, 200
Transtympanic electrodes, 186, **187**, 209
Transtympanic summating potential, **181**
Trapezoid body
  description of, 8
  medial nucleus of, 8–11
Tympanic membrane electrodes, 186, **187**
Type II fibers, 4

U

Unresolved complex sounds, 287–290
Upper brainstem lesions, 161–162

V

VAS. *See* Ventral acoustic stria
VCN. *See* Ventral cochlear nucleus
VEMPs. *See* Vestibular evoked myogenic potentials
Ventral acoustic stria, 8, **8**
Ventral cochlear nucleus, 7
Ventral nucleus of lateral lemniscus, **6**, 8, **8**, 11, **11**
Vestibular evoked myogenic potentials, 184
Vestibular schwannoma, 140, **140**, **203**, **207**
Videonystagmography, 184
VNG. *See* Videonystagmography
VNLL. *See* Ventral nucleus of lateral lemniscus
Vocoded speech sounds, 318–319, **320**
Voltage-gated calcium channels, **23**
Volume conduction
  in EEG domain, 24
  factors that affect, 24
von Bekesy's experiments, 2

W

Waveform morphology, of auditory brainstem responses, 48, **48**
Weighted average, 44
Whole-nerve compound action potential, 184–190

Z

Zwislocki coupler, 35